Don Sundean

ANTI-INFECTIVE THERAPY

ANTI-INFECTIVE THERAPY

Edited by

GERALD L. MANDELL, M.D.
Professor of Medicine
Owen R. Cheatham Professor of the Sciences
Head, Division of Infectious Diseases
University of Virginia School of Medicine
Charlottesville, Virginia

R. GORDON DOUGLAS, JR., M.D.
E. Hugh Luckey Distinguished Professor in Medicine
Professor and Chairman, Department of Medicine
Cornell University Medical College
Physician-in-Chief
The New York Hospital
New York, New York

JOHN E. BENNETT, M.D.
Head, Clinical Mycology Section
Laboratory of Clinical Investigation
National Institute of Allergy and Infectious Diseases
National Institutes of Health
Bethesda, Maryland

A WILEY MEDICAL PUBLICATION
JOHN WILEY & SONS
New York • Chichester • Brisbane • Toronto • Singapore

Library of Congress Cataloging in Publication Data:

Main entry under title:

Anti-infective therapy.

(A Wiley medical publication)
Includes index.
1. Anti-infective agents. I. Mandell, Gerald L.
II. Douglas, R. Gordon (Robert Gordon), 1934–
III. Bennett, John E. (John Eugene), 1933–
IV. Series
RM262.A56 1985 616.9'0461 85–3135
ISBN 0–471–80442–8

Printed in the United States of America

10 9 8 7 6 5 4 3 2 1

CONTRIBUTORS

Robert H. Alford, M.D.
Professor of Medicine
Vanderbilt University School of Medicine
Chief, Infectious Diseases
Veterans Administration Medical Center
Nashville, Tennessee

Vincent T. Andriole, M.D.
Professor of Medicine
Chief, Infectious Diseases Section
Yale University School of Medicine
New Haven, Connecticut

John E. Bennett, M.D.
Head, Clinical Mycology Section
Laboratory of Clinical Investigation
National Institute of Allergy and Infectious Diseases
Bethesda, Maryland

R. Gordon Douglas, Jr., M.D.
E. Hugh Luckey Distinguished Professor of Medicine
Professor and Chairman, Department of Medicine
Cornell University Medical College
Physician-in-Chief
The New York Hospital
New York, New York

Barry Farr, M.D.
Assistant Professor of Medicine
Division of Epidemiology and Virology
University of Virginia School of Medicine
Charlottesville, Virginia

Robert Fekety, M.D.
Professor of Internal Medicine
Head, Division of Infectious Diseases
Department of Internal Medicine
University of Michigan Medical School
Chief, Adult Infectious Diseases Service
University Hospitals
Ann Arbor, Michigan

Sydney M. Finegold, M.D.
Professor of Medicine, Microbiology and Immunology
University of California School of Medicine
Chief, Infectious Disease Section
Veterans Administration Wadsworth Medical Center
Los Angeles, California

Frederick G. Hayden, M.D.
Associate Professor of Internal Medicine and Pathology
Director, Clinical Virology Laboratory
University of Virginia School of Medicine
Charlottesville, Virginia

Calvin M. Kunin, M.D.
Pomerene Professor
Department of Medicine
Ohio State University School of Medicine
Columbus, Ohio

Paul S. Leitman, M.D.
Wellcome Professor of Clinical Pharmacology
Director, Division of Clinical Pharmacology
The Johns Hopkins University School of Medicine
Baltimore, Maryland

Gerald L. Mandell, M.D.
Professor of Medicine
Owen R. Cheatham Professor of the Sciences
Head, Division of Infectious Diseases
University of Virginia School of Medicine
Charlottesville, Virginia

J. Joseph Marr, M.D.
Professor of Medicine and Biochemistry
Director, Infectious Diseases
Department of Medicine-Infectious Diseases
University of Colorado
Health Sciences Center
Denver, Colorado

Kenneth Mayer, M.D.
Assistant Professor of Medicine
Division of Infectious Disease
Brown University
Memorial Hospital
Pawtaucket, Rhode Island

Robert C. Moellering, Jr., M.D.
Professor of Medicine
Shields Warren-Mallinckrodt Professor of Clinical Research
Harvard Medical School
Physician-in-Chief
New England Deaconess Hospital
Boston, Massachusetts

Harold C. Neu, M.D.
Professor of Medicine and Pharmacology
Chief, Division of Infectious Diseases and Epidemiology
Columbia University
College of Physicians and Surgeons
New York, New York

Sandra Norris, Pharm.D.
Instructor, Department of Medicine
University of Virginia School of Medicine
Charlottesville, Virginia

Harold C. Standiford, M.D.
Associate Professor of Medicine
University of Maryland School of Medicine
Chief, Section of Infectious Diseases
Baltimore Veterans Administration Hospital
Baltimore, Maryland

Neal H. Steigbigel, M.D.
Professor of Medicine
Albert Einstein College of Medicine
Head, Division of Infectious Diseases
Montefiore Medical Center
Bronx, New York

Stephen H. Zinner, M.D.
Professor of Medicine
Head, Division of Infectious Diseases
Department of Medicine
Brown University
Roger Williams General Hospital
Providence, Rhode Island

PREFACE

This book fills an urgent need for a comprehensive, well-referenced, up-to-date book on antibacterial agents, antivirals, and antifungal agents. Although a number of sources for such drugs are available ranging from tabular summaries of information to detailed treatises of basic pharmacology, a book by infectious disease physicians emphasizing thorough discussion of the commonly and not so commonly used drugs is lacking.

Anti-infective Therapy is organized by drugs or groups of drugs. There is complete coverage of currently licensed (U.S.), soon to be licensed, and promising anti-infective agents written from the point of view of the practicing infectious diseases consultant. Experts in their fields will find the information contained here essential to their practice. The treatment of each agent is up-to-date, comprehensive, and extensively referenced. In addition, chapters are devoted to such topics as principles of anti-infective therapy, pharmacokinetics, the use and abuse of antibiotics, and cost issues related to antibiotic therapy. It is not a "cookbook" manual. The book is scholarly yet highly practical because of the physician authorship and the liberal use of tables and charts to help the reader find key or often used information concerning each of the major drugs. Specific tables on the pharmacology of anti-infective agents should prove especially useful. A complete list of tables and their location is included in the front matter, and a special index has been prepared for easy access to information on specific clinical problems. This work, a reproduction of the section on anti-infective therapy from the complete infectious disease textbook *Principles and Practices of Infectious Diseases,* will be helpful to internists, family practitioners, pediatricians, surgeons, obstetrician-gynecologists, and pharmacists.

We are grateful to our contributors for their skillful handling of the material, to our secretaries for their careful work, to our wives and children for their continued support, and to Andrew Ford and others at John Wiley & Sons for their support and encouragement in this project.

Gerald L. Mandell
R. Gordon Douglas, Jr.
John E. Bennett

CONTENTS

LIST OF TABLES

Chapter 5

Chapter 6

Chapter 7

Chapter 8

Chapter 9

Chapter 17

Chapter 18

Chapter 19

Chapter 20

Tables of Antimicrobial Agent Pharmacology by Family

ANTI-INFECTIVE THERAPY

1

PRINCIPLES OF ANTI-INFECTIVE THERAPY

ROBERT C. MOELLERING, JR.

Although the discovery of effective agents to prevent and treat infection caused by bacteria and other pathogenic microorganisms is one of the most important developments of modern medicine, the use of such agents has not been limited to the present era. Substances with anti-infective potential have been applied medically for thousands of years. Indeed, more than 2500 years ago the Chinese were aware of the therapeutic properties of moldy soybean curd applied to carbuncles, boils, and other infections (1), and the ancient Greek physicians, including Hypocrates, routinely used substances with antimicrobial activity including wine, myrrh, and inorganic salts in their treatment of wounds (2). Until the discovery of the microbiologic basis of infections in the nineteenth century, however, the therapy for infections remained strictly empiric. Heavy metals such as arsenic and bismuth were found to be useful against a number of infections, including syphilis, in the early 1900s; but the modern era of chemotherapy did not really begin until the discovery and initial clinical use of the sulfonamides in 1936 (1). This was followed in the 1940s by the discovery of the therapeutic value of penicillin and streptomycin, and by 1950 the "golden age" of antimicrobial chemotherapy was well underway.

It is the result of the relatively recent work in this area since 1936 that forms the basis for this and each of the succeeding chapters on anti-infective therapy. The major emphasis in this chapter is on antibacterial agents because there are more data available on these drugs. However, many of the principles to be discussed can also be applied to the use of antifungal, antiviral, and, to some extent, antiparasitic drugs.

CHOICE OF THE PROPER ANTIMICROBIAL AGENT

In choosing the appropriate antimicrobial agent for the therapy of a given infection, a number of important factors must be considered. First, the identity of the infecting organism must be known or, at the very least, it must be possible to arrive at a reasonable statistical guess as to its identity, based on clinical information. Second, we must have as accurate information as possible about the antimicrobial susceptibility (or potential susceptibility) of the infecting organism. Finally, a series of so-called host factors must be taken into consideration to arrive at the optimal choice of antimicrobial agent. Each of these items will be considered in this book.

Identification of the Infecting Organism

Several methods for the rapid identification of pathogenic bacteria in clinical specimens are available. A Gram's stain preparation is perhaps the simplest, least expensive, and most useful of all the "rapid methods" of identification of bacterial (and some fungal) pathogens. This technique can be used to identify the presence and morphologic features of microorganisms in body fluids that are normally sterile (cerebrospinal fluid, pleural fluid, synovial fluid, peritoneal fluid, urine). On occasion, Gram's stain of a buffy-coat preparation of blood will reveal phagocytosed organisms in the polymorphonuclear leukocytes of patients with bacteremia or fungemia. Similar preparations of sputum will also be helpful in revealing the nature of the infecting organism in patients with bacterial bronchitis or pneumonia. Gram's stain of a stool specimen may also produce useful information. In patients with staphylococcal enterocolitis, the Gram's stain reveals sheets of gram-positive cocci replacing the normal stool flora. The presence of polymorphonuclear leukocytes in the stool also provides a helpful clue to the cause of certain cases of diarrhea. Polymorphonuclear leukocytes are not found in normal stools. When present, they suggest the possibility of a bacterial gastroenteritis such as shigellosis, salmonellosis, or *Campylobacter,* or invasive *Escherichia coli* gastroenteritis. Polymorphonuclear leukocytes are not found in the stools of patients with viral gastroenteritis, food poisoning, cholera, and diarrhea due to noninvasive toxigenic *E. coli* (3). *Campylobacter* may be identified in the stools of patients by its characteristic gull-wing appearance on smears of stool (4).

Immunologic methods for antigen detection [such as enzyme-linked immunoabsorbent assay (ELISA) or latex agglutination] may also provide clues for the rapid identification of the infecting pathogens. Final and definitive identification of pathogenic organisms usually requires cultural techniques. It is thus imperative that appropriate specimens be obtained for culture before beginning antimicrobial therapy. Once anti-infective agents have been started, cultures often are rendered sterile, even though viable organisms remain in the host.

In most cases, it may be impossible to determine the exact nature of the infecting organisms before the institution of antimicrobial therapy. In these cases, the use of bacteriologic statistics may be particularly helpful (5,6). The term *bacteriologic statistics* refers to the application of knowledge of the organisms most likely to cause infection in a given clinical setting. For example, a person with normal host defense mechanisms who develops cellulitis of the arm after a minor abrasion most likely has an infection due to *Staphylococcus aureus* or group A streptococci, and antimicrobial therapy should be tailored accordingly, even though there is no material available for examination with Gram's stain. Similarly, a young child with acute otitis media almost certainly has an infection due either to a virus or to one of four major bacterial pathogens: *Hemophilus influenzae, Streptococcus pneumoniae, Branhamella catarrhalis,* or a group A streptococcus.

Determination of Antimicrobial Susceptibility of Infecting Organism

Since different organisms vary in their susceptibility to antimicrobial agents, it is imperative that we have some means for determining the antimicrobial susceptibility of the actual (or presumed) infecting organism(s). If the pathogen is isolated from a culture, it can be subjected to direct susceptibility testing. A number of methods for determining antimicrobial susceptibility is available. The commonly used disk-diffusion method is simple to perform and is relatively inexpensive, but it provides at best only semiquantitative or qualitative data about the susceptibility of a given organism to a given agent. It is not useful for slow-growing or fastidious organisms and has not been standardized for anaerobes. Nonetheless, if the test is carefully done, it provides data that are clinically useful. Quantitative data are provided by methods that incorporate serial dilutions of antimicrobials in agar-containing or broth culture media. The lowest concentration of the antimicrobial agent that prevents visible growth after an 18- to 24-hour incubation period is known as the minimal inhibitory concentration (MIC). The minimal bacterial concentration (MBC) or minimal lethal concentration (MLC) may be determined in broth dilution tests by subculturing the containers that show no growth onto antibiotic-free agar-containing media. The lowest concentration of antimicrobial that totally suppresses growth on antibiotic-free media (or results in a 99.9 percent or greater decline in colony count) after overnight incubation is known as the MBC (or MLC).

Susceptibility testing is particularly important for certain organisms such as *S. aureus* and the various facultative and aerobic gram-negative bacilli. The widespread clinical and agricultural use of antibiotics since the 1930s and 1940s has resulted in the emergence of many strains of bacteria resistant to one or more antimicrobial agents (7). In most cases in which adequate studies have been done, it appears that the role of antimicrobial agents is to exert selective pressure that results in the emergence of resistant organisms. In some cases the organisms are naturally resistant to the antibiotic used. Examples of this include gram-positive organisms such as staphylococci and streptococci, which are naturally resistant to the polymyxins. Many gram-negative bacilli are naturally resistant to penicillin G, erythromycin, and clindamycin. In other cases the resistant bacterial strains have acquired R factors or plasmids, which enable them to resist antimicrobial inhibition. These plasmids may provide the organisms with the ability to synthesize enzymes that modify or inactivate the antimicrobial agent; they may result in changes in the bacterial cell's ability to accumulate the antimicrobial agent; or may permit the cell to produce metabolic enzymes resistant to inhibition by the antimicrobial agent (7). Examples of each of these mechanisms of resistance are well known. Most strains of *S. aureus* that are resistant to penicillin contain plasmids that enable them to produce an extracellular β-lactamase that hydrolyzes and inactivates penicillin G (7). Many gram-negative bacilli that are resistant to aminoglycosidic aminocyclitol antibiotics such as streptomycin, kanamycin, tobramycin, gentamicin, and even amikacin contain plasmids that code for the production of periplasmic enzymes that catalyze a modification of the aminoglycosidic aminocyclitols by phosphorylation, acetylation, or adenylylation (7). R-factor-mediated tetracycline resistance in both gram-negative bacilli and *S. aureus* involves an inducible decrease in uptake of tetracycline, although the actual mechanism for this decreased uptake is not yet understood (7). *Escherichia coli* resistant to trimethoprim have been found to contain R factors that enable them to synthesize a new dihydrofolate reductase (the enzyme specifically inhibited by trimethoprim) that is 10,000 times less susceptible to the in vitro effects of trimethoprim than is the host bacteria's own chromosomal enzyme (7).

The above-mentioned developments provide the rationale for performing tests of antimicrobial susceptibility whenever there is reasonable doubt about the susceptibility of a given organism. There are certain cases in which routine susceptibility testing need not be done, but they make up an ever-diminishing list. All group A streptococci remain susceptible to the penicillins and cephalosporins; meningococci likewise are universally susceptible to ampicillin and chloramphenicol; virtually all anaerobes except *Bacteroides* species are susceptible to penicillin G. Thus, testing these organisms against the agents listed need not be routinely carried out at the present time. Even a statement such as this is fraught with a certain amount of danger. The recent discoveries of penicillin-resistant pneumococci in South Africa, the emergence of penicillin-resistant gonococci in Asia and Africa, the rapid spread of ampicillin-resistant (and even chloramphenicol-resistant) strains of *H. influenzae* in the United States and Europe make us realize that, in time, strains of virtually any organism may be found that are resistant to antimicrobial agents that previously had been effective against them (7).

It is important to consider geographic differences in patterns of susceptibility of organisms when choosing antimicrobial agents. In many cases, there may be variations in susceptibility patterns between hospitals and the community or among hospitals themselves. The recent emergence of gram-negative bacilli that are resistant to gentamicin is a good example of this. At present, most of the aminoglycoside-resistant organisms are found in hospitals, whereas majority of isolates from nonhospitalized patients remains susceptible to gentamicin (7,8).

The possibility of significant geographic variations in antimicrobial susceptibility must be remembered as we examine Table 1, which is a compendium of antimicrobial agents of choice for various commonly encountered infectious agents. The data in this table are based on material accumulated primarily in the United States and are similar in many aspects to data published periodically in the *Medical Letter on Drugs and Therapeutics* (9).

Host Factors

It is of obvious importance to determine the identity and antimicrobial susceptibility of the organism(s) causing a given infection. However, optimal therapy is impossible unless we also consider a number of host factors that may influence the efficacy and toxicity of antimicrobial agents (10).

History of Previous Adverse Reactions to Antimicrobial Agents. Simply obtaining an adequate history of previous adverse reactions to drugs may prevent the inadvertent administration of an antimicrobial agent to which the patient is allergic. Failure to do so can have serious (and sometimes fatal) consequences.

Age. The age of the patient is a major factor to consider in the choice of antimicrobial agents. Gastric acidity varies with age. The pH of gastric secretions is higher in young children and does not reach adult levels of acidity until approximately the age of 3. At the other end of the age spectrum, there is also a decline in gastric acidity so gastric achlorhydria is found in 5.3 percent of people 20–29 years of age, in 16 percent of those 40–49, and in 35.4 percent of those over 60 (10). The absorption of a number of antimicrobials via the oral route depends on their acid stability and on the pH of gastric secretions. Penicillin G is an excellent example of this phenomenon. The oral absorption of penicillin G is markedly reduced by gastric acid. However, in young children and in older achlorhydric patients, the absorption of the drug is markedly enhanced. As a result, various orally administered penicillins will produce high serum levels in young children and in elderly patients who have achlorhydria. It makes no sense to give such a patient the more expensive acid-resistant forms of penicillin such as phenoxymethyl penicillin (penicillin V) since these drugs will not be absorbed any better than the less expensive penicillin G. Absorption of other orally administered β-lactam antibiotics is probably also enhanced in achlorhydric patients; however, evidence is convincing only in the case of the penicillins (11). Gastric acidity does not always have a negative influence on the absorption of antimicrobials. Drugs that are weak acids such as ketoconazole may be better absorbed at low pH. Thus, absorption of ketoconazole is impaired by the administration of antacids, cimetidine, or even food (12).

Renal function, likewise, varies with age. It is relatively diminished in premature and newborn children, reaching "adult levels" between 2 and 12 months of age (10). Thus the serum half-lives of drugs that are primarily excreted by the kidneys may be considerably increased in neonates. As a result, doses of

TABLE 1. Antimicrobial Agents of Choice

Organism	*Antimicrobial of Choice*	*Alternative Agents*
Gram-positive cocci		
Staphylococcus aureus		
Nonpenicillinase producing	Penicillin	A cephalosporin[a], vancomycin, clindamycin, erythromycin
Penicillinase producing	A penicillinase-resistant penicillin[b]	A cephalosporin[a], vancomycin, clindamycin, erythromycin
β-Streptococci (groups A,B,C,G)	Penicillin	A cephalosporin[a], erythromycin
α-Streptococci (*Streptococcus viridans*)	Penicillin	A cephalosporin[a], vancomycin, erythromycin
Streptococcus bovis	Penicillin	A cephalosporin[a], vancomycin, erythromycin
Enterococci		
(Endocarditis or other serious infection)	Penicillin (or ampicillin) plus gentamicin or streptomycin	Vancomycin plus gentamicin or streptomycin
Uncomplicated urinary tract infection	Ampicillin or amoxicillin	Erythromycin, nitrofurantoin
Streptococcus pneumoniae	Penicillin	A cephalosporin[a], erythromycin, chloramphenicol
Gram-negative cocci		
Neisseria meningitidis	Penicillin	Chloramphenicol, a sulfonamide
Neisseria gonorrhoeae	Penicillin or a tetracycline	Spectinomycin, ampicillin, amoxicillin, cefoxitin, cefotaxime, moxalactam, erythromycin
Gram-negative bacilli		
Acinetobacter sp. (*Mima, Herellea*)	Tobramycin or kanamycin (± carbenicillin)	Sulfisoxazole, trimethoprim-sulfamethoxazole[c], ticarullin, mezlocillin, piperacillin, doxycycline
Brucella sp.	Tetracycline (± streptomycin)	Chloramphenicol (± streptomycin)
Campylobacter sp.	Erythromycin	Tetracycline, chloramphenicol, gentamicin
Enterobacter sp.	Gentamicin or tobramycin	Carbenicillin, ticarcillin, mezlocillin, piperacillin, netilmicin, amikacin, cefotaxime, moxalactam, tetracycline
Escherichia coli		
Uncomplicated urinary tract infection	Ampicillin, amoxicillin, or sulfisoxazole	A cephalosporin[a], a tetracycline
Systemic infection	Gentamicin or tobramycin	Ampicillin, a cephalosporin[a], carbinicillin or ticarcillin, kanamycin, amikacin, netilmicin
Francisella tularensis	Streptomycin	Tetracycline, chloramphenicol

Hemophilus influenzae		
Meningitis	Chloramphenicol, cefotaxime, or moxalactam	Ampicillin
Other infections	Ampicillin	Trimethoprim-sulfamethoxazole, chloramphenicol, tetracycline, cefamandole
Klebsiella pneumoniae	Gentamicin or tobramycin	A cephalosporin[a], cefotaxime, moxalactam, cefoxitin, cefuroxime, cefamandole, amikacin, netilmicin, chloramphenicol, trimethoprim-sulfamethoxazole[c]
Legionella sp.	Erythromycin	Rifampin plus erythromycin
Proteus mirabilis	Ampicillin	Gentamicin or tobramycin, a cephalosporin[a]
Other *Proteus* sp. (*P. rettgeri, M. morganii, P. vulgaris*)	Gentamicin or tobramycin	Cefotaxime, moxalactam, carbenicillin, ticarcillin, mezlocillin, piperacillin, amikacin, kanamycin, netilmicin
Providencia sp.	Gentamicin or tobramycin	Cefotaxime, moxalactam, amikacin, kanamycin, netilmicin, carbenicillin, ticarcillin, mezlocillin, piperacillin
Pseudomonas aeruginosa	Tobramycin or gentamicin, ± ticarcillin, carbenicillin, azlocillin, or piperacillin	Amikacin, a polymyxin
Salmonella sp.	Chloramphenicol	Ampicillin or amoxicillin, trimethoprim-sulfamethoxazole[c]
Serratia marcescens	Gentamicin or amikacin	Cefotaxime, moxalactam, carbenicillin or ticarcillin, tobramycin, netilmicin
Shigella sp.	Trimethoprim-sulfamethoxazole[c]	Ampicillin, chloramphenicol
Yersinia pestis	Streptomycin	Tetracycline, chloramphenicol
Anaerobes		
Anaerobic streptococci	Penicillin	Clindamycin, erythromycin, chloramphenicol, tetracycline
Bacteroides sp.		
Oropharyngeal strains	Penicillin	Clindamycin, tetracycline, chloramphenicol, metronidazole, cefoxitin
Gastrointestinal strains	Clindamycin	Chloramphenicol, metronidazole, cefoxitin, moxalactam, carbenicillin, ticarcillin, piperacillin, mezlocillin
Clostridium sp.	Penicillin	Chloramphenicol, clindamycin, metronidazole

[a] The term *cephalosporin* refers to the first-generation cephalosporins: cephalothin, cefazolin, cephapirin, cephradine, cephalexin, cefaclor, cefadroxil.
[b] Methicillin, nafcillin, oxacillin, cloxacillin, or dicloxacillin.
[c] Not approved for this indication by the U.S. Food and Drug Administration.

antimicrobial agents such as penicillin G and its various semisynthetic derivatives as well as the aminoglycosides must be altered in neonates.

Aging results in the decline of a number of physiologic processes, including renal function (11). It is especially important to realize that creatinine clearance may be significantly reduced in elderly patients even though they have normal blood urea nitrogen (BUN) or serum creatinine concentrations. In view of this, high doses of the penicillins or cephalosporins must be given with caution to elderly patients to prevent the development of excessively high serum levels that may produce severe neurotoxic reactions such as myoclonus, seizures, and coma (10,11). It is likewise possible that other adverse reactions to the penicillins such as reversible neutropenia may be dose related and may occur with increased frequency when high doses of such drugs are given to elderly patients with physiologic renal impairment (11). This, however, has not been proven. Impaired renal excretion of the aminoglycoside antibiotics may result in elevated serum concentrations, which, in turn, may be associated with an increasing incidence of ototoxicity in elderly patients (13).

In addition to the toxicity that may result from impaired renal excretion in neonates and elderly patients, other adverse effects of antimicrobial agents may also be age related (12). Hepatic function in the neonate is underdeveloped by adult standards. This can result in difficulties if such patients are given drugs that are normally excreted or inactivated by the liver. Chloramphenicol is inactivated by conjugation to the glucuronide form in the liver. However, in the neonate, hepatic levels of glucuronyl transferase are relatively insufficient. Thus when neonates are given large doses of chloramphenicol, high serum levels of unconjugated chloramphenicol result. Such high concentrations of unconjugated chloramphenicol are toxic and can result in shock, cardiovascular collapse, and death (the so-called gray syndrome) (10,15). For this reason, chloramphenicol should be avoided if possible in the neonate. If it is necessary to use the drug, however, it may be safely administered if given in a dosage that has been reduced appropriately for the patient's age (15,16).

The sulfonamides compete with bilirubin for binding sites on serum albumin. When given to neonates, they produce increased serum levels of unbound bilirubin that predispose the child to kernicterus (15,16). For this reason, these agents should not be given to neonates. Hyperbilirubinemia per se may be associated with the administration of novobiocin to neonates (15). This is due to the ability of this drug to inhibit hepatic glucuronyl transferase, which in turn diminishes the ability of the liver to conjugate and excrete bilirubin. Hence, novobiocin should be avoided in newborn infants.

The tetracyclines are avidly bound to developing bone and tooth structures. As they bind to developing teeth, tetracyclines may cause a number of adverse effects, ranging from purplish to brownish discoloration of the teeth to actual enamel hypoplasia (10,15). The tetracyclines readily cross the placenta (17). Thus, when administered during the latter half of pregnancy or from birth to the age of 6 months, they may cause these effects on the deciduous teeth of the infant. From the age of 6 months to 6–8 years, similar damage to the permanent teeth may occur. In view of this, tetracycline should be avoided, if possible, in young children.

Adverse effects due to a number of antimicrobial agents have been noted to occur with increased incidence in the elderly (11). In some cases (and perhaps in all if adequately studied), this relationship may be shown to be due to specific disease states or to impairment of physiologic processes associated with aging as noted above. However, in certain cases no specific factors other than age can be identified. The hepatotoxicity associated with isoniazid administration is a good example of this. A small percentage of patients receiving isoniazid develop toxic hepatitis that may be fatal if not recognized in time (18). Liver damage from isoniazid almost never occurs in patients under 20 years of age. In patients 20–34 years of age, the incidence of isoniazid hepatotoxicity is 0.3 percent, rising steadily with age to reach 2.3 percent in patients 50 years of age or more. Because of this, it is currently recommended that routine prophylactic use of isoniazid for patients discovered to have positive tuberculin tests be limited to people under the age of 35 (19).

Nephrotoxic reactions to certain antimicrobial agents, likewise, appear to be more frequent or to occur with lower doses of drugs among the elderly. This has been demonstrated to occur with cephaloridine (20) and colistin (10,21) and may be true for other nephrotoxic antimicrobials as well.

Finally, hypersensitivity reactions to antimicrobial agents also appear to be more common in elderly than in younger patients (10). This appears to be due to the fact that older patients are more likely to have been previously exposed to and, thus, sensitized to these agents. In addition, prior exposure to drugs such as the aminoglycosidic aminocyclitols which produce irreversible cochlear damage can result in cumulative toxicity on repeat exposure (11).

Genetic or Metabolic Abnormalities. The presence of genetic or metabolic abnormalities may also have significant effect on the use or toxicity of a given antimicrobial agent. The rate at which isoniazid is conjugated and biologically inactivated by acetylation in the liver is genetically determined (10). Rapid acetylators are more commonly found among Oriental populations, whereas 45–65 percent of U.S. and North European populations are slow acetylators. Several studies have suggested that polyneuritis is seen more frequently as a complication of isoniazid therapy in slow than in rapid acetylators (10). It was once thought that hepatotoxicity due to isoniazid is related to the conversion of isoniazid to acetyl hydrazine and other related hepatotoxic derivatives and is more common among rapid acetylators (22), but this does not appear to be true.

A number of antimicrobial agents has been shown to be capable of provoking hemolysis in patients with glucose-6-phosphate dehydrogenase (G6PD) deficiency, including the sulfonamides, nitrofurantoin, furazolidine, diaminodiphenylsulfone, and chloramphenicol (10). Sulfonamides may, likewise, cause hemolytic reactions in the presence of certain hemoglobin opathies, including hemoglobin Zurich and hemoglobin H (10).

The presence of metabolic disorders such as diabetes mellitus may also pose problems in antimicrobial therapy. Certain agents such as the sulfonamides (especially the long-acting types) and chloramphenicol can potentiate the hypoglycemic activity of sulfonylurea hypoglycemic agents such as tolbutamide and chlorpropamide (11). In the case of the sulfonamides, this action may be related to their structural simularity to the sulfonylurea drugs. Chloramphenicol inhibits microsomal enzyme activity in the liver and this impairs metabolism of the sulfonylurea hypoglycemic agents. The dextrose load infused with intravenous antibiotics dissolved in dextrose-containing vehicles may be sufficient to produce hyperglycemia and glucosuria in diabetic patients. Another kind of "glucosuria" can occur in patients receiving antimicrobial agents. The cephalosporins, chloramphenicol, isoniazid, nalidixic acid, nitrofurantoin, penicillin, streptomycin, sulfanilimide, and the tetracyclines can all cause false-positive test results when urine sugar is determined by a method (such as Benedict's test or Clinitest) that measures reducing substances in the urine (23). Tests that are specific for glucose (i.e., that use glucose oxidase) such as Dextrostix or Labstix, are not affected by antimicrobial agents.

Absorption of intramuscularly administered antibiotics may be impaired in diabetic patients. Diabetics with bacterial endocarditis who failed to respond to intramuscular penicillin have been described (10). Administration of the same dose of penicillin by the intravenous route, however, resulted in cure (10). Because of the potential impaired absorption of intramuscularly administered antimicrobial agents, it is probably prudent to initiate therapy by the intravenous route when using drugs such as the aminoglycosides to treat diabetic patients with gram-negative bacteremia (especially if accompanied by hypotension) or other serious infections.

Concomitant administration of chloramphenicol has been noted to delay the reticulocyte response to vitamin B_{12} or iron therapy in patients with pernicious anemia or iron deficiency anemia (10). As noted previously, patients with pernicious anemia and gastric achlorydria may exhibit enhanced serum levels of antimicrobials such as penicillin G when given by the oral route.

Rifampin may increase the hepatic metabolism and therefore decrease the effect of oral anticoagulants, oral contraceptives, and barbiturates. See Ref. 24 for a comprehensive list of drug interactions.

Pregnancy. Patients who are pregnant and nursing mothers also pose certain problems in the selection of appropriate antimicrobial agents. All antimicrobial agents cross the placenta in varying degrees (25,26). Thus, the use of such agents in pregnant women provides direct exposure of the fetus to the adverse effects of the drug. Although there are little solid data on the teratogenic potential of most antimicrobial agents in humans, experience suggests that certain drugs such as the penicillins [with the possible exception of ticarcillin (27)], the cephalosporins, and erythromycin are unlikely to be teratogenic and are safe to use in pregnant women (15,25,26). Metronidazole and ticarcillin have been shown to be teratogenic in rodents and thus should be avoided in pregnancy (27,28). The teratogenic potential of many other drugs in humans, including rifampin and trimethoprim, is simply unknown.

A number of antimicrobials has been shown to be deleterious in pregnancy. Tetracycline heads the list. The possible adverse effects of this drug on fetal dentition have already been noted. In addition, pregnant women receiving tetracycline are particularly vulnerable to certain toxic effects, including acute fatty necrosis of the liver, pancreatitis, and probably renal damage (10). The liver damage may be severe and can result in death. When given to patients with impaired renal function, these effects may be magnified, particularly if the agent is one of the tetracyclines that is primarily excreted by the kidneys. These adverse effects are dose related and may be more frequent after intravenous administration. Although it has been suggested that tetracyclines may be given to pregnant women by the oral route in doses of 1 g or less per 24 hours, it is probably safer to avoid these agents entirely in pregnancy (10,15).

The aminoglycosidic aminocyclitol antibiotics cross the placenta. So far fetal toxicity has been reported only for streptomycin when used to treat tuberculosis in pregnant women. Even in that setting, the toxicity has been mild, detectable only by formal vestibular testing or by audiogram (29). Psychomotor retardation, myoclonus, and convulsions have been reported in a small uncontrolled series of children whose mothers received isoniazid for tuberculosis during pregnancy (30). This observation has not been confirmed to date.

Another aspect of drug therapy in pregnancy has recently been examined. It has been found that serum levels after a given dose of ampicillin are lower in pregnant than in nonpregnant women (31). This is related to more rapid clearance of the drug and to a greater volume of distribution (probably due to increased plasma volume) in pregnancy. Thus, higher doses of ampicillin are required to achieve therapeutic blood levels in pregnancy. It is likely that these observations will also apply to other antimicrobial agents, but data on this are not presently available.

Virtually all antimicrobial agents appear in measurable concentrations in breast milk when administered in therapeutic doses to nursing women (32). The amount of drug excreted into breast milk depends on its degree of ionization, its molecular weight, and its solubility in fat and water. Under usual circumstances, the concentrations of antibiotics found in breast milk are quite low. However, even these small amounts may cause significant adverse reactions in the nursing infant. Nalidixic acid and the sulfonamides in breast milk have been shown to cause hemolysis in infants with G6PD deficiency. Sulfonamides in breast milk may be dangerous to premature babies because even small doses of ingested sulfonamides may produce increased levels of unbound bilirubin by displacing bilirubin from its albumin binding sites. As noted previously, this predisposes the child to kernicterus (32). The possibility that antimicrobial agents in breast milk can sensitize newborn children is a theoretical one, but it has not been convincingly demonstrated to date. Although tetracycline is excreted in breast milk, it is unlikely to produce damage to the nursing child's bones or teeth because the calcium in the milk forms an insoluble chelate with tetracyclines, which is not absorbable by the oral route (32).

Renal and Hepatic Function. The ability of the patient to metabolize or excrete antimicrobial agents is one of the most important host factors to consider, especially when high serum or tissue concentrations of the administered drugs are potentially toxic. From a practical point of view, this means that we must carefully assess the patient's renal and hepatic function since these organs serve as the major (and in most cases the *only*) routes of excretion and/or inactivation of antimicrobials. Renal excretion is the most important route of elimination for the majority of antimicrobial agents (33–37). Table 2 lists those drugs that must be used with particular care in patients with decreased renal function. Doses for these drugs may be found in the chapters dealing with the individual agents. In general those agents that require no dosage change in impaired renal function are excreted effectively by extrarenal routes (usually the hepatobiliary system) in patients with renal failure. Their use in normal doses does not result in the appearance of toxic serum levels in this situation, although the urine levels of a number of these agents such as doxycycline and chloramphenicol may be significantly diminished.

Toxic serum levels of the remaining agents may develop if they are used without dosage modification in patients with impaired renal function. Excessive serum levels of penicillin G or carbenicillin may be associated with neuromuscular hyperexcitability, myoclonus, seizures, or coma (10). Excessive serum levels of semisynthetic penicillins such as carbenicillin and ticarcillin or of cephalothin or moxalactam may cause hemostatic defects in patients with impaired renal failure because of interference with platelet function (38,39). Elevated serum levels of aminoglycosidic aminocyclitol antibiotics or vancomycin may result

TABLE 2. Antimicrobial Use in Patients With Varying Degrees of Impaired Renal Function

Antimicrobial agents requiring no dosage change regardless of renal function
Erythromycin, clindamycin, chloramphenicol, doxycycline, cefoperazone, oxacillin, cloxacillin, dicloxacillin, nafcillin, nalidixic acid, rifampin, amphotericin B,[a] sulfadimidine
Antimicrobial agents requiring dosage change only with severe renal failure
Penicillin G, amoxicillin, ampicillin, methicillin, cephalothin, cephalexin, cefamandole, cefoxitin, cefotaxime, ceftizoxime, piperacillin, lincomycin, isoniazid, ethambutol, trimethoprim-sulfamethoxazole
Antimicrobial agents requiring dosage change with impaired renal function
Carbenicillin, ticarcillin, cefazolin, moxalactan, streptomycin, kanamycin, gentamicin, tobramycin, sisomicin, amikacin, nefilmicin, polymyin B, colistin, vancomycin, flucytosine
Antimicrobial agents contraindicated in renal failure
Tetracyclines (except doxycycline and possibly minocycline), nitrofurantoin, cephaloridine, long-acting sulfonamides, methenamine, para-aminosalicyclic acid

[a] Even though amphotericin B is excreted primarily by nonrenal means, this drug must be used with caution in patients with impaired renal function because of its nephrotoxicity.

in eighth nerve damage (13,37). Neurotoxic reactions, including respiratory arrest and death, may occur in patients with excessive serum levels of certain aminoglycosidic aminocyclitols or of the polymyxins (10,21). Bone marrow suppression may occur in patients with renal failure who receive inappropriately high doses of 5-fluorocytosine (40). In all the above situations, the possibility of toxic reactions can be significantly lessened or eliminated if the doses of the antimicrobial agents are appropriately reduced in the presence of renal insufficiency.

The tetracyclines (except doxycycline and possibly minocycline) are contraindicated in patients with impaired renal function because the elevated serum levels that result may produce a significant worsening of the uremic state due to their antianabolic effect. Moreover, they may cause enhanced hepatotoxicity in this situation (10). Cephaloridine and the long-acting sulfonamides should be avoided in this situation because they are potentially nephrotoxic.

Certain antimicrobial agents, including erythromycin, chloramphenicol, lincomycin, and clindamycin, should be used with caution in patients with impaired hepatic function. These drugs are primarily excreted or detoxified in the liver. Bone marrow suppression due to chloramphenicol is much more likely to occur in patients with impaired hepatic function; because of this, it has been suggested that the dose of chloramphenicol be cut at least in half in patients with cirrhosis and other severe liver disease (41). Serum half-lives of clindamycin and lincomycin are increased in patients with severe liver disease; because of this, the doses of both drugs should be decreased in this situation. The tetracyclines may produce elevations in serum transaminase levels in patients recovering from viral hepatitis (10). They should be avoided or used with extreme caution in patients with underlying liver disease. The serum half-lives of both rifampin and isoniazid are prolonged in patients with cirrhosis (42). Hepatobiliary disease influences antimicrobic therapy in still another way. The biliary concentrations of many antimicrobial agents, including ampicillin and nafcillin, normally excreted in high concentration in the bile may be significantly reduced in patients with liver disease or biliary obstruction (10).

Site of Infection. Of all the host factors to be considered in the choice of an antimicrobial agent, none is more important than the site of infection. The locus of the infectious process determines not only the choice of the agent but also its dose and the route by which it should be administered. For antimicrobial therapy to be effective, an adequate concentration of the drug must be delivered to the site of infection. In most cases, this means that the local concentration of the antimicrobial agent should at least equal the minimal inhibitory concentration of the infecting organism. Concentrations representing multiples of the MIC are generally felt more likely to be efficacious, but in many cases such local concentrations may be difficult or impossible to achieve. Failure to achieve local concentrations of antibiotics higher than the MIC of the infecting organism may not always be disastrous, however, because there is evidence that subinhibitory concentrations of drugs may produce antimicrobial effects that aid the host defenses against infections. It has been clearly demonstrated that subinhibitory concentrations of antibiotics can alter bacterial morphology (43), adherence properties (44), and opsonic requirements (45), can enhance phagocytosis (46), and can even aid intracellular killing of bacteria by polymorphonuclear leukocytes (47). This may explain the clinical observation that on occasion doses of antimicrobials that produce seemingly inadequate serum levels may still result in clinical cure. In spite of such observations, most infectious disease clinicians feel that optimal therapy requires concentrations of antimicrobials that are above the MIC.

Serum concentrations of antimicrobial agents are relatively easy to determine and therefore are often used as a guide in the therapy. However, except in cases of bacteremia, antimicrobial efficacy is more likely determined by the tissue concentration than by blood level, as noted earlier. Binding to serum proteins may affect both the tissue distribution and the activity of antimicrobial agents in the blood. Although much careful investigation has been done on protein binding, the precise clinical significance of this phenomenon remains to be determined. For example, it has been shown that only the unbound form of a given antimicrobial agent is active in vitro (and presumably also in vivo) against infecting organisms (48). However, since protein binding is rapidly reversible (49), the activity of even highly protein-bound agents may not be absolutely limited by protein binding. The penetration of antimicrobial agents into interstitial fluid and lymph is related to protein binding, since only the free form of the agent is able to pass through the capillary wall (48). Penetration of antibiotics into fibrin clots (which may be analogous to the penetration of the drugs to reach the site of infection in patients with bacterial endocarditis) is, likewise, related to the amount of unbound antibiotic in the surrounding fluid (50). Nevertheless, it is often difficult to correlate therapeutic outcome with in vitro susceptibility and protein binding unless several variables are carefully controlled (51,52). The reason for this is simply that it is the concentration of antibiotic at the site of infection that is the major determinant in the successful therapy. Such concentrations are often difficult to assess because they are the result of a complex interaction between local factors that may bind, inactivate, or enhance the activity of a given antimicrobial agent. The ability of an antibiotic to pass through membranes by nonionic diffusion is related to its lipid solubility. Thus, lipid soluble agents such as chloramphenicol, rifampin, trimethoprim, and isoniazid are all more adept at penetrating membranes than the more highly ionized compounds (48). These agents rapidly cross the blood-brain barrier and produce better cerebrospinal fluid levels than more highly ionized compounds such as the aminoglycosidic aminocyclitols. Except in neonates, none of the aminoglycosides produces effective cerebrospinal fluid levels when given parenterally. To be effective for the treatment of meningitis, they must be given via the intrathecal or intraventricular route in adults (53). This is an excellent example of the importance of the site of infection in determining the most efficacious antimicrobial therapy. For the treatment of bacterial meningitis in adults, we either must choose agents, such as chloramphenicol or the third-generation cephalosporins (e.g., cefotaxime, ceftriaxone, or moxalactam) that cross the blood-brain barrier reasonably well or we must use high concentrations of parenteral doses of drugs such as penicillin G, ampicillin, or nafcillin that penetrate into the cerebrospinal fluid only with difficulty. Agents, such as the aminoglycosidic aminocyclitols and first-generation cephalosporins that produce inadequate cerebrospinal fluid levels even after high-dose parenteral therapy must be administered directly into the cerebrospinal fluid or must be avoided entirely.

The vegetations of bacterial endocarditis, bones, and devitalized tissue represent examples of other areas in which the penetration of antimicrobial agents to the site of infection may be borderline or inadequate. Because of this, high-dose and prolonged parenteral therapy is usually required for the effective treatment of bacterial endocarditis and osteomyelitis. In some cases, we may take advantage of the physiologic handling of antimicrobials to achieve therapeutic success. Agents that are excreted by the liver and are concentrated in the bile, such as ampicillin or doxycycline, may be more effective in treating cholangitis than agents, such as the first-generation cephalosporins or aminoglycosidic aminocyclitols that are not greatly concentrated in bile.

Even the achievement of "therapeutic concentrations" of antimicrobial agents at the site of infection may not be sufficient for cure. The reason for this is that a number of local factors may influence the activity of antimicrobial agents. These, too, must be considered in designing an appropriate therapeutic regimen. Aminoglycosidic aminocyclitols and the polymyxins are bound to and inactivated by purulent material (54). This is one of many reasons why surgical drainage is imperative when treating abscesses with agents such as these. Interestingly, carbenicillin does not lose activity in pus (54). Although carbenicillin (and other penicillins) may be more active in purulent material, clinical experience strongly suggests that appropriate drainage procedures greatly enhance the efficacy of these agents as well. Although penicillin G, like carbenicillin, is not inactivated by purulent material per se (48), recent studies suggest that the presence of β-lactamase-producing organisms such as *Bacteroides fragilis* in abscesses may result in local inactivation of penicillin G (55).

Penicillins and tetracyclines are also bound by hemoglobin and thus may be less effective in the presence of significant hematoma formation (48). In vitro *Pseudomonas aeruginosa* is protected from the action of the aminoglycosidic aminocyclitols and polymyxins by high concentrations of calcium or magnesium in the culture medium (56). The clinical significance of this observation, if any, remains to be determined. Local decreases in oxygen tension such as occur in abscesses and intraperitoneal infections may also have an effect on the activity of certain antimicrobial agents. The aminoglycosidic aminocyclitols, for example, are inactive against anaerobes and may also be less effective against facultative organisms under anaerobic conditions because oxygen is required for transport of these agents into the bacterial cell (57).

Local alterations in pH such as occur in abscesses and especially in the urine may have an important effect on the activity of a number of antimicrobial agents. Methenamine, nitrofurantoin, novobiocin, and chlortetracycline are more active at acid pH, whereas alkalinization enhances the activity of erythromycin, lincomycin, clindamycin, and the aminoglycosidic aminocyclitol antibiotics. Indeed, the aminoglycosidic aminocyclitols show marked loss of activity at low pH. These observations have been used in treating patients with urinary tract infections, a situation in which the local pH can be altered by the addition of acidifying or alkalinizing agents (58,59).

The presence of foreign bodies also has a profound effect on the activity of antimicrobial agents. Thus, it is often necessary to remove the foreign material to cure an infection in the vicinity of a prosthetic heart valve or joint implant (60). The mechanism by which foreign bodies potentiate infection is not clear, but they probably cause localized impairment of host defense mechanisms (61). It has also been demonstrated that antimicrobial agents, themselves, may cause alterations in host defenses. Clinically achievable concentrations of many different agents have been shown to have adverse effects on leukocyte chemotaxis, lymphocyte transformation, monocyte transformation, delayed hypersensitivity, antibody production, phagocytosis, and the microbicidal action of polymorphonuclear leukocytes (62–67). It is not clear, however, whether any of these effects (largely demonstrated by in vitro studies) are of clinical significance. Nonetheless, the possibility that antimicrobial agents can cause immunosuppression exists, and this fact should discourage the indiscriminate use of antibiotics, especially in patients who are already immunosuppressed because of their underlying disease or because of their concomitant drug therapy (66).

ANTIMICROBIAL COMBINATIONS

The majority of infections in humans can be treated with a single antimicrobial agent, but there are clear-cut (as well as borderline) indications for the use of combinations (usually two) of antimicrobials. Because combinations may provide more broad-spectrum coverage than single agents, the physician is often tempted to use combinations for the sense of security they provide, even in situations in which they are not indicated. Such inappropriate use of antimicrobial combinations may have significantly deleterious effects. In this section we will examine the indications for the use of combinations and the potential disadvantages of this approach to therapy.

In Vitro Results of Combination Therapy

When two antimicrobial agents are combined, they may have one of three types of activity against a given organism in vitro: (*1*) additive effect (sometimes called an indifferent effect), (*2*) synergism, (*3*) antagonism (68). Two drugs are said to be additive when the activity of the drugs in combination is equal to the sum (or a partial sum) of their independent activities when studied separately. The combined effect of a synergistic pair of antimicrobials is greater than the sum of their independent activities when measured separately. If two drugs are antagonistic, the activity of the combination is less than the sum of their independent effects when measured alone. These concepts are illustrated by "time-kill curves" in Figure 1. A discussion of the various methods used to determine the in vitro effects of antibiotic combinations is beyond the scope of this chapter but has recently been reviewed in detail (69).

Indications for the Clinical Use of Antimicrobial Combinations

Five reasons have been advanced to justify the use of antimicrobial combinations. The first three of these are discussed in detail elsewhere and, therefore, will be given only brief mention here.

Prevention of the Emergence of Resistant Organisms. Although the use of antimicrobial agents to prevent the emergence of resistant organisms would seem to be a major indication for the use of such therapy, combination therapy has been clearly documented as effective in preventing resistance only during the treatment of tuberculosis (see Chapter 15). There is somewhat less epidemiologic evidence in support of this concept as it applies to the use of rifampin for the treatment of nonmycobacterial infections, but it nonetheless appears that one of the major benefits of using rifampin in combination with a second agent for treating staphylococcal infections, for example, is that the combination prevents the rapid emergence of resistance to rifampin, which is evident when this drug is used alone (70,71).

Polymicrobial Infections. In the majority of infections, even those due to more than one organism, a single effective agent can be found. For example, cellulitis due to *S. aureus* and group A streptococci can be treated with a penicillinase-

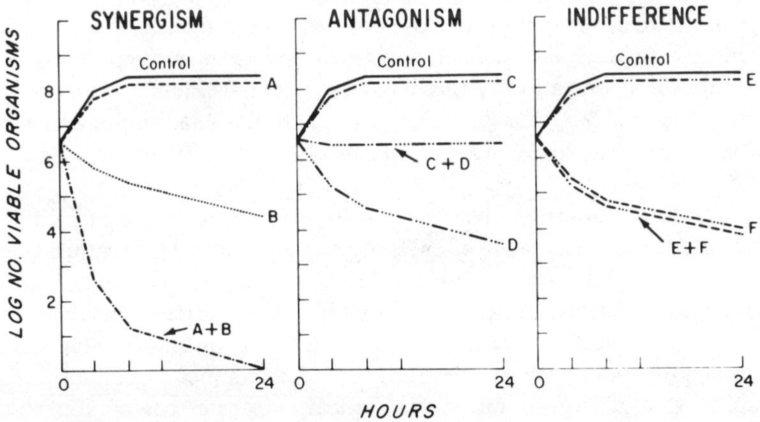

FIGURE 1. Antibacterial effects of antibiotic combinations. *Left* (A and B): synergism; center (C and D): antagonism; *right* (E and F): indifference (additive). [Used with permission from Moellering (74).]

resistant penicillin alone. However, there are certain types of infections due to such a broad variety of organisms that more than one antimicrobial agent may be required to provide adequate coverage. Examples of such infections include intraperitoneal and pelvic infections due to mixed bowel flora and certain brain abscesses.

Initial Therapy. In neutropenic patients or other patients with presumed infection in whom the nature of the infection is not clear, it is reasonable to begin broad-spectrum coverage, usually with two agents such as nafcillin or carbenicillin plus gentamicin or tobramycin while awaiting the results of cultures. In this setting, it is often possible to discontinue one of the agents or to switch to an alternate single drug after the results of cultures are available. The continued development of new drugs with broad spectra of activity may eventually make it possible to use a single agent for most cases of initial therapy, but it would be premature to advocate general application of this concept at present.

Decreased Toxicity. Many of the drugs used in the therapy for infections are potentially toxic (e.g., aminoglycosidic aminocyclitols). Therefore, a major goal of combination therapy has been to reduce the amount of drug required for treatment and, thus, to reduce dose-related toxicity. Unfortunately, at present there are no data from clinical trials that establish beyond doubt that combination therapy with different agents permits a reduction of drug dose sufficient to reduce dose-related toxicity. There is evidence that the use of a mixture of similar agents (e.g., triple sulfonamides) can reduce the incidence of a dose-related complication: crystalluria with stone formation (72). The explanation for this effect is that the solubility of each component (sulfadiazine, sulfamerazine, sulfamethazine) in urine is independent of the others, although their antibacterial activity is cumulative.

Synergism. The use of synergistic combinations of antimicrobial agents to treat infections due to resistant or relatively resistant organisms represents one of the most appealing ways to use these agents. There are numerous examples of in vitro synergism, but thus far synergistic antimicrobial combinations have proven more effective than single agents in only a limited number of clinical settings (73,74).

Perhaps the best known application of synergistic combinations of antimicrobial agents is for the treatment of enterococcal endocarditis. Treatment of this disease with penicillin alone results in an unacceptable relapse rate because enterococci are relatively resistant to penicillin (75). Indeed, penicillin alone seems to act as a bacteriostatic and not a bactericidal agent (76). The addition of an aminoglycoside, such as streptomycin or gentamicin, results in both in vitro and in vivo synergism and yields clinical cure rates comparable to those achieved for endocarditis caused by less resistant streptococci (75,76). Penicillin enhances the uptake of aminoglycosides by enterococci; the result of this interaction is the synergistic killing of the organisms (77). In recent years some enterococci have been found to be resistant to penicillin-streptomycin, penicillin-kanamycin, and penicillin-amikacin synergism due to high-level resistance (MIC > 2000 μg/ml) to streptomycin, and/or to kanamycin (78). Strains may resist synergism if they are ribosomally resistant to streptomycin (79) or if they contain plasmid-mediated enzymes that inactivate streptomycin, kanamycin, or amikacin (80). The exact clinical significance of these in vitro observations remains to be proven; but because of this a number of physicians feel that penicillin-gentamicin combinations are preferred to penicillin-streptomycin for enterococcal endocarditis (especially if the infection is caused by a strain that is highly resistant to streptomycin). The recent discovery of enterococci with plasmid-mediated high-level gentamicin resistance is particularly disconcerting (81). Fortunately, such isolates are relatively rare at the present time in the United States, but their existence means that in vitro testing for synergism or at least for high-level aminoglycoside resistance should be performed before the use of combination therapy for serious enterococcal infections.

Penicillin-streptomycin combinations are also synergistic against *Streptococcus viridans* and have been used for the treatment of endocarditis due to these organisms (65). However, *S. viridans* are usually very susceptible to penicillin, and penicillin alone has been used successfully for treatment of this kind of endocarditis (66).

A similar type of synergism occurs when semisynthetic penicillinase-resistant penicillins such as nafcillin or oxacillin are combined with gentamicin against *S. aureus* (67). So far there are no data to document that the use of combination therapy for *S. aureus* infections in humans has any advantage over therapy with a penicillin or cephalosporin alone (85).

Combinations of carbenicillin, ticarcillin mezlocillin, azlocillin, or piperacillin with gentamicin, tobramycin, or amikacin exhibit synergism against many strains of *P. aeruginosa* (86,87). Although it has not been studied in detail, it is likely that the mechanism of synergism in this setting is similar to that described for enterococci (i.e., enhanced uptake of the aminoglycoside in the presence of the antipseudomonal penicillin). Studies with experimental animals demonstrate convincingly the superiority of such combinations for the treatment of serious *Pseudomonas* infections (88). Although the information available from limited human trials to date is also consistent with enhanced activity of these combinations for *Pseudomonas* infections, this form of therapy has not been subjected to definitive controlled study (69).

Synergism occurs by a different mechanism when sulfonamides are combined with trimethoprim. In this case, the two agents are synergistic because they act to inhibit sequential steps in the microbial pathway of folic acid metabolism (89). As a result, combinations of sulfonamides with trimethoprim are often useful for the treatment of infections due to organisms that may be resistant to sulfonamides alone. A fixed combination of sulfamethoxazole and trimethoprim is available for clinical use and has been shown effective for the treatment and prevention of chronic urinary tract infections, even when due to sulfonamide-resistant organisms (90). The combination has also been shown to be useful for the treatment of typhoid fever and shigellosis caused by organisms resistant to ampicillin and/or chloramphenicol and for the treatment of infections due to ampicillin-resistant *H. influenzae* (69,91,92).

Combinations of amphotericin B with a number of other agents including 5-fluorocytosine, rifampin, and tetracycline have been shown to result in enhanced antimicrobial activity against fungi (93). The mechanism of synergism seems to involve damage to the fungal cell envelope by amphotericin B with resultant enhanced intracellular penetration of 5-fluorocytosine and other agents (93). Flucytosine and low-dose amphotericin B have been used successfully in treating candidiasis and cryptococcosis when the patients' isolate was susceptible to both drugs (94,95).

Synergism and Infections in Impaired Hosts. The clinical applications of antimicrobial combinations discussed thus far have all represented attempts to use a synergistic interaction for enhanced efficacy in the treatment of infections due to relatively resistant organisms. Another use of such therapy is to obtain enhanced antimicrobial activity in the treatment of infections due to susceptible organisms occurring in patients with abnormalities of host defense systems. Several groups have conducted randomized trials of various combinations of two agents chosen from among carbenicillin, ticarcillin, piperacillin, the cephalosporins, gentamicin, tobramycin, and amikacin for the treatment of severe infections in patients with impaired host defense mechanisms. Both Lau et al. (96) and Klastersky et al. (97) have demonstrated improved survival rates in such patients treated with combinations that were synergistic against the infecting organisms compared with patients receiving nonsynergistic combinations. These studies add strong support to the concept that synergistic combinations of antimicrobials may be an important determinant of success in the treatment of serious infections, especially when due to gram-negative organisms in patients with impaired host defenses.

Disadvantages of the Inappropriate Use of Antimicrobial Combinations

Whereas the clinical use of synergistic combinations of antimicrobial agents may have beneficial results as noted above, the inappropriate use of antimicrobial combinations may have important adverse effects, three of which will be discussed below.

Antagonism. The medical literature contains a large number of reports of in vitro antagonism between antimicrobial agents (73,74). In view of this, it is surprising that there are only a few well-documented clinical examples of antagonism. Perhaps the most impressive is the study of Lepper and Dowling, who demonstrated conclusively in 1951 that penicillin is more effective than the combination of penicillin with chlortetracycline for the treatment of pneumococcal meningitis (98). The fatality among patients treated with penicillin alone was 21 percent, whereas that among patients treated with penicillin plus chlortetracycline was 79 percent. A study of childhood meningitis has also demonstrated the superiority of single drug therapy. Mathies et al. treated a group of children suffering from bacterial meningitis with either ampicillin alone or a combination of ampicillin, chloramphenicol, and streptomycin (99). The mortality among 140 children treated with ampicillin alone was 4.3 percent, whereas the mortality among 124 children receiving the antibiotic combination was 10.5 percent, a difference that reached statistical significance. There are several other reports of the influence of antagonism on the treatment of urinary tract infections and streptococcal pharyngitis, but none are particularly impressive (74). Considering the extensive clinical use of antimicrobial combinations and especially in view of the large number of reports of in vitro antagonism, it is surprising that there are so few reports of in vivo antagonism. This may be due in part to the paucity of well-controlled studies in this area, or to the reluctance of investigators to report adverse results. Another possible explanation is simply that clinically significant antagonism is not a common event. In most cases, in vitro antagonism results in the loss or partial loss of activity of the most active drug (e.g., the bactericidal activity of such an agent may be reduced to simple bacteriostasis), but the combination still retains some antimicrobial activity. As long as the patient receiving such therapy has normal host defense mechanisms, it is unlikely that adverse effects will be seen. This has been the case in studies using an antagonistic combination of antibiotics (chloramphenicol plus gentamicin) to treat experimental infections due to *Proteus mirabilis* in mice (100). In healthy mice, in vivo antagonism could not be demonstrated; but after irradiation to render the animals neutropenic, gentamicin alone was more effective than gentamicin plus chloramphenicol. This combination has also been shown to be antagonistic in experimentally produced meningitis due to *P. mirabilis* in rabbits (101). Thus, it seems that clinically important antagonism is most likely to be manifest in patients with generalized impairment of host defense mechanisms (such as seen in leukemia, cancer patients who are neutropenic, etc.) or in patients with infections such as meningitis or endocarditis where localized host defenses may be inadequate.

The observation of in vivo antagonism in the treatment of bacterial meningitis raises some questions about the present recommendations for the use of ampicillin plus chloramphenicol in the initial treatment of childhood meningitis. Chloramphenicol has been added to the former ampicillin regimen because of the emergence of ampicillin-resistant strains of *H. influenzae* (7). Combinations of penicillin plus chloramphenicol have been shown to exhibit in vitro antagonism against pneumococci and other organisms (73). However, this antagonism takes the form of lessened bactericidal activity of penicillin in the presence of chloramphenicol. Since chloramphenicol alone is quite active against the organisms likely to cause childhood meningitis (*H. influenzae, S. pneumoniae, Neisseria meningitidis*) and since there is no evidence that penicillin or ampicillin antagonizes the activity of chloramphenicol, it seems unlikely that the current recommendations for pediatric meningitis will result in in vivo antagonism when used to treat meningitis due to the organisms listed above (73).

Recent studies documenting the effectiveness of some of the newer cephalosporins such as cefuroxime and ceftriaxone (102,103) for childhood meningitis may ultimately make it unnecessary to continue to use combination therapy in this setting.

There has been a recent upsurge of interest in the use of the newer broad-spectrum β-lactams in combination with each other to obtain broad-spectrum coverage without exposing the patient to the possible toxicity of an agent such as chloramphenicol or an aminoglycosidic aminocyclitol (104). For the most part, this seems reasonable. However, there is in vitro and in vivo evidence that some β-lactam–β-lactam combinations may be antagonistic against certain organisms such as *Enterobacter, Serratia,* or *Pseudomonas.* This antagonism seems to be the result of the induction of β-lactamase production by one of the agents, resulting in the inactivation of the second (105). The exact clinical significance of this phenomenon is not presently clear, but it must be kept in mind when we consider the clinical use of such combinations.

Most of the examples of in vitro antagonism are the result of interactions of the antimicrobial agents as they react at a subcellular level on a given microorganism. However, another type of antagonism should also be included in this discussion. This may result from the direct interaction of drugs before they reach the microorganism. If chloramphenicol and erythromycin are inadvertently mixed together in the same parenteral infusion solution, they form insoluable precipitates and hence lose activity. In recent years, it has become clear that the mixing of penicillins (especially carbenicillin or ticarcillin) with aminoglycosides results in the inactivation of the aminoglycoside (106). Because the reaction occurs slowly, this is usually not a problem in vivo, provided the drugs are given by separate routes of administration. However, in uremic patients in whom the serum half-life of aminoglycosides is greatly prolonged, in vivo inactivation can occur (107). The clinical significance of this observation, however, has not yet been elucidated.

Cost. With the possible exception of penicillin G and certain of the tetracyclines and sulfonamides, antimicrobials are expensive drugs. Thus the inappropriate use of antimicrobial combinations (when a single agent would be adequate) can add greatly to the cost of the patient's illness. This important consideration is discussed in greater detail in Chapter 19.

Adverse Effects. It has been estimated that approximately 5 percent of the patients receiving a given antibiotic in the hospital will experience some sort of adverse reaction (12,108). Obviously the possibility of such adverse reactions (including hypersensitivity reactions and direct toxic effects) is increased without any enhanced therapeutic benefit when we inappropriately use combinations of antimicrobial agents. Moreover, when an adverse reaction occurs in a patient receiving more than one drug, it is often difficult to be certain of the agent that caused the reaction. This may mean that several or all drugs must be stopped. If combination drug therapy is to be used in such a patient, each drug must be tested carefully before use to make certain that it was not the cause of the original adverse reaction. This is time consuming and expensive and may needlessly deprive the patient of the benefits of a useful agent.

CHOICE OF APPROPRIATE ROUTE OF ADMINISTRATION OF ANTIMICROBIAL AGENTS AND EVALUATION OF EFFICACY

Route of Administration

Once the physician has determined the most appropriate drug or drugs with which to treat a given infection, he or she must decide which route of administration to use to obtain maximum benefits from the therapy. In most cases this is a choice between oral and parenteral routes. In general, the oral route of administration is chosen for those infections that are mild and that can be treated on an outpatient basis. Not all antibiotics can be administered in this way. Drugs such as vancomycin, the polymyxins, the aminoglycosidic aminocyclitols, and amphotericin B are absorbed so poorly from the gastrointestinal tract that they cannot be administered orally to treat systemic infections. When drugs are administered by the oral route, the physician must ascertain that the patient will reliably take them as ordered. The absorption of certain agents such as penicillin G is markedly impaired if taken with meals, whereas the absorption of acid-stable penicillins such as penicillin V is not affected by food or gastric acidity. The concomitant administration of antacids or iron-containing preparations may severely impair the absorption of tetracycline since this drug forms insoluble chelates in the presence of Mg^{2+}, Ca^{2+}, or Fe^{2+} ions. More detailed information on the oral absorption of antimicrobial agents may be found in the chapters on the individual drugs.

The parenteral route of administration is used for agents that are inefficiently absorbed from the gastrointestinal tract and for the treatment of patients with serious infections in whom high serum concentrations of antimicrobial agents are required. The aminoglycosidic aminocyclitols and polymyxins are usually given by intramuscular injection and are well tolerated when given this way. For most infections, adequate serum concentrations are achieved after intramuscular administration of these drugs. However, in life-threatening infections, especially in the presence of shock (or in diabetic patients as discussed earlier) intravenous administration is preferred. Intravenous administration allows large doses of drugs to be given with a minimum of discomfort to the patient when high serum concentrations are required for the effective treatment of disease processes such as meningitis, endocarditis, and osteomyelitis. Whether intravenously administered drugs should be given by continuous infusion or by intermittent bolus infusion remains a matter of controversy. The former method has the advantage of simplicity; because pulses containing very high concentrations of drugs are avoided, it may result in less venous irritation and phlebitis. Studies in animal models suggest that the concentration of drugs such as penicillins and cephalosporins in fibrin clots is related to the peak serum levels achieved. Thus, greater concentrations of drugs are achieved in the clots in the face of intermittent bolus therapy (109). It has been suggested that this data may be applicable to the therapy for infective endocarditis and other infections in which high tissue concentrations of antibiotics are required. Convincing clinical proof of this concept, however, does not exist.

As discussed earlier, the intrathecal or intraventricular route of administration may be necessary for the treatment of meningeal infections with drugs such as the aminoglycosidic aminocyclitols, polymyxins, bacitracin, and possibly vancomycin, all of which cross the blood-brain barrier with considerable difficulty. Parenteral administration of antimicrobial agents results in adequate concentrations in pleural, peritoneal, pericardial, and synovial fluid (110,111). Thus, direct installation of antibiotics into these areas is not necessary.

Monitoring the Response of the Patient to Antimicrobial Therapy

Although several laboratory tests are available to assist in the monitoring of antimicrobial therapy, clinical assessment remains the most important method for determining the efficacy of treatment. It is not uncommon to see patients fail to respond in the face of laboratory studies that suggest adequate therapy and vice versa. The reasons for this may usually be found among the many host factors that affect therapy as described earlier.

Nonetheless, measurement of serum concentrations of antimicrobial agents and determination of serum bactericidal titers are often of considerable use. The major value of the direct determination of serum concentrations of antimicrobial agents is to avoid toxicity from excessive levels of agents such as the aminoglycosidic aminocyclitols and vancomycin, especially in patients with impaired renal or hepatic function. These tests are also useful for determining inadequate serum levels due to insufficient dosing or unusually rapid clearance.

Another method used to monitor the effectiveness of antimicrobial therapy is the serum bactericidal titer (sometimes called the serum antimicrobial dilution titer). This test was originally described by Schlichter and MacLean as a guide for effective therapy for subacute bacterial endocarditis (112). Subsequently this test has been used to monitor therapy in patients with infective endocarditis, osteomyelitis, septic arthritis, empyema, and bacteremia (97,113). In this test, serial dilutions of the patient's serum are incubated with an inoculum of the infecting organism; after incubation, the highest dilution that inhibits and/or kills the organism is determined. Most investigators feel that a serum bactericidal titer of at least 1:8 can be correlated with a successful therapeutic outcome

(97,112,114). However, lack of standardization and lack of consistency in specifying the point (peak, trough, or midpoint serum levels) at which the test should be done have hindered attempts at more widespread application and evaluation of this test (116,117).

CONCLUSION

Optimal use of antimicrobial agents demands consideration of a large number of important factors that may influence the choice of an appropriate agent and that determine the most effective dose and route of administration of a drug. A number of these factors has been outlined in this chapter. In the final analysis, sound clinical judgment remains the most important determinant of a successful outcome.

REFERENCES

1. Weinstein L: General considerations, in Goodman LS and Gilman A (eds): *The Pharmacological Basis of Therapeutics.* New York, The Macmillan Company, 1970, p 1154.
2. Majno G: *The Healing Hand: Man and Wound in the Ancient World.* Cambridge, Mass, Harvard University Press, 1975, pp 154 and 215.
3. Harris JC, Dupont HL, Hornick RB: Fecal leukocytes in diarrheal illness. *Ann Intern Med* 76:697, 1972.
4. Ho D, Ault MJ, Ault MA, et al: Campylobacter enteritis. Early diagnosis with Gram's stain. *Arch Intern Med* 142:1858, 1982.
5. Weinstein L: Common sense (clinical judgment) in the diagnosis and antibiotic therapy of etiologically undefined infections. *Pediatr Clin North Am* 15:141, 1968.
6. Moellering RC Jr: A rational approach to the choice of antimicrobial agents in bacterial infections. Seminar on Gram-Negative Infections, St. Louis, 1974, p 5.
7. Murray BE, Moellering RC Jr: Patterns and mechanisms of antibiotic resistance. *Med Clin North Am* 62:899, 1978.
8. Moellering RC Jr, Kunz LJ, Poitras JW, et al: Microbiologic basis for the rational use of antibiotics. *South Med J* 70(suppl):8, 1977.
9. Abramowicz M (ed): The choice of antimicrobial drugs. *The Medical Letter* 1984.
10. Weinstein L, Dalton AC: Host determinants of response to antimicrobial agents. *N Engl J Med* 279:467, 1968.
11. Moellering RC Jr: Factors influencing the clinical use of antimicrobial agents in elderly patients. *Geriatrics* 33:83, 1978.
12. Mannisto PT, Mantyla R, Nykanen S, et al: Impairing effect of food on ketoconazole absorption. *Antimicrob Agents Chemother* 21:730, 1982.
13. Jackson GG, Arcieri G: Ototoxicity of gentamicin in man: A survey and controlled analysis of clinical experience in the United States. *J Infect Dis* 119:432, 1969.
14. Calderwood S, Moellering RC Jr: Common adverse effects of antibacterial agents on major organ systems. *Surg Clin North Am* 60:65, 1980.
15. Moellering RC Jr: Antimicrobial agents in pregnancy and the postpartum period. *Clin Obstet Gynecol* (in press).
16. McCracken GH Jr: Pharmacologic basis for antimicrobial therapy in newborn infants. *Am J Dis Child* 128:407, 1974.

17. Kline AH, Blattner RJ, Lunin M: Transplacental effect of tetracyclines on teeth. *JAMA* 118:178, 1964.
18. Garibaldi RA, Drusin RE, Ferebee SH, et al: Isoniazid-associated hepatitis. *Am Rev Respr Dis* 106:357, 1972.
19. Anonymous: Preventive therapy of tuberculous infection. *Morbidity and Mortality Weekly Report* 24:71, 1975.
20. Foord RD: Cephaloridine, cephalothin and the kidney. *J Antimicrob Chemother* 1(suppl):119, 1975.
21. Koch-Weser J, Sidel VW, Federman EB, et al: Adverse effects of sodium colistimethate. *Ann Intern Med* 72:857, 1970.
22. Van Scoy RE: Antituberculous agents. *Mayo Clin Proc* 52:694, 1977.
23. Young DS, Thomas DW, Friedman RB, et al: Effects of drugs on clinical laboratory tests. *Clin Chem* 18:1041, 1972.
24. Rizack MA, Hilman CDM: *The Medical Letter Handbook of Drug Interactions,* New Rochelle, NY, The Medical Letter, 1983.
25. Sabath LD: Antibiotics in obstetric practice, in Charles D, Finland M (eds): *Obstetric and Perinatal Infections.* Philadelphia, Lea & Febiger, 1973, p 563.
26. Monif GRG: *Infectious Diseases in Obstetrics and Gynecology.* Hagerstown, Md, Harper & Row, 1974, p 18.
27. Anonymous: Ticarcillin. *The Medical Letter* 19:17, 1977.
28. Anonymous: Is Flagyl dangerous? *The Medical Letter* 17:53, 1975.
29. Conway N, Birt BD: Streptomycin in pregnancy: Effect in foetal ear. *Br Med J* 2:260, 1965.
30. Monnet P, Kalb JC, Pujol M: Toxic influence of isoniazid on fetus. *Lyon Med* 218:431, 1967.
31. Philipson A: Pharmakokinetics of ampicillin during pregnancy. *J Infect Dis* 136:370, 1977.
32. Vorherr H: Drug excretion in breast milk. *Postgrad Med* 56:97, 1974.
33. Jackson EA, McLeod DC: Pharmacokinetics and dosing of antimicrobial agents in renal impairment, part i. *Am J Hosp Pharm* 31:36, 1974.
34. Jackson EA, McLeod DC: Pharmacokinetics and dosing of antimicrobial agents in renal impairment, part ii. *Am J Hosp Pharm* 31:137, 1974.
35. Cheigh J: Drug administration in renal failure. *Am J Med* 62:555, 1977.
36. Bennett WM, Singer I, Coggins CJ: A guide to drug therapy in renal failure. *JAMA* 230:1544, 1974.
37. Appel GB, Neu HC: The nephrotoxicity of antimicrobial agents. *N Engl J Med* 296:663, 722, 1977.
38. Natelson EA, Brown CH III, Bradshaw MW, et al: Influence of cephalosporin antibiotics on blood coagulation and platelet function. *Antimicrob Agents Chemother* 9:91, 1976.
39. Neu HC: Adverse effects of new cephalosporins. *Ann Intern Med* 98:415, 1983.
40. Kaufman CA, Frame PT: Bone marrow toxicity associated with 5-fluorocytosine therapy. *Antimicrob Agents Chemother* 11:244, 1977.
41. Suhrland LG, Weisberger AS: Choramphenicol toxicity in liver and renal disease. *Arch Intern Med* 112:747, 1963.
42. Pessayre D, Allemand H, Benhamou J-P: Effets des maladies du foie et des voies biliaires sur le métabolisme des médicaments. *Nouv Presse Med* 35:3209, 1977.
43. Lorian V, Atkinson B: Killing of oxacillin-exposed staphylococci in human polymorphonuclear leukocytes. *Antimicrob Agents Chemother* 18:807, 1980.
44. Ofek IE, Beachey H, Eisenstein BI, et al: Suppression of bacterial adherence by subminimal inhibitory concentration of β-lactam and aminoglycoside antibiotics. *Rev Infect Dis* 1:832, 1979.
45. Gemmell CG, Peterson PK, Schmeling DJ, et al: Potentiation of oponization and phagocytosis of *Streptococcus pyogenes* following growth in the presence of clindamycin. *J Clin Invest* 67:1249, 1981.
46. Friedman H, Warren GH: Enhanced susceptibility of penicillin-resistant staphylococci to phagocytosis after in vitro incubation with low dose of nafcillin. *Proc Soc Exp Biol Med* 146:707, 1974.

47. Elliott GR, Peterson PK, Verbrugh HA, et al: Influence of subinhibitory concentrations of penicillin, cephalothin, and clindamycin on *Staphyloccus aureus* growth in human phagocytic cells. *Antimicrob Agents Chemother* 22:781, 1982.
48. Craig WA, Kunin CM: Significance of serum protein and tissue binding of antimicrobial agents. *Ann Rev Med* 27:287, 1976.
49. Peterson LR, Gerding DN: Interaction of cephalosporins with human and canine serum proteins. *J Infect Dis* 137:452, 1978.
50. Barza M, Samuelson T, Weinstein L: Penetration of antibiotics into fibrin loci in vivo. II. Comparison of nine antibiotics: effect of dose and degree of protein binding. *J Infect Dis* 129:66, 1974.
51. Kunst MW, Mattie H: Cefazolin and cephradine: Relationship between antibacterial activity in vitro and in mice experimentally infected with *Escherichia coli. J Infect Dis* 137:391, 1978.
52. Merrikin DJ, Briant J, Rolinson GN: Effect of protein binding on antibiotic activity in vivo. *J Antimicrob Chemother* 11:233, 1983.
53. Kaiser AB, McGee ZA: Aminoglycoside therapy of gram-negative bacillary meningitis. *N Engl J Med* 293:1215, 1975.
54. Bryant RE, Howard D: Interaction of purulent material with antibiotics used to treat *Pseudomonas* infections. *Antimicrob Agents Chemother* 6:702, 1974.
55. O'Keefe JP, Tally FP, Barza M, et al: Inactivation of penicillin G during experimental infection with *Bacteroides fragilis. J Infect Dis* 137:437, 1978.
56. Zimelis VM, Jackson GG: Activity of aminoglycoside antibiotics against *Pseudomonas aeruginosa:* Specificity and site of calcium and magnesium antagonism. *J Infect Dis* 127:663, 1973.
57. Bryan LE, Van Den Elzen HM: Streptomycin accumulation in susceptible and resistant strains of *Escherichia coli* and *Pseudomonas aeruginosa. Antimicrob Agents Chemother* 9:928, 1976.
58. Zinner SH, Sabath LD, Casey JI, et al: Erythromycin and alkalinization of the urine in the treatment of urinary tract infections due to gram-negative bacilli. *Lancet* 1:1267, 1971.
59. Sabath LD, Gerstein DA, Leaf CD, et al: Increasing the usefulness of antibiotics: Treatment of infections caused by gram-negative bacilli. *Clin Pharmacol Ther* 11:161, 1970.
60. Karchmer AW, Dismukes WE, Buckley MJ, et al: Late prosthetic valve endocarditis. *Am J Med* 64:99, 1978.
61. Zimmerli W, Waldvogel FA, Vaudaux P, et al: Pathogenesis of foreign body infection: Description and characteristics of an animal model. *J Infect Dis* 146:487, 1982.
62. Forsgren A, Schmeling D, Quie PG: Effect of tetracycline on the phagocytic function of human leukocytes. *J Infect Dis* 130:412, 1974.
63. Seklecki MM, Quintiliani R, Maderazo EG: Aminoglycoside antibiotics moderately impair granulocyte function. *Antimicrob Agents Chemother* 13:552, 1978.
64. Chaperon EA, Sanders WE Jr: Suppression of lymphocyte responses by cephalosporins. *Infect Immun* 19:378, 1978.
65. Mandell LA: Effects of antimicrobial and antineoplastic drugs on the phagocytic and microbicidal function of the polymorphonuclear leukocyte. *Rev Infect Dis* 4:683, 1982.
66. Hauser WE, Remington JS: Effect of antibiotics on the immune response. *Am J Med* 72:711, 1982.
67. Manzella JP, Clark JK: Effects of moxalactam and cefuroxime on mitogen-stimulated human mononuclear leukocytes. *Antimicrob Agents Chemother* 23:360, 1983.
68. Jawetz E: Combined antibiotic action: Some definitions and correlations between laboratory and clinical results. *Antimicrob Agents Chemother* 1967, 1968, p 203.
69. Krogstad, DJ, Moellering RC Jr: Combinations of antimicrobial agents: Mechanisms of interaction against bacteria, in Lorian V (ed): *Antibiotics in Laboratory Medicine.* Baltimore, Williams and Wilkins (in press).
70. VanderAuwera P, Meunier-Carpentier F, Klastersky J: Clinical study of combination therapy with oxacillin and rifampin for staphylococcal infections. *Rev Infect Dis* 5 (suppl 3):S515, 1983.
71. Karchmer AW, Archer GL, Dimukes WE: Rifampin treatment of prosthetic valve endocarditis due to *Staphyloccus epidermidis. Rev Infect Dis* (suppl 3):S543, 1983.

72. Lehr D: Inhibition of drug precipitation in the urinary tract by the use of sulfonamide mixtures. I. Sulfathiazole-sulfadiazine mixture. *Proc Soc Exp Biol Med* 58:11, 1945.

73. Rahal JJ Jr: Antibiotic combinations: The clinical relevance of synergy and antagonism. *Medicine* 57:179, 1978.

74. Moellering RC Jr: Use and abuse of antibiotic combinations. *R I Med J* 55:341, 1972.

75. Mandell GL, Kaye D, Levison ME, et al: Enterococcal endocarditis. An analysis of 38 patients observed at the New York Hospital-Cornell Medical Center. *Arch Intern Med* 125:258, 1970.

76. Moellering RC Jr, Wennersten C, Weinberg AN: Studies on antibiotic synergism against enterococci: I. Bacteriologic studies. *J Lab Clin Med* 77:821, 1971.

77. Moellering, RC Jr, Weinberg AN: Studies on antibiotic synergism against enterococci: II. Effect of various antibiotics on the uptake of ^{14}C-labelled streptomycin by enterococci. *J Clin Invest* 50:2580, 1971.

78. Moellering RC Jr, Wennersten CBG, Medrek T, et al: Prevalence of high-level resistance to aminoglycosides in clinical isolates of enterococci. *Antimicrob Agents Chemother 1970,* 1971, p 335.

79. Zimmermann RA, Moellering RC Jr, Weinberg AN: Mechanism of resistance to antibiotic synergism in enterococci. *J Bacteriol* 105:873, 1971.

80. Krogstad DJ, Korfhagen TR, Moellering RC Jr, et al: Aminoglycoside-inactivating enzymes: An explanation for resistance to penicillin-aminoglycoside synergism in enterococci. *J Clin Invest* 62:480, 1978.

81. Mederski-Samoraj BD, Murray BE: High-level resistance to gentamicin in clinical isolates of enterococci. *J Infect Dis* 147:751, 1983.

82. Wolfe JC, Johnson WD Jr: Penicillin-sensitive streptococcal endocarditis. *Ann Intern Med* 81:178, 1974.

83. Karchmer AW, Moellering RC Jr, Maki D, et al: Single antibiotic therapy of streptococcal endocarditis. *JAMA* 241:1801, 1979.

84. Watanakunakorn C, Glotzbecker C: Enhancement of the effects of antistaphylococcal antibiotics by aminoglycosides. *Antimicrob Agents Chemother* 6:802, 1974.

85. Korzeniowski O, Sande MA: The National Collaborative Endocarditis Study Group: Combination antimicrobial therapy for *Staphylococcus aureus* endocarditis in patients addicted to parenteral drugs and in nonaddicts. *Ann Intern Med* 97:496, 1982.

86. Smith CB, Dans PE, Wilfert JN, et al: Use of gentamicin in combination with other antibiotics. *J Infect Dis* 119:370, 1969.

87. Eliopoulos GM, Moellering RC Jr: Azlocillin, mezlocillin and piperacillin: New broad-spectrum penicillins. *Ann Intern Med* 97:755, 1982.

88. Andriole VT: Antibiotic synergy in experimental infection with *Pseudomonas:* II. The effect of carbenicillin, cephalothin or cephanone combined with tobramycin or gentamicin. *J Infect Dis* 129:124, 1974.

89. Then R: Synergism between trimethoprim and sulfonamides. *Science* 197:1301, 1977.

90. Harding GKM, Ronald AR: A controlled study of antimicrobial prophylaxis of recurrent urinary tract infections in women. *N Engl J Med* 291:597, 1974.

91. Gilman RN, Terminel M, Levine MM, et al: Comparison of trimethoprim-sulfamethoxazole and amoxicillin in therapy of chloramphenicol-resistant and chloramphenicol-sensitive typhoid fever. *J Infect Dis* 132:630, 1975.

92. Chang MJ, Dunkle LM, Van Reken D, et al: Trimethoprim-sulfamethoxazole compared to ampicillin in the treatment of shigellosis. *Pediatrics* 59:726, 1977.

93. Kwan CN, Medoff G, Kobayashi G, et al: Potentiation of the anti-fungal effects of antibiotics by amphotericin B. *Antimicrob Agents Chemother* 2:61, 1972.

94. Titsworth E, Grunberg E: Chemotherapeutic activity of 5-fluorocytosine and amphotericin B against *Candida albicans* in mice. *Antimicrob Agents Chemother* 4:306, 1973.

95. Bennett J, Dismukes W, Duma R, et al: Comparison of amphotericin B alone with amphotericin B plus flucytosine in cryptococcal meningitis. Abstracts 16th Interscience Conference on Antimicrobial Agents and Chemotherapy, 1976, p 307.

96. Lau WK, Young LS, Block RE, et al: Comparative efficacy and toxicity of amikacin/carbenicillin versus gentamicin/carbenicillin in leukopenic patients. *Am J Med* 62:959, 1977.

97. Klastersky J, Hensgens C, Meunier-Carpentier F: Comparative effectiveness of combinations of amikacin with penicillin G and amikacin with carbenicillin in gram-negative septicemia: Double-blind clinical trial. *J Infect Dis* 134 (suppl):S433, 1976.
98. Lepper MH, Dowling HF: Treatment of pneumococcic meningitis with penicillin compared with penicillin plus aureomycin. *Arch Intern Med* 88:489, 1951.
99. Mathies AW Jr, Leedom JM, Ivler D, et al: Antibiotic antagonism in bacterial meningitis. *Antimicrob Agents Chemother* 7:218, 1967.
100. Sande MA, Overton JW: In vivo antagonism between gentamicin and chloramphenicol in neutropenic mice. *J Infect Dis* 128:247, 1973.
101. Strausbaugh LJ, Sande MA: Factors influencing the therapy of experimental *Proteus mirabilis* meningitis in rabbits. *J Infect Dis* 137:251, 1978.
102. Swedish Study Group: Cefuroxime versus ampicillin and chloramphenicol for the treatment of bacterial meningitis. *Lancet* 1:295, 1982.
103. Del Rio MDL, Chrane D, Shelton S, et al: Ceftriaxone versus ampicillin and chloramphenicol for treatment of bacterial meningitis in children. *Lancet* 1:1241, 1983.
104. Moellering RC Jr: Rationale for the use of antibiotic combinations. *Am J Med* (amdinocillin symposium):4, 1983.
105. Sanders CC: Novel resistance selected by the new expanded spectrum cephalosporins: A concern. *J Infect Dis* 147:585, 1983.
106. McLaughlin JE, Reeves DS: Clinical and laboratory evidence for inactivation of gentamicin by carbenicillin. *Lancet* 1:261, 1971.
107. Riff LJ, Jackson GG: Laboratory and clinical conditions for gentamicin inactivation by carbenicillin. *Arch Intern Med* 130:887, 1972.
108. Seidl LG, Thornton GF, Smith SW, et al: Studies on epidemiology of adverse drug reactions. III. Reactions in patients on general medical service. *Bull Johns Hopkins Hosp* 119:299, 1966.
109. Barza M, Brusch J, Bergeron M, et al: Penetration of antibiotics into fibrin loci in vivo. III. Intermittent versus continuous infusion and the effect of probenicid. *J Infect Dis* 129:73, 1974.
110. Nelson JD: Antibiotic concentrations in septic joint effusions. *N Engl J Med* 284:349, 1971.
111. Gerding DN, Hall WH: The penetration of antibiotics into peritoneal fluid. *Bull NY Acad Med* 51:1016, 1975.
112. Schlichter JG, MacLean H: A method of determining the effective therapeutic level in the treatment of subacute bacterial endocarditis with penicillin. *Am Heart J* 34:209, 1947.
113. Reller LB, Stratton CW: Serum dilution test for bactericidal activity. II. Standardization and correlation with antimicrobial assays and susceptibility tests. *J Infect Dis* 136:196, 1977.
114. Carrizosa J, Kaye D: Antibiotic concentrations in serum, serum bactericidal activity, and results of therapy of streptococcal endocarditis in rabbits. *Antimicrob Agents Chemother* 12:479, 1977.
115. Levy J, Klastersky J: Serum bactericidal test: a review with emphasis on its role in the evaluation of antibiotic combination, in Klastersky J, Staquet MJ (eds). *Combination Antibiotic Therapy in the Compromised Host.* New York, Raven Press, 1982, p 43.
116. Pien FD, Vosti KL: Variation in performance of the serum bactericidal test. *Antimicrob Agents Chemother* 6:330, 1974.
117. Stratton CW, Reller LB: Serum dilution test for bactericidal activity. I. Selection of a physiologic diluent. *J Infect Dis* 136:187, 1977.

2

PHARMACOKINETICS OF ANTIMICROBIAL AGENTS

PAUL S. LIETMAN

The pharmacokinetics of antimicrobial agents should be considered in terms of the time-dependent interactions with both microorganisms and humans.

The time-dependent interactions of antimicrobial agents with microorganisms are important to the effectiveness of the drug. This effectiveness is influenced by both the kinetics of microbial growth and the drug concentration in the environment of the microbe. Usually, the drug concentration in the environment of the microbe changes over time, with peaks and troughs that roughly parallel the plasma levels when intermittent doses are administered. Although much is unknown about the interplay between microbial growth kinetics and constantly changing drug concentrations in the microbial environment, some generalizations can be made. Penicillin G (and probably other penicillins, β-lactams, and inhibitors of cell wall synthesis) can inhibit bacterial cell growth and can produce cell lysis even though the concentration of antibiotic drops quite low during some of each dosing interval if the target organism is *Staphylococcus* sp., *Streptococcus pyogenes,* or *Streptococcus pneumoniae* (1). With these organisms and drugs, the physician does not need to keep the level of these antibiotics above the minimum bacteriostatic concentration (MIC) throughout all of each dosing interval. Although there is insufficient evidence about any other drugs and these organisms, it can be assumed that the level of drug in the environment of these bacteriae should be maintained above the MIC throughout each dosing interval. The MIC should be considered as the lowest concentration, which, if constantly maintained adjacent to the bacterium, will prevent bacterial growth. β-lactam antibiotics behave quite differently with gram-negative bacilli, and there is mounting evidence that bacterial regrowth begins as soon as the concentration of drug falls below the MIC (1,2). In these situations, the β-lactam level should be maintained above the MIC throughout each dosing interval. Aminoglycoside antibiotics also appear to be dependent on the bacterial species being treated. When aminoglycosides interact with *Pseudomonas aeruginosa*, there is a significant lag between the time the bacteria begin to regrow and the time the antibiotic concentration falls below the MIC (1). With *Escherichia coli*, however, and probably other Enterobacteriaceae as well, bacterial regrowth commences very quickly after the adjacent antibiotic concentration falls below the MIC (1). Since data exist for only a very few combinations of antimicrobial agents and microbes, the physician is often forced to act without the benefit of adequate information. Thus, a dosing regimen that would maintain the drug level above the MIC throughout each entire dosing interval would be the conservative approach.

The time-dependent interactions of antimicrobial agents with humans are important to both effectiveness and toxicity. The interactions of drugs and microorganisms depend on attaining antibiotic concentrations immediately adjacent to bacteria, and consequently these levels depend on human drug interactions including absorption, distribution, metabolism, and excretion. In addition, the plasma and tissue concentrations of drugs may correlate with dose-related toxicities. The time-dependent interactions with humans can also be used to construct dosing regimens.

Although the precise description of the pharmacokinetics of any drug can be exceedingly complex, the clinician can benefit considerably from approximations that are reasonably accurate and yet comprehensible. The goal of this chapter is to provide a foundation of pharmacokinetics of chemotherapeutic agents that is useful in the construction of therapeutic regimens and in the modification of these regimens for individualization of antimicrobial therapy. More extensive discussions of pharmacokinetics can be found in several excellent books (3,4,5).

VOLUME OF DISTRIBUTION (V_D)

The volume of distribution (V_D) of a drug is defined as that volume in which the total amount of drug in the body (A) would have to be uniformly distributed in order to give the observed plasma concentration (C_P).

$$V_D = \frac{A}{C_P} \tag{1}$$

Thus if 140 mg of gentamicin were given to a 70 kg patient and the plasma concentration was found to be 8 μg/ml (= 8 mg/liter), then the volume of distribution would be (140 mg) ÷ (8 mg/ liter) = 17.5 liters.

The volume of distribution is often expressed in terms of the body weight, liters/kg. If expressed as liters/kg, then the actual V_D is obtained simply by multiplying the volume of distribution per kg by the body weight.

By rearranging Equation 1, the dose (or amount) necessary to produce any desired plasma concentration can be calculated with a drug whose volume of distribution is known or the plasma concentration that can be expected with any chosen dose. Thus, if the goal is to produce a plasma gentamicin concentration of 10 μg/ml (= 10 mg/liter) in a 70 kg man and the V_D is known to be 0.25 liter/kg, then the dose must = $(V_D)(C_P)$ = (0.25 liter/kg)(70 kg)(10 mg/liter) = 175 mg.

The volume of distribution need not and usually does not correspond to any actual anatomic or physiologic space. It is simply a mathematical tool.

Most antimicrobial agents have volumes of distribution of between 0.15 liter/kg and 0.40 liter/kg. However, a few have larger volumes of distribution. For example, flucytosine, isoniazid, and erythromycin have volumes of distribution of 0.6 liter/kg to 0.7 liter/kg while chloramphenicol, doxycycline, nafcillin, and tetracycline have volumes of distribution of about 1 liter/kg. A few antimicrobial agents have volumes of distribution that exceed the body weight. Trimethoprim, ethambutol, and rifampin have volumes of distribution of 1.6 liters/kg to 1.8 liters/kg, and amphotericin B has a V_D of 4 liters/kg.

The important clinical use of the V_D is that it provides an initial or loading dose that promptly provides a therapeutic plasma concentration. The V_D is also useful, as is described below, in calculating subsequent or maintenance doses to achieve therapeutic and yet safe plasma concentrations.

HALF-LIFE ($T_{1/2}$)

The half-life of a drug is defined as the time required for the plasma concentration to fall to one-half its former value as it is being eliminated from the body.

It is usually assumed that the half-life associated with a drug is the half-life of the predominant phase of drug elimination, that absorption of the drug is completed, and that the distribution of the drug throughout the entire volume of distribution has been completed. It is also assumed that the fall in the plasma concentration parallels the fall in the total amount of drug in the body.

The half-life of a drug remains constant over time if there has been no change in the processes of drug elimination. During each half-life, 50 percent of the total amount of drug in the body is eliminated, and the plasma concentration falls by 50 percent. Generally, a constant percentage (or fraction) of drug is eliminated from the body in any constant period of time.

The half-lives of antimicrobial agents vary considerably. All of the currently marketed β-lactam antibiotics have very short half-lives (usually $<$1.5 hours). The aminoglycosides have somewhat longer half-lives (2–3 hours). Chloramphenicol, flucytosine, sulfisoxazole, and vancomycin have half-lives of 3–6 hours. Sulfamethoxazole, tetracycline, and trimethoprim have half-lives of 6–12 hours. Doxycycline has a relatively long half-life of 20 hours.

The usually quoted half-life of a drug is applicable as a generalization to young adults without renal or hepatic dysfunction. Clinically significant prolongation of a drug's half-life often accompanies renal dysfunction and occasionally occurs with hepatic dysfunction. The half-life may also be influenced by age with prolongations of the half-life in the newborn and the elderly and with shortened half-lives in young children when compared with young adult values. Other drugs administered concomitantly can also alter a drug's half-life as, for example, probenecid prolongs the half-life of many β-lactam antibiotics.

The half-life data are used to calculate continuing (or maintenance) doses of a drug and provide important information about oscillations of plasma concentrations of a drug given intermittently and repetitively.

REPETITIVE DOSING: THE PLATEAU PRINCIPLE

With repetitive dosing of a drug at regular intervals, the maximal or peak plasma concentrations and the minimal or trough plasma concentrations rise to a steady-state or plateau, and after such a plateau is reached, the peak and trough plasma concentrations remain constant if the dose remains constant and if there is no change in the rate of drug elimination. The attainment of a plateau is also applicable to continuous dosing at a constant rate where the plasma concentrations climb until a plateau is reached and then remain constant.

The rate at which the plateau is attained is a function exclusively of the half-life of drug elimination and is independent of the rate of drug administration. Thus, giving twice as much drug per dose or per unit of time ultimately provides a higher plasma concentration at the plateau but the plateau is still reached at the same time. A useful concept is that the plateau is reached after four half-lives. Actually, after one half-life the peak and trough or mean plasma concentrations are about 50 percent of the plateau concentrations, after 2 half-lives 75 percent, after 3 half-lives 88 percent, and after 4 half-lives 94 percent of the ultimate plateau levels. Similarly, when a dosage change is made or when a drug is discontinued, the new plateau is reached after about four half-lives.

The plateau principle is especially important in antimicrobial chemotherapy where the physician often wishes to provide therapeutic levels of the antimicrobial agent very promptly and where waiting four half-lives to achieve a desired level may be disastrous. In such situations an initial, or loading dose, of the drug should be given in order to achieve quickly the desired therapeutic level of the antimicrobial agent. As mentioned above, the loading dose is determined exclusively by the volume of distribution and not by the half-life.

Clearly, the plateau principle has greater clinical significance when a half-life is several hours or longer than when the half-life is an hour or less. As a generalization in antimicrobial chemotherapy, a loading dose should be considered whenever the half-life of the chosen drug in the patient is estimated to be longer than 3 hours and whenever a delay of 12 hours or longer to achieve a therapeutic level is unacceptable. A loading dose should also be considered whenever the half-life of the chosen drug is estimated to be prolonged beyond 3 hours by renal or hepatic dysfunction.

It is often useful to estimate the peak and trough plasma concentrations that can be expected with a chosen dose and dosing interval. This can be easily calculated if the volume of distribution and half-life are known. At steady state the minimal plasma concentrations (C_{min}) or trough levels are related to the V_D, $T_{1/2}$ and dose (D) by the following equation where n equals the dosing interval expressed in half-lives.

$$C_{min} = \frac{D}{(V_D)(2^n - 1)} \tag{2}$$

Thus, if a 6 g dose of carbenicillin ($V_D = 0.18$ liter/kg; $T_{1/2} = 1.0$ hour) is given every 6 hours (i.e., every 6 half-lives; $n = 6$) to an 80 kg man, the minimal or trough plasma concentration can be anticipated to be (6000 mg) ÷ (0.18 liter/kg)(80 kg)($2^6 - 1$) = 6.6 mg/liter = 6.6 μg/ml.

The relationship between the maximal plasma concentrations (C_{max}) or peak levels and the minimal plasma concentrations (C_{min}) or trough levels is given by Equation 3 where n is again the dosing interval expressed in half-lives.

$$\frac{C_{max}}{C_{min}} = 2^n \tag{3}$$

Thus, to continue with the example of carbenicillin given above, the drug was to be given every six half-lives and the ratio of C_{max} to C_{min} = 2^6 or 64. Thus, the peak plasma levels at steady state will be 64 times the trough levels or (64)(6.6 μg/ml) = 422 μg/ml. The oscillations during every dosing interval of 6 hours at steady state will be from a peak of 422 μg/ml to a trough of 6.6 μg/ml.

It may be desirable to give an antimicrobial agent by continuous intravenous infusion rather than intermittently. In such a case a plateau can be reached in about four half-lives as with intermittent dosing but there will be no peaks and troughs but only a plasma concentration at steady state (C_{ss}). The plasma concentration can also be easily estimated from a fourth simple equation.

$$C_{ss} = \frac{\text{Dose per half-life}}{(0.693)(V_D)} \tag{4}$$

Thus to extend the example of carbenicillin cited above, assume that the same total daily dose (i.e., 24 g) is given by continuous intravenous infusion without a loading dose. The dose per half-life is then 1 g/hour, and the plasma concentration at steady state will be 1000 mg ÷ (0.693)(V_D) = 1000 mg ÷ (0.693)(0.18 liter/kg)(80 kg) = 100 mg/liter = 100 μg/ml.

By rearranging Equations 3 or 4, it is easy to solve for the dose that needs to be given to achieve any desired plasma concentration or alternatively the dosing interval that can provide any desired oscillation from peak to trough level.

DOSE-RELATED KINETICS

Most antimicrobial agents behave pharmacokinetically in a manner that can be described with reasonable accuracy by the above four equations. However, Equations 2, 3, and 4 all used the half-life, and we have stated that the half-life is constant over time. This constancy of the half-life is dependent on there being no process of elimination (renal, hepatic, or other) that is saturable at the concentrations of drug realized. If, however, the concentration of drug begins to exceed that which can be removed from the body, then the drug is said to exhibit dose-related kinetics. With dose-related kinetics, it is as if the half-life of the drug were not constant. Although it is theoretically possible to exceed the renal secretory mechanism or the renal reabsorption mechanism, this is rarely, if ever, seen in clinical practice. The hepatic drug metabolizing capacity is, however, occasionally exceeded, in which case the drug may exhibit dose-related kinetics. A specific example is chloramphenicol where at high plasma concentrations the half-life is prolonged. This is especially pertinent to the newborn or the patient with hepatic disease.

ALTERATIONS OF DOSE WITH RENAL OR LIVER DISEASE

In general, antibiotics are eliminated from the body either into the gut after secretion into the bile or into the urine. In either case, the drug may be eliminated unchanged or may be metabolized, usually by the liver, before excretion. Thus, liver disease can impair drug elimination either as a result of impaired drug metabolism or impaired drug secretion into the bile. Kidney disease can impair drug elimination as a result of impaired glomerular filtration or, occasionally, impaired tubular secretion. The extent to which renal or hepatic processes are rate-limiting is quite variable for different drugs and is pivotal in the construction of a dosing regimen in the presence of reduced renal or hepatic function. In the presence of liver disease, the elimination of a few antimicrobial agents is slowed, that is, the half-life is prolonged. There are, however, no clear and useful correlations between any test of liver structure or function and the rate of drug elimination from the body. Thus, in a patient with known liver disease, the examiner cannot predict how the half-life of any drug will be affected, and the patient must be monitored, either clinically or with plasma drug levels, in order to be provided with safe and effective dosing.

In the presence of renal disease the elimination of many antimicrobial agents is slowed and the half-life prolonged. The prolongation of the half-life can often be estimated, however, and rational dosing adjustments can be calculated.

REFERENCES

1. Bundtzen RW, Gerber AU, Cohn DL, et al: Postantibiotic suppression of bacterial growth. *Rev Infect Dis* 3:28, 1981.

2. Rolinson, GN: Plasma concentrations of penicillin in relation to the antibacterial effect, in Davies DS, Pritchard BNC (eds): *Biological Effects of Drugs in Relation to Their Plasma Concentrations.* Baltimore, University Park Press, 1973, p 183.
3. Gladtke E, von Hattingberg HM: *Pharmacokinetics: An Introduction.* New York, Springer-Verlag, 1979.
4. Rowland M, Tozer TN: *Clinical Pharmacokinetics: Concepts and Applications.* Philadelphia, Lea & Febiger, 1980.
5. Tedrell T, Dedrick RL, Condliffe PG: *Pharmacology and Pharmacokinetics.* New York, Plenum Press, 1974.

3

PENICILLINS

HAROLD C. NEU

Penicillin was isolated from *Penicillium notatum* by Fleming in 1929. The fortuitous isolation of this compound did not bear fruit until the work of Florey, Chain, and associates in 1941 made possible the commercial production of penicillin G. In 1928 Fleming found that the mold *Penicillium* produced a substance, which he named penicillin, that inhibited the growth of *Staphylococcus aureus* (1). Fleming was not successful in attempts to obtain significant amounts of the agent and let the matter rest while he continued his work on lysozyme. In 1939 Florey at the Sir William Dunn School of Pathology began to work out the isolation, structure, and properties of the compound. In 1940 his group showed that penicillin protected mice experimentally infected with streptococci, and by 1941 they had produced enough penicillin to treat a few patients, the first of whom was a British policeman infected with both staphylococci and streptococci. As a result of the war, production of penicillin was undertaken in the United States. Initial clinical trials at Yale and the Mayo Clinic were so successful that the U.S. Army began to use the material and used it to treat streptococcal, gonococcal, and treponemal infections. As fermentation techniques improved, production of large amounts of pure drug became possible, and by the end of the 1940s penicillin G was available for general use in the United States.

Initial production of penicillin was from *P. notatum,* but it was discovered that greater yields could be achieved from *Pencillium chrysogenum* and from growing the organism in different media. It was soon apparent that the growth medium affected the type of natural penicillin produced. Although a number of penicillins were found, for example, F, X, N, K, none of these were superior to the benzylpenicillin that was designated as penicillin G.

CHEMISTRY

The basic structure of the majority of commercially available penicillins is a nucleus that consists of three components—a thiazolidine ring, the β-lactam

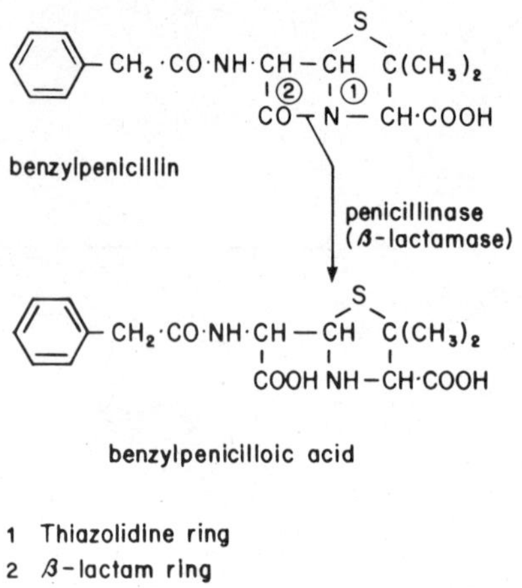

FIGURE 1. Structure of penicillin and site of β-lactamase attack.

ring, and a side chain (Fig. 1). The side chain determines in large part the antibacterial spectrum and pharmacologic properties of a particular penicillin. The penicillin nucleus is a condensation of alanine and β-dimethylcysteine. Penicillins currently in use are dextrorotatory and usually exist as salts combined with alkaline earth metals such as sodium or potassium. The penicillin nucleus itself is essential for antibacterial activity. Although biosynthesis of penicillin has been achieved, it has not proved to be a useful technique, and fermentation remains the method of production of penicillin.

The appearance of β-lactamase-producing organisms, particularly of *S. aureus,* prompted studies to develop compounds with resistance to hydrolysis by β-lactamases and also to find agents that had increased activity over that of penicillin G against gram-negative species. In 1959 Batchelor et al. (2) isolated the penicillin nucleus 6-amino-penicillanic acid from a precursor-depleted fermentation of *P. chryogeneum.* This made possible the production and testing of numerous semisynthetic penicillins, the first of which was methicillin, active against β-lactamase-producing *S. aureus;* followed by ampicillin, active against selected gram-negative bacilli; and in 1957 by carbenicillin, which had activity against *Pseudomonas aeruginosa.* The past few years have seen the development of a score of agents with different pharmacologic and antimicrobial properties, which will be discussed subsequently in this chapter.

MECHANISM OF ACTION OF PENICILLINS

It can be stated that we do not know precisely how penicillins kill bacterial cells. Study of the action of penicillins has elucidated many aspects of bacterial physiology, but recent advances suggest that the concept that penicillin inhibited the last step in cell wall synthesis is a simplistic one. The cell wall of bacteria is assembled in a series of enzymatic steps that involve at least 30 enzymes.

Bacterial Cell Walls

The cell walls of both gram-positive and gram-negative bacteria are held in a rigid manner protecting against osmotic rupture by the peptidoglycan, also called murein sacculus (3,4). The cell wall of gram-positive bacteria is a large, 50–100 molecular layer, whereas the peptidoglycan component of gram-negative bacteria is only 1 or 2 molecules thick.

There is an outer lipopolysaccharide layer on top of the peptidoglycan in gram-negative species such as Enterobacteriaceae and the pseudomonads, which is absent in gram-positive species.

All peptidoglycans are long polysaccharide chains in which *N*-acetylglucosamine (NAG) and *N*-acetylmuramic (NAM) acid alternate in a linear form. These long chains are cross-linked by short peptides linked in amide linkage to the D-alanyl group of the *N*-acetylmuramic acid. In gram-negative species the 6-amino group of diaminopimelic acid is linked to the carboxyalanine terminus of another chain (4). Interestingly, cross-linking is less common in *Escherichia coli* (25 percent), compared to the 90 percent cross-linking in *S. aureus* (5).

Peptidoglycan synthesis has been divided into three stages. The first is the synthesis of the nucleotide precursors with uridine diphosphate (UDP) by cytoplasmic enzymes to make UDP-*N*-acetylmuramyl-LAra-Disglu-LX-DAla-Dala and UDP-*N*-acetylglucosamine. The "X" in gram-negative species is diaminopimelic acid. The next step is the translocation of the NAM-pentapeptide and NAG across the cytoplasmic membrane by a lipid-soluble carrier, which is a C_{55} isoprenyl alcohol phosphate. Transglycosylation into peptidoglycan polymer occurs at this stage. The final reaction is to incorporate new peptidoglycan into the existing peptidoglycan. In this final reaction a free amino group on the third amino acid of the NAM-pentapeptide of one strand displaces the terminal D-alanine from a pentapeptide of a second strand in a transpeptidation reaction. This final step was the step thought to be the sole penicillin-sensitive reaction, but we now realize that the other earlier steps also can be inhibited.

It has been shown that penicillin can inhibit transpeptidation without altering transglycosylation of the disaccharide units. There appear to be distinct transpeptidases that provide for anchoring of new peptidoglycan to old, that cross-link special structures, and that make the cell wall septum. Although there are other penicillin-susceptible reactions, such as the effects on carboxypeptidase, these reactions do not seem to be critical in gram-negative species. The most telling argument that penicillin inactivates transpeptidases was the stereo chemistry modeling of Strominger's group (6), which supports an acylenzyme intermediate because of the structural similarity of penicillin and the acyl-D-alanyl-D-alanine.

Penicillin-Binding Proteins

In 1972 Suginaka and Blumberg and Strominger detected penicillin-binding proteins (PBPs). Subsequently Spratt's studies (7,8) of the PBPs in *E. coli* provided the biggest advance in our understanding of the effect of β-lactams on cell walls. Since then the PBPs of almost all species have been studied.

The PBPs of a given organism are numbered in order of decreasing molecular weight, for example, PBP-1 weighs about 120,000 and PBP-6 weighs 40,000. The particular number of a PBP will not readily relate from one species to another, and the PBP numbering system of gram-positive bacteria bears no relation to the PBP numbering of gram-negative bacteria. The PBPs probably account for only 1 percent of the membrane protein.

The PBPs vary greatly in the amount present. High molecular weight PBPs, that is, 1, 2, 3, are in low amounts compared to the PBPs 5 and 6, which account for 78 percent of the PBPs in *E. coli.* The PBPs also vary greatly in their affinity for certain β-lactams. In general, the affinity of a β-lactam to a particular PBP has been expressed as the concentration of antibiotic needed to reduce the ^{14}C-penicillin G binding to that PBP. The PBPs bind β-lactams covalently. It is believed that penicillins bind to PBPs through the carbonyl as a penicilloyl moiety and the binding of penicilloyl moiety is to a serine residue in the PBP via a bimolecular reaction.

Since the 1940s it has been known that low concentrations of penicillins cause filamentation of *E. coli;* whereas, at high concentrations lysis occurs. It seems most likely that binding of a β-lactam to PBP-1Bs, or its substitute enzyme PBP-1A, results in rapid cell lysis and that this PBP is the most important protein for cell elongation (8).

The role of PBP-2 in cell shape of bacteria was delineated by the availability of amdinocillin (mecillinam). *Escherichia coli* in the presence of amdinocillin form osmotically stable large round forms (9). After several hours in the presence of amdinocillin, these bacteria lyse. It is probable that PBP-2 catalyzes a specific topologically restricted transpeptidase or carboxypeptidase reaction during a particular part of the cell cycle.

The third major PBP is PBP-3, which is important in cell division of *E. coli* and other Enterobacteriaceae. The PBP-3 is activated upon completion of DNA replication and subsequently catalyzes a carboxypeptidase reaction needed for the special peptidoglycan synthesis that ensues when cells divide. The other low molecular weight PBPs have been thought to lack importance in the killing events associated with β-lactam binding to the proteins since mutants lacking PBP-4, -5, -6 have been isolated and grow well (10).

The PBPs that are important in gram-positive organisms are PBPs-1, -2, and -4, since their antibiotic susceptibility closely resembles the effect of the agents on whole organisms (11). In general, low molecular PBP-5, the carboxypeptidases, are not killing targets. Analysis of the lack of activity of β-lactams such as amdinocillin or aztreonam shows that these agents fail to bind to PBPs of gram-positive species (12).

The high activity of penicillins such as penicillin G against staphylococci can be correlated with binding to essential PBPs in these agents. Alteration of PBPs in gram-positive species has been correlated with resistance of *Streptococcus pneumoniae* to penicillin and of some *S. aureus* to penicillins.

"Unleashing" of bacterial autolysins by β-lactam antibiotics may be responsible for cell death in certain species.

BACTERIAL RESISTANCE TO PENICILLINS

Since there are many components involved in cell wall synthesis, variation in the composition of the wall components among bacteria accounts for some of the differences in sensitivity of individual bacterial strains to a particular penicillin. The differential binding of specific penicillins to target sites also accounts for differences in activity of different penicillins against a single organism or species. Mutation in a gene that specifies a binding site may lead to resistance to a penicillin, but this has been rare since most penicillins attack more than one of the peptidoglycan targets, and a coordinated mutation in a number of genes is an unlikely event.

Some organisms are resistant to penicillins because the penicillin fails to reach its receptor site. Failure of a penicillin to reach its target is unlikely to be a mechanism of resistance in gram-positive species since the peptidoglycan layer lies outside the bacterial membrane (13). But in gram-negative bacteria, two membranes compose the cell envelope, and the peptidoglycan lies inside the outer membrane. Thus in gram-negative bacteria a penicillin must pass through the outer membrane to reach its target site. Formerly it was supposed that lipophilicity of a molecule determined its activity. We now know that the protein layers on the outer surface of the bacterial membrane are held together by protein molecules that pass through the structure from one surface to the other. It is probable that penicillins that conform to the structural and charge properties of these stability proteins pass through to their receptor sites, whereas those β-lactam antibiotics that are structurally "different" do not enter the envelop and hence fail to reach a receptor site. Changes in structural protein components of the outer membrane due to mutations yield organisms more sensitive or less sensitive to penicillins. It is uncommon for naturally occurring resistant bacterial strains to owe their resistance to an alteration in membrane properties that interferes with the particular penicillin from reaching its target.

The most important mechanism of bacterial resistance to penicillins is enzymatic hydrolysis of the β-lactam bond by β-lactamases with loss of antibiotic activity of the molecule (14). In gram-positive bacteria such as staphylococci, β-lactamase production is plasmid mediated. The enzyme is both inducible and is an exoenzyme; that is, it is liberated into the surrounding medium in which it carries out its protective role by destroying the penicillins in the environment before they reach the cell surface. This mechanism of production of an exoenzyme is a protective one for bacteria such as staphylococci since they produce a large amount of enzyme with a very high affinity for penicillins.

On the other hand, β-lactamases of gram-negative bacteria are located in the periplasmic space that lies between the inner and outer membranes of gram-negative bacteria. Thus the enzyme is strategically located to protect the β-lactam target. Gram-negative β-lactamases may be either chromosomally or plasmid mediated, constitutive or inducible enzymes, with an affinity for penicillins or for cephalosporins or both types of compounds. It is probable that all gram-negative species contain small amounts of a β-lactamase. The activity of the β-lactamase stable compounds, methicillin, and the isoxazolyl penicillins against staphylococci, is due to their β-lactamase stability. Differences in β-lactamase stability also account for some of the differences in activity of different penicillins against gram-negative bacteria. For example, carbenicillin is destroyed at a much slower rate than is ampicillin by *Enterobacter cloacae* or *Morganella morganii.*

Increased β-lactamase stability may decrease overall antibacterial activity since addition of bulky side chains that prevent β-lactamase hydrolysis also interfere with passage of the molecule across the outer membrane of gram-negative bacteria (15). In general, increased activity of penicillins against β-lactamase-producing gram-negative bacteria is not associated with stability against β-lactamase hydrolysis but with affinity to penicillin receptor proteins and with increased entry into the bacterial cell. The one exception is temocillin, which contains a methoxy group on the β-lactam ring.

One final mechanism of resistance to penicillins seen in some gram-positive species is that of tolerance. This has been reported primarily for *S. aureus* and *S. pneumoniae.* Bacterial loss of viability, that is, cell death, is the result of secondary responses to inhibition of cell wall assembly. In some organisms the lytic effect of β-lactam antibiotics can be eliminated by inactivation of peptidoglycan hydrolyases (autolysins). For example, in pneumococci, lipoteichoic acids inhibit amidases. These acids are secreted into the surrounding milieu when penicillins are present. Suppression of autolytic activity protects the bacterium from the lytic effect of cell wall inhibition by penicillin. Thus an isolate that lacks autolysins will be inhibited but not killed by penicillin, that is, it is tolerant (12a). At certain pHs the cellular autolysins are inactive and the bacteria although inhibited are not killed. The relevance of these observations to clinical situations is unclear.

CLASSIFICATION OF PENICILLINS

Penicillins can be conveniently divided into classes on the basis of antibacterial activity (Table 1). Great overlaps do exist among the groups, but differences within a group usually are of a pharmacologic nature, although one compound in a group may be more active than another.

The susceptibility patterns of various species of microorganisms are given in Tables 2, 3, and 4. Gram-positive bacteria inhibited by natural penicillins in general are more susceptible to these penicillins than to semisynthetic penicillins (16–21). Penicillin V (used orally) can be substituted for penicillin G, except against gram-negative species since it is less active than penicillin G against *Neisseria* and *Hemophilus.* Semisynthetic penicillinase-resistant penicillins are

TABLE 1. Classification of Penicillins

	Routes of Use	*Trade Names*
Natural penicillins		
Penicillin G	po	Pfizerpen, Pentids, Kesso-Pen
	IM	Procaine—Wycillin, Duracillin, Crysticillin
	IV	Benzatrine—Permapen, Bicillin
Penicillin V	po	Ledercillin, Compocillin, Betapen, V-cillin, Veetids, Uticillin, S-K penicillin, Robicillin, Pen-Vee, Penapar
Phenethicillin	po	Broxil, Syncillin, Maxipen, Pensig
Penicillanase-resistant penicillins		
Methicillin	IM, IV	Staphcillin, Celbenin
Nafcillin	IM, IV	Unipen
Isoxazolyl penicillins		
Cloxacillin	po	Tegopen
Dicloxacillin	po	Veracillin, Pathocil, Dynapen
Flucloxacillin	po	
Oxacillin	po, IM, IV	Prostaphlin, Bactocill
Aminopenicillins		
Ampicillin	IM, IV	Alpen, Amcill, Pen A/N, Omipen, Totacillin, Supen, S-K ampicillin, Principen, Probampcin, Polycillin, Pensyn, Penbritin
Amoxicillin	po	Amoxil, Larotid, Polymox
Bacampicillin	po	Spectrobid
Cyclacillin	po	Cyclapen
Epicillin	po	
Hetacillin	po	Versapen
Pivampicillin	po	
Antipseudomonas penicillins		
Azlocillin	IM, IV	Azlin
Carbenicillin	IM, IV	Pyopen, Geopen
Indanylcarbenicillin	po	Geocillin
Ticarcillin	IM, IV	Ticar
Extended-spectrum penicillins		
Mezlocillin	IM, IV	Mezlin
Piperacillin	IM, IV	Pipral, Pipracil
Amidino penicillins		
Amdinocillin	IM, IV	
Pivamdinocillin	po	
Stable against gram-negative β-lactamases		
Temocillin	IM	
	IV	

TABLE 2. Usual Minimal Inhibitory Concentrations of Penicillins Against Cocci

	Mean Minimum Inhibitory Concentration (μg/ml)							
	Penicillin G	*Penicillin V*	*Ampicillin, Amoxicillin*	*Methicillin*	*Oxacillin, Cloxacillin Dicloxacillin*	*Nafcillin*	*Carbenicillin, Ticarcillin*	*Azlocillin Mezlocillin, Piperacillin*
Streptococcus pneumoniae	0.01 [a]	0.02 [a]	0.02 [a]	0.1 [a]	0.04	0.02	0.4	0.02
Streptococcus pyogenes	0.005	0.01	0.02	0.2	0.04	0.02	0.2	0.02
Streptococcus agalactiae	0.005	0.01	0.02	0.2	0.06	0.02	0.2	0.15
Streptococcus viridans	0.01	0.01	0.05	0.1	0.1	0.06	0.2	0.12
Streptococcus fecalis	3.0	6.0	1.5 [c]	>25	>25	>25	50	1.5
Peptostreptococcus	0.2	0.5	0.2	2.0	0.6	0.5	0.4	0.8
Staphylococcus aureus								
Penase negative	0.02	0.02	0.05	1.0	0.3	0.25	1.2	0.8
Penase positive	>25	>25	>25	2.0	0.4	0.25	25	25
Staphylococcus epidermidis	0.02 [b]	0.02 [b]	0.05 [b]	0.8 [b]	0.2 [b]	0.2 [b]	0.8 [b]	1.6 [b]
Neisseria gonorrhoeae [d]	0.01	0.1	0.03	12.0	12.0	12.0	0.3 [b]	0.05
Neisseria meningitidis	0.05	0.25	0.05	6.0	6.0	6.0	0.1 [b]	0.05

[a] Rare isolates resistant to penicillins have been found MIC >5 μg/ml.
[b] Many isolates resistant.
[c] Amoxicillin has a mean MIC of 0.4.
[d] Can range from 0.005 to 100.

TABLE 3. Activity of Penicillins Against Selected Bacilli and Anaerobic Organisms

	Mean Minimum Inhibitory Level (μg/ml)				
Organism	*Penicillin G*	*Ampicillin, Amoxicillin*[a]	*Oxacillin*[b]	*Carbenicillin, Ticarcillin*[a]	*Azlocillin, Mezlocillin, Piperacillin*[a]
Clostridium perfringens	0.5	0.05	0.5	0.5	0.05
Corynebacterium diphtheriae	0.1	0.02	0.1	0.1	1.0
Listeria monocytogenes	0.2	0.5	1.25	4	0.5
Hemophilus influenzae[c]	0.8	0.5	25	0.5	0.1
Bacteroides melaninogenicus	0.5	0.5	>100	0.5	0.2
Fusobacterium nucleatum	0.5	0.1	>100	0.5	0.5
Bacteroides fragilis	32	32	>500	64	16

[a] Minor differences do occur.
[b] Oxacillin is used as representative of isoxazoyl penicillins.
[c] β-lactamase-producing strains occur and are resistant to the penicillins.

TABLE 4. Activity of Penicillins Against Enterobacteriaceae and Pseudomonas

	Mean Minimum Inhibitory Levels (μg/ml)						
	Penicillin G	*Ampicillin, Amoxicillin*	*Oxacillin*[a]	*Carbenicillin, Ticarcillin*	*Azlocillin,*[d] *Mezlocillin, Piperacillin*	*Amdinocillin*	*Temocillin*
Escherichia coli[b]	100	3	>1000	6	10	0.4	10
Proteus mirabilis	50	3	>1000	1.5	0.8	25	5
Klebsiella	>400	200	>1000	>400	6	1.5	10
Enterobacter	>500	>500	>1000	50	3	1.5	10
Citrobacter diversus	>500	>100	>1000	12	6	1.5	2.5
Citrobacter freundii	>500	50	>1000	12	6	1.5	2.5
Serratia	>500	>500	>1000	100	25	100	25
Salmonella[b]	10	1.5	>1000	3	3	0.8	5
Shigella[b]	20	1.5	>1000	3	6	0.8	5
Proteus vulgaris	>500	>500	>1000	12	12	100	2.5
Providencia	>500	>500	>1000	12	6	100	2.5
Morganella	>500	200	>1000	25	6	6	2.5
Pseudomonas, other	>500	>500	> 500	>100	>100	>100	<100
Acinetobacter	>500	250	>1000	25	12	400	>100
Pseudomonas aeruginosa	>500	>500	>1000	50[c]	3[e]	100	>100

[a] Used as representative antistaphylococcal penicillin.

[b] Amoxicillin is twofold more active against *Salmonella* and twofold less active against *Shigella*. Strains containing the TEM plasmid β-lactamase are resistant except to temocillin.

[c] Ticarcillin two- to fourfold more active.

[d] Some isolates, particularly *Klebsiella,* are resistant to azlocillin but susceptible to mezlocillin and piperacillin.

[e] Mezlocillin is less active than azlocillin or piperacillin.

the drugs of choice only for penicillin-resistant *S. aureus* and *Staphylococcus epidermidis,* even though they will inhibit streptococci at concentrations below that needed to inhibit staphylococci (17,18). Carboxypenicillins such as carbenicillin and ticarcillin are less active than the ureidopenicillins against streptococcal and *Hemophilus* species. The susceptible gram-negative organisms that are members of the Enterobacteriaceae or *Pseudomonas* vary from hospital to hospital and from community to community. Most of the anaerobic gram-positive bacteria are susceptible to all the penicillins. Gram-negative anaerobic bacteria are susceptible to most penicillins with the exception of isolates of *Bacteroides fragilis,* which are inhibited by high levels of penicillin G or the semisynthetic antipseudomonas agents—azlocillin, carbenicillin, mezlocillin, piperacillin, and ticarcillin (20). *Fusobacterium varium* often are resistant to all penicillins.

PHARMACOLOGIC PROPERTIES IN GENERAL

Penicillins differ markedly in their oral absorption (Table 5). Penicillin G is not stable to acid and has a half-life of less than 20 minutes at pH 2. In contrast, at pH 4 it has a half-life of an hour. The other penicillins, which are acid liable, are methicillin and all the antipseudomonas penicillins. However, acid stability is not a guarantee of oral absorption, and there are major differences in oral absorption of compounds within a group. Penicillin V is well absorbed even when ingested with food, and the greatest absorption of penicillin V is with the potassium salt (22). The semisynthetic penicillins, with the exception of nafcillin, are well absorbed. Ampicillin is only partially absorbed, 30–60 percent (17); whereas amoxicillin and the "proampicillins"—bacampicillin and pivampicillin—are almost totally absorbed (21,23). The pivaloyl ester of amdinocillin is absorbed. Although carbenicillin is not absorbed, esters of the compound such as indanyl carbenicillin are adequately absorbed to provide urinary concentration to treat urinary tract infections (24).

The majority of penicillins are absorbed so they yield peak levels 1–2 hours after ingestion. When ingested with food, absorption is delayed to yield peak serum levels 2–3 hours after ingestion, and peak levels are lower, except for the pivaloyl esters and amoxicillin.

Repository forms of penicillin G are available. These are procaine penicillin G and benzathine penicillin G. These are absorbed more slowly from intramuscular sites than are the crystalline salts. Procaine or lidocaine can also be used as a diluent for intramuscular injection of antipseudomonas penicillins, but the half-life of these drugs is not prolonged by this maneuver.

Penicillins are bound to protein in varying degrees from 17 percent for the aminopenicillins to 97 percent for dicloxacillin (Table 5). The major protein to which they bind is albumin (17). Only an unbound (free) drug exerts antibacterial activity, since the bound drug cannot reach a receptor site within the bacteria. However, protein binding is a reversible process, and it is possible for bound penicillin to be released and to kill bacteria in tissue or in the blood

TABLE 5. Pharmacokinetic Properties of Penicillins

					Serum Level[a]		Serum $T_{1/2}$ (hr)[b]		
Antibiotic	*Oral Adsorption (%)*	*Food Decreases Adsorption*	*Protein Binding (%)*	*Percentage of Dose Metabolized (%)*	*Total Drug (μg/ml)*	*Free Drug (μg/ml)*	*Normal ($C_{cr} > 90$ ml/min)*	*Renal Failure ($C_{cr} < 10$ ml/min)*	*Liver Impairment Increases ($T_{1/2}$)*
Penicillin G	20	Yes	55	20	2	0.9	0.5	10	+
Penicillin V	60	No	80	55	4	0.8	1	4	
Methicillin	Nil		35	10			0.5	4	
Oxacillin	30	Yes	93	45	6	0.4	0.5	1	
Cloxacillin	50	Yes	94	20	10	0.6	0.5	1	++
Dicloxacillin	50	Yes	97	10	15	0.45	0.5	1.5	++
Nafcillin	Erratic	Yes	87				0.5	1.5	+++
Ampicillin[c]	40	Yes	17	10	3.5	2.9	1	8	++
Amoxicillin	75	No	17	10	7.5	6.2	1	8	+
Carbenicillin	Nil		50	2			1.1	15	++, 18–20 hr
Indanyl carbenicillin	30	No	50		15	7.5	1.1	15	++
Ticarcillin	Nil		50	15			1.2	15	++, 18–20 hr
Amdinocillin	Nil		20				0.8	4	+
Pivamdinocillin	50	No	20		3		1	4	+
Mezlocillin	Nil		50				1.1	4	++
Piperacillin	Nil		50				1.3	4	++
Azlocillin	Nil		20				0.8	4	++
Temocillin	Nil		85	10			4	17	++

[a] After 500 mg dose taken fasting.

[b] Values have been rounded off to approximate values.

[c] Proampicillins (bacampicillin, pivampicillin) are absorbed twice as well as ampicillin and food does not decrease absorption, but other properties are those of the parent ampicillin. Bacampicillin would give a serum level of 9 μg/ml after 500 mg.

stream. Penicillins are metabolized to a minor degree (25). However, differences in metabolism explain the differences in half-lives in the presence of renal failure. The major mechanism by which they are removed from the body is by excretion as intact molecules via the kidney (26). Biliary excretion of penicillins does occur, but it probably is important only for nafcillin and the antipseudomonas penicillins (27).

The mechanism of excretion of penicillins is via renal tubular cells. Penicillins are rapidly excreted into urine, and hence they have a short half-life, ranging from less than 30 minutes for penicillin to 72 minutes for carbenicillin. The one exception is a new agent, temocillin, that has a half-life of 4 hours in healthy people (28). The ability of the renal tubular cells to excrete penicillin varies with the agents, but up to 4 g/hr of penicillin G can be excreted. This excretion can be blocked by probenecid, which prolongs the serum half-life of all the penicillins (29). Probenecid also competes for binding sites on albumin; hence, there is more free drug in the presence of probenecid. Renal excretion of all penicillins by the newborn is markedly less than in older children since tubular function is not fully developed. Hence, the dosage programs for penicillins must be modified when given to newborns or low birth weight infants.

Reduction in renal function is an important consideration in the administration of certain penicillins, namely, carbenicillin, ticarcillin and temocillin. If the creatinine clearance is greater than 10 ml/min, it is necessary to make only minor adjustments in the dosage of other penicillins. In the presence of anuria, reduction in total daily dose of the natural penicillins, of many of the penicillinase-resistant penicillins, and of the aminopenicillins is necessary (30) (Table 6).

Peritoneal dialysis removes variable amounts of the penicillins. In general, after peritoneal dialysis only the dosage programs of carbenicillin and ticarcillin need to be adjusted. After hemodialysis it is necessary to replace the dialyzed penicillin G, ampicillin, amoxicillin, carbenicillin, ticarcillin, azlocillin, mezlocillin, piperacillin and temocillin, but not nafcillin or the isoxazolyl penicillins (19).

Penicillins are well distributed to most areas of the body such as lung, liver, kidney, muscle, bone, and placenta. The levels of penicillins in abscesses, middle ear, and pleural, peritoneal, and synovial fluids are sufficient in the presence of inflammation to inhibit most susceptible bacteria (31–35). Most penicillins are relatively insoluble in lipid and so do not penetrate cells, including polymorphonuclear cells. Distribution of all the penicillins to eye, brain, cerebrospinal fluid, or prostate are nil in the absence of inflammation (36). Inflammation alters normal barriers permitting entry of penicillins, but more importantly it interferes with the anion pump that removes penicillins from areas such as cerebrospinal fluid. Low protein-bound penicillins reach levels in fetal serum equivalent to levels in maternal serum 30–60 minutes after injection. In contrast, the highly protein-bound semisynthetic penicillins achieve low concentrations in both amniotic fluid and fetal serum (37).

Urinary concentrations of all penicillins are high, even in the presence of moderately reduced renal function, but in people with creatinine clearances

TABLE 6. Antibiotic Dosage Change in Renal Disease and After Dialysis

	Dosage Change in Renal Failure[a]		
Agent	*Creatinine Clearance (30–50 ml/min)*	*Creatinine Clearance (<10 ml/min)*	*Dosage After Hemodialysis*
Penicillin G	NC[c]	1.6×10^6 units/6 hr	Yes (1.6×10^6 units)
Penicillin V	NC	250 mg/6 hr	Yes (250 mg)
Methicillin	NC	2 g/8 hr	Slight (2 g)
Oxacillin	NC	NC	Slight (as in uremia)
Cloxacillin	NC	NC	Slight (as in uremia)
Dicloxacillin	NC	NC	Slight (as in uremia)
Nafcillin	NC	NC	Slight (as in uremia)
Ampicillin[d]	NC	0.5–1 g/8 hr	Yes (500 mg)
Amoxicillin	NC	500 mg/12 hr	Yes (250 mg)
Carbenicillin	3 g/4 hr	2 g/8 hr	Yes (2 g)
Ticarcillin	2 g/4 hr	2 g/12 hr	Yes (2 g)
Indanyl carbencillin	NC	Avoid	
Azlocillin	NC	3 g/8–12 hr	Yes (2 g)
Mezlocillin	NC	3 g/8–12 hr	Yes (2 g)
Piperacillin	NC	3 g/8–12 hr	Yes (2 g)
Temocillin	1 g/24 hr	1 g/48 hr	Yes (1 g)
Amdinocillin	NC	1 g/8 hr	Yes (1 g)

[a] Refers to maximum dose used.
[b] Only carbenicillin and ticarcillin need adjustment of dosage after peritoneal dialysis.
[c] NC: no change.
[d] Dosage adjustments of "pivampicillins" should be the same as those of amoxicillin.

below 10 ml/min the urinary levels may not exceed those in the blood. Cortical and medullary concentrations of penicillins during normal hydration and in hydropenia exceed serum levels (38).

Most penicillins are actively secreted into the bile, yielding biliary concentrations well in excess of those in serum. The levels of penicillin G, ampicillin, and amoxicillin are at least 10 times those in the serum, and the levels of nafcillin and mezlocillin are as high as 100 times the simultaneous serum level. In the presence of common duct obstruction, the levels of all penicillins in bile are markedly reduced. Since the biliary transport system is a saturable one, at very high serum levels the biliary levels are not significantly increased over those obtained at lower serum levels.

UNTOWARD REACTIONS TO PENICILLINS

The major adverse effects of the penicillins are hypersensitivity reactions, which range in severity from rash to immediate anaphylaxis (Table 7) (39,40). Penicillins are capable of acting as haptens to combine with proteins contaminating the solution or with human protein after the penicillin has been administered

TABLE 7. Adverse Reactions to Penicillins

Type of Reaction	Frequency	Occurs Most Frequently with[a]
Allergic		
IgE antibody	0.004–0.4%	Penicillin G
Anaphylaxis		
Early urticaria (<72 hr)		
Cytotoxic antibody	Rare	Penicillin G
Hemolytic anemia		
Ag-Ab complex disease	Rare	Penicillin G
Serum sickness		
Delayed hypersensitivity	4–8%	Ampicillin
Contact dermatitis		
Idiopathic	4–8%	Ampicillin
Skin rash		
Fever		
Late onset urticaria		
Gastrointestinal	2–5%	
Diarrhea	25%	Ampicillin
Enterocolitis	<1%	Ampicillin
Hematologic		
Hemolytic anemia	Rare	Penicillin G
Neutropenia	1–4%	Penicillin G Oxacillin Piperacillin
Platelet dysfunction	3%	Carbenicillin
Hepatic		
Elevated SGOT level	1–4%	Oxacillin Nafcillin Carbenicillin
Electrolyte Disturbance		
Sodium overload	Variable	Carbenicillin
Hypokalemia	Variable	Carbenicillin
Hyperkalemia—acute	Rare	Penicillin G
Neurologic		
Seizures	Rare	Penicillin G
Bizarre sensations		Procaine Penicillin
Renal		
Interstitial nephritis	1–2%	Methicillin
Hemorrhagic cystitis	Rare	Methicillin

[a] All the reactions can occur with any of the penicillins.

to humans. The most important antigenic component of penicillins is the penicolloyl determinant, which is produced through opening of the β-lactam ring, thereby allowing amide linkage to body proteins (Fig. 2). Penicillanic acid and derivatives of penicillanic acid are produced when reconstituted penicillins break down in solution due to acidity or temperature elevation. The penicillolyl and penicillanic derivatives are the major determinants of penicillin allergy. Minor

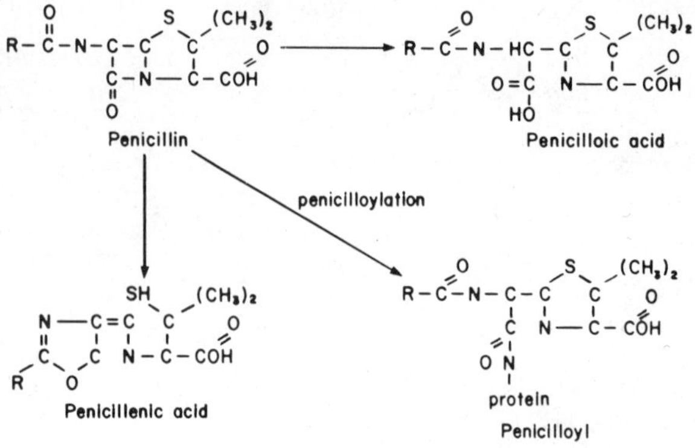

FIGURE 2. Mechanisms for formation of antigens from penicillins.

determinants of allergy are benzyl penicillin itself or sodium benzyl penicilloate, which can act either as sensitizing agents or of their own elicit an allergic reaction (39,40). Both major and minor determinants may be involved in anaphylactic reactions, as well as in urticarial reactions. These reactions are mediated by IgE antibody. Minor determinants are the major cause of anaphylactic reactions. When a person has been sensitized by the hapten-carrier complex, he or she can have a reaction to penicillin alone or to penicillin that has formed dimers or polymers in solution. Anaphylactic reactions to penicillins are uncommon, occurring in only 0.2 percent of 10,000 courses of treatment, with 0.001 percent out of 100,000 cases resulting in fatality (41). People with atopic dermatitis or allergic rhinitis appear not to be at increased risk of a penicillin reaction (42).

Serum sickness does occur with penicillins, but it is very uncommon today. It probably is due to IgG antibodies to the benzyl penicilloyl hapten. The illness is characterized by fever, urticaria, joint pains, and angioneurotic edema. Exfoliative dermatitis and Stevens-Johnson syndrome are rare forms of allergic reactions to penicillins. The morbilliform eruptions that develop after penicillin therapy probably are due to IgM antibody to the benzyl penicilloyl hapten and to the minor determinants. In many patients these rashes will disappear, even if the penicillin is continued, due to the production of IgG blocking antibody. There is a risk, however, that the rash could progress to generalized desquamation.

Skin testing with benzyl penicilloyl-polylysine (prePen), benzyl penicillin G, and sodium benzyl penicilloylate will probably detect antibodies to both determinants (42). Benzyl penicillin G should be used at a concentration such that only 5 units are administered intradermally in a volume no larger than 0.05 ml. Benzyl penicilloylate is prepared by diluting benzyl penicillin with 0.1 N sodium hydroxide and subsequently diluting in normal saline to yield a solution that contains 5 units in 0.05 ml. Failure to develop an immediate reaction to these agents makes it highly unlikely (less than 5 percent) that a person will have an immediate or accelerated reaction to penicillins. If an allergic reaction does occur, epinephrine given intramuscularly or intravenously will usually abort the reaction. Antihistamines and corticosteroids have not been shown to be of benefit. Desensitization to penicillins can be accomplished (see below) but, except in rare cases, it is preferable to select an agent in another class.

Another allergic reaction to penicillins is that of allergic vasculitis with development of cutaneous and visceral lesions similar to that found with periarteritis nodosa. This reaction is extremely rare.

Hematologic toxicity is rare, although neutropenia has been encountered with the use of all types of penicillins, particularly when large doses are used (43). The mechanism of the neutropenia is unknown, and white blood cell counts return to normal rapidly if the offending agent is discontinued. Coombs-positive hemolytic anemia occurs rarely (44). All penicillins at high concentrations, but particularly carbenicillin and ticarcillin, bind to the adenosine diphosphate receptor site in platelets preventing normal platelet aggregation. A clinically significant bleeding disorder occurs relatively infrequently (45).

Renal toxicity from penicillins has varied from allergic angiitis to interstitial nephritis (46,47). Interstitial nephritis has occurred most commonly with the use of methicillin, but it has been seen with all penicillins. The clinical syndrome is one of fever, macular rash, eosinophilia, proteinuria, eosinophiluria, and hematuria. Initially the reaction is one of nonoliguric renal failure with a decrease in creatinine clearance and a rise in serum urea nitrogen and serum creatinine concentrations. This reaction can progress to anuria and renal failure. Biopsy specimens of the kidney show an interstitial infiltrate of mononuclear and eosinophilic cells with tubular damage but no glomerular lesions. Discontinuation of the penicillin will result in the return of renal function to normal in the majority of situations (48).

Administration of massive doses of any penicillin, but most often carbenicillin and ticarcillin, may result in hypokalemia due to the large dose of nonreabsorbable anion presented to the distal renal tubules (46).

Central nervous system toxicity in the form of myoclonic seizures can follow administration of massive doses of penicillin G, ampicillin, carbenicillin, or methicillin. If there is reduced renal function, the drugs accumulate and this toxicity is more likely (49). Direct instillation of small doses of methicillin, oxacillin, or nafcillin into the ventricles at the time of surgery for placement of atrioventriculo shunts has not resulted in seizures. Direct application of penicillin to the cortex will provoke seizure activity.

Gastrointestinal disturbances have followed the use of any of the oral forms but have been most pronounced with ampicillin. Enterocolitis due to *Clostridium difficile* has followed the use of penicillin V, ampicillin, and indanyl carbenicillin. All the penicillins used at high doses for prolonged periods will abolish normal bacterial flora with resulting colonization with resistant gram-negative bacilli and/or with fungi such as *Candida.* Abnormalities in hepatic function tests such as elevation of the alkaline phosphatase and serum glutamic-oygloacetic transaminase (SGOT) levels have been reported most often after the use of oxacillin and carbenicillin (43,50). The pathogenesis of the hepatic reaction is unknown. Major hepatic injury is very uncommon.

Penicillin Desensitization

Desensitization of a patient to penicillin is based on the theory that small amounts of penicillin given parenterally over a period of time will result in minor anaphylactic discharge so a major anaphylactic reaction will not occur (51). In recent years tolerance to therapeutic doses of penicillin has been achieved by use of the following program. Penicillin is administered intracutaneously in the lower arm at 60–90-minute intervals beginning with 5 units, then with 10, 100, and 1000 units. Subsequently, doses of 10,000 and 50,000 units are given subcutaneously; if this is tolerated, intravenous penicillin is begun.

Evaluation of penicillin desensitization as a useful clinical maneuver is impossible because of the unpredictability of the history of penicillin allergy and of the small number of patients allegedly desensitized. Since a large number of patients who report that they are allergic to penicillin do not have adverse reactions when given penicillin, the efficacy of desensitization remains in doubt. The procedure is not innocuous since death due to laryngeal edema has been reported during desensitization. Since there are many effective alternative antimicrobial agents available today, desensitization should be used with extreme caution and used only if no alternative agents can be given.

Antihistamines or steroids will suppress some of the late allergic reactions to penicillins and allow the use of therapeutic doses of penicillins to complete the therapy for an illness. Again, however, the merits of continued penicillin therapy versus use of another agent should be carefully considered.

CLINICAL USE

In the nonallergic person a pencillin should usually be the drug of choice to treat infections caused by susceptible organisms (Table 8). This is particularly true if the person has a defect of host defense such as neutropenia. Penicillin G remains the primary agent for treatment of *Streptococcus pyogenes* and *S. pneumoniae* infections (regardless of the site). None of the newer penicillins or agents in other classes has been shown to be more effective. *Streptococcus pneumoniae* resistant to penicillin have been isolated in South Africa and the United States, but these are rarely encountered. Recently in the United States *S. pneumoniae* of relative resistance to penicillin, minimum inhibitory concentration (MIC) values of 0.1–1 μg/ml, have been seen. Much higher doses of penicillin are required to kill these organisms. All *Neisseria meningitidis* strains are susceptible to penicillin G. *Neisseria gonorrhoeae* vary in susceptibility to penicillin G from the highly susceptible forms that cause the disseminated forms of the disease to isolates that contain a plasmid-mediated β-lactamase and are

TABLE 8. Antimicrobial Spectrum of Penicillins[a]

Organisms	*Penicillin of Choice*	*Alternate Acceptable Penicillin*	*Frequency of Resistance to Penicillins*
Gram-positive cocci			
Streptococcus pneumoniae	G	V	Rare, <1%
Streptococcus pyogenes (A)	G	V	None
Streptococcus agalactiae (B)	G	Ampicillin	None
Streptococcus viridans	G		None
Streptococcus bovis (D)	G		None
Streptococcus fecalis (*enterococcus*)	Ampicillin	Mezlocillin	<0.1%
Staphylococcus aureus (*nonpenicillinase*)	G	Penase-resistant	80%
Staphylococcus aureus (*penicillinase*)	Penase-resistant		
Staphylococcus aureus (*methicillin resistant*)	None	None	100%
Staphylococcus epidermidis	Penase-resistant		80%
Staphylococcus epidermidis (*methicillin-resistant*)	None	None	100%
Gram-negative cocci			
Neisseria meningitidis	G	Ampicillin	None
Neisseria gonorrhoeae	G	Ampicillin	1–10%
Gram-positive bacilli			
Bacillus anthracis	G		None
Corynebacterium diphtheriae	G		None
Listeria monocytogenes	Ampicillin	G	None
Anaerobic species			
Peptostreptoccocci	G	Ampicillin	None
Actinomyces israelii	G	V	None
Bacteroides melaninogenicus	G	CT	10%
Fusobacteria	G	Ampicillin	<1%
Bacteroides fragilis	M, PA		50%
Clostridia	G	Ampicillin	<1%

TABLE 8. (Continued)

Organisms	*Penicillin of Choice*	*Alternate Acceptable Penicillin*	*Frequency of Resistance to Penicillins*
Gram-negative bacilli			
Hemophilus	Ampicillin	G	5–30%
Escherichia coli	Ampicillin		30%
Proteus mirabilis	Ampicillin	G	<5%
Salmonella typhi	Ampicillin		20%
Salmonella, other sp.	Ampicillin		20%
Klebsiella	None		95%
Enterobacter	MPTC		20%
Citrobacter freundii	M, P, T		20%
Proteus, indole positive	MPTC		20%
Serratia	MPTC		80%
Pseudomonas aeruginosa	A, P, T		20–30%
Pseudomonas, other	None		95%
Acinetobacter	T	A, M, P	50%
Providencia	M, P, TC		20–30%
Other organisms infrequently encountered			
Erysipelothrix	G	Ampicillin	None
Pasturella multocida	G		Rare, <1%
Streptobacillus moniliformis	G		None
Spirillum minus	G		None
Fusospirochetes	G	Ampicillin	None
Treponema pallidum	G		None

[a] In each case it is assumed that a route of administration would be used that would achieve levels in serum and tissue to erradicate the organism. If there is no entry in the alternate column, it means that an antibiotic in another class would be a more appropriate choice. Amoxicillin can be used in place of ampicillin in all situations except with *Shigella*.

[b] a: azlocillin; C: carbenicillan; M: mezlocillin, P: piperacillin; T: ticarcillin.

completely resistant. Penicillin G is the drug of choice for treponemal infection in all its forms. Puerperal infections due to anaerobic streptococci or group B streptococci (*Streptococcus agalactiae*), as well as genital clostridial infections, are best treated with penicillin G. Infections produced by anaerobic mouth flora including gram-positive and gram-negative cocci and the *Actinomyces* can be treated with penicillin G, although *Bacteroides melaninogenicus* resistant to penicillin is being encountered.

PROPHYLACTIC USE OF PENICILLIN

Penicillins have been used in a number of situations for prevention of infection. Oral administration of 200,000 units of penicillin G or penicillin V every 12 hours has resulted in a significant reduction in recurrences of rheumatic fever. Because of the problems with compliance with oral therapy, intramuscular injections of 1.2 or 2.4 million units of benzathine penicillin given once each month has also been used with excellent results.

Outbreaks of streptococcal infection due to *S. pyogenes* have been aborted by the use of oral penicillin G or V given twice a day for 5 days, by single injections of procaine penicillin daily, or by administration of benzathine penicillin.

One of the most important prophylactic uses of penicillin is for prevention of bacterial endocarditis.

Penicillins may be used prophylactically at the time of implantation of an artificial joint or heart valve. These agents should be given just before the surgery, during the procedure, and in the immediate postoperative period. There are no studies that deliniate the best penicillin agent for such procedures, and many physicians prefer to use a cephalosporin.

Ampicillin or amoxicillin has been administered to asplenic children or to children with agammaglobulinemia to prevent infections caused by *H. influenzae* and *S. pneumoniae* but proof of efficacy is lacking.

Penicillin prophylaxis has not been of benefit in prevention of meningococcal infection, bacterial infection after viral respiratory infection, or pneumonia after coma, shock, or congestive heart failure.

PROPERTIES OF INDIVIDUAL PENICILLINS

Dosages of penicillins are given in Tables 9 and 10.

Natural Penicillins

Penicillin G. Penicillin G or benzylpenicillin G (Fig. 3) is available in oral, parenteral, and repository salts. Oral salts are either the sodium or potassium forms, which are available as suspensions for pediatric use or as tablets in doses

TABLE 9. Dosage of Penicillins

Compound	*Oral*	*Intramuscular*	*Intravenous*
Penicillin G			25,000–500,000 units/kg/day, 6 doses
Procaine		300,000–600,000 units every 12 hr	
Benzathine		1.2–2.4 mega units every 15–20 days	
Penicillin V	Infant: 50 mg/kg/day, 3 doses 125–500, 4 doses		
Ampicillin[a]	25–200 mg/kg/day, 4 doses	100–200 mg/kg/day, 4 doses	100–400 mg/kg/day, 6 doses
Amoxicillin	25–50 mg/kg/day, 3 doses		
Methicillin, Oxacillin, Nafcillin		100 mg/kg/day, 4 doses	100–300 mg/kg/day, 6 doses
Cloxacillin	25–100 mg/kg/day, 4 doses		
Dicloxacillin	12–25 mg/kg/day, 4 doses		
Carbenicillin		50–100 mg/kg/day, 4 doses	50–500 mg/kg/day, 6 doses
Ticarcillin		50–100 mg/kg/day, 4 doses	50–300 mg/kg/day, 6 doses
Indanylcarbenicillin	50–65 mg/kg/day, 4 doses		
Azlocillin		50–100 mg/kg/day, 4 doses	200–300 mg/kg/day, 4 doses
Mezlocillin		50–100 mg/kg/day, 4 doses	200–300 mg/kg/day, 4 doses
Piperacillin		50–100 mg/kg/day, 4 doses	200–300 mg/kg/day, 4 doses

[a] Proampicillins are given at the same dose as amoxicillin.

TABLE 10. Dosage of Antibiotics in Newborn Infants

	Infants Less than 1 Week Old		*Infants 1 Week–1 Month Old*	
Compound	*Dose (per kg/day)*	*Interval Between Doses (in hours)*	*Dose (per kg/day)*	*Interval Between Doses (in hours)*
Penicillin G	50,000–100,000 units	12	100,000 units	8
Ampicillin	100 mg	12	200 mg	6
Oxacillin	100 mg	12	200 mg	6
Methicillin	100 mg	12	300 mg	6
Nafcillin	100 mg	12	200 mg	6
Carbenicillin	250 mg	8	400 mg	6
Ticarcillin	150 mg	8	300 mg	6
Mezlocillin	75 mg	12	300 mg	6
Azlocillin	75–100 mg	12	300 mg	6

of 50,000 to 1 million units (200,000 units equals 125 mg). Penicillin G should be used orally only if it is taken 1 hour before or 2 hours after a meal to prevent its destruction by gastric acid. There is little reason to use oral penicillin G for acute infection at the present time, and penicillin V should be the oral preparation used.

Crystalline penicillin G in aqueous solution has been used intramuscularly, subcutaneously, intravenously, and intrathecally. It is available either as the potassium or sodium salt. The sodium salt is much more expensive than the potassium salt, and it rarely needs to be used since the amount of potassium present in 6 million units, an amount a patient with reduced renal function would receive, is less than 10 mEq. Given intramuscularly as an aqueous solution, penicillin G is very rapidly cleared from the body, and it is preferable to use a repository form. It is available as sterile dry powder in ampules or vials

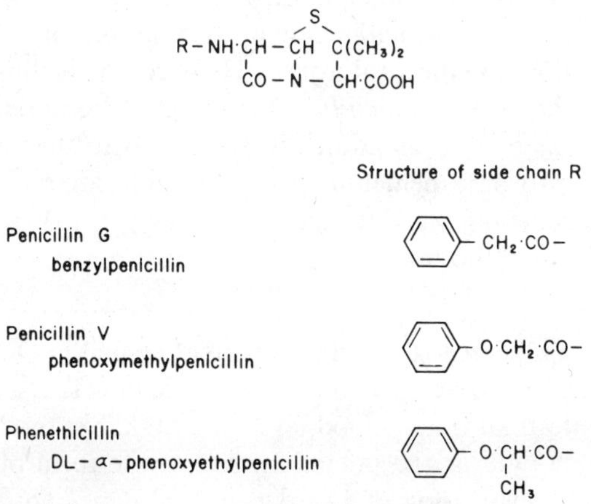

FIGURE 3. Structure of penicillin G, penicillin V, and phenethicillin.

containing 200,000–20 million units per vial. Each million units of penicillin G contains 1.7 mEq of sodium or potassium.

Repository penicillins provide tissue depots from which the drug is absorbed over hours in the case of procaine penicillin or over days in the case of benzathine penicillin. Repository penicillins are only for intramuscular use and cannot be used intravenously or subcutaneously or to irrigate wounds. Procaine penicillin is a mixture of equal molar parts of procaine and penicillin. Thus 300,000 units contains 120 mg of procaine. Use of this suspension delays the peak of activity but provides serum and tissues levels for at least 12 hours. Doubling the dose of procaine penicillin given at a single injection site does not double the serum level. To increase the peak level it is necessary to use two body sites as is done in the treatment of gonorrhea, for example, with 2.4 million units of procaine penicillin given in each buttock. Marketed procaine penicillin preparations are of two types: One is an aqueous solution of the crystalline salt, and the other contains 2 percent aluminum monosterate as a dispensing agent. The preparations are marketed in cartridges and vials in doses of 300,000, 500,000, and 600,000 units in 1–4 ml and as 2.4 million units/4 ml.

Benzathine penicillin is a repository form of penicillin, which is a combination of 1 mole of penicillin and 2 moles of an ammonium base. It is available for intramuscular injection in 10-ml vials containing 300,000 units/ml and as prefilled syringes containing 600,000 units/ml in 1-, 2-, and 4-ml sizes. It provides detectable serum levels of 15–30 days depending on the size of the dose. Concentrations of penicillin G in the spinal fluid after use of benzathine penicillin probably are inadequate to treat treponemal infections of the nervous system.

Penicillin V. Phenoxymethyl penicillin (Fig. 3) is available only for oral use as sodium or potassium salts in suspension or tablets in doses of 125 mg, 250 mg, and 500 mg. The potassium salt produces higher blood levels than the other salts. Serum levels are from two to five times those obtained with penicillin G. Absorbed penicillin V is handled in the body similarly to penicillin G. Penicillin V can be substituted for penicillin G in most situations in which it is reasonable to treat an infection by the oral route. However, penicillin V is less active than penicillin G against *Hemophilus, Neisseria,* and enteric organisms. Blood levels after 500 mg given to an adult are equivalent to the levels achieved with 600,000 units of procaine penicillin given intramuscularly. The usual dosage for children is 25–50 mg/kg/day and for adults, of 1–4 g/day. The interval between dosages is 6–8 hours.

Phenethicillin. This phenoxyethyl analogue of penicillin G (Fig. 3) has microbiologic properties similar to penicillin G. It is acid stable and better absorbed from the gastrointestinal tract. Blood levels are high, but food delays its absorption. It is available only as the potassium salt in the form of 125- and 250-mg tablets and an oral suspension of 125 mg in 5 ml. Once absorbed it is handled in the body the same way as is penicillin G.

Propicillin. This is a phenoxypropyl penicillin similar in antibacterial activity to penicillin G. About 30 percent undergoes conversion in the body to an active metabolite, which is also excreted in the urine. The compound offers no advantage over penicillin V.

Phenbenicillin. This is the phenoxybenzyl penicillin that has lower in vitro activity than penicillin G or penicillin V but is much better absorbed. Superiority of this form to penicillin V has not been demonstrated.

Penicillinase-Resistant Penicillins (Fig. 4)

Methicillin. Methicillin (2,6-dimethoxyphenylpenicillin) is a penicillin resistant to staphylococcal β-lactamase (34). Its activity against staphylococci is low, with most strains inhibited by 2–3 μg/ml. Methicillin-resistant *S. aureus* are resistant not because of β-lactamase activity but by virtue of altered penicillin-binding proteins. These organisms have become a serious problem in some parts

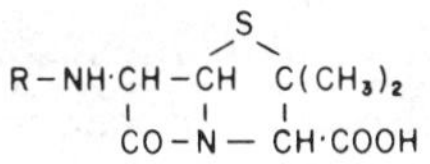

Structure of side chain R

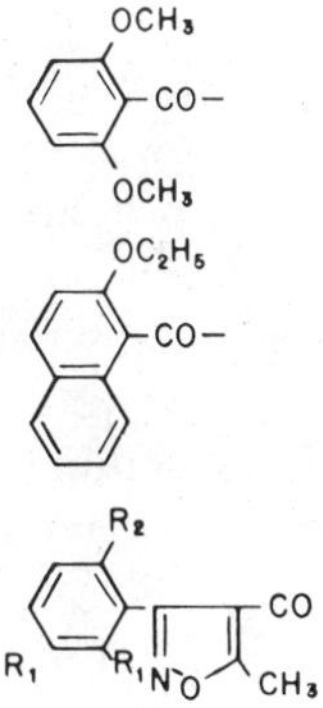

methicillin
2,6-dimethoxyphenylpenicillin

nafcillin
2-ethoxy-1-naphthylpenicillin

	R_2	R_1
oxacillin 3-phenyl-5-methyl-4-isoxazolylpenicillin	H	H
cloxacillin 3-(2-chlorophenyl)-5-methyl-4-isoxazolylpenicillin	Cl	H
dicloxacillin 3-(2,6-dichlorophenyl)-5-methyl-4-isoxazolylpenicillin	Cl	Cl
flucloxacillin 3-(2-chloro-6-fluorophenyl)-5-methyl-4-isoxazolylpenicillin	Cl	F

FIGURE 4. Antistaphylococcal penicillins.

of the United States. Methicillin inhibits *S. pyogenes* and *S. pneumoniae* at levels of 0.2 μg/ml, but it has no activity against *Streptococcus fecalis* and gram-negative bacilli. Methicillin is acid unstable and must be given parenterally. Absorption after an intramuscular injection is rapid, as is excretion, with peak levels after 1 g of 17 μg/ml but subinhibitory levels by 4 hours. Methicillin is less protein bound than the other antistaphylococcal penicillins, and although its intrinsic activity is less than the other antistaphylococcal penicillins, it is as active in the presence of serum as are the more intrinsically active oxacillin and nafcillin. Methicillin is available as a sodium salt, but since it is unstable in acidic media, it is used as a buffered solution. It is packaged as 1-, 4-, and 6-g vials and can be diluted with sodium chloride or dextrose in water. When diluted, buffered solutions are stable at room temperature for 8 hours. It is preferable to administer the drug every 4 hours if used intravenously. Methicillin should be used only for the treatment of penicillin-G-resistant staphylococcal infections. Toxicity is that seen with any penicillin, although interstitial nephritis may be more common. The usual dosage is 4–12 g/day for adults and 200–300 mg/kg/day for children given in 4 or 6 doses.

Nafcillin. Nafcillin (2-ethoxy-1-naphthylpenicillin) has more intrinsic activity than methicillin against both staphylococci and streptococci but is not active against gram-negative bacteria. Nafcillin is highly protein bound, and in the presence of serum its activity is similar to methicillin. Although nafcillin is absorbed when taken by mouth, absorption is erratic whether the drug is taken fasting or with food, and hence serum levels are low (34). Levels after intramuscular injection are low, and the preferred route of administration is intravenously. The antibiotic is primarily excreted by the liver and to a lesser extent by the kidney. Serum levels are elevated and the half-life is prolonged by probenecid. Although available as capsules (250 mg) and a suspension, one of the other agents in this class would be preferred for oral use. Sterile vials of 500 mg/1, 2, or 4 g of the sodium salt can be reconstituted in most solutions and are stable for up to 4 hours at room temperature. The usual dosage of nafcillin is 4–9 g/day, depending on the severity of the infection, and 100–200 mg/kg/day for children.

Isoxazolyl Penicillins. All these agents are stable to staphylococcal β-lactamase and inhibit both penicillin-sensitive and penicillin-resistant staphylococci at mean concentrations of 0.2–0.4 μg/ml. Methicillin-resistant *S. aureus* is resistant to these penicillins. Recently an increasing number of *S. epidermidis* isolates resistant to these penicillins has been found as the cause of serious infections. The mechanism of resistance is altered PBPs. Isoxazolyl penicillins inhibit streptococci and pneumococci but are virtually inactive against gram-negative bacilli. All are absorbed after oral administration, but absorption is adversely affected by food. There are differences in serum levels among the drugs after oral ingestion, with the serum level of cloxacillin twice that of oxacillin and the levels of dicloxacillin and flucloxacillin twice that of cloxacillin; all the drugs are highly bound to serum proteins; oxacillin, cloxacillin, and flucloxacillin are equally, bound but dicloxacillin is bound to a greater extent. Thus, actual free serum concentrations of the drugs is greatest for flucloxacillin followed by cloxacillin and dicloxacillin as equals and oxacillin the least (Table 5). After intravenous infusion of 1 g over 15 minutes, peak serum levels are 70–100 μg/ml, with levels of 25 μg/ml at 1 hour and less than 1 μg/ml at 6 hours. The isoxazolyl penicillins undergo some metabolism but are excreted primarily by the kidney with slight biliary excretion. Oxacillin undergoes more rapid degradation in the body than does cloxacillin or dicloxacillin.

OXACILLIN. Oxacillin is available as a sodium salt for oral use in 250- and 500-mg capsules and as a powder for suspension at 250 mg/5 ml. It should be taken 1–2 hours before meals. The daily dosage for adults is 1–4 g taken in four parts. The dosage for children is 50–100 mg/kg/day taken in four parts. Oxacillin sodium for injection may be given intramuscularly or intravenously. It is available in 500-mg and 1-, 2-, or 4-g vials and is stable in most saline and dextrose solutions for 6 hours at room temperature. Adult dosage is 2–12 g/day and for children, 100–300 mg/kg/day given every 4–6 hours.

CLOXACILLIN. Cloxacillin sodium is available in the United States only as an oral solution (125 mg/5ml) or capsules of 250 and 500 mg. Dosage for children is 50–100mg/kg/day given as four equal doses. Dosage for adults is 1–4g/day given as four equal doses. In Europe cloxacillin is available as a parenteral for intramuscular or intravenous administration in 250-mg vials. It yields serum levels similar to those achieved with oxacillin.

DICLOXACILLIN. Dicloxacillin sodium is available as a suspension (62.5 mg/5 ml) and as capsules of 125 and 250 mg. The dosage for children less than 40 kg is 25 mg/kg/day given as four doses. Some authorities recommend doses as above for cloxacillin. For adults, a dosage of 250 mg–1 g every 6 hours can be given, depending on the severity of the infection.

FLUCLOXACILLIN. Flucloxacillin sodium is not available in the United States. It is available in Europe in the form of suspension and capsules similar to the forms of cloxacillin, 250-mg capsules, and for parenteral use in 250-mg vials.

Aminopenicillins (Fig. 5)

The antibacterial activity of all these penicillins is similar (52). They are not stable to β-lactamases of either gram-positive or gram-negative bacteria. The aminopenicillins are only slightly less active than penicillin G against *S. pyogenes, S. pneumoniae,* and *S. agalactiae.* They are more active against group D streptococci (e.g., *S. fecalis*). Activity of the compounds against clostridial species, *Actinomyces,* corynebacteria, and *N. meningitidis* is equal to that of penicillin G. They are more active than penicillin G against *Listeria monocytogenes.* Sensitivity of *N. gonorrhoeae* (see Chapter 172) varies from highly sensitive to completely resistant strains that bear a plasmid-mediating production of a β-lactamase. *Hemophilus influenzae* (both typeable and nontypeable strains) and *Hemophilus parainfluenzae* are usually susceptible, except for the isolates that

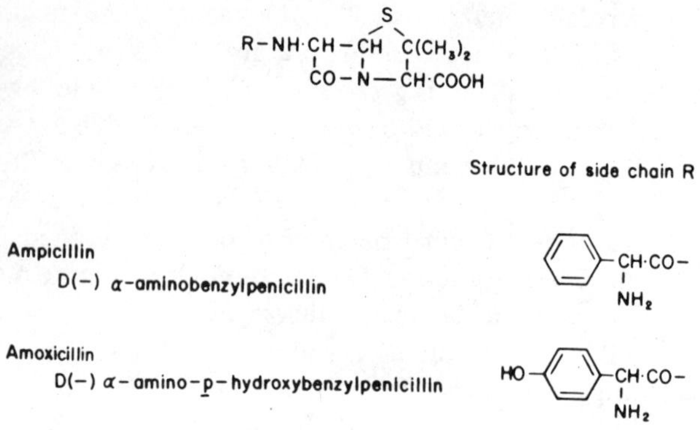

FIGURE 5. Aminopenicillins.

produce β-lactamases. Although most domiciliary *E. coli* are sensitve to aminopenicillins, plasmid resistance is common in hospital isolates. *Shigella sonnei,* many salmonellae, including many *Salmonella typhi* are resistant because of β-lactamases. Most *Klebsiella, Serratia, Acinetobacter,* indole-positive *Proteus, Pseudomonas,* and *Bacteroides fragilis* are resistant to the penicillins of this class.

Ampicillin. Ampicillin is moderately well absorbed after oral administration, but peak levels are delayed and lowered if it is ingested with food. Peak blood levels of 3 μg/ml occur 1–2 hours after ingestion of 0.5 g. Drug can be detected in the serum for 4–6 hours. After intramuscular injection of 0.5 g peak levels of 10 μg are achieved in 1 hour and persist for 4 hours. Probenecid increases the height of peak levels and prolongs the period in which the drug can be detected in serum. Ampicillin is well distributed to body compartments and achieves therapeutic concentrations in cerebrospinal fluid (CSF) and in pleural, joint, and peritoneal fluids in the presence of inflammation after parenteral administration. Urinary levels are high even in the presence of markedly reduced renal function. Peritoneal dialysis is ineffective in removing the drug, but hemodialysis removes approximately 40 percent in a 6-hour period.

Ampicillin is available for oral use as the sodium salt or as the trihydrate in capsules of 125, 250, and 500 mg as a suspension of 125 and 250 mg/5 ml, as drops of 100 mg/ml, and as 125-mg chewable tablets. It is also prepared as a suspension, which contains 3.5 g of ampicillin trihydrate and 1 g of probenecid. It is available as ampicillin trihydrate in 2.5-g vials only for intramuscular use. As a sodium salt in vials of 0.125, 0.5, 2, and 4 g it can be used either intramuscularly or intravenously. It is stable in sodium chloride for 8 hours at concentrations up to 30 mg/ml, but for intravenous use at concentrations greater than 2 mg/ml it is stable at room temperature for less than 4 hours and hence would preferably be administered by "piggy back" within 0.5–1 hour. Dosage varies with the age of the patients, the status of renal function, and the severity of the disease. For children above 1 month of age the oral dosage is 50–100 mg/kg/day in four doses; the intramuscular or intravenous dosage is 100–400 mg/kg/day in four or six doses. For adults the oral dosage is 2–4 g/day given in a dose every 6 hours. For severe infection the parental dosage is 6–12 g/day given in divided doses every 4 hours.

Hetacillin. This is a condensation product of ampicillin and acetone that is rapidly hydrolyzed to ampicillin either as it crosses the gastrointestinal mucosa or in the serum. A number of studies has shown that peak antibiotic blood levels are equal to or lower than those achieved with a comparable dose of ampicillin, although minimally higher blood levels are present 6 and 8 hours after oral administration of hetacillin. Administration of hetacillin by intramuscular injection produces lower blood levels than does administration of ampicillin (53). It is available as a potassium salt in a suspension of 112.5 and 225 mg/5 ml, as pediatric drops, and as capsules of 255 and 450 mg. It offers no advantage over ampicillin.

Pivampicillin. The pivaloyloxymethyl ester of ampicillin—pivampicillin—is stable in aqueous acid but undergoes rapid hydrolysis in serum and tissue (54). Pivampicillin is absorbed intact and is rapidly hydrolyzed by nonspecific esterases in cells and blood to yield pivalic acid and the hydroxyl methyl ester of ampicillin, which are rapidly hydrolyzed to ampicillin and formaldehyde. At no time does the concentration of ester in the blood exceed 2 percent of the ampicillin, and within 15 minutes more than 99 percent of the compound has been converted to ampicillin. Pivampicillin is more rapidly absorbed than ampicllin with peak levels at 1 hour, and serum levels are approximately twice those achieved with a comparable oral dose of ampicillin and are equal to those achieved with a comparable intramuscular dose of ampicillin. Urinary recovery and levels are twice those achieved with the same dose of ampicillin. In terms of distribution in the body, the compound is identical to ampicillin. Side effects due to the drug are those encountered with ampicillin, although there may be more gastric intolerance than with ampicillin, especially if not taken with food, but diarrhea is less. The drug is not available in the United States. In Europe it is available in capsules of 178 and 358 mg, which contain 125 and 250 mg of ampicillin. An advantage for the drug has not been established.

Bacampicillin. Bacampicillin is the hydrochloride of the 1-ethoxycarboxyloxyethyl ester of ampicillin. It has no antibacterial activity, but when it is administered orally it is totally hydrolyzed to free ampicillin. It is better absorbed in the presence of food, with peak serum levels occurring earlier than with ampicillin and approximately from one and a half to two times greater than that achieved with an equimolar dose of ampicillin. Peak serum levels of 9 μg/ml follow a dose of 500 mg, and serum levels exceed those of ampicillin and amoxicillin for 2.5 hours, but thereafter serum levels of ampicillin from bacampicillin are equivalent to those of amoxicillin (23). Clinical studies have shown efficacy similar to that of ampicillin (55). Bacampicillin is available as an oral suspension containing 125 mg per 5 ml as 400-mg tablets, which is the equivalent of 280 mg of ampicillin.

Talampicillin. This is the phthalidyl ester of ampicillin. It has no antibacterial activity but is hydrolyzed to free ampicillin as it is absorbed. It produces serum levels earlier and three times those achieved with equimolar doses of ampicillin. It is not available in the United States, and studies have been too few to determine if it has any merit over ampicillin.

Epicillin. Epicillin is a compound in which the benzene ring has been replaced by a 1,4-cyclohexadienyl ring. It has a bacterial spectrum similar to ampicillin. It is acid stable and has oral absorption, serum binding, excretion, and tissue distribution similar to ampicillin. It has been effective in treatment of a variety of infections. It is not available in the United States.

Cyclacillin. Cyclacillin, 6-(1-aminocyclohexande carboxy- amido) penicillanic acid, is an acid-stable aminopenicillin with antibacterial activity similar to ampicillin. It is the most rapidly absorbed aminopenicillin, with levels of 10–18 μg/ml 30 minutes after ingestion of 500 mg—levels four times that of ampicillin. However, it is extremely rapidly cleared, and levels at 2 hours are less than those achieved with a comparable dose of ampicillin. Probenecid causes appreciably less delay in excretion than with other penicillins.

Amoxicillin. Amoxicillin differs from ampicillin only in the presence of a hydroxyl group in the paraposition of the benzene side chain. It has in vitro activity similar to ampicillin. It is significantly better absorbed when given by mouth than is ampicillin (21). Peak blood levels are from two to two and a half times those achieved with a similar dose of ampicillin, and food does not decrease absorption. Oral amoxicillin produces blood levels similar to those produced by intramuscularly administered sodium ampicillin or ampicillin trihydrate. Urinary excretion of amoxicillin is greater than that of ampicillin. Tissue distribution is similar to that of ampicillin. Clinical studies with amoxicillin have been extensive, and it has been used in the treatment of otitis media, bronchitis, pneumonia, typhoid, gonorrhea, and urinary tract infections (56). It has been used as a single 3-g dose for therapy for bacterial cystitis in women (57). It is not useful as treatment of shigellosis. Side effects of amoxicillin are similar to those seen with ampicillin, although diarrhea may be less common than with ampicillin. It is available as the trihydrate in suspension of 125 and 250 mg/5 ml, as drops of 50 mg/ml, and as capsules of 250 and 500 mg. Usual dosage for children is 20–40 mg/kg/day given in three doses every 8 hours, and for adults the dosage is 250 mg every 8 hours, although it has been used in doses up to 1 g every 4 hours. It has been useful in pediatric infections, except for shigellosis, and may be preferred to ampicillin. In adult infections its use would depend on cost factors and tolerance.

Carboxy Penicillins (Fig. 6)

Carbenicillin. Carbenicillin was the first penicillin with activity against *P. aeruginosa* and certain indole-positive *Proteus* species that were not susceptible to other penicillins or to the cephalosporins (35). It is destroyed by β-lactamases of both gram-positive and gram-negative organisms, but it is more stable against hydrolysis by the β-lactamases of species such as *Pseudomonas, Enterobacter,*

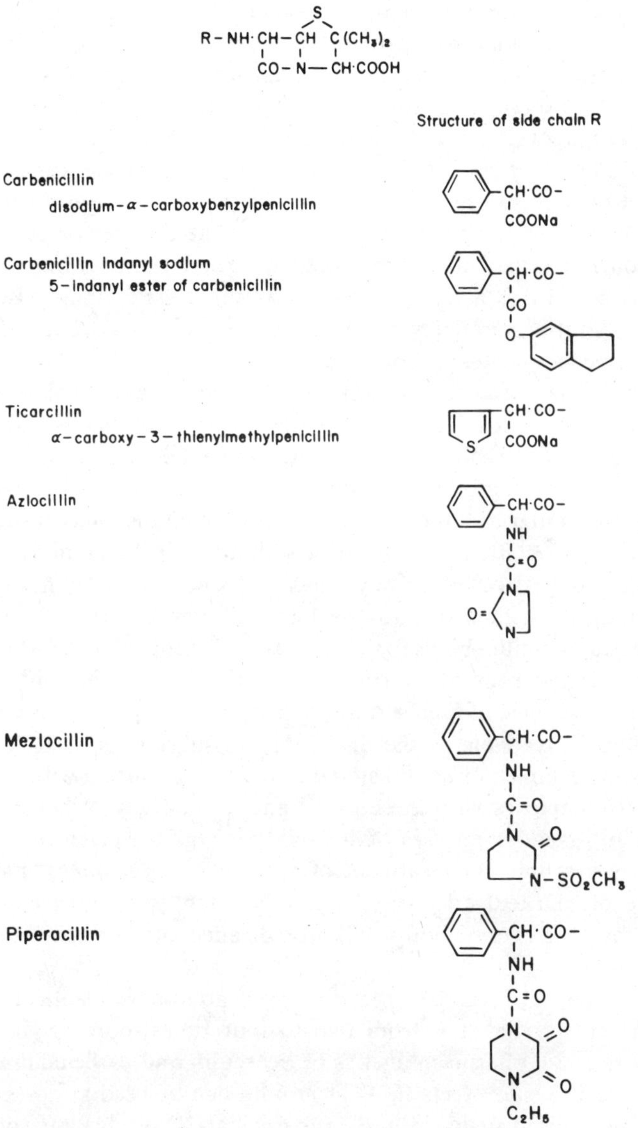

FIGURE 6. Penicillins active against gram-negative bacteria.

Morganella, and *Proteus-Providencia,* which function primarily as cephalosporinases. Carbenicillin is less active than ampicillin against *S. pyogenes, S. pneumoniae,* and *S. fecalis.* It is less active than the ureidopenicillins against streptococcal species. Its activity against *Hemophilus, N. gonorrhoeae,* and *N. meningitidis* is similar to ampicillin. It has gram-negative activity similar to ampicillin against *E. coli, Proteus mirabilis, Salmonella* species, and *Shigella* species, but it is inactive against *Klebsiella.* It inhibits some *Enterobacter* and *Serratia* strains and many *B. fragilis,* although high concentrations are required. Carbenicillin acts synergistically with amikacin, gentamicin, and tobramycin to inhibit *P. aeruginosa.* Carbenicillin is not absorbed by mouth but can be given by intramuscular or intravenous administration. After an intramuscular dose of 1 g, peak serum levels of 20 μg/ml are reached in 1 hour, but the drug is not detectable at 4 hours. These levels are not adequate for treatment of tissue *Pseudomonas* infections, but levels of 2000–4000 μg/ml are achieved in the urine, and, therefore, it could be used by this route for urinary infections. Serum levels of 150–200 μg/ml will be maintained when it is given at dosages of 70–100 mg/kg over 1–2 hours. Carbenicillin is excreted by renal tubules, but since less is converted to penicilloic acid, its half-life (72 minutes) is longer than that of penicillin G, and it accumulates in the presence of renal failure (35,58). Greater accumulation occurs if there is combined hepatic and renal dysfunction. Hemodialysis reduces plasma concentrations. Probenecid delays renal excretion and increases serum concentrations. Tissue distribution is similar to ampicillin but concentrations in the cerebrospinal fluid often are not adequate for *Pseudomonas* due to the high levels needed to inhibit these organisms. Side effects due to carbenicillin are similar to those seen with other penicillins. Since it is a disodium salt and each gram contains 4.7 mEq of sodium, when administered at doses of 30–40 g/day congestive failure may occur. Carbenicillin causes more hypokalemia than other penicillins due to the load of nonreabsorbable anion in the distal tubule. Carbenicillin binds to the adenosine 5′-dephosphate (ADP) receptor site on platelets and prevents normal contraction; hence, bleeding occurs on occasion in the presence of high serum levels such as may occur in renal failure.

Carbenicillin is available as the disodium salt in vials of 1, 2, 5, and 10 g. It should never be mixed or administered in the same solution with aminoglycosides, since it complexes with these drugs and the activity of both compounds is inhibited. Intravenous dosages of 400–600 mg/kg/day given over 1–2 hours every 4 hours are used for treatment of systemic *Pseudomonas* infections. In the presence of markedly decreased renal function (creatinine clearance less than 10 ml/min) 2 g every 8 hours will provide adequate levels without toxicity.

Ticarcillin. The antibacterial spectrum of ticarcillin is identical to that of carbenicillin, except that it is from two to four times more active against *P. aeruginosa* (59). The pharmacokinetics of ticarcillin and carbenicillin are virtually identical as are side effects (60). Ticarcillin can be used at dosages of 200–300 mg/kg/day. It is available in 1-, 3-, and 6-g vials. One advantage of ticarcillin over carbenicillin would be that in certain situations the same dose as carbenicillin will inhibit some *Pseudomonas* that could not be inhibited by the concentrations of carbenicillin that could be achieved with safety (61). Another advantage would be the use of a reduced dose of ticarcillin (with the same therapeutic efficacy) to deliver a lower sodium load and result in less platelet dysfunction.

Oral Antipseudomonas Penicillins

Indanyl carbenicillin. Indanyl carbenicillin (carindacillin) is an α-carboxy ester of carbenicillin. It has no intrinsic activity of its own, but as a sodium ester it is highly acid stable and relatively well absorbed from the gastrointestinal tract. Ingestion with food may actually enhance absorption. The ester is immediately hydrolyzed to free carbenicillin, and only trace amounts of ester are found in serum or urine. Peak serum levels after 1 g taken orally are 10 μg at 1–2 hours. Urine levels are 300–1000 μg/ml with 30 percent of a dose recovered in the first 6 hours. The compound does not provide adequate serum or tissue levels for systemic infections, and it is useful only for the treatment of urinary tract infections. In the presence of decreased renal function, urine levels are lower and may be inadequate to treat *Pseudomonas* infections. Side effects are those of all the penicillins, but gastrointestinal irritation has been a problem in some people. It is available as 500-mg capsules (containing 382 mg of carbenicillin). The usual dosage is 1 g every 6 hours for adults.

Carfecillin. Carfecillin is the phenyl ester of carbenicillin. It is also well absorbed and rapidly hydrolyzed to yield carbenicillin. Serum levels are similar to those of the indanyl ester. It is useful only to treat urinary infections due to *Pseudomonas.* It has been better tolerated due to a less bitter taste. It is not available in the United States.

Ureidopenicillins

Azlocillin. Azlocillin is an acylureido penicillin that is 8–16 times more active than carbenicillin against *P. aeruginosa* and is less active against indole-positive *Proteus* species. It has the same activity as ampicillin against streptococcal species (62). It is destroyed by β-lactamases of both gram-positive and gram-negative bacteria. It is not orally absorbed and must be given by the intravenous route to provide adequate serum levels to treat *Pseudomonas* infection. The half-life is approximately 50 minutes, and administration of 4 g yields peak levels of 285 μg/ml.

Azlocillin shows nonlinear pharmacokinetics. The peak serum concentrations and the area under the drug curve are not proportional; that is, a 4- or 5-g dose produces serum levels that are greater than four or five times the 1-g dose (63). The drug thus could be administered in larger doses at intervals of 6 hours rather than the 4-hour intervals used for carbenicillin. Azlocillin also does not accumulate in renal failure to the same degree as do carbenicillin and ticarcillin since its half-life rises only to 4 hours with creatinine clearances below 7 ml/min (64,65). Azlocillin enters the cerebrospinal fluid in the presence of meningeal inflammation, but levels are only 10 percent of the serum level. Azlocillin also causes less increase in bleeding time than does carbenicillin since it apparently has less affinity for the ADP receptor site. Azlocillin is used primarily to treat *Pseudomonas* infections. It has proved to be a useful drug in a variety of clinical situations (65). It is available as 1-, 2-, 3-, and 4-g vials, which contain 2.17 mEq sodium per gram of drug.

Mezlocillin. Mezlocillin is an acylureido penicillin similar in antibacterial spectrum to carbenicillin and ticarcillin but with some significant differences (62). It is more active in vitro against streptococci, particularly *Streptococcus faecalis,* than either of the above-mentioned agents. It inhibits about 75 percent of *Klebsiella* species at a concentration of 25 μg/ml, whereas less than 5 percent would be inhibited by 100 μg/ml of carbenicillin (66). It is also more active than carbenicillin or ticarcillin against *H. influenzae* and is more active than carbenicillin against *B. fragilis.* It is, however, not more stable to β-lactamase hydrolysis than is carbenicillin; hence its greater intrinsic activity is due to other factors such as greater affinity for penicillin-binding proteins and better entry into the bacterial periplasmic space. It acts synergistically against gram-negative bacteria when combined with aminoglycosides. The drug must be given parenterally. Its pharmacokinetics are different from carbenicillin since, like azlocillin and piperacillin, it shows dose-related nonlinear kinetics. Peak serum levels, half-life, and area under the time curve are greater with larger doses. Administration of 4 g produces peak levels of 300 μg/ml. Its half-life increases only to 4 hours in patients in renal failure. Mezlocillin is the least likely of the broad-spectrum penicillins to alter bleeding times. Clinical studies in the United States and Europe have shown that it is effective therapy for respiratory, urinary, gynecologic, and surgical infections (67–70). It causes less increase in bleeding time than does carbenicillin. Usual doses have been 12–18 g/day for adults. It is available as 1-, 2-, 3-, and 5-g vials, which contain 1.85 mEq of sodium per gram.

Piperacillin. Piperacillin is an acylureido penicillin derivative that is similar in activity to ampicillin against gram-positive species (71). It has excellent activity against streptococcal species and against *Neisseria* and *Hemophilus* and many *Enterobacteriaceae.* It also has excellent activity against both cocci and bacilli anaerobic species. It inhibits 60 percent of *Pseudomonas* species at 3 μg/ml and 90 percent at 12 μg/ml (71,72). It is hydrolyzed by plasmid-mediated β-lactamases of gram-positive and gram-negative bacteria. Its acts synergistically against *Pseudomonas* and against some of the Enterobacteriaceae when combined with aminoglycosides (71). The human pharmacology of piperacillin is similar to that of azlocillin and mezlocillin (73,74). Administration of 4 g by the intravenous route produces peak serum levels of 300 μg/ml. It shows kinetics that are dose dependent. It accumulates in renal failure to a lesser degree than does carbenicillin, and its half-life is only 4 hours in renal failure (75). It is removed by hemodialysis. Piperacillin has shown adverse reactions similar to those of the other penicillins noted earlier. After prolonged administration at high doses neutropenia has been reported. Alteration of bleeding time and hypokalemia occur but less frequently than with carbenicillin. Clinical studies have shown that it is a useful agent in treatment of a variety of infections (76–79). It is administered in daily doses to adults of 12–18 g. It is available in vials of 2, 3, and 4 g, which contain 1.85 mEq of sodium per gram of drug.

Amidinopenicillanic Acid Derivatives

Amdinocillin, formerly called mecillinam, is a 6-β-acylaminopenicillanic acid. It has unusual antibacterial properties for a penicillin (80,81). It has poor anti-gram-positive activity. In situations in which 0.01 μg/ml of penicillin G inhibits *S. pyogenes,* 6 μg/ml of amdinocillin are needed to inhibit streptococci. It does not bind to the penicillin binding proteins of gram-positive species. It has poor activity against *Hemophilus* and *Neisseria.* However, it is extremely active against *E. coli,* inhibiting many β-lactamase-containing strains even though it is hydrolyzed by the plasmid-mediated β-lactamases. The reason for this activity is that it binds only to PBP-2 in Enterobacteriaceae, and this protein is critical in cell wall production in these species. Amdinocillin is active against many ampicillin-resistant *Shigella* and *Salmonella* species. In contrast to ampicillin, it is active against many *Klebsiella, Enterobacter,* and *Citrobacter* species. It has variable activity against *Proteus,* both *P. mirabilis* and the indole-positive *Proteus,* and it fails to inhibit *Pseudomonas* and anaerobic species such as *B. fragilis.* Amdinocillin acts synergistically with other penicillins such as ampicillin or carbenicillin and also with cephalosporins (81). It does not act synergistically with aminoglycosides nor is its activity inhibited by chloramphenicol.

Amdinocillin is not acid stable and cannot be used orally except in the form of a pivaloyl ester. This ester is well absorbed, immediately hydrolyzed, yielding free compound in the serum. Serum levels of pivamdinocillin after ingestion are equivalent to those obtained with pivampicillin (see above), and absorption is improved in the presence of food. Amdinocillin administered parenterally as a sodium salt yields serum levels comparable to those achieved with equimolar doses of ampicillin (82). The compound is renally excreted similarly to ampicillin and is distributed within the body in the same manner as ampicillin. Clinical studies have shown the compound to be effective in the treatment of infections caused by susceptible microorganisms (83,84). It is available in Europe as the pivaloyl ester for oral use and as the sodium salt for parenteral administration.

6-Methoxy Penicillin Derivatives

Temocillin is a 6-α-methoxy derivative of ticarcillin. The presence of the methoxy group on the β-lactam ring renders the compound extremely resistant to hydrolysis by both plasmid and chromosomally mediated β-lactamases. However, there has been a marked loss in activity against gram-positive species and *Pseudomonas*

(85). Temocillin inhibits the majority of *E. coli, Klebsiella, Enterobacter* species, *Proteus, Serratia,* and *Citrobacter* species at 10 μg/ml or less. *Hemophilus* and *Branhamella* are inhibited by less than 1 μg/ml. *Bacteroides* species are resistant. Temocillin is not hydrolyzed by the common chromosomal and plasmid β-lactamases. Although it does not inhibit *Pseudomonas,* this is due to failure to cross the outer cell wall.

Peak serum concentrations of temocillin after 500 mg and 1 g are administered by the intramuscular route average 50 and 70 μg/ml, respectively (28). Serum half-life of temocillin after intramuscular administration ranges from 4 to 6 hours. After bolus intravenous administration of temocillin peak serum concentrations have been 75 μg/ml for 500 mg and 170 μg/ml for 1 g. Serum half-life after intravenous administration averages 4½ hours. Urinary recovery of temocillin is 70–80 percent, with urine concentrations of 100–500 μg/ml for 12 hours after a 500-mg intramuscular injection. Temocillin accumulates in the presence of renal failure with serum half-life reaching 15–20 hours (28). It is partially removed by hemodialysis but not by peritoneal dialysis. Temocillin has been used in Europe to treat urinary infections and tissue infections due to gram-negative bacilli. It is not available in the United States.

REFERENCES

1. Fleming A: On the antibacterial action of cultures of a penicillium, with special reference to their use in the isolation of *B. influenzae. Br J Exp Pathol* 10:226, 1929.
2. Batchelor FR, Doyle FP, Naylor JHC, et al: Synthesis of penicillin: 6-aminopenicillanic acid in penicillin fermentations. *Nature* 183:257, 1959.
3. Tipper DJ, Wright A: The structure and biosynthesis of bacterial cell walls, in Sokatch JR, Ornstein LA (eds): *The Bacteria.* New York, Academic Press, 1979, vol 7, p 291.
4. Strominger JL: Penicillin-sensitive enzymatic reactions in bacterial cell wall synthesis. *Harvey Lect* 64:179, 1970.
5. Mirelman D: Biosynthesis and assembly of cell wall peptidoglycan, in Inouye M (ed): *Bacterial Outer Membranes.* New York, John Wiley & Sons, 1980, p 166.
6. Waxman DL, Yocum RR, Strominger JL: Penicillins and cephalosporins are active site-directed acylating agents: Evidence in support of the substrate analogue hypothesis. *Philos Trans R Soc Lond [Biol]* 289:257, 1980.
7. Spratt BG: Distinct penicillin binding proteins involved in the division, elongation and shape of *Escherichia coli,* K 12. *Proc Natl Acad Sci USA* 72:2999, 1975.
8. Spratt BG: Biochemical and genetical approaches to the mechanism of action of penicillin. *Philos Trans R Soc Lond (Biol)* 289:273, 1980.
9. Tamaki S, Nakajima S, Matsuhashi M: Thermosensitive mutation in *Escherichia coli* simultaneously causing defects in penicillin-binding protein 1Bs and in enzyme activity for peptidoglycan synthesis in vivo. *Proc Natl Acad Sci USA* 74:5472, 1977.
10. Suzuki H, Nishimuka Y, Hirota Y: On the process of cellular division in *Escherichia coli:* A series of mutants of *E. coli* altered in penicillin-binding proteins. *Proc Natl Acad Sci USA* 75:664, 1978.
11. Yocum RR, Waxman DW, Strominger JL: The mechanism of action of penicillin. *J Biol Chem* 255:3977, 1980.
12. Georgopapadakou NH, Liu FY: Binding of β-lactam antibiotics to penicillin-binding proteins of *Staphylococcus aureus* and *Streptococcus faecalis* in relation to antibacterial activity. *Antimicrob Agents Chemother* 18:834, 1980.

12a. Tomasz A, Holtje JV: Murein hydrolases and the lytic and killing action of penicillin, in Schlessinger D (ed): *Microbiology—1977.* Washington DC, American Society for Microbiology, 1977, p 209.
13. Neu HC: Penicillins: New insights into their mechanisms of activity and clinical use. *Bull NY Acad Med* 58:681, 1982.
14. Sykes RB, Matthew M: The β-lactamases of gram-negative bacteria and their role in resistance to β-lactam antibiotics. *J Antimicrob Agents Chemother* 2:115, 1976.
15. Neu HC: Structure-activity relations of new β-lactam compounds and in vitro activity against common bacteria. *Rev Infect Dis* 5(suppl):319, 1983.
16. Barber M, Waterworth PM: Antibacterial activity of the penicillins. *Br Med J* 1:1159, 1962.
17. Rolinson GN, Sutherland R: Semisynthetic penicillins. *Adv Pharmacol Chemother* 11:152, 1973.
18. Marcy SM, Klein JO: The isoxazolyl penicillins: Oxacillin, cloxacillin and dicloxacillin. *Med Clin North Am* 54:1127, 1970.
19. Finland M, Garner C, Wolcox C, et al: Susceptibility of pneumococci and *Haemophilus influenzae* to antibacterial agents. *Antimicrob Agents Chemother* 9:274, 1976.
20. Sutter VL, Finegold SM: Susceptibility of anaerobic bacteria to 23 antimicrobial agents. *Antimicrob Agents Chemother* 10:736, 1976.
21. Neu HC: Antimicrobial activity and human pharmacology of amoxicillin. *J Infect Dis* 129(suppl):123, 1974.
22. McCarthy CG, Finland M: Absorption and excretion of four penicillins: Penicillin G, penicillin V, phenethicillin and phenylmercaptomethyl penicillin. *N Engl J Med* 263:315, 1960.
23. Neu HC: The pharmacokinetics of bacampicillin. *Rev Infect Dis* 3:110, 1981.
24. Butler K, English AR, Briggs B, et al: Indanyl carbenicillin: Chemistry and laboratory studies with a new semisynthetic penicillin. *J Infect Dis* 127(suppl):97, 1973.
25. Cole M, Kening MD, Hewitt VA: Metabolism of penicillins to penicilloic acidosis and 6-aminopenicillanic acid in man and its significance in assessing penicillin absorption. *Antimicrob Agents Chemother* 3:463, 1973.
26. Eagle H, Newman E: Renal clearance of penicillin F, G, K, and X in rabbits and man. *J Clin Invest* 26:903, 1947.
27. Acocella G, Mattiussi R, Nichols FB, et al: Biliary excretion of antibiotics in man. *Gut* 9:536, 1968.
28. Bodaert J, Daneels R, Schurgers M, et al: The pharmacokinetics of temocillin in patients with normal and impaired renal function. *J Antimicrob Chemother* 11:349, 1983.
29. Gilbaldi M, Swartz MA: Apparent effect of probenecid on the distribution of penicillins in man. *Clin Pharmacol Ther* 9:345, 1968.
30. Appel GB, Neu HC: Infections and antibiotic usage in patients with renal diseases, in Martinez-Maldonado M (ed): *Handbook of Renal Therapeutics.* New York, Plenum, 1983, p 227.
31. Parker RH, Schmid FR: Antibacterial activity of synovial fluid during therapy of septic arthritis. *Arthritis Rheum* 14:96, 1971.
32. Barza M, Weinstein L: Penetration of antibiotics into fibrin loci in vivo. I. Comparison of penetration of ampicillin into fibrin clots, abscesses and interstitial fluid. *J Infect Dis* 129:59, 1974.
33. Pancoast SJ, Neu HC: Antibiotic levels in human bone and synovial fluid. *Orthopedics Rev* 9:49, 1980.
34. Neu HC: Antistaphylococcal penicillins. *Med Clin North Am* 66:51, 1982.
35. Neu HC: Carbenicillin and ticarcillin. *Med Clin North Am* 66:61, 1982.
36. Fishman RA: Blood-brain and CSF barriers to penicillin and related organic acids. *Arch Neurol* 15:13, 1966.
37. Depp R, Kind AC, Kirby WMM, et al: Transplacental passage of methicillin and dicloxacillin into the fetus and amniotic fluid. *Am J Obstet Gynecol* 197:1054, 1970.
38. Whelton A, Carter GG, Bryant HH, et al: Carbenicillin concentrations in normal and diseased kidneys. A therapeutic consideration. *Ann Intern Med* 78:659, 1973.
39. Levine BB, Redmond AP, Feller MF, et al: Penicillin allergy and the heterogeneous immune response of man to benzylpenicillin. *J Clin Invest* 45:1895, 1966.

40. Saxon A: Immediate hypersensitivity reactions to β-lactam antibiotics. *Rev Infect Dis* 5(suppl 2):368, 1983.
41. Idsoe O, Gothe T, Wilcox RR, et al: Nature and extent of penicillin side reactions with particular reference to fatalities from anaphylactic shock. *Bull WHO* 38:159, 1968.
42. Green GR, Rosenblum A: Report of the penicillin study group, American Academy of Allergy. *J Allergy Clin Immunol* 48:331, 1971.
43. Parry MF, Neu HC: The safety and tolerance of mezlocillin. *J Antimicrob Chemother* 9(suppl A):273, 1982.
44. Kerr RO, Cardamone J, Dalmasso AP, et al: Two mechanisms of erthrocyte destruction in penicillin-induced hemolytic anemia. *N Engl J Med* 287:1322, 1972.
45. Brown CH, Natelson EA, Bradshaw W, et al: The hemostatic defect produced by carbenicillin. *N Engl J Med* 291:265, 1974.
46. Appel GB, Neu HC: The nephrotoxicity of antimicrobial agents. *N Engl J Med* 296:63, 1977.
47. Appel GB, Neu HC: Acute interstitial nephritis induced by β-lactam antibiotics, in Fillastre JP (ed): *Nephrotoxicity-Ototoxicity of Drugs.* Inserum Publ de l'Universite de Rouen, 1981, p 195.
48. Baldwin DS, Levine BB, McCluskey RT, et al: Renal failure and interstitial nephritis due to penicillin and methicillin. *N Engl J Med* 279:1245, 1968.
49. Bloomer HA, Barton LJ, Maddock RJ Jr: Penicillin-induced encephalopathy in uremic patients. *JAMA* 200:121, 1967.
50. Wilson FM, Belamavic J, Lauter CB, et al: Anicteric carbenicillin hepatitis. Eight episodes in four patients. *JAMA* 232:818, 1967.
51. Sullivan TJ: Antigen-specific densitization of patients allergic to penicillin. *J Allergy Clin Immunol* 69:50, 1982.
52. Neu HC: Aminopenicillins: Clinical pharmacology and use in disease states. *Int J Clin Pharmacol Biopharm* 11:132, 1975.
53. Tuano SB, Johnson LD, Brodie JL, et al: Comparative blood levels of hetacillin, ampicillin and penicillin G. *N Engl J Med* 275:635, 1966.
54. Daehne W von, Godfredsen WO, Rotrott K, et al: Pivampicillin, a new orally active ampicillin ester. *Antimicrob Agents Chemother* 10:431, 1971.
55. Scheife RT, Neu HC: Bacampicillin hydrochloride: Chemistry, pharmacology and clinical use. *Pharmacotherapy* 2:313, 1982.
56. Prince AS, Neu HC: New penicillin and their use in pediatrics. *Pediatr Clin North Am* 30:3, 1983.
57. Fang LST, Tolokoff-Rubin NE, Rubin RH: Efficacy of single-dose and conventional amoxicillin therapy in urinary tract infection localized by antibody-coated bacteria technique. *N Engl J Med* 298:413, 1978.
58. Hoffman TA, Cestero R, Bullock WE: Pharmacodynamics of carbenicillin in patients with hepatic and renal failure. *Ann Intern Med* 73:173, 1970.
59. Fuchs PC, Thornsberry C, Barry AL, et al: Ticarcillin: A collaborative in vitro comparison with carbenicillin against 9,000 clinical bacterial isolates. *Am J Med Sci* 274:255, 1977.
60. Neu HC, Garvey GG: Comparative in vitro activity and clinical pharmacology of ticarcillin and carbenicillin. *Antimicrob Agents Chemother* 8:457, 1975.
61. Parry MF, Neu HC: Ticarcillin for treatment of serious infections with gram-negative bacteria. *J Infect Dis* 134:476, 1976.
62. Fu KP, Neu HC: Azlocillin and mezlocillin: New ureido penicillins. *Antimicrob Agents Chemother* 13:930, 1978.
63. Bergen T: Review of the pharmacokinetics and dose dependency of azlocillin in normal subjects and patients with renal insufficiency. *J Antimicrob Agents* 11(suppl B):101, 1983.
64. Whelton A, Stout RL, Delgado FA: Azlocillin kinetics during extracorporeal haemodialysis and peritoneal dialysis. *J Antimicrob Chemother* 11(suppl B):89, 1983.
65. Schacht P, Arcieri G, Bruck H, et al: International experience with azlocillin. *J Antimicrob Chemother* 11(suppl B):215, 1983.
66. Parry MF, Folta D: The in vitro activity of mezlocillin against community hospital isolates

in comparison to other penicillins and cephalosporins. *J Antimicrob Chemother* 11(suppl C):97, 1983.

67. Pancoast SJ, Jahre JA, Neu HC: Mezlocillin in the therapy of serious infections. *Am J Med* 67:747, 1979.
68. Issell BF, Bodey GP: Mezlocillin for treatment of infections in cancer patients. *Antimicrob Agents Chemother* 17:1008, 1980.
69. Melikian V, Wise R, Allum WH, et al: Mezlocillin and gentamicin in the treatment of infections in seriously ill and immunosuppressed patients. *J Antimicrob Chemother* 7:657, 1981.
70. Ramirez-Ronda CH, Gotierrez J, Bermudez RH: Comparative effectiveness, safety and tolerance of mezlocillin and ticarcillin: A prospective randomized trial. *J Antimicrob Chemother* 9(suppl A):125, 1982.
71. Fu KP, Neu HC: Piperacillin, a new penicillin active against many bacteria resistant to other penicillins. *Antimicrob Agents Chemother* 13:358, 1978.
72. Verbist L: Comparison of the activities of the new ureido-penicillins—piperacillin, mezlocillin, azlocillin and Bay K4999—against gram-negative organisms. *Antimicrob Agents Chemother* 16:115, 1979.
73. Bergen T: Overview of acylureidopenicillin pharmacokinetics. *Scand J Infect Dis* 29:33, 1981.
74. Tjandramaga TB, Mollie A, Verbesselt R, et al: Piperacillin pharmacokinetics after intravenous and intramuscular administration. *Antimicrob Agents Chemother* 14:829, 1978.
75. Francke EL, Appel GB, Neu HC: Pharmacokinetics of intravenous piperacillin in patients undergoing chronic hemodialysis. *Antimicrob Agents Chemother* 16:788, 1979.
76. Winston DJ, Murphy W, Young LS, et al: Piperacillin therapy for serious bacterial infections. *Am J Med* 69:255, 1980.
77. Wade JC, Schimpff SC, Newman KA, et al: Piperacillin or ticarcillin plus amikacin: A double blind prospective comparison of emperic antibiotic therapy for febrile granulocytopenic cancer patients. *Am J Med* 71:983, 1981.
78. Pancoast SJ, Prince AS, Francke EL, et al: Clinical evaluation of piperacillin for therapy of infection. *Arch Intern Med* 141:1447, 1981.
79. Prince AS, Neu HC: Use of piperacillin, a semisynthetic penicillin in the therapy of acute exacerbations of pulmonary disease in patients with cystic fibrosis. *J Pediatr* 97:148, 1980.
80. Neu HC: Mecillinam, a novel penicillanic acid derivative with unusual activity against gram-negative bacteria. *Antimicrob Agents Chemother* 9:793, 1976.
81. Neu HC: Mecillinam: An amdinocillin which acts synergistically with other β-lactam compounds. *J Antimicrob Chemother* 3(suppl B):43, 1977.
82. Neu HC, Srinivasan S, Francke EL, et al: Pharmacokinetics of amdinocillin and pivamdinocillin in normal volunteers. *Am J Med* 75(suppl 2A):60, 1983.
83. Demos CH, Green E: Review of clinical experience with amdinocillin monotherapy and comparative studies. *Am J Med* 75(suppl 2A):72, 1983.
84. King JW, Beam TR Jr, Neu HC, et al: Systemic infections treated with amdinocillin in combination with other beta-lactam antibiotics. *Am J Med* 75(suppl 2A):90, 1983.
85. Jules K, Neu HC: Antibacterial activity and β-lactamase stability of temocillin. *Antimicrob Agents Chemother* 22:453, 1982.

4

CEPHALOSPORINS

GERALD L. MANDELL

Most of the new antibiotics introduced for clinical use in recent years are cephalosporins. These agents are now the most prescribed of all antimicrobials and account for a large segment of the health care budget. It all started in 1945 when Professor Giuseppe Brotzu began searching for antibiotic-producing microorganisms. He hypothesized that the process of self-purification of water might be due in part to substances produced by certain organisms inhibiting other microbes. He isolated a fungus, *Cephalosporium acremonium,* from seawater near a sewage outlet in Kaglara, Sardinia, and found that this organism inhibited the growth of a variety of gram-positive and gram-negative bacteria. Broth cultures produced a filtrate that showed some antibacterial effect on infections in animals and later in patients.

Professor Brotzu sent a culture of his organism to Oxford in 1948, and attempts were made by several workers, led by Professor Edward P. Abraham, to isolate the active antibacterial factors. Several different antibiotic fractions were isolated from these broth cultures. These included cephalosporin C, which is the parent substance from which the first cephalosporins for clinical use were derived. In addition to its fairly broad range of antimicrobial activity, it had the interesting features of being relatively acid stable and resistant to penicillinase (1).

CHEMISTRY

The three active fermentation products of *Cephalosporium* were identified as cephalosporin C, cephalosporin N, and cephalosporin P. Cephalosporin N is

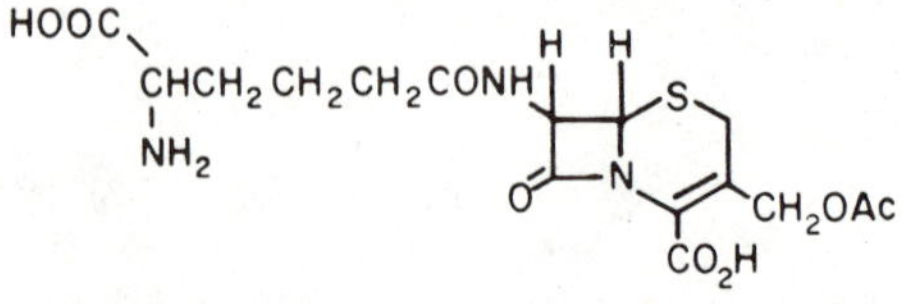

FIGURE 1. Structure of cephalosporin C.

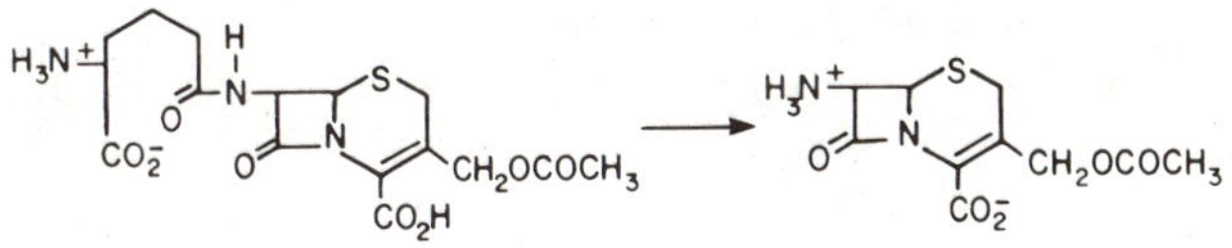

FIGURE 2. Preparation of 7-ACA from cephalosporin C.

actually a penicillin, with an aminocarboxybutyl side chain. Cephalosporin P is a steroid with a very narrow range of antibacterial activity. Cephalosporin C is the major product, and it is the basis for the new cephalosporins. Cephalosporin C resembles a penicillin since it has a β-lactam structure, but the five-member thiazolidine ring characteristic of the penicillins is replaced by a six-member dihydrothiazine ring (Fig. 1). Previous experience has shown that the potency of penicillins was improved by substitution of different groups at the 6-acylamido function adjacent to the β-lactam ring. Attempts were made to cleave the side chain off enzymatically, but these failed. Acid treatment, however, did hydrolyze cephalosporin C to 7-aminocephalosporanic acid (7-ACA) (Fig. 2). This compound has been subsequently modified with different side chains to create a whole family of cephalosporin antibiotics. It appears that modifications at position 7 of the 7-aminocephalosporanic acid nucleus are associated with alteration in antibacterial activity, and substitutions at position 3 of the dihydrothiazine ring are associated with changes in the pharmacokinetics and the metabolic parameters of the drug (Fig. 3) (2,3). Hepatic metabolism occurs at the 3-acetoxymethyl position. There has been an association made with certain adverse side effects such as disulfuram-like (Antabuse) reactions, and the potential for bleeding associated with the methylthiotetrazole group at position 3 of the dihydrothiazoladine ring (4). Molecules with a methoxy group in position 7 of the 7-aminocephalosporanic acid nucleus are called cephamycins.

MECHANISM OF ACTION

The mechanism of action of the β-lactam antibiotics could be explained with confidence and precision several years ago. It was thought that all β-lactam antibiotics had the same mechanism of action and that this was related to interference with cell wall structure. A brilliant series of experiments by a number

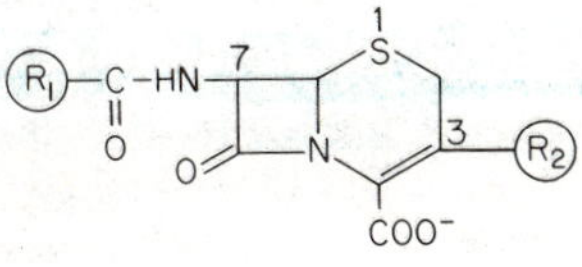

FIGURE 3. Basic structure of a cephalosporin.

of investigators identified the particular step in the cross-linking of the peptidoglycan polymer that was interfered with by the β-lactam antibiotics (5). It was thought that these weak or defective cell walls then allowed for growth of bizarre bacterial forms with subsequent lysis and death of bacterial cells.

More recent information suggests that this explanation of the mechanism of action of the β-lactam antibiotics appears to be oversimplified. Some of the penicillins and cephalosporins have clearly different morphologic effects on bacterial cells. Certain β-lactam antibiotics produce lytic effects such as those seen with cephalothin or benzyl penicillin on *Staphylococcus aureus.* Long filamentous forms are noted when cephalexin interacts with *Escherchia coli,* and amdinocillin (mecillinam) tends to produce osmotically fragile round forms.

Several β-lactam antibiotic binding proteins have been isolated from bacterial cells. These tend to be associated with the cell membrane and bind tightly to β-lactam antibiotics. There are at least seven binding sites in bacteria; it is thought that these binding sites are enzymes, probably transpeptidases and carboxypeptidases, that are important for the biosynthesis of the peptidoglycan component of bacterial cell walls. The binding pattern varies with different antibiotics. When β-lactam antibiotics bind to these proteins, a complex series of events is initiated. These involve inhibition of protein synthesis and the loss from the cell of an inhibitor of an enzyme that functions as an autolysin. Bacterial cells containing the autolysins are often lysed by the activity of the β-lactam antibiotics. Bacterial cells not containing the autolysin may develop bizarre forms, and their growth may be only inhibited. Thus the β-lactam exhibits a bacteristatic effect rather than a bactericidal effect.

Some of the newer concepts of the mechanism of action of the β-lactam antibiotics may be of clinical importance. In the past it was thought that there would be no reason to combine β-lactam antibiotics, since it was thought that they all worked in an identical fashion and thus true synergism would not be seen. However, since these agents may bind to different proteins in the bacterial cell, it may be feasible to use two (or even more) β-lactam antibiotics together to achieve a synergistic effect (6).

CLASSIFICATION

Cephalosporins may be classified by their chemical structure, major differences in clinical pharmacology, β-lactamase resistance, or their antibacterial spectrum. The well-accepted generations scheme is a somewhat arbitrary but useful way to classify these agents (Table 1). *Generations* are based on general features of antimicrobial activity. The first-generation cephalosporins, characterized by cephalothin and cefazolin, have good gram-positive activity and relatively modest gram-negative activity. Most gram-positive cocci (with the exception of enterococci, methicillin-resistant *S. aureus,* and *Staphylococcus epidermidis*) are suscep-

TABLE 1. Selected Cephalosporins, Generic, and Proprietary Names (U.S.), and Serum Half-Life

Generic Name	*Proprietary Name*	*Adult Dose for Serious Infection*	*Serum Half-Life (H)*
First Generation			
Cefadroxil	Duricef, Ultracef	1 g q12h p.o	1.5
Cefazolin	Ancef, Kefzol	2 g q8h	1.5
Cephalexin	Keflex	1 g q6h p.o	1.3
Cephalothin	Keflin	2 g q4h	0.6
Cephapirin	Cefadyl	2 g q4h	0.6
Cephaloridine		1 g q6h	1.3
Cephradine	Velosef, Anspor	2 g q6h	1.3
		1 g q6h p.o	1.3
Second generation			
Cefaclor	Ceclor	1 g q8h p.o	0.8
Cefamandole	Mandol	2 g q4h	0.8
Cefmetazole		2 g q4h	0.8
Cefonacid	Monicid	2 g q24h	4.4
Ceforanide	Precef	1 g q12h	3.0
Cefotiam		2 g q4h	0.8
Cefoxitin	Mefoxin	2 g q4h	0.8
Cefuroxime	Zinacef	3 g q8h	1.5
Third generation			
Cefbuperazone			1.6
Cefmenoxime	Cefmax	2 g q4h	1.0
Cefotaxime	Claforan	2 g q4h	1.1
Cefotetan		2 g q12h	4.0
Ceftizoxime	Cefizox	4 g q8h	1.7
Ceftriaxone	Rocephin	1 g q12h	8.0
Moxalactam	Moxam	4 g q8h	1.0
Third generation with good antipseudomonas activity			
Cefoperazone	Cefobid	3 g q6h	1.9
Cefpiramide		2 g q12h	4.4
Cefsulodin	Cefomonil	3 g q6h	1.8
Ceftazadime	Fortaz	2 g q8h	4.4

tible. Activity against *E. coli, Klebsiella pneumoniae,* and *Proteus mirabilis* is good.

The second-generation cephalosporins have somewhat increased activity against gram-negative organisms but are much less active than the third-generation agents.

Third-generation cephalosporins are generally less active than first-generation cephalosporins against gram-positive cocci but are much more active against the Enterobacteriaceae, including penicillinase-producing strains. A subset of the third-generation agents is also active against *Pseudomonas aeruginosa* (Table 2) (7–10).

TABLE 2. In Vitro Activities of Selected Cephalosporins[a]

	S. aureus	*S. epidermidis*	*H. influenzae*	*S. pyogenes*	*E. coli*	*K. pneumoniae*	*S. marcesens*	*P. aeruginosa*	*B. fragilis*
First generation									
Cefazolin	1.0	0.8	10	0.1	5.0	6.0	>100	>100	>100
Cephalothin	1.0	0.5	10	0.1	5.0	32	>100	>100	>100
Second generation									
Cefamandole	1.0	2.0	1.0	0.06	4.0	8.0	>100	>100	>100
Cefoxitin	3.0	12.5	6.0	0.7	8.0	5.0	>100	>100	16
Cefotiam	1.0	1.6	2.0	0.1	0.4	0.4	>100	>100	>100
Cefuroxime	2.0	1.0	2.0	0.06	4.0	4.0	>100	>100	>100
Ceforanide	4.0	4.0	4.0	0.05	2.0	2.0	>100	>100	>32
Third generation									
Cefotaxime	3.0	6.3	0.01	0.05	0.6	0.6	10	>100	>100
Moxalactam	16	16	0.1	2.0	0.5	0.5	10	64	32
Ceftizoxime	1.0	16	0.03	0.05	.25	0.1	4.0	>100	50
Ceftriaxone	6.0	>100	0.01	0.03	1.0	0.1	16	>100	>100
Cefmenoxime	2.0	4.0	0.01	.10	.10	0.8	6.0	28	32
Third generation with good antipseudomonas activity									
Cefoperazone	4.0	8.0	0.03	0.4	40	2.0	26	16	>100
Ceftazidime	12	32	0.06	0.3	0.5	0.7	1.0	4	>100
Cefsulodin	6.0	2.0	24	2.0	>64	>64	>100	7	>100

SOURCE: Values are approximations and are derived from Refs. 3, 7, 10, 78–80.

[a] Minimum Inhibitory Concentration (MIC) for 90% of strains.

MECHANISM OF BACTERIAL RESISTANCE TO THE CEPHALOSPORINS

One reason for bacterial resistance to the cephalosporins may be related to inability of the antibiotic to reach the site of the binding protein. A second possible explanation for resistance could be alterations in antibiotic binding proteins such that binding does not take place. Bacteria also have the ability to produce enzymes—β-lactamases (or cephalosporinases) that can disrupt the β-lactam ring and render the cephalosporin inactive.

Gram-negative cell walls appear to be a potential barrier to the penetration of the β-lactam antibiotics. Cell wall deficient mutants seem to be especially susceptible to β-lactam antibiotics. In addition, β-lactam antibiotics more avidly inhibit peptidoglycan synthesis in cell fractions than in intact bacteria. Gram-positive bacteria have relatively exposed sites of peptidoglycan synthesis, and thus a barrier effect is unlikely with these organisms.

If the antibiotic binds to only one binding site and therefore inactivates only one enzyme, it is possible that a mutation in the gene coding for that enzyme (binding site) may lead to resistance. This is probably not a common cause of resistance to the cephalosporins since most of these agents appear to bind to several different sites. Bacteria may destroy cephalosporins by hydrolysis of the β-lactam ring. If this ring is broken, the molecule loses its antibiotic activity. Many gram-positive organisms release relatively large amounts of β-lactamase into the surrounding medium. Although gram-negative organisms seem to produce less β-lactamase, the location of their β-lactamase in the periplasmic space may make this enzyme more effective in destroying cephalosporins as they attempt to reach their target on the inner membrane (11).

The cephalosporins have variable susceptibility to β-lactamase. Cephaloridine is the most sensitive to both gram-positive and gram-negative β-lactamases, and thus more antibiotic is hydrolyzed by the enzyme. Cefazolin is more susceptible to hydrolysis by β-lactamases from *S. aureus* than is cephalothin (12). Cefoxitin, cefuroxime, and the third-generation cephalosporins are the most resistant to hydrolysis by the β-lactamases produced by gram-negative organisms (13). However, the correlation between antimicrobial activity and β-lactamase resistance is not linear. Some bacterial strains that fail to hydrolyze the antibiotics are nevertheless resistant. Conversely, some bacteria with β-lactamases that can destroy cephalosporins are susceptible to the cephalosporins (14). The cephalosporins can protect a penicillin from hydrolysis by β-lactamases by binding to these enzymes in vitro.

Certain bacterial strains may resist the bactericidal activities of the penicillins and the cephalosporins, although the growth of these organisms is inhibited. This phenomenon has been called tolerance. Tolerance has been shown in some cases to be related to the deficiency of autolytic enzymes in the cells, thus the lethal action of the β-lactam antibiotic is converted to a bacteriostatic action. This may be important in certain patients with endocarditis.

Although most of the third-generation cephalosporins are relatively resistant to hydrolysis by bacterial β-lactamases, there have been reports of development of resistance to the third-generation cephalosporins by *Enterobacter, Serratia,* and *Pseudomonas* species (13). Sanders and Sanders (15) have suggested that the derepression of β-lactamase enzymes in these organisms has resulted in the production of β-lactamases that have a high affinity for the antibiotics although they cannot hydrolyze them. They propose that the third-generation cephalosporins are tightly bound to the β-lactamases and thus are prevented from binding to the target penicillin binding proteins (15). This hypothesis is unproven, but certain gram-negative rods have developed resistance to multiple β-lactam agents during therapy with third-generation cephalosporins, thus the potential for an increase in the number of these multiple-resistant strains exists.

It is important to remember that none of the available (or even investigational) cephalosporins has reliable activity or effectiveness against the following organisms: penicillin-resistant *Streptococcus pneumoniae,* methicillin-resistant *S. aureus,* methicillin-resistant *S. epidermidis, Streptococcus faecalis, Listeria monocytogenes, Legionella pneumophila, Legionella micdadei, Clostridium difficile, Pseudomonas maltophilia, Pseudomonas putida, Campylobacter jejuni,* and, of course, *Candida albicans.*

PHARMACOLOGY

The details of pharmacology will be discussed under each drug. Cephalexin, cephradine, cefaclor, and cefadroxil are all absorbed by mouth.

Cephalothin and cephapirin are painful after intramuscular injection and thus are usually restricted to intravenous administration. Most of the others can be administered intramuscularly or intravenously.

Several cephalosporins penetrate into cerebrospinal fluid in sufficient amounts to be useful for treating meningitis. These include cefuroxime, moxalactam, cefotaxime, ceftriaxone, and cefoperazone. All the cephalosporins except cefoperazone (which is primarily excreted in the bile) are primarily excreted by the renal route; therefore, doses should be altered in patients with renal insufficiency. Probenecid slows excretion of cephalosporins.

Agents with the acetyl group at the R2 position, including cephalothin, cephapirin, and cefotaxime (Figs. 4,5) undergo in vivo metabolism to the desacetyl forms, which have less biologic activity than the parent compounds. The desacetyl form is also excreted by the kidneys. None of the other cephalosporins appears to undergo appreciable degradation.

Cephalosporins are found in high concentrations across the placenta and in synovial (16) and pericardial fluid. Penetration into the aqueous humor of the eye after the systemic administration is relatively good for third-generation cephalosporins, but vitreous penetration is poor. There is some evidence that therapeutic levels for eye infections due to gram-positive and certain gram-negative organisms can be achieved after systemic administration. Bile levels are usually high, with those after cefoperazone administration being the highest.

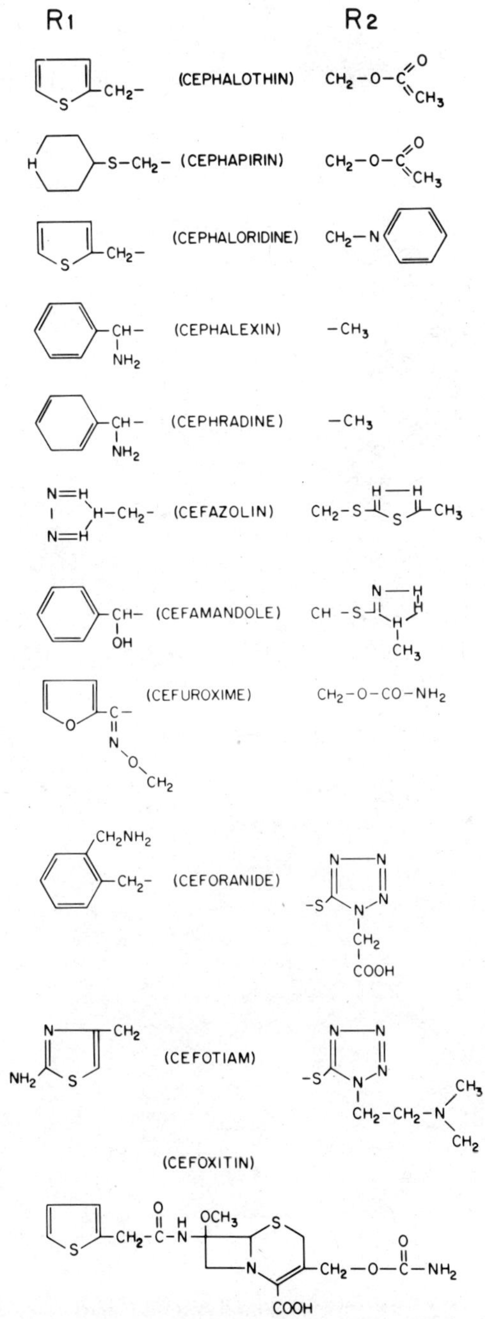

FIGURE 4. Structures of selected first- and second-generation cephalosporins (see Fig. 3).

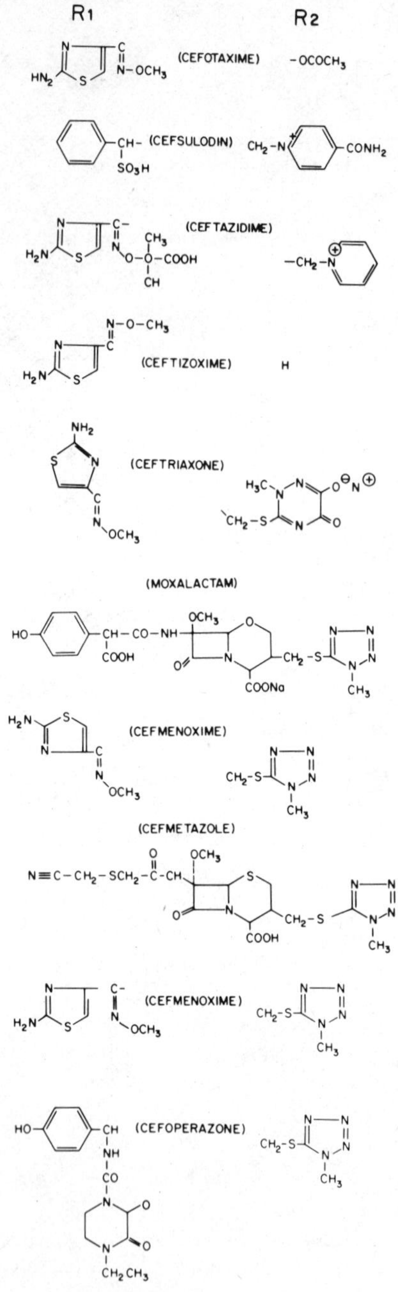

FIGURE 5. Structures of selected third-generation cephalosporins (see Fig. 3).

ADVERSE REACTIONS

The cephalosporins are relatively safe drugs. Thrombophlebitis occurs with intravenous administration of all the cephalosporins. There are no conclusive data indicating significant differences (17,18).

Hypersensitivity reactions related to the cephalosporins are the most common systemic side effects (19). There is no evidence that any one of the cephalosporins is more likely to cause hypersensitivity reactions than any of the others. The reactions appear to be identical to those caused by the penicillins, and this may be related to the shared β-lactam structure of both groups of antibiotics. Immediate reactions of anaphylaxis, bronchospasm, and urticaria have been reported. More commonly, patients develop maculopapular rash, usually after several days of therapy. Patients may or may not have fever and eosinophilia. Fever and lymphadenopathy have been associated with cephalosporin administration without other manifestations of allergic phenomena (20).

Because of the similarity in structure of the penicillins and cephalosporins, it is felt that patients who are allergic to the penicillins may manifest cross-reacting allergy when a cephalosporin is administered. Immunologic studies have found cross-reactivity in as many as 20 percent of penicillin-allergic patients (21), but clinical reports seem to demonstrate a lower range (5–10 percent) of cephalosporin reactions in penicillin-allergic patients. There are no cephalosporin skin tests that can reliably predict whether or not a patient will show an allergic reaction to the cephalosporins (22).

It appears that patients with a history of a mild or temporally distant penicillin reaction are at low risk of developing a rash or other allergic reaction on the administration of a cephalosporin. However, patients who have had a recent severe immediate reaction should be given a cephalosporin with great caution, if at all. A positive Coombs reaction appears frequently in patients receiving large doses of cephalosporin drugs. Hemolysis is not usually associated with this phenomenon, although it has been reported. Rare cases of bone marrow depression characterized by granulocytopenia have been reported.

The cephalosporins have been implicated as potentially nephrotoxic agents, although they are not nearly as toxic to the kidney as are the aminoglycosides or the polymyxins (23). Renal tubular necrosis has been described with cephaloridine in doses greater than 4 g/day. Other cephalosporins are much less toxic and, in recommended doses, rarely produce significant renal toxicity when used by themselves. High doses of cephalothin have produced acute tubular necrosis in certain cases, and usual doses (8–12 g/day) have been nephrotoxic in patients with preexisting renal disease (24). There is fairly good evidence that the combination of cephalothin plus gentamicin or tobramycin is synergistically nephrotoxic (25). Interstitial nephritis, identical to that occuring during therapy with semisynthetic penicillins, may result from cephalosporin therapy. This is especially marked in patients over 60 years of age. Diarrhea has been reported with cephalosporin administration and may be more frequent with cefoperazone, perhaps because of its greater biliary excretion. Alcohol intolerance (a disulfuram-like reaction) has been noted with cefamandole, moxalactam, and cefoperazone. Serious bleeding related to hypoprothrombinemia, thrombocytopenia, and/or platelet dysfunction has been reported with several β-lactam agents (26). This appears to be a particular problem with certain patients (elderly, poorly nourished, those with renal insufficiency) receiving moxalactam.

MODIFICATION OF DOSE WITH RENAL INSUFFICIENCY

The cephalosporins, although largely excreted by the kidney, require only moderate dose reduction in patients with renal insufficiency (see Chapter 20). An exception is cephaloridine, which should be avoided because of its nephrotoxic potential.

CLINICAL USES

The cephalosporins are widely used antibiotics. Clinical studies have shown them to be effective as prophylactic agents and as therapy. In the past it was stated that cephalosporins were not drugs of first choice for any indication. However, they are effective and well tolerated, and indications appear to be changing with the rapid development of new second- and third-generation agents (27,28). Cephalosporins, either with or without aminoglycosides, have been considered to be the drugs of choice for serious *Klebsiella* infections. Surgical prophylaxis is another area in which cephalosporins have found wide use. There are several indications for which first-generation cephalosporins have been shown to be safe and effective prophylaxis. The third-generation cephalosporins are presently the drugs of choice for gram-negative enteric rod meningitis because of their in vitro activity, good cerebrospinal fluid penetration, and record of clinical successes. Therapeutic trials are in progress evaluating the role of these agents in community-acquired meningitis, and it appears that some second- or third-generation cephalosporins may be equivalent to two-drug (ampicillin plus chloramphenicol) therapy.

Cephalosporins are still useful as alternatives to penicillins in a variety of infections in patients who cannot tolerate penicillins. These include streptococcal and staphylococcal infections. The role of the third-generation cephalosporins in the treatment of serious gram-negative rod infections outside of the central nervous system is unclear. Those relatively uncommon organisms that are resistant to other agents frequently will be sensitive to third-generation cephalosporins, and clearly these drugs should be used in those situations. In other cases, organisms may be sensitive to a variety of antibiotics, but third-generation cephalosporins may be the most active in vitro. Whether this increased in vitro activity translates to increased clinical success is unclear, but some infectious disease physicians use the highly active third-generation cephalosporins for serious infections caused by gram-negative organisms.

Anaerobic infections are often treated with combinations of antibiotics, since the infections are usually caused by both aerobic and anaerobic organisms. Cefoxitin and several of the third-generation cephalosporins have good antianaerobic activity and are useful alternatives to combination therapy under certain conditions. Penicillinase-producing gonococcal infections can be treated effectively with several of the penicillinase-resistant second- or third-generation cephalosporins. The spectrum of activity of some of the second- or third-generation cephalosporins appears to be excellent for the treatment of community-acquired pneumonia, that is, that caused by pneumococci, *Hemophilus influenzae* (including β-lactamase positive strains), or staphylococci.

Nosocomial infections are frequently caused by organisms resistant to many of the commonly used agents, such as first-generation cephalosporins, ampicillin, and some of the aminoglycosides. Third-generation cephalosporins have been useful additions to therapy in these situations. Patients who are severely neutropenic have been treated successfully with either third-generation cephalosporins plus aminoglycosides or a third-generation cephalosporin (e.g., ceftazadime) that is active against *Pseudomonas* without aminoglycosides.

The role of cephalosporins in therapy must be modified as experience with these agents is obtained and as new agents are developed and tested (29).

SPECIFIC AGENTS (Table 1)

First-Generation Cephalosporins

Cephalothin (Keflin) is not well absorbed orally and is available only in parenteral form. Because of pain on intramuscular injection, it is rarely administered via that route. After intravenous use, cephalothin has a large volume of distribution indicating wide dispersal throughout body tissues and fluids. Peak serum levels after 1 g intramuscularly are about 20 μg/ml. Cephalothin has a short half-life (30–40 minutes) and is actively metabolized in addition to being excreted. From 20 to 30 percent of cephalothin is excreted as the desacetyl metabolite (30,31). Unmetabolized active cephalothin does not appreciably enter the cerebrospinal fluid, and thus this drug should not be used for the treatment of meningitis. Meningitis due to cephalothin-sensitive organisms has been reported to have developed while cephalothin was being administered. Since cephalothin is the cephalosporin most impervious to attack by staphylococcal β-lactamase, some authorities consider it to be the cephalosporin of choice in severe staphylococcal infections such as endocarditis.

Cephapirin (Cefadyl) is very similar to cephalothin. Like cephalothin it is painful after intramuscular injection. Also like cephalothin, it is metabolized as the desacetyl derivative, which is about half as active as the parent compound. The half-life and excretion pattern of cephapirin are like that of cephalothin (32).

Cephaloridine is the most nephrotoxic of the available cephalosporins, and although toxicity can be avoided with care, the use of this compound is not recommended (33).

The antibacterial spectrum of *cefazolin* (Ancef and Kefzol) is similar to cephalothin. However, cefazolin is more active against *E. coli* and *Klebsiella* species (34). Cefazolin is somewhat more sensitive to staphylococcal penicillinase than is cephalothin (35,36). Serum levels of cefazolin are higher after intramuscular (64 μg/ml after 1 g) and intravenous injections than are levels of either cephaloridine or cephalothin. This is related in part to a smaller volume of distribution. The half-life is also appreciably longer, being 1.8 hours as compared with 0.5 hour for cephalothin (37). The renal clearance of cefazolin is lower than that of cephalothin. This is probably related to the fact that cefazolin is excreted by glomerular filtration, whereas cephalothin is also excreted by the kidney tubule. Cefazolin is highly (about 80 percent) protein bound. Cefazolin is relatively well tolerated after intramuscular or intravenous injection. It is the usually preferred first-generation cephalosporin since it can be administered less frequently because of its longer half-life (38).

Cephradine (Anspor—oral, Velosef—oral and parenteral) is similar in structure to cephalexin, and its in vitro activity is almost identical. Cephradine is unmetabolized and after rapid oral absorption is excreted unchanged in the urine. Cephradine can be administered intramuscularly or intravenously. When administered by mouth the clinical pharmacology of cephradine is very much like that of cephalexin, and some authorities feel that these two drugs can be used interchangeably. Because cephradine is so well absorbed, the serum levels after an oral or intramuscular dose are nearly equivalent (about 10–18 μg/ml after 0.5 g orally or intramuscularly). The peak serum level for the oral dose is actually higher, but the area under the curve for both routes of administration is equivalent (39).

Cefadroxil monohydrate (Duricef, Ultracef) is the parahydroxy analogue of cephalexin. Serum and urine concentrations of cefadroxil are somewhat more sustained than those noted with cephalexin. The drug may be used once or twice a day for treatment of urinary tract infections. In vitro activity is similar to that of cephalexin (40).

Cephalexin (Keflex) is a cephalosporin for oral use that has the same antibacterial spectrum as other first-generation cephalosporins. It is somewhat less active, however, against penicillinase-producing staphylococci. Oral cephalexin therapy results in peak serum levels of 16 μg/ml after 0.5 g by mouth, which are adequate for the inhibition of many cephalosporin-sensitive gram-positive and gram-negative pathogens. The drug is unmetabolized, and more than 90 percent is excreted in the urine (41).

Second-Generation Cephalosporins

Cefamandole (Mandol) is more active than the first-generation cephalosporins against certain species of gram-negative organisms. This is especially evident for *H. influenzae* (42), *Enterobacter* species, indole-positive *Proteus* species, *E. coli,* and *Klebsiella* species (43). Heavy bacterial inocula show decreased susceptibility, and this appears to be related to destruction of the antibiotic by β-lactamase. Most gram-positive cocci are susceptible to cefamandole. The half-life is 32 minutes, and the drug is excreted unchanged in the urine. Serum levels are 20–36 μg/ml after a 1 g intramuscular dose (44,45).

Cefoxitin (Mefoxin) is a cefamycin produced by *Streptomyces lactamdurans.* It is highly resistant to β-lactamases produced by gram-negative rods (46). This antibiotic is more active than cephalothin against certain gram-negative organisms, although it is less active than cefamandole against *Enterobacter* species and *H. influenzae.* It is also less active than both cefamandole and the older cephalosporins against gram-positive bacteria. Cefoxitin is more active than other first- or second-generation agents against anaerobes, especially *Bacteroides fragilis.* Its activity is similar to that of moxalactam and better than other third-generation cephalosporins. After a 1-g intramuscular dose serum levels are about 22 μg/ml. The half-life is about 50 minutes. Cefoxitin's special role seems to be for treatment of certain anaerobic and mixed aerobic–anaerobic infections such as pelvic inflammatory disease and lung abscess (47–49). It is an effective agent for gonorrhea caused by penicillinase-producing organisms (50).

Cefaclor (Ceclor) is a cephalosporin for oral administration. The serum levels after an oral dose are about 50 percent of those achieved after equivalent oral doses of cephalexin. However, cefaclor is more active against gram-negative bacilli. This may be especially important for *H. influenzae, E. coli,* and *P. mirabilis,* although some β-lactamase-producing strains of *H. influenzae* may be resistant (51).

Ceforanide (Precef) is similar in structure and antimicrobial activity to cefamandole. However, it is less active against strains of *H. influenzae.* Peak plasma concentrations after 1 g given intramuscularly are approximately 65 μg/ml. Ninety percent of a dose is excreted unchanged in the urine, and the half-life is approximately 3 hours. The drug has been effective when administered every 12 hours (52).

Cefonacid (Monicid) has similar in vitro activity to cefamandole. The plasma half-life of the drug is about 4½ hours, and one dose a day has been effective for certain infections caused by susceptible organisms (53).

Cefuroxime (Zinacef) is very similar to cefamandole in structure and in vitro antibacterial activity (54). It is relatively more stable to β-lactamases than is cefamandole, its serum half-life is longer (1.5 vs. 0.5 hours), and the drug can be given every 8 hours. Cerebrospinal fluid penetration is about 10 percent, and the drug is effective for meningitis due to *H. influenzae* (including ampicillin-resistant strains), *Neisseria meningitidis,* and *S. pneumoniae* (55).

Cefotiam is a second-generation cephalosporin with a half-life of 0.8 hour and in vitro activity similar to cefamandole (56).

Cefmetazole is a second-generation agent with poor activity against *Enterobacter* species but is otherwise similar to cefoxitin (57).

Third-Generation Cephalosporins

Cefotaxime sodium (Claforan) was the first of the third-generation cephalosporins to become available in the United States. Cefotaxime is highly resistant to bacterial β-lactamases and has good activity against gram-positive organisms, with the exception of enterococci and *L. monocytogenes,* and to gram-negative aerobic organisms, with the exception of all strains of *Pseudomonas.* Activity against *B. fragilis* is poor compared to agents such as clindamycin and metronidazole (58). Cefotaxime has a serum half-life of about 1 hour, and for serious infections doses should be administered every 4–6 hours. The drug is metabolized in vivo to desacetyl cefotaxime, and this metabolite is less active than the parent compound. Cefotaxime has been effective therapy for gram-negative meningitis (59,60). It is generally well tolerated and has the typical cephalosporin spectrum of adverse reactions (61).

Moxalactam (Moxam) has a unique structure (designated oxa-β-lactam), which is created by the substitution of an oxygen for the sulfur atom in the six-membered ring of the cephem nucleus (see Fig. 5). Moxalactam has the broad antimicrobial activity characteristic of the third-generation cephalosporins (62). In comparison to cefotaxime, it is less active against gram-positive organisms including streptococci and staphylococci. It is somewhat less active against *H. influenzae* and has very similar activity against most of the *Enterobacteraceae.* It is slightly more active against *Pseudomonas* and appreciably more active against *B. fragilis* than is cefotaxime. Moxalactam has a serum half-life of approximately 2 hours, and the drug is excreted in the urine unmetabolized (63). Clinically significant bleeding has been described with moxalactam administration (64), and it appears that moxalactam can interfere with hemostasis through either hypoprothrombinemia, platelet dysfunction, or more rarely, immune-mediated thrombocytopenia. It is recommended by the U.S. Food and Drug Administration that patients who receive moxalactam be given 10 mg of vitamin K per week prophylactically. Since platelet dysfunction is dose related, it is suggested that bleeding times be monitored in patients (with normal renal function) who receive more than 4 g of moxalactam per day for more than 3 days.

Ceftizoxime (Cefizox) has an in vitro spectrum of activity very similar to that of cefotaxime. The serum half-life is somewhat longer, 1.7 hours, and thus the drug can be administered every 8 hours for serious infections. Ceftizoxime is not metabolized and is excreted unchanged in the urine. Adverse reactions appear to follow the usual cephalosporin pattern. Ceftizoxime protein binding is low, but the clinical significance of that observation is unknown (65).

Ceftriaxone (Rocephin) has in vitro activity very similar to that of ceftizoxime and cefotaxime. A serum half-life of about 8 hours is its outstanding feature. Twice daily therapy has been effective for patients with meningitis (66), and once daily therapy has been effective for patients with other infections (67). Sixty percent of the drug can be recovered from the urine, and about 40 percent appears to be eliminated by biliary secretion. It has been effective as single-dose therapy (125 mg) for gonorrhea caused by penicillinase-negative or penicillinase-producing organisms (68,69).

Cefotetan is a 7-α-methoxy cephalosporin (a cephamycin). Cefotetan has in vitro activity against gram-negative bacilli similar to that of cefotaxime and moxalactam; however, it is less active against *Enterobacter aerogenes* and has no useful activity against *Pseudomonas*. Gram-positive activity is similar to moxalactam, but cefotetan is significantly less active against the pneumococcus. Its activity against anaerobes is similar to that of cefotaxime (70). The half-life is 3.3 hours (71).

Cefbuperazone is a third-generation agent that is a cephamycin. Activity is similar to moxalactam, and half-life is about 100 minutes.

Cefmenoxime (Cefmax) has a spectrum of in vitro activity very similar to that of cefotaxime. Half-life is 1 hour.

Third-Generation Cephalosporins with Good Antipseudomonas Activity

Cefoperazone (Cefobid) is less active than cefotaxime against gram-positive organisms and is less active than cefotaxime or moxalactam against many species of gram-negative organisms. However, it is more active than both of these agents against *P. aeruginosa*. Activity against *B. fragilis* is similar to that of cefotaxime. Only 25 percent of a dose of cefoperazone can be recovered from the urine, and most of the drug is eliminated by biliary excretion. The serum half-life is about 2 hours. Cefoperazone bile levels are higher than that achieved with any other cephalosporin. Blood levels are higher than those found with cefotaxime by about 2 or 3 times. The dose does not have to be altered in renal insufficiency, but hepatic dysfunction or biliary obstruction affects clearance. Cefoperazone can cause bleeding due to hypoprothrombinemia, which can be reversed by administration of vitamin K. A disulfiram-like (Antabuse) reaction has been reported in patients drinking alcohol while taking cefoperazone. Cefoperazone is slightly less stable to β-lactamases than are the cefotaxime-like or 7-methoxycephem drugs (72).

Ceftazidime (Fortaz) is about half as active by weight against gram-positive organisms as is cefotaxime. Its activity against the *Enterobacteriaceae* is very similar, but its major distinguishing feature is good activity against *Pseudomonas* with a minimum inhibitory concentration (MIC) 90 of about 8 μg/ml. Ceftazidime has poor activity against *B. fragilis* (73). The serum half-life is 1.8 hours, and the drug is not metabolized. Ceftazidime was found to be more active in vitro against *Pseudomonas* than was cefsulodin, cefoperazone, or piperacillin (74,75).

Cefpiramide is a third-generation agent with good activity against pseudomonas and gram-positive organisms (76). The half-life is about 4 hours.

Cefsulodin (Cefomonil) has good anti-*Pseudomonas* and modest antistaphylococcal activity but is relatively inactive against most other organisms (77).

REFERENCES

1. Abraham EP, Loder PB: Cephalosporin C, in Flynn EH (ed): *Cephalosporins and Penicillins*. New York, Academic Press, 1972, p 2.

2. Huber FM, Chauvette RR, Jackson BG: Preparative methods for 7-aminocephalosporanic acid and 6-aminopenicillanic acid, in Flynn EH (ed): *Cephalosporins and Penicillins.* New York, Academic Press, 1972, p 27.
3. Neu HC: Structure-activity relations of new beta-lactam compounds and in vitro activity against common bacteria. *Rev Infect Dis* 5(suppl 2):S319, 1983.
4. Neu HC: The new beta-lactamase-stable cephalosporins. *Ann Intern Med* 97:408, 1982.
5. Strominger JL: How penicillin kills bacteria: A short history, in Schlessinger D (ed): *Microbiology 1977.* Washington, DC, ASM Publications, 1977, p 177.
6. Tomasz A: Penicillin-binding proteins in bacteria. *Ann Intern Med* 96:502, 1982.
7. Neu HC: The in vitro activity, human pharmacology, and clinical effectiveness of new beta-lactam antibiotics. *Annu Rev Pharmacol Toxicol* 22:599, 1982.
8. Schumacher GE: Pharmacokinetic and microbiologic evaluation of dosage regimens for newer cephalosporins and penicillins. *Clin Pharm* 2:448, 1983.
9. Garzone P, Lyon J, Yu VL: Third-generation and investigational cephalosporins: I. Structure-activity relationships and pharmacokinetic review. *Drug Intell Clin Pharm* 17:507, 1983.
10. Garzone P, Lyon J, Yu VL: Third-generation and investigational cephalosporins: II. Microbiologic review and clinical summaries. *Drug Intell Clin Pharm* 17:615, 1983.
11. Richmond MH, Sykes RB: The β-lactamases of gram-negative bacteria and their possible physiological role. *Adv Microb Physiol* 9:31, 1973.
12. Farrar WE, Jr, O'Dell NM: Comparative beta-lactamase resistance and antistaphylococcal activities of parenterally and orally administered cephalosporins. *J Infect Dis* 137:490, 1978.
13. Sykes RB, Bush K: Interaction of new cephalosporins with beta-lactamases and beta lactamase-producing gram-negative bacilli. *Rev Infect Dis* 5(suppl 5):S356, 1983.
14. Farrar WE, Krause JM: Relationship between β-lactamase activity and resistance of enterobacter to cephalothin. *Infect Immun* 2:610, 1970.
15. Sanders CC, Sanders EW: Emergence of resistance during therapy with the newer beta-lactam antibiotics: Role of inducible beta-lactamases and implications for the future. *Rev Infect Dis* 5(4):639, 1983.
16. Nelson JD: Antibiotic concentration in septic joint effusion. *N Engl J Med* 284:349, 1971.
17. Berger S, Ernest E, Barza M: Comparative incidence of phlebitis due to buffered cephalothin, cephapirin and cefamandole. *Antimicrob Agents Chemother* 9:575, 1976.
18. Carrizosa J, Levison ME, Kaye D: Double-blind controlled comparison of phlebitis produced by cephapirin and cephalothin. *Antimicrob Agents Chemother* 3:306, 1973.
19. Petz LD: Immunologic cross-reactivity between penicillins and cephalosporins: A review. *J Infect Dis* 137(suppl):S74, 1978.
20. Sanders WE, Johnson JE, Taggart JG. Adverse reactions to cephalothin and cephapirin. *N Engl J Med* 290:424, 1974.
21. Levine B: Antigenicity and cross reactivity of penicillins and cephalosporins. *J Infect Dis* 128(suppl):S364, 1973.
22. Saxon A: Immediate hypersensitivity reactions to beta-lactam antibiotics. *Rev Infect Dis* 5(suppl 2):S368, 1983.
23. Barza M: The nephrotoxicity of cephalosporins: An overview. *J Infect Dis* 137(suppl):S60, 1978.
24. Pasternack DP, Stephens BG: Reversible nephrotoxicity associated with cephalothin therapy. *Arch Intern Med* 135:599, 1975.
25. Wade JC, Petty BG, Conrad G, et al: Cephalothin plus an aminoglyside is more nephrotoxic than methicillin plus an aminoglycoside. *Lancet* 2:604, 1978.
26. Bank NU, Kammer RB: Hematologic complications associated with beta-lactam antibiotics. *Rev Infect Dis* 5(suppl 2):S380, 1983.
27. Brooks GF, Barriere SL: Clinical use of the new beta-lactam antimicrobial drugs. *Ann Intern Med* 98:530, 1983.
28. Neu HC: Clinical uses of cephalosporins. *Lancet* 252, 1982.
29. Kunin CM: Beta-lactam efficacy: Introduction. *Rev Infect Dis* 5(suppl 2):S317, 1983.
30. Chang TW, Weinstein L: In vitro biological activity of cephalothin. *J Bacteriol* 85:1022, 1963.

31. Klein JO, Eickhoff TC, Tilles JG, et al: Cephalothin: Activity in vitro, absorption and excretion in normal subjects and clinical observations in 40 patients. *Am J Med Sci* 248:640, 1964.
32. Renzini G, Ravagnan G, Oliva B: In vitro and in vivo microbiological evaluation of cephapirin, a new antibiotic. *Chemotherapy* 21:289, 1975.
33. Mandell GL: Cephaloridine. *Ann Intern Med* 79:561, 1973.
34. Sabath LD, Wilcox C, Garner C, et al: In vitro activity of cefazolin against recent clinical bacterial isolates. *J Infect Dis* 128(suppl):S320, 1973.
35. Regamey C, Libke RD, Engelking ER, et al: Inactivation of cefazolin, cephaloridine, and cephalothin by methicillin-sensitive and methicillin-resistant strains of *Staphylococcus aureus. J Infect Dis* 131:291, 1975.
36. Fong IW, Engelking ER, Kirby WMM: Relative inactivation by *Staphylococcus aureus* of eight cephalosporin antibiotics. *Antimicrob Agents Chemother* 9:939, 1976.
37. Bergeron MG, Brusch JL, Barza M, et al: Bactericidal activity and pharmacology of cefazolin. *Antimicrob Agents Chemother* 4:396, 1973.
38. Quintiliani R, Nightingale CH: Cefazolin: Diagnosis and treatment. *Ann Intern Med* 89:650, 1978.
39. Neiss E: Cephradine: Summary of preclinical studies and clinical pharmacology. *J Irish Med Assoc* 66(suppl):1, 1973.
40. Hartstein AI, Patrick KE, Jones SR, et al: Comparison of pharmacological and antimicrobial properties of cefadroxil and cephalexin. *Antimicrob Agents Chemother* 12:93, 1977.
41. Meyers BR, Kaplan K, Weinstein L: Cephalexin microbiological effects and pharmacologic parameters in man. *Clin Pharmacol Ther* 10:810, 1969.
42. Delgado DG, Brau CJ, Cobbs CG, et al: Clinical and laboratory evaluation of cefamandole in the therapy of *Haemophilus* spp. Bronchopulmonary infections. *Antimcrob Agents Chemother* 15(6):807, 1979.
43. Meyers BR, Hirschman SZ: Antibacterial activity of cefamandole in vitro. *J Infect Dis* 137(suppl):S25, 1978.
44. Fong I, Ralph E, Engelking F, et al: Clinical pharmacology of cefamandole as compared with cephalothin. *Antimicrob Agents Chemother* 9:65, 1976.
45. Neu HC: Comparison of the pharmacokinetics of cefamandole and other cephalosporin compounds. *J Infect Dis* 137(suppl):S80, 1978.
46. Kass EH, Evans DA: Future prospects and past problems in antimicrobial therapy: The role of cefoxitin. *Rev Infect Dis* 1:1, 1979.
47. Chow AW, Bednorz D: Comparative in vitro activity of newer cephalosporins against anaerobic bacteria. *Antimicrob Agents Chemother* 14:668, 1978.
48. Sutter VL, Finegold SM: Susceptibility of anaerobic bacteria to carbenicillin, cefoxitin, and related drugs. *J Infect Dis* 131:417, 1975.
49. Back VT, Roy I, Thadepalli H: Susceptibility of anaerobic bacteria to cefoxitin and related compounds. *Antimicrob Agents Chemother* 11:912, 1977.
50. Greaves WL, Kraus SJ, McCormack WM, et al: Cefoxitin vs. penicillin in the treatment of uncomplicated gonorrhea. *Sex Transm Dis* 10:53, 1983.
51. Silver MS, Counts GW, Zeleznik D, et al: Comparison of in vitro antibacterial activity of three oral cephalosporins: Cefaclor, cephalexin, and cephradine. *Antimicrob Agents Chemother* 12:591, 1977.
52. Barriere SL, Mills J: Ceforanide: Antibacterial activity, pharmacology, and clinical efficacy. *Pharmacotherapy* 2(6):322, 1982.
53. Gremillion DH, Winn RE, Vandenbout E: Clinical trial of cefonicid for treatment of skin infections. *Antimicrob Agents Chemother* 23(6):944, 1983.
54. Smith BR, LeFrock JL: Cefuroxime: Antimicrobial activity, pharmacology, and clinical efficacy. *Therapeutic Drug Monitoring* 5:149, 1983.
55. Swedish Study Group (Johansson Ö, Cronberg S, Hoffstedt B, et al): Cefuroxime versus ampicillin and chloramphenicol for the treatment of bacterial meningitis. *Lancet* 1:295, 1982.
56. Bodey G, Fainstein V, Hinkle A: Comparative in vitro study of new cephalosporins. *J Antimicrob Agents Chemother* 20:226, 1981.

57. Goto SM, Ogawa M, Tsuji A, et al: Bacteriological evaluation of a new cephamycin substance, CS-1170: Comparison with antibacterial action of cephalosporins and cefoxitin. *Chemotherapy* 26(S):1, 1978.
58. Neu HC, Aswapokee N, Aswapokee P, et al: HR756: A new cephalosporin active against gram-positive and gram-negative aerobic and anaerobic bacteria. *Antimicrob Agents Chemother* 15(2):273, 1979.
59. Landesman SH, Corrado ML, Shah PM, et al: Past and current roles for cephalosporin antibiotics in treatment of meningitis. *Am J Med* 71:693, 1981.
60. Mullaney DT, John JF: Cefotaxime therapy. *Arch Intern Med* 143:1705, 1983.
61. Cherubin CE, Neu HC, Turck M: Current status of cefotaxime sodium: A new cephalosporin. *Rev Infect Dis* 4:5281, 1982.
62. Moellering RC, Young LS: Moxalactam international symposium. *Rev Infect Dis* 4:S489, 1982.
63. Olson DA, Hoeprich PS, Nolan SM, et al: Successful treatment of gram-negative bacillary meningitis with moxalactam. *Ann Intern Med* 95:302, 1981.
64. Weitekamp MR, Aber RC: Prolonged bleeding times and bleeding diathesis associated with moxalactam administration. *JAMA* 249(1):69, 1983.
65. Neu HC, Turck M, Phillips I: Ceftizoxime: A broad-spectrum beta-lactamase stable cephalosporin. *J Antimicrob Chemother* 10(suppl C):1, 1982.
66. Del Rio MA, Chrane D, Shelton S, et al: Ceftriaxone versus ampicillin and chloramphenicol for treatment of bacterial meningitis in children. *Lancet* 1:1241, 1983.
67. Baumgartner J, Glauser MP: Single daily dose treatment of severe refractory infections with ceftriaxone. *Arch Intern Med* 143:1868, 1983.
68. Handsfield HH, Murphy VL: Comparative study of ceftriaxone and spectinomycin for treatment of uncomplicated gonorrhoea in men. *Lancet* 2:67, 1983.
69. Rajan VS, Sng EH, Thirumoorthy T, et al: Ceftriaxone in the treatment of ordinary and penicillinase-producing strains of *Neisseria gonorrhoeae. Br J Vener Dis* 58:314, 1982.
70. Ayers LW, Jones RN, Barry AL, et al: Cefotetan: A new cephamycin: Comparison of in vitro antimicrobial activity with other cephems, beta-lactamase stability, and preliminary recommendations for disk diffusion testing. *Antimicrob Agents Chemother* 22(5):859, 1982.
71. Phillips I, Wise R, Leigh DA: Cefotetan: A new cephamycin. *J Antimicrob Chemother* 11(suppl A): 1983.
72. Klein JO, Neu HC: Empiric therapy for bacterial infections: Evaluation of cefoperazone. *Rev Infect Dis* 5:S1, 1983.
73. Hamilton-Miller JMT, Brumfitt W: Activity of ceftazidime (GR20263) against nosocomially important pathogens. *Antimicrob Agents Chemother* 19(6):1067, 1981.
74. Neu HC, Labthavikul P: Antibacterial activity and beta-lactamase stability of ceftazidime: An Aminothiazolyl cephalosporin potentially active against *Pseudomonas aeruginosa. Antimicrob Agents Chemother* 21(1):11, 1982.
75. Neu HC: In-vitro activity of ceftazidime: A beta-lactamase stable cephalosporin. *J Antimicrob Chemother* 8(suppl B):131, 1981.
76. Kato M, Inoue M, Mitsuhashi S: Antibacterial activities of SM-1652 compared with those of other broad-spectrum cephalosporins. *Antimicrob Agents Chemother* 22(5)721, 1982.
77. King A, Shannon K, Phillips I: In-vitro antibacterial activity and susceptibility of cefsulodin, an antipseudomonal cephalosporin, to beta-lactamases. *Antimicrob Agents Chemother* 17:165, 1980.
78. Fass RJ: Comparative in vitro activities of third-generation cephalosporins. *Arch Intern Med* 143:1743, 1983.
79. Muytjens HL, van der Ros-van de Repe J: Comparative activities of 13 beta-lactam antibiotics. *Antimicrob Agents Chemother* 21(6):925, 1982.
80. Bodey GP, Fainstein V, Hinkle AM: Comparative in vitro study of new cephalosporins. *Antimicrob Agents Chemother* 20(2):226, 1981.

5

OTHER BETA-LACTAM ANTIBIOTICS

HAROLD C. NEU

Several antimicrobial agents belonging to the β-lactam class of antibiotics have been developed in recent years. Since these agents differ widely in their antibacterial and pharmacologic properties, they will be discussed as separate entities.

THIENAMYCINS

Imipenem is the prototype drug of this class of compounds. In the early 1970s scientists in Spain discovered a new streptomyces species called *Streptomyces cattleya,* which produced a carbapenem compound subsequently named thienamycin (1).

Chemistry

Figure 1 shows the chemical structure of the *N*-formimidoyl derivative of thienamycin. Unfortunately, the presence of an azetidiome group caused thienamycin to undergo aminolysis of the β-lactam ring through reaction of the amino group of one molecule with another. *N*-formimidoyl thienamycin, which is variously referred to in the antimicrobial literature as MK-0787 or imipemide, is now called imipenem.

Thienamycins possess novel stereochemical features that differentiate them from penicillin and cephalosporins. They are in a transconfiguration, and the endocyclic sulfur is replaced with a methylene group, with the sulfur atom adjacent to the bicyclic ring system. Biochemically they are carbapenems.

Antibacterial Activity

Imipenem has excellent in vitro activity against aerobic gram-positive species such as the hemolytic streptococci of the Lancefield classifications A,B,C,G,

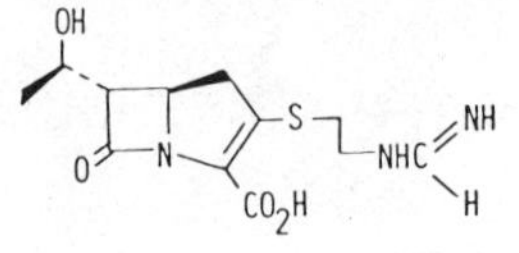

FIGURE 1. Imipenem (*N*-formimidoyl thienamycin).

with minimal inhibitory values (MIC) of 0.2 μg/ml or less (Table 1) (2,3). *Streptococcus pneumoniae* are inhibited by less than 0.1 μg/ml, and *S. pneumoniae* resistant to penicillin (MIC values >4 μg/ml) are inhibited 1 μg/ml or less, of imipenem. *Streptococcus faecalis* are inhibited by less than 1.5 μg/ml, but there is a discrepancy between inhibitory and bactericidal levels just as there exists one for ampicillin and vancomycin, and *S. faecalis* and *S. faecium* resistant to ampicillin are resistant to imipenem. *Staphylococcus aureus* and *Staphylococcus epidermidis* are inhibited by less than 0.2 and 1.5 μg/ml, respectively. Methicillin-resistant staphylococci at 30°C have MIC values of 8–64 μg/ml. *Listeria* and *Bacillus* sp. are also inhibited by less than 1 μg/ml.

The majority of the Enterobacteriaceae are inhibited by concentrations of imipenem less than or equal to 1 μg/ml. Some *Proteus* sp. have MIC values of 2–4 μg/ml. *Hemophilus influenzae* and *Neisseria gonorrhoeae,* including β-lactamase-producing isolates, are inhibited by less than 0.25 μg/ml.

Pseudomonas aeruginosa, including strains resistant to penicillins such as piperacillin and to cephalosporins such as ceftazidime and cefsulodin, are inhibited by 1–6 μg/ml. *Pseudomonas cepacia* are inhibited by imipenem, but *Pseudomonas maltophilia* are resistant. Most *Acinetobacter* sp. are inhibited by less than 1 μg/ml.

Imipenem inhibits most anaerobic species, including *Bacteroides fragilis* and some isolates resistant to moxalactam and cefoxitin, at concentrations of less than 0.5 μg/ml (4,5). Most *Clostridium* sp. are inhibited by 1 μg/ml or less, with the exception of *Clostridium difficile,* which requires 6–8 μg/ml. *Fusobacterium, Actinomyces, Campylobacter,* and *Yersinia* are inhibited by imipenem, and many *Nocardia asteroides* are inhibited by 1 μg/ml.

Mechanism of Action

Imipenem binds to penicillin-binding protein-2 (PBP-2) 2 of gram-negative aerobic bacteria and to critical PBPs in *S. aureus* and *S. faecalis.* Unlike the situation with amdinocillin, imipenem causes rapid death of bacteria and there is no major discrepancy between inhibitory and bactericidal activity.

Imipenem is not hydrolyzed by the majority of β-lactamases, penicillinases, cephalosporinases, plasmid or chromosomally mediated, of *S. aureus, Escherechia coli, Enterobacter cloacae, Citrobacter freundii, Proteus rettgeri, Serratia marcescens, Proteus vulgaris, Klebsiella oxytoca, P. aeruginosa, P. cepacia* and *B. fragilis.* It is partially hydrolyzed by a *P. maltophilia* β-lactamase.

TABLE 1. Activity of Imipenem, *N*-formimidoyl Thienamycin

Organism	MIC_{90} (μg/ml)
Staphylococcus aureus[a]	0.1
S. epidermidis[a]	0.2
Streptococcus pyogenes	0.1
S. agalactiae	0.1
Viridans streptococci	0.1
S. pneumoniae	0.01
S. bovis	0.1
S. faecalis	0.8
Hemophilus influenzae	0.1
Neisseria gonorrhoeae	0.1
N. meningitidis	0.02
Listeria monocytogenes	0.02
Clostridium sp.	0.05
Klebsiella pneumoniae[a]	0.4
Enterobacter cloacae[a]	1.6
E. aerogenes[a]	0.2
E. agglomerans[a]	0.4
E. hafnia[a]	0.4
Escherichia coli[a]	0.4
Klebsiella oxytoca[a]	0.2
Arizona hinshawii[a]	0.1
Aeromonas hydrophila[a]	0.1
Citrobacter freundii[a]	1.6
C. diversus[a]	0.2
Serratia marcescens[a]	6.3
Proteus mirabilis	1.6
Morganella morganii[a]	1.6
Proteus rettgeri[a]	1.6
P. vulgaris[a]	0.6
Providencia stuartii[a]	1.6
Salmonella	0.1
Shigella	0.2
Acinetobacter	0.8
Pseudomonas aeruginosa[a]	12.5
P. maltophilia	>50
P. cepacia	>50
Bacteroides fragilis, group[a]	0.2
B. fragilis ssp. *fragilis*	0.2

[a] Both β-lactamase- and non-β-lactamase-containing strains.

Pharmacology

Imipenem cannot be absorbed after oral ingestion due to instability of the molecule in gastric acid. Although initial studies of imipenem after intravenous infusion showed high serum levels, urinary recovery was only 6–38 percent of an administered dose (6). In contrast to many other drugs, extrarenal metabolism is minimal. A renal peptidase, dehydropeptidase-1, which hydrolyzes L-L and

L-D dipeptides, is located on the brush border of the proximal renal tubules. After imipenem is removed from the circulation by glomerular filtration and secretion, it is hydrolyzed.

Imipenem in the circulation is not destroyed and is widely distributed to various body compartments (7). There is virtually no biliary secretion of imipenem. In the absence of meningeal inflammation only minor amounts of imipenem enter the cerebrospinal fluid. In the presence of meningeal inflammation cerebrospinal fluid levels of 1–5 μg/ml have been recorded. Imipenem has cured meningitis due to *S. pneumoniae* and *H. influenzae* in a rabbit model of meningitis.

To overcome the problem of destruction of imipenem in urine, a dehydropeptidase inhibitor was synthesized. This molecule, called cilastatin, is administered in equal amounts to imipenem. Cilastatin has no antibacterial activity nor does it alter the antibacterial activity of imipenem. Cilastatin does not affect zinc metalloenzyme peptidases or angiotensin-converting enzymes.

After 20–30 minutes of infusion of 250 mg imipenem plus 250 mg cilastatin, mean peak serum levels of imipenem are 13 μg/ml. After 500 mg, mean peak serum levels are 33 μg/ml; the half-life of imipenem is 1 hour in healthy people. Serum half-life increases with fall in creatinine clearance with a T½ of 4 hours in patients whose creatinine clearance is less than 10 ml/min. Imipenem is not removed from the body by hemodialysis. Cilastatin serum concentrations parallel those of imipenem, and it also is not removed by dialysis.

In the presence of cilastatin, urinary recovery of imipenem is 70 percent with 25–29 percent recovery of metabolites. Fecal elimination of imipenem is less than 1 percent.

Adverse Reactions

The number of patients treated with imipenem has been only several thousand, so the precise incidence of clinical adverse reactions or abnormal laboratory tests is unknown (8). No major adverse effects such as diarrhea, pseudomembranous colitis, coagulation abnormalities, nephrotoxicity, or hepatotoxicity have been reported. Rapid infusion of imipenem has produced nausea and emesis in about 1 percent of patients. About 2–4 percent of imipenem-treated patients will have from a one to twofold elevation of serum glutamic-oxaloacetic transaminase and/or serum glutamic-pyruvic transaminase (SGOT, SGPT) values. Leukopenia has also been reported. No drug interactions have been reported.

Clinical Use

Imipenem plus cilastatin has the proprietary name of Primaxin. The precise clinical role of imipenem has not been established. Imipenem has been used to treat bacteremia, respiratory infections, intra-abdominal infections, bone and joint infections, endocarditis, skin and soft-tissue infections, and urinary tract infections (9). It has eradicated bacteria resistant to aminoglycosides and to penicillin and cephalosporins. Doses used have been 250–750 mg of imipenem plus 250–750 mg of cilastatin, four times daily by the intravenous route infused over 30–60 minutes.

MONOBACTAMS

The development of new methods by Sykes and his colleagues (10) to screen large numbers of organisms for production of β-lactam antibiotics showed that a number of species, particularly *Gluconobacter* and *Acinetobacter*, produced monocyclic β-lactam antibiotics with antibacterial activity. From a *Chromobacterium violaceum* a monocyclic compound was isolated and the structure confirmed. This compound was subsequently modified to yield a highly active therapeutic agent, aztreonam.

Chemistry

Aztreonam is a monocyclic β-lactam (Fig. 2) in which there is a sulfate group afixed to the nitrogen at position 1, an acyl side chain at position 3, which consists of an aminothiazolyl nucleus and an iminocarboxypropyl group, and a methyl group at position 4 of the ring.

Mechanism of Action

Aztreonam has no appreciable antibacterial activity against gram-positive or anaerobic bacteria. This is because it does not bind to penicillin-binding proteins in these species. Aztreonam binds primarily to PBP-3 in Enterobacteriaceae, *Pseudomonas*, and other gram-negative aerobic species. It produces long filamentous structures that are not viable. Aztreonam readily passes through the outer wall of gram-negative species, and it is not hydrolyzed by most plasmid and chromosomal β-lactamases, with the exception of slight hydrolysis by the K-1 β-lactamases of some *K. oxytoca* and β-lactamases of some *P. cepacia.*

Antibacterial Activity

Aztreonam inhibits most Enterobacteriaceae at concentrations below 0.5 μg/ml (Table 2); some *P. aeruginosa, E. cloacae,* and *C. freundii* are resistant.

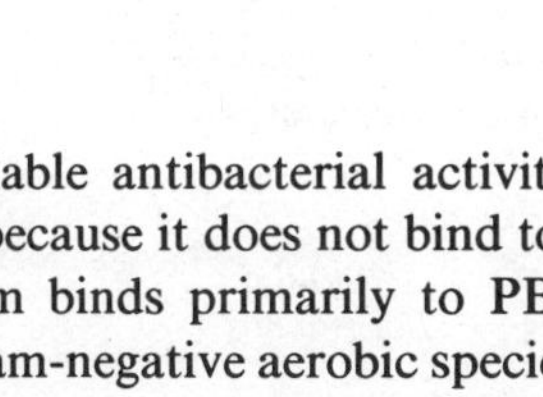

FIGURE 2. Aztreonam.

TABLE 2. In Vitro Activity Aztreonam

Organism	MIC_{90} (μg/ml)
Escherichia coli	0.2
Klebsiella pneumoniae	0.8
K. oxytoca	0.4
Enterobacter cloacae	25
E. aerogenes	12.5
E. agglomerans	0.4
Citrobacter freundii	0.4
C. diversus	0.2
Serratta marcescens	3.1
Proteus mirabilis	0.01
P. vulgaris	0.1
P. rettgeri	0.1
Morganella morganii	0.2
Providencia	0.025
Salmonella enteritidis	0.2
Shigella	0.1
Arizona hinshawii	0.1
Aeromonas hydrophila	0.1
A. shigelloides	0.1
Yersinia enterocolitica	3.1
Pasteurella multocida	0.1
Salmonella typhi	0.1
Hemophilus influenzae	0.1
Neisseria gonorrhoeae	0.2
N. meningitidis	0.025
Pseudomonas aeruginosa	25
P. maltophila	>100
Pseudomonas, other (*P. cepacia, P. diminuta, P. stutzeri, P. fluorescens*)	>100

Most *P. aeruginosa* are inhibited by less than 16 μg/ml. Its antibacterial activity against *P. aeruginosa* is similar to that of ceftazidime. Most *P. cepacia* and *P. maltophilia* are resistant as are many *Acinetobacter* sp; *Hemophilus,* and *Neisseria,* including β-lactamase-producing isolates, are inhibited by less than 0.2 μg/ml. *Yersinia* and *Aeromonas* are inhibited by less than 0.5 μg/ml. In general, the antibacterial activity is minimally affected by inoculum size except for *P. aeruginosa,* and there is no major difference between MIC and minimum bactericidal concentration (MBC) values (11,12).

Pharmacology

Aztreonam is not absorbed after oral ingestion. Administration of aztreonam by intravenous bolus over 5 minutes, in doses of 500, 1000, and 2000 mg produced peak serum levels of 58, 125, and 242 μg/ml, respectively (13). Serum half-life by these methods is 1.7 hours with an apparent volume of distribution of 0.18 liter/kg. After intravenous infusion of 1 and 2 g over 30 minutes, peak serum levels of 164 and 255 μg/ml, respectively, are achieved; after infusion over 8.5 hours, serum levels of 3 and 8.5 μg/ml, respectively, are achieved, with an approximated half-life of 2 hours (14). Peak serum levels after 500 mg intramuscularly are 20 μg/ml and after 1 g are 40 μg/ml. There is no accumulation of the drug in healthy people. Urinary excretion averages 60 percent, with urine levels averaging 1000 μg/ml for the first 2 hours after 500 mg are administered intravenously. Urine levels above 10 μg/ml persist for 12 hours after 500 mg intravenously or intramuscularly. About 6 percent of a dose is excreted as the open β-lactam ring hydrolysis product of aztreonam.

In the presence of renal failure there is accumulation of aztreonam, with serum half-life increasing to 6 hours. The compound is removed by hemodialysis to an extent of 50 percent (15). Peritoneal dialysis will alter the serum half-life to 3 hours.

A dosage program of 1 g every 24 hours has been proposed for renal failure; adjustment is necessary when hemodialysis is performed.

Adverse Reactions

No new major adverse reactions to aztreonam have been reported. Skin rashes have occurred. Neither anaphylaxis nor rashes have followed its use in patients with positive skin tests to penicillins. About 2–4 percent of patients will have increases in serum transaminase values two times above normal when receiving aztreonam. No hematologic, gastrointestinal, nephrotoxic, or neurotoxic reactions have been noted with this agent.

Clinical Use

Aztreonam has been used to treat a variety of serious infections due to gram-negative aerobic species such as *E. coli, Klebsiella, Serratia,* and *Pseudomonas.* Preliminary studies have shown that the compound is effective in treatment of gram-negative aerobic pulmonary infection, septicemia, osteomyelitis, and urinary tract infections. It has been combined with clindamycin, semisynthetic antistaphylococcal penicillins, metronidazole, and vancomycin to treat mixed infections.

β-LACTAMASE INHIBITORS

Clavulanic Acid

Clavulanic acid (Fig. 3) is a β-lactamase inhibitor. This compound was found in cultures of *Streptomyces clavuligerus.* It showed only a low level of antibacterial action, but when the compound was combined with penicillin G, inhibition of a *Klebsiella* isolate normally resistant to penicillin was noted. Clavulanic

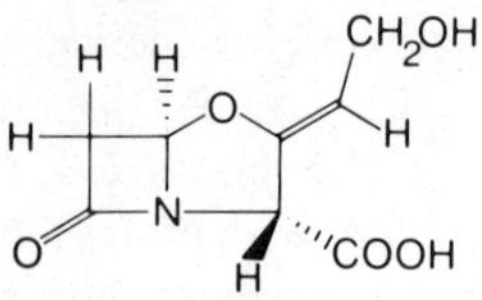

FIGURE 3. Clavulanic acid.

acid has subsequently been shown to inhibit β-lactamases from a number of clinically important gram-positive and gram-negative organisms (16,17).

Mechanism of Action

β-lactamases account for the major form of resistance to penicillins and cephalosporins. These enzymes hydrolyze the cyclic amide bond in β-lactam-containing molecules. When the β-lactam ring is hydrolyzed an inactive penicilloate is produced, or, in the case of cephalosporins, because of the unsaturated bond between carbons 3 and 4, both rings decompose to smaller fragments.

β-lactamases of gram-positive species are exoenzymes, and in *S. aureus* the enzyme is plasmid mediated and inducible. Generally endemic hospital *S. aureus* produces large amounts of β-lactamase. The β-lactamases of gram-negative bacteria, aerobic and anaerobic, are situated in the periplasmic space and are either of chromosomal or plasmid origin. Richmond and Sykes developed a classification for gram-negative β-lactamases which lists them as I–V (18). The most important chromosomal β-lactamases, most of which fall into class I, are present in *Acinetobacter, Citrobacter, Enterobacter, Proteus* species, *Pseudomonas,* and *Serratia.* These are inducible enzymes and are not inhibited by clavulanic acid except at very high concentrations, which are only possible in test tube conditions. β-lactamases constitutively are produced by some *Enterobacter, E. coli,* and *Shigella.* These are not inhibited by clavulanic acid. Conversely, β-lactamases of *Legionella* and *Bacteroides* are inhibited by clavulanic acid. Another important chromosomally mediated β-lactamase is the class IV enzymes produced by *Klebsiella.* These are also inhibited by clavulanic acid.

Plasmid-mediated β-lactamases are of a number of types. The most common is TEM-I, so-called for the initials of the original patient from whom the *E. coli* β-lactamase-containing isolate was derived. There is also TEM-2, oxacillin-hydrolyzing enzymes, OXA 1,2,3, sulfhydro-inhibited enzymes SHV-1 and HMS, and finally PSE 1, PSE-2, PSE-3, and PSE-4, originally felt to be enzymes found only in *Pseudomonas* but now found occasionally in *E. coli.* All of these plasmid enzymes are inhibited by clavulanic acid (Table 3). Concentrations needed to inhibit bacteria are shown in Table 4.

Since clavulanic acid inhibits β-lactamases, it has been shown to act synergistically with amoxicillin, ampicilin, piperacillin, mezlocillin, and cefoperazone, all of which can be destroyed by *Staphylococcus, Klebsiella,* or plasmid-mediated β-lactamases. Currently clavulanic acid is combined with amoxicillin and referred to as Augmentin.

TABLE 3. Inhibition of β-lactamases by β-lactam Inhibitors

β-lactamases	*Name*	*Organisms*	*Inhibited by Clavulanic acid–Sulbactam*
Plasmid		*S. aureus*	Yes
Plasmid	TEM-1	*E. coli* *Hemophilus* *N. gonorrhoeae* *Salmonella* *Shigella*	Yes
Plasmid	TEM-2	*E. coli*	Yes
Plasmid	SHV-1	*Klebsiella*	Yes
Plasmid	OXA 1,2,3	*E. coli*	Variable
Plasmid	PSE 1,2,3	*Pseudomonas*	Variable
Chromosomal	Type Ia[a]	*Enterobacter* *Morganella* *Citrobacter* *Serratia*	No
Chromosomal	Type Id[a]	*Pseudomonas*	No
Chromosomal	Type IV,K1[a]	*Klebsiella*	Yes
Chromosomal		*Bacteroides*	Yes
Chromosomal		*Legionella*	Yes

[a] Richmond-Sykes classification (18).

The mode of inhibition of a β-lactamase by clavulanic acid is characteristic of the particular enzyme studied. Although competitive inhibition is seen, clavulanic acid most often acts as a suicide inhibitor, which, after forming an acyl enzyme intermediate with the enzyme, causes distruction of the enzyme.

Pharmacology

Clavulanic acid is moderately well absorbed from the gastrointestinal tract, with peak serum levels occurring 40–120 minutes after ingestion. Mean peak serum levels for 62.5 mg are 1 μg/ml, for 125 mg are 4 μg/ml, and for 250

TABLE 4. Antibacterial Activity of Augmentin

Organism	*Concentration to Inhibit (μg/ml)*[a]
S. aureus	2
H. influenzae	2
N. gonorrhoeae	2
B. catarrhalis	2
E. coli	16
Klebsiella	8
Proteus	16
B. fragilis	16

[a] Ratio 1:1.

mg are 6 μg/ml (19,20). Combining clavulanic acid with amoxicillin does not significantly alter the pharmacologic parameters of either drug. The pharmacokinetics of orally administered clavulanic acid in children in terms of peak serum levels and plasma half-lives of the drug are similar to those in adults (21).

The absorption of clavulanic acid in the adult is unaffected by the simultaneous administration of food, milk, or aluminum hydroxide containing antacids. After intravenous infusion of clavulanic combined either with amoxicillin or ticarcillin, the drug is rapidly distributed. Peak serum concentration are approximately 11 μg/ml after a 200-mg intravenous dose, with drug detectable to levels of 0.2 μg/ml at 6 hours. Peak serum concentrations of clavulanic acid in children receiving 5 mg/kg have been 19 μg/ml, with less than 1 μg/ml present at 3 hours (21).

The serum half-life of clavulanic acid is slightly less than that of amoxicillin, 0.76–1.4 hours. No accumulation of clavulanic acid occurs until creatinine clearances fall below 10 ml/min. Dose adjustment usually is made on adjustment for amoxicillin or ticarcillin. Clavulanic acid has been shown to be degraded in vivo in animals with metabolites being excreted via lung, feces, and urine and only 20–60 percent appearing unchanged in urine 6 hours after an oral dose. Following a dose of 125 mg of clavulanic acid urine levels are 115–508 μg/ml for 0–2 hours and 45–74 μg/ml for 4–6 hours.

Concentrations less than 1 μg/ml of clavulanic acid are achieved in sputum after oral administration of amoxicillin–clavulanic acid, but pleural fluid levels are 46–91 percent of peak serum levels. There is rapid penetration of clavulanic acid into peritoneal fluid, with mean peritoneal fluid levels of clavulanic acid 66 percent of serum levels (22). After 200 mg of clavulanic acid, peritoneal fluid levels fall below 5 μg/ml after about 0.5 hours and below 1 μg/ml after about 3 hours. Clavulanic acid does not penetrate noninflamed meninges, but after large intravenous doses in patients with meningitis, cerebrospinal fluid levels of clavulanic acid have been in the range of 1 μg/ml. Clavulanic acid produces therapeutic levels in bile, middle ear fluid, and tonsil tissue.

Clavulanic acid crosses the placenta and may be found in the cord blood of newborns and in the amniotic fluid, but no clavulanic acid can be detected in breast milk.

Adverse Reactions

No new or major adverse reactions to the use of clavulanic acid combined with amoxicillin or of clavulanic acid combined with ticarcillin have been reported. The incidence of skin reactions has been similar to that of penicillin used alone. Diarrhea has followed the use of 250 mg clavulanic acid given three times daily, and some nausea has occurred with this dose program.

AMOXICILLIN–CLAVULANIC ACID (AUGMENTIN)

Augmentin (amoxicillin–clavulanic acid) has proved to be a successful treatment of skin-structure infections due to β-lactamase-producing staphylococci, otitis due to *H. influenzae,* and urinary infections due to β-lactamase-producing *E. coli* and *Klebsiella.* The situations in which this combination would be preferred to other β-lactams has not been fully clarified.

TICARCILLIN–CLAVULANIC ACID (TIMENTIN)

Timentin is a combination of 3 g ticarcillin and 100 or 200 mg clavulanic acid. Pharmacology of both agents is the same as previously noted. Studies on the use of this combination are in progress.

SULBACTAM

Sulbactam (Fig. 4) is a 6-desaminopenicillin sulfone that resembles clavulanic acid structurally by lack of substitution at C-6 of the β-lactam ring and by the presence of an activated center at C-5. Sulbactam has weak antibacterial activity against most gram-positive cocci, Enterobacteriaceae, and *Pseudomonas,* but has reasonable activity against *Neisseria* sp. and *Bacteroides* sp. (23,24).

Sulbactam acts similarly to clavulanic acid as a suicide inhibitor of certain plasmid and chromosomally mediated β-lactamases. It does not inhibit β-lactamases of the Richmond-Sykes type Ia classification. These are chromosomally mediated β-lactamases of *Enterobacter, Citrobacter freundii,* and the indole-positive *Proteus-Providencia* organisms.

Sulbactam acts synergistically with penicillin and cephalosporins, which are degraded by β-lactamases. In the presence of concentrations of 8 μg/ml of sulbactam and 16 μg/ml of ampicillin, the majority of staphylococci, *Klebsiella, Hemophilus, E. coli,* and *Bacteroides* sp, which would normally be resistant to ampicillin, would be inhibited (24) (Table 5).

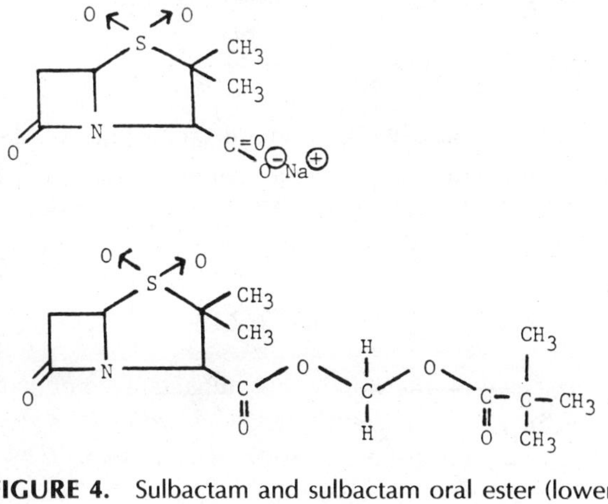

FIGURE 4. Sulbactam and sulbactam oral ester (lower).

TABLE 5. In Vitro Activity of Ampicillin–Sulbactam

Organism	*Ampicillin*[a] *MIC*$_{90}$	*Ampicillin–Sulbactam*[a] *MIC*$_{90}$[b]
S. aureus		
Ampicillin resistant	>128	2
S. aureus		
Methicillin resistant	>128	>16
S. epidermidis	64	2
B. fragilis	>128	16
H. influenzae		
Ampicillin resistant	>64	1
E. coli	>128	16
K. pneumoniae	>128	8
K. oxytoca	>128	16
E. cloacae	>128	>64
Serratia sp.	>128	32
Citrobacter sp.	>128	>32
Proteus sp.	>128	8

[a] Values in micrograms per milliliter (μg/ml).
[b] Ratio 1:1.

Pharmacology

Sulbactam has pharmacokinetics in humans similar to ampicillin or amoxicillin (25). After intravenous administration the sulbactam half-life is 1 hour. Peak serum levels after intramuscular injection of 0.250 g are 7 μg/ml and of 0.5 g are 13 μg/ml, with a serum half-life of 1.1–1.3 hours. After intravenous infusion of 0.5 g, peak serum levels of 30 μg/ml are achieved and after 1 g, 68 μg/ml are achieved. Serum half-life is 1 hour. Sulbactam is excreted by the kidney with urinary recovery of 70–80 percent of a dose. Concentrations of sulbactam in interstitial fluid and peritoneal secretions are comparable to levels in serum. Penetration of sulbactam into inflamed meninges is low, with levels of 0.1–10 μg/ml found in the cerebrospinal fluid after a 1 g infusion.

Adverse Reactions

Few clinical studies of the combination of sulbactam plus ampicillin have been reported. But no major hematologic, renal, hepatic, or central nervous system reactions have occurred. Diarrhea has not been a major problem after intravenous use, but is serious when the drug is used orally.

Clinical Use

Experience with the use of the ampicillin–sulbactam combination is limited. Successful therapy for β-lactamase-producing *H. influenzae, N. gonorrheae, B. fragilis,* and *S. aureus* infections is well documented. Few patients with β-lactamase-producing Enterobacteriaceae infections treated with sulbactam–ampicillin are recorded in the literature.

REFERENCES

1. Kahan JS, Kahan FM, Goegleman R, et al: Thienamycin, a new β-lactam antibiotic. 1. Discovery, taxonomy, isolation and physical properties. *J Antibiot* 32:1, 1979.
2. Neu HC, Labthavikul P: Comparative in vitro activity of N-formimidoyl thienamycin against gram-positive and gram-negative aerobic and anaerobic species and its β-lactamase stability. *Antimicrob Agents Chemother* 21:180, 1982.
3. Wise R, Andrews JM, Patel N: N-formimidoyl thienamycin a novel β-lactam: An in-vitro comparison with other β-lactam antibiotics. *J Antimicrob Chemother* 7:521, 1981.
4. Broron JE, Del Benes VE, Collins CD: In vitro activity of N-forminmidoyl thienamycin, moxalactam and other new beta-lactam agents against *Bacteroides fragilis:* Contribution of beta-lactamase to resistance. *Antimicrob Agents Chemother* 19:248, 1981.
5. Kesado T, Hashizume T, Ashi Y, et al: Susceptibilities of anaerobic bacteria to N-formimidoyl thienamycin (MK0787) and to other antibiotics. *Antimicrob Agents Chemother* 21:1016, 1982.
6. Norby SR, et al: Urinary recovery of N-formimidoyl thienamycin (MK0787) as affected by coadministration of N-formimidoyl thienamycin dehydropeptidase inhibitors. *Antimicrob Agents Chemother* 23:300, 1983.
7. Norby SR, et al: Pharmacokinetics and tolerance of N-formimidoyl thienamycin (MK0787) in humans. *Antimicrob Agents Chemother* 23:293, 1983.
8. Calandra GB, Ricci FM, Wang C, et al: Safety and tolerance comparison of imipenen-cilstatin to cephalothin and cefazolin. *J Antimicrob Chemother* 12(suppl D), 1983, p. 125.
9. Neu HC: Clinical perspectives on imipenem. *J Antimicrob Chemother* 12(suppl D), 1983, p. 149.
10. Sykes RB, et al: Monocyclic β-lactam antibiotics produced by bacteria. *Nature* 291:489, 1981.
11. Neu HC, Labthavikul P: Antibacterial activity of a monocyclic β-lactam SQ 26, 776. *J Antimicrob Chemother* 8(suppl E): 111, 1981.
12. Sykes RB, Bonner DP, Bush K, et al: Aztreonam (SQ 26, 776): A synthetic monobactam active against aerobic gram-negative bacteria. *Antimicrob Agents Chemother* 21:85, 1982.
13. Swabb EA, Sugferiman A, Platt TB, et al: Single-dose pharmacokinetics of the monobactam aztreonam (SQ 26, 776) in healthy subjects. *Antimicrob Agents Chemother* 21:944, 1982.
14. Scully BE, Swabb EA, Neu HC: Pharmacology of aztreonam after intravenous infusion. *Antimicrob Agents Chemother* 24:18, 1983.
15. Mihindu JCL, Scheld M, Bolton ND, et al: Pharmacokinetics of aztreonam in patients with various degrees of renal dysfunction. *Antimicrob Agents Chemother* 24:252, 1983.
16. Neu HC, Fu KP: Clavulanic acid: A novel inhibitor of β-lactamases. *Antimicrob Agents Chemother* 14:650, 1978.
17. Reading C, Cole M: Clavulanic acid: A beta-lactamase-inhibiting beta-lactam from *Streptomyces clavuligerus. Antimicrob Agents Chemother* 11:852, 1977.
18. Richmond MM, Sykes RB: The β-lactamases of gram-negative bacteria and their possible physiological role. *Adv Microb Physiol* 9:31, 1973.
19. Munch P, Luthy R, Blaser J, et al: Human pharmacokinetics and CSF penetration of clavulanic acid. *J Antimicrob Chemother* 8:29, 1981.
20. Adam D, Visser I, Koeppe P: Pharmacokinetics of amoxicillin and clavulanic acid administered alone and in combination. *Antimicrob Agents Chemother* 22:353, 1982.
21. Schaad UB, Casey PA, Copper DL: Single-dose pharmacokinetics of intravenous clavulanic acid with amoxicillin in pediatric patients. *Antimicrob Agents Chemother* 23:252, 1983.
22. Bennett S, Wise R, Weston D, et al: Pharmacokinetics and tissue penetration of ticarcillin combined with clavulanic acid. *Antimicrob Agents Chemother* 23:831, 1983.

23. Aswapokee N, Neu HC: A sulfone, β-lactam compound which acts as a β-lactamase inhibitor. *J Antibiot* 31:1238, 1978.
24. Retsema VA, English AR, Girard AE: CP-45, 899 in combination with penicillin or ampicillin against penicillin-resistant *Staphylococcus, Haemophilus influenzae* and *Bacteroides. Antimicrob Agents Chemother* 17:615, 1980.
25. Foulds G, Stankewich JP, Marshall DC, et al: Pharmacokinetics of sulbactam in humans. *Antimicrob Agents Chemother* 23:692, 1983.

6

AMINOGLYCOSIDES AND SPECTINOMYCIN: AMINOCYCLITOLS

PAUL S. LIETMAN

Since the introduction of streptomycin in the mid-1940s, one or another of the aminoglycosides has been a mainstay in our therapeutic armamentarium. Their bactericidal activity against aerobic gram-negative bacilli, their coverage of pseudomonas species, and their antitubercular activity are their three most acclaimed attributes. However, their dose-related toxicity is a major consideration limiting their dosage and making them prime targets for competition by other, and presumably safer, classes of antibiotics. Nevertheless, they continue to be widely used in serious infections.

HISTORY

Waksman and colleagues derived streptomycin from *Streptomyces griseus* in 1943. This drug was used for tuberculosis but resistance rapidly emerged when used alone. In 1949 neomycin was isolated from *Streptomyces fradiae.* The agent proved to be too toxic for systemic administration. Kanamycin was isolated by Japanese investigators in 1957 and became the dominant aminoglycoside until its replacement by newer agents, including gentamicin, tobramycin, and amikacin.

STRUCTURES

The family of aminoglycoside antibiotics is defined by the presence of two or more aminosugars linked by glycosidic bonds to an aminocyclitol ring (1–3). The six-membered aminocyclitol ring is either streptidine (as in streptomycin) or 2-deoxystreptamine (as in neomycin, kanamycin, gentamicin, tobramycin, amikacin, and netilmicin). Spectinomycin is often included as a member of the family although it contains no aminosugar and no glycosidic bond. Since spectinomycin does contain an aminocyclitol ring, as do the aminoglycosides, a general term that includes both aminoglycosides and spectinomycin is *aminocyclitol antibiotics.* However, the term *aminoglycoside* is sanctioned by common usage.

Streptomycin, neomycin, kanamycin, and tobramycin have each been isolated from a different species of streptomyces, whereas the gentamicins and netilmicin have been isolated from a micromonospora species. The spelling of gentamicin and netilmicin with -micin rather than -mycin denotes this difference in origin. The two newest aminoglycosides, amikacin and netilmicin, are semisynthetic aminoglycosides since they are both artificial derivatives of naturally occurring aminoglycosides. Amikacin is the 1-*N*-hydroxyaminobutyric acid derivative of kanamycin A, and netilmicin is the 1-*N*-ethyl derivative of sisomicin, a naturally occurring aminoglycoside derived from a micromonospora species (4).

The structure–activity relationships of the aminoglycosides are incompletely understood, but the importance of the several hydroxyl and amino groups attached to the various rings is established by the loss of antibacterial activity when these groups are modified, either by synthetic chemists or by numerous bacterial enzymes (4,5). Numerous intriguing similarities between aminoglycosides and polyamines such as spermine and spermidine suggest that aminoglycosides might be viewed as unusual polyamines both with respect to their interactions with bacteria and humans.

The groups of aminoglycosides differ from one another in the nature of the aminosugars that are linked to the central aminocyclitol ring. Structures of the aminoglycosides currently marketed in the United States are shown in Figure 1.

Although most of the aminoglycosides are unique chemical entities, gentamicin consists of a mixture of roughly equal amounts of three individual components, gentamicin C_1, C_{1a} and C_2, and neomycin consists of roughly equal amounts of neomycin B and neomycin C. The inherent difficulties in separating the closely related gentamicins and neomycins have accounted for the inclusion of two or three components in the commercial formulations of each.

INTERACTIONS WITH MICROBES

Mechanism of Action

The precise biochemical mechanism of action of the aminoglycosides remains enigmatic in spite of an enormous amount of sophisticated attention. The difficulty lies in an inability to correlate the known biochemical effects of aminoglycosides with their lethal action. Aminoglycosides clearly inhibit bacterial protein synthesis, and this effect appears to be a necessary component of the lethal event. However, inhibition of bacterial protein synthesis is not a sufficient expla-

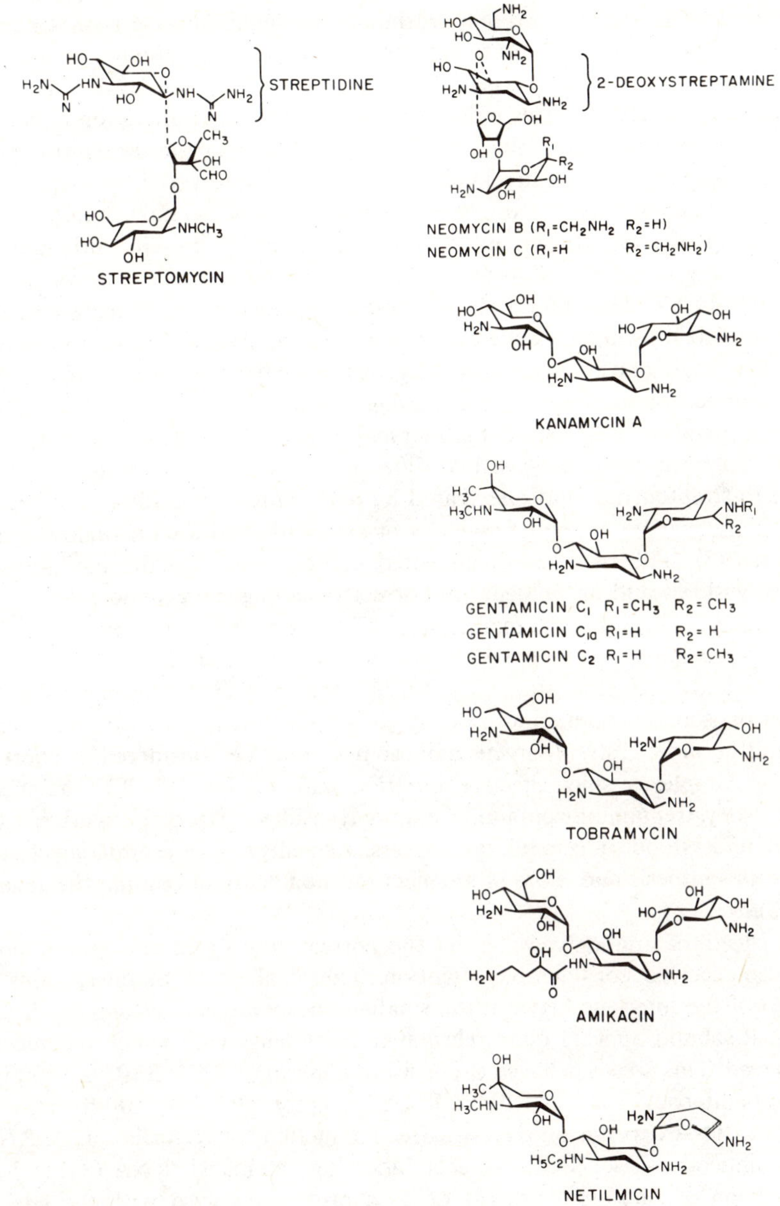

FIGURE 1. Structures of aminoglycosides.

nation for aminoglycoside lethality, and a second target for aminoglycoside effect appears to be necessary. The second target has remained elusive (6,7).

Aminoglycosides inhibit protein synthesis after interacting with one or more ribosomal binding sites. The interactions appear to be specifically localized to the interface between the smaller ribosomal subunit and the larger ribosomal subunit, an area that includes individual proteins of the smaller ribosomal unit (S3, S4, S5, and S12), as well as at least one protein of the larger ribosomal subunit (L6) (8–12). Streptomycin binds specifically, rapidly, tightly, and reversibly in a 1 : 1 stoichiometric ratio with the smaller 30s ribosomal subunit (13,14). The binding of streptomycin is dependent on the S12 protein, although the actual binding is not to this protein but to an adjacent area in the vicinity of S3 and S5 (15,16). The other aminoglycosides that have been studied (including neomycin, kanamycin, gentamicin, and tobramycin) appear to bind to multiple ribosomal binding sites on both the larger and smaller ribosomal subunits and fail to compete with streptomycin binding to the smaller subunit (13). Thus, the exact site of aminoglycoside binding may differ among the aminoglycosides, and there appear to be at least two different types of ribosomal binding, one unique to streptomycin and one shared by other aminoglycosides.

The consequences of the interactions of aminoglycosides with ribosomes are numerous (7). The two best-documented consequences are the inhibition of protein synthesis and an infidelity in correctly reading the genetic code.

Streptomycin prevents the maintenance of polysomal function by stimulating polysome breakdown to monosomes, thereby precluding effective peptide bond formation and chain elongation (17). These "streptomycin monosomes" dissociate into ribosomal subunits more slowly than do normally released monosomes (18). Furthermore, "streptomycin monosomes" may be considered as abortive initiation complexes, since effective initiation cannot occur (18–20). The effects of the deoxystreptamine-containing aminoglycosides on protein synthesis are less well understood. In general, there is less of an effect of these aminoglycosides on protein synthesis and more of an effect on the fidelity of reading the genetic code (8).

The effects of aminoglycosides on the correct reading of the genetic code have also received considerable attention. The localization of interactions to the area of the interface between the smaller ribosomal subunit and the larger ribosomal subunit appears quite relevant to the fidelity with which the genetic code is read. This area is believed to consist of messenger-RNA (mRNA) binding sites and aminoacyl-transfer-RNA (tRNA) acceptor sites. The faithful translation of the RNA depends on the error-free interaction between ribosomes, RNA and the anticodon associated with each incoming aminoacyl-tRNA (8–11). The identification of ribosomal protein L6 as a protein involved with the fidelity of codon–anticodon recognition and its function in terms of determining aminoglycoside sensitivity or resistance suggests an important role for this protein in the process of aminoglycoside-induced misreading of the genetic code (10). As a result of faulty codon–anticodon recognition, "fraudulent" proteins and proteins of abnormal length are synthesized in the presence of aminoglycosides.

These effects of aminoglycosides are less prominent with streptomycin and more prominent with deoxystreptamine-containing members of the family.

Unfortunately, the relationship between either of the two prominent ribosomal effects of aminoglycosides and aminoglycoside lethality remains inconclusive (7). Other antibacterial agents inhibit protein synthesis at least as effectively as do the aminoglycosides and yet fail to cause a lethal event, that is, produce only bacteriostasis. Thus, the inhibition of protein synthesis appears insufficient to explain the bactericidal effect of aminoglycosides. Similarly, the production of "fraudulent" proteins correlates imperfectly with lethality. Based on the inadequacy of either of these two ribosomal effects to explain lethality, other targets for aminoglycide action must be considered. Hancock has recently provided a thoughtful review of the issues involved in identifying the second target for aminoglycoside lethality (7). Its nature, however, remains speculative.

Although the precise biochemical events leading to aminoglycoside lethality remain to be defined, it is clear that an essential element in the process leading to lethality is the transport of aminoglycosides from the external milieu across the cell membrane and into the interior of the bacterium (6,7,21,22). Aminoglycoside transport by bacteria results in the accumulation of aminoglycosides inside bacterial cells to concentrations far in excess of the external concentrations. Ineffective transport precludes aminoglycoside lethality.

The transport process is energy dependent, and the energetics of transport depend on an electrochemical gradient of protons (designated $\Delta\mu_{H+}$) that is generated by proton extrusion during respiration or adenosine 5′-triphosphate (ATP) hydrolysis (23,24). The electrochemical gradient of protons is composed of both an electrical potential (designated $\Delta\Psi$) and a chemical component (designated as Δ pH), which represents the difference in proton concentrations across a membrane. The transport of aminoglycosides is well correlated with the electrical potential ($\Delta\Psi$), and the effects of several situations in which aminoglycoside transport is impaired can be rationalized by considering this component of the electrochemical gradient of protons (23,24). For example, anaerobiasis is associated with a low magnitude of $\Delta\Psi$ and impaired aminoglycoside transport, a low external pH is associated with a diminution of $\Delta\Psi$ and impaired aminoglycoside transport, an increase in the osmolarity of the environment is associated with a lower $\Delta\Psi$ and less aminoglycoside transport, and bacterial mutants that are unable to maintain a proton gradient are unable to generate a $\Delta\Psi$ and are unable to transport aminoglycosides. In each of these situations in which the electrical potential ($\Delta\Psi$) is diminished, aminoglycoside transport is impaired and relative aminoglycoside resistance is seen.

The transport of aminglycosides also appears to involve a transporter molecule to which the aminoglycosides bind during their internalization. Although the nature of this putative carrier molecule has not been defined, it seems likely that both divalent calcium or magnesium and polyvalent polyamines bind to the same carrier (6,7,22,25). This competition could explain the fact that high external concentrations of calcium, magnesium, or polyamines prevent aminoglycoside transport. The interactions with calcium and magnesium are particularly relevant to the creation of appropriate and consistant media for the in vitro assessment of minimal inhibitory (MIC) or minimal bacteriocidal (MBC) concentrations of aminoglycosides.

Aminoglycoside transport is also blocked by low and clinically relevant concentrations of chloramphenicol (22,26). Thus, in the presence of chloramphenicol the aminoglycosides will be ineffective, at least in those organisms sensitive to chloramphenicol. Whether or not the same phenomenon exists in bacteria resistant to chloramphenicol is unknown.

Mechanisms of Resistance

The usefulness of aminoglycosides depends on their selective toxicity to bacteria as opposed to eucaryotic (including human) cells. This selective toxicity to bacterial cells or, conversely, this selective resistance of eucaryotic cells is due to the inability of the cells of most human organs to transport aminoglycosides and to the failure of aminoglycosides to interact with eucaryotic cytosolic ribosomes (8). Although mitochondrial ribosomes are sensitive to aminoglycosides, mitochondria cannot transport aminoglycosides and mitochondrial protein synthesis is probably unaffected in vivo, even in the few tissues (such as the proximal renal tubule and cochlea) that can internalize aminoglycosides.

Bacterial resistance to aminoglycosides can occur by at least three different mechanisms: ribosomal resistance, ineffective transport, or enzymologic modification of the aminoglycoside.

Ribosomal resistance to streptomycin is dependent on one specific aberrant protein (S12) in the smaller ribosomal subunit. A mutation in S12 leads to loss of ribosomal binding of streptomycin and to very high levels of resistance in a single mutational event (15). At a clinical level, this type of streptomycin resistance is very uncommon in gram-negative bacilli. Ribosomal resistance can also exist for the deoxystreptamine group of aminoglycosides. In contrast to the ribosomal resistance to streptomycin, however, this resistance requires multiple mutational events before high-level resistance is seen, suggesting that more than one site must be altered (10–12). This type of ribosomal resistance is also exceedingly uncommon clinically.

Resistance due to ineffective transport appears to be uncommon in most geographic areas, although a few centers have reported this to be the most common mechanism for aminoglycoside resistance. Genetic defects associated with ineffective transport can be localized to any of numerous proteins, having in common an involvement in bacterial electron transport or adenosine triphosphatase (ATPase) activity (6,7). An inability to maintain the requisite electrical potential appears to be pivotal to each of the known mutants. It is fortunate that this mechanism for aminoglycoside resistance is uncommon, since these transport mutants are defective in the transport of all aminoglycosides.

The most common mechanism for aminoglycoside resistance involves the conjugation of the aminoglycoside with one of three groups, an acetyl group, an adenylyl group, or a phosphoryl group, thereby rendering the aminoglycoside inactive (27,28). The conjugation, in each case, is catalyzed by an enzyme that is produced in the bacterial cell from information contained in an extrachromasomal plasmid. Plasmid-mediated resistance is particularly worrisome because the responsible plasmids can infect other gram-negative bacteria, even of different species, and because information for multiple-resistance mechanisms involving other antibacterial classes can be simultaneously introduced into bacterial cells. A very large number of individual enzymes has been identified, each of which catalyzes the addition of one of the above groups onto a specific site on one or more than one aminoglycoside. The overlapping substrate specificities of the individual inactivating enzymes leads to a bewildering array of possibilities for cross resistance to several aminoglycosides (27,28). For example, an enzyme capable of acetylating an aminoglycoside at the 6 prime position (i.e., the 6 position on one of the aminosugar rings adjacent to the deoxystreptamine ring) can inactivate neomycin, kanamycin, tobramycin, amikacin, and netilmicin but not streptomycin or gentamicin. An enzyme capable of phosphorylating the 3 prime position, however, can inactivate only neomycin and kanamycin. To complicate the picture even further, isoenzymes have been identified for many of the specific enzymatic functions. Thus, there may be several unique isoenzymes, each capable of catalyzing the addition of an acetyl group to the 6 prime position of an aminoglycoside but each possessing different substrate specificity so that one might inactivate kanamycin whereas another might inactivate tobramycin. Thus, an incredible multiplicity of possibilities exists for cross resistance to multiple aminoglycosides.

The prevalence of individual aminoglycoside-inactivating enzymes varies widely both with respect to place and time. Thus, whereas the 2-double prime adenyltransferase, 3-acetyltransferase, and 6-prime acetyltransferase are predominant in that order in the United States, the 6-prime acetyltransferase is most common in Japan and the 3-acetyltransferase is most common in Chile (28). Further geographic variability exists between hospitals in any one country, state, or city and even between wards in one hospital. The reasons for this variability have remained an enigma. A simple relationship to patterns of aminoglycoside usage does not exist. This may be explicable in part by the overlapping of aminoglycoside resistance generated by each of the inactivating enzymes. Thus, the prevalence of resistance to amikacin might be expected to be lessened by the infrequent use of amikacin and the consequent diminished genetic pressure for the emergence of amikacin-inactivating enzymes. This may well be partially negated by the continued use of other aminoglycosides that can also be inactivated by the same enzymes that are capable of inactivating amikacin. For example, the continued use of kanamycin, tobramycin, or netilmicin should provide genetic pressure for the emergence of a 6-prime acetylating enzyme; the continued use of kanamycin or tobramycin should provide pressure for the emergence of a 4-prime adenylating enzyme; and the continued use of any of the available deoxystreptamine-containing aminoglycosides should provide pressure for the emergence of a 2-double prime phosphorylating enzyme.

At a clinical level, there are several conclusions that are justifiable by the current information on aminoglycoside resistance.

First, we cannot predict the precise enzymologic mechanism responsible for aminoglycoside resistance in an individual patient. Although resistance patterns may be known for a particular time and place, these patterns can be helpful only in the selection of an initial aminoglycoside to be used before the determination of the specific sensitivity of the individual patient's pathogen.

Second, it is seldom feasible to determine the precise enzymologic mechanism responsible for aminoglycoside resistance, and we must rely on more general tests of sensitivity and resistance such as the MIC or MBC.

Third, it may be futile to reserve an individual aminoglycoside for future use in hopes of delaying the emergence of resistance, since the continued use of other aminoglycosides that are inactivated by the same enzymes may provide sufficient genetic pressure for the emergence of the enzyme that can inactivate the reserved drug.

Spectrum of In Vitro Activity

The spectrum of in vitro activity of the aminoglycosides includes primarily aerobic and facultative gram-negative bacilli and *Staphylococcus aureus.* A representative summary of MICs at which 75 or 100 percent of the strains of various bacteria are sensitive in one laboratory is shown in Table 1 (29). Some hospitals have more aminoslycoside resistance than that shown in the table. In general, aminoglycosides are not often used for known staphylococcal infections since a number of alternative antibiotics has considerably more data backing their clinical efficacy. Aminoglycosides are considered excellent choices for serious infections caused by aerobic or facultative gram-negative bacilli and especially those caused by *Pseudomonas aeruginosa.* For these latter infections, in spite of some in vitro differences in MICs, there is no clinical evidence to substantiate an advantage for any one of the aminoglycosides in treating an infection due to a susceptible organism. Thus, although the percentage of resistant strains in a given locale may dictate the most rational initial aminoglycoside to be used, equivalent effectiveness should be expected from any of this group in treating a patient with a sensitive organism. Nevertheless, differences in in vitro activity do exist with respect to some bacteria. Streptomycin has the greatest in vitro activity against *Mycobacterium tuberculosis,* is considered the drug of choice for *Francisella tularensis* and *Yersinia pestis,* and is often used in brucellosis (30). Streptomycin is seldom used for aerobic or facultative gram-negative bacillary infections due to the frequency of resistance (30). Kanamycin is limited in its spectrum, compared to the other 2-deoxystreptamine-containing aminoglycosides, because of the common resistance of *P. aeruginosa* (30). Kanamycin is also inactivated by a large number of the plasmid-mediated enzymes and consequently kanamycin resistance among other gram-negative bacilli is prevalent in many locales. Gentamicin and tobramycin share very similar in vitro profiles, although gentamicin is somewhat more potent in vitro against *Serratia* species and tobramycin somewhat more potent against *P. aeruginosa* (29). However, these minor differences in in vitro potencies have not been demonstrated to correlate with greater in vivo effectiveness. Since gentamicin and tobramycin

TABLE 1. In Vitro Susceptibility of Various Bacteria to Five Aminoglycosides[a]

	Kanamycin		*Gentamicin*		*Tobramycin*		*Amikacin*		*Netilmicin*	
Organism (No.)	*75%*	*100%*	*75%*	*100%*	*75%*	*100%*	*75%*	*100%*	*75%*	*100%*
Staphylococcus aureus (25)	1.6	3.1	≤0.2	0.8	≤0.2	6.2	1.6	3.1	0.4	0.8
Enterococci (20)	12.5	>50	3.1	6.2	6.2	12.5	25	50	3.1	6.2
Neisseria gonorrhoeae (20)	12.5	25	6.2	12.5	6.2	12.5	25	50	6.2	12.5
Escherichia coli (40)	12.5	>50	1.6	6.2	3.1	12.5	6.2	12.5	1.6	6.2
Klebsiella sp. (20)	3.1	>50	0.4	1.6	0.4	1.6	1.6	6.2	0.4	0.8
Enterobacter sp. (40)	3.1	>50	0.8	1.6	1.6	6.2	1.6	6.2	0.4	6.2
Citrobacter sp. (15)	12.5	25	1.6	6.2	1.6	1.6	3.1	6.2	0.8	3.1
Serratia sp. (15)	3.1	6.2	1.6	1.6	3.1	6.2	3.1	6.2	1.6	3.2
Proteus mirabillis (20)	3.1	25	1.6	3.1	1.6	3.1	6.2	12.5	1.6	3.1
Morganella morganii (29)	3.1	6.2	0.8	0.8	0.8	1.6	3.1	6.2	0.8	1.6
Proteus vulgaris (6)	6.2	6.2	1.6	1.6	1.6	3.1	3.1	6.2	0.8	0.8
Providencia rettgeri (6)	3.1	3.1	3.1	6.2	3.1	6.2	1.6	1.6	12.5	12.5
Providencia stuartii (8)	1.6	3.1	3.1	6.2	3.1	12.5	3.1	3.1	3.1	12.5
Pseudomonas aeruginosa (40)	ND	ND	0.8	3.1	≤0.2	1.6	0.8	12.5	0.8	6.2

SOURCE: Data derived from Ref. 29.

[a] MIC (μg/ml) for percent of strains indicated.

are both susceptible to the same enzymologic modifications (save for a few uncommon enzymes that can inactivate gentamicin and not tobramycin), the percentage of resistant strains to these two aminoglycosides is also quite similar (29). Amikacin has a clear advantage over gentamicin or tobramycin as a result of its resistance to many of the common plasmid-mediated enzymes. Consequently, the percentage of strains susceptible to amikacin is significantly greater for amikacin compared to gentamicin or tobramycin (29). The in vitro potency of amikacin with respect to many of the gram-negative bacilli is less than that of gentamicin or tobramycin, but the dose that is allowed by its lesser toxicity (i.e., three to four times the dose of gentamicin or tobramycin) compensates for this lesser potency. Again, there is no clinical evidence to suggest lesser or greater effectiveness against sensitive bacteria. Netilmicin shares the spectrum of gentamicin and tobramycin in general. However, netilmicin is resistant to aminoglycoside-adenylylating enzymes and as a result some *Escherichia coli, Klebsiella, Enterobacter,* and *Citrobacter* isolates that are resistant to gentamicin remain sensitive to netilmicin (31). Gentamicin-resistant *Serratia, Proteus, Providencia,* and *Pseudomonas* strains are, however, usually also netilmicin resistant (32).

In vitro sensitivity and resistance to aminoglycosides is usually determined as a minimal inhibitory concentration. Since the minimal bactericidal concentration is nearly always close to the MIC, there is no advantage associated with this more cumbersome technique. The MIC is most frequently assessed by a disk diffusion method but may be more accurately quantified by either agar dilution or broth dilution methods (30). For the disk diffusion method, standards have been set for the aminoglycoside content of the individual disks, zone diameters, and agar composition (33). Standardization of agar diffusion and broth dilution methods is also important since several variables in the media can significantly influence the MIC, especially pH and cation concentration (34). These variables affect the MIC determinations primarily by affecting transport of the aminoglycosides into the bacteria. An acid pH of the media will provide erroneously high MICs, whereas an alkaline pH will give an erroneously low MIC. The pH of the agar or broth should be kept at pH 7.3–7.5. High concentrations of cations, especially calcium, magnesium, and sodium, yield erroneously high MICs, especially with *P. aeruginosa* (34). Standardization of the calcium salt concentration at about 50 μg/ml and the magnesium salt concentration at about 25 μg/ml has been proposed (34). The number of bacteria used should also be standardized, although the "inoculum effect" is far less important with aminoglycosides than with β-lactams (30). The relative lack of inoculum effect is attributable to the failure of aminoglycoside-inactivating enzymes to be released into the medium. Thus, the concentration of aminoglycoside in the medium will remain nearly constant, even with large inocula of resistant bacteria.

Time Course of Antibacterial Effects

Each of the routine methods of determining an MIC provides a constant concentration of antibiotic adjacent to the bacterium for the entire period of incubation.

Thus, the MIC should be interpreted as the lowest concentration that inhibits bacterial growth *if constantly adjacent to the bacterium.*

Recent interest has focused on more sophisticated systems to assess the in vitro effects of changing concentrations of antibiotics (35–41). Although these systems are not feasible for the routine definition of in vitro activity of antibiotics, they contribute significantly to an understanding of the complex interrelationships between the pharmacokinetics of the antibiotic and the kinetics of bacterial growth. In these systems with continously decreasing aminoglycoside concentrations adjacent to continuously growing bacteria, there is a rapid resumption of the inhibited bacterial growth as the aminoglycoside concentration drops below a level approximating the MIC for *E. coli* or *S. aureus* (40–44). The same may also be true for *P. aeruginosa,* although the evidence appears to be conflicting on the persistence of an aminoglycoside effect in this species (40,44). These results would seem to suggest that the aminoglycoside level adjacent to the bacteria should not be allowed to drop below the MIC for very long, at least with respect to *E. coli* and *S. aureus.*

Synergism

Aminoglycosides frequently exhibit synergism with other antibiotics. Especially noteworthy is the synergism usually found in enterococcal species between penicillin or vancomycin and the aminoglycosides (45). The mechanism of this synergism involves the enhancement of aminoglycoside uptake into cells whose wall has been damaged by the cell wall inhibitor (46). Numerous other synergistic combinations involving an aminoglycoside also exist.

INTERACTIONS WITH HUMANS

Pharmacokinetics

The pharmacokinetics of all of the aminoglycosides are quite similar. Subtle differences among individual members of the family may have importance with respect to the pathophysiology of their toxicities, but these minor differences are unimportant with respect to rational dosing.

Absorption. The extent of absorption of oral aminoglycosides is unpredictable but always low (47–51). Consequently, aminoglycosides are generally considered as nonabsorbable antibiotics and are occasionally used to alter the gut flora. In the presence of impaired elimination, however, even a small amount of absorbed aminoglycoside may accumulate to toxic levels (52–55).

Absorption after intramuscular aminoglycoside administration is both complete and rapid, with maximal plasma levels achieved between 30 and 90 minutes (56,57). Impaired tissue perfusion, as in shock, delays the absorption of intramuscular aminoglycosides.

Intravenous aminoglycoside administration is frequently used in patients with serious infections, and the dose is completely delivered to the vascular space. When the intravenous infusion lasts for 20–30 minutes, the plasma levels are similar to those achieved by intramuscular administration.

Topical aminoglycosides generally either are not absorbed or only minimally absorbed. Exceptions include patients with extensive epidermal loss due to burns or epidermolysis and patients with open wounds in which significant absorption can occur (58,59).

Intraperitoneal or intrapleural aminoglycosides are rapidly absorbed, quickly providing plasma levels that are dependent on the concentration of drug instilled into the peritoneal or pleural fluid (60,61). Administration of large amounts of aminoglycosides can result in very high plasma levels and toxicity.

Bladder irrigation is not associated with significant aminoglycoside absorption (62), intratracheal or aerosolized aminoglycosides are poorly absorbed (63,64), and intrathecal or intraventricular aminoglycosides produce negligible plasma levels (65).

Distribution. Aminoglycosides are freely distributed in the vascular space and relatively freely distributed in the interstitial spaces of most tissues. Although the mean aminoglycoside concentration in interstitial fluids approximates the mean plasma concentration at steady state with repetitive dosing, the peak concentrations are lower, the oscillations between peak and trough concentrations are less, and the rate of elimination is slower from interstitial fluids (66).

Because of their size and polycationic charge, aminoglycosides cross biologic membranes that lack transport mechanisms very poorly. This accounts for their low intracellular concentrations in nearly all human tissues. An exception is the proximal renal tubular cell, which appears to have a unique transport mechanism and can concentrate aminoglycosides to levels far in excess of plasma or interstitial fluid levels (67).

Aminoglycosides enter bronchial secretions poorly, attaining mean levels approximately 20 percent of mean plasma levels (68). Intermittent administration produces higher peak levels in bronchial secretions than does continuous infusion, but areas under the concentration versus time curves are similar (68,69). Neither mode of delivery produces high aminoglycoside levels in bronchial secretions, however, and the direct intratracheal administration of aminoglycosides to patients with serious gram-negative pneumonitis has been advocated on the basis of higher levels in bronchial secretions and greater clinical effectiveness (69).

Intravenous or intramuscular administration of aminoglycosides to adults produces very low aminoglycoside levels in the cerebrospinal fluid (65,70,71). In newborns cerebrospinal fluid levels are higher relative to plasma levels (72). Intrathecal administration in the lumbar area produces high lumbar cerebrospinal fluid levels but poor intraventricular levels, whereas intraventricular administration produces high levels in both ventricular fluid and lumbar cerebrospinal fluid (70). Based on these findings, intraventricular aminoglycoside administration has been proposed for gram-negative bacillary meningitis in adults (70,71). In the newborn, intraventricular aminoglycoside administration has been shown to be no more effective and possibly more toxic than intravenous administration alone (72).

Aminoglycoside distribution in the eye has been studied after repetitive intramuscular or continuous intravenous dosing in the rabbit. The cornea and aqueous fluids attain levels approximating serum levels, whereas entry into vitreous fluid is slow and mean vitreous levels are only about 40 percent of serum levels over a 12-hour period (73). Subconjunctival injection produces high aqueous fluid levels of aminoglycosides in humans (74). However, neither systemic nor subconjunctival aminoglycoside administration in single doses produces reliable levels in the vitreous humor of humans, and intravitreal injection has been advocated in the treatment of endophthalmitis (75).

Aminoglycosides enter the synovial fluid rather easily and achieve levels only modestly less than simultaneously measured plasma levels (76–80).

Aminoglycosides penetrate into prostatic fluid poorly, and levels are low compared to plasma levels (81).

Aminoglycosides do not enter saliva (82).

The biliary concentrations of aminoglycosides are significantly less than the plasma levels (83,84).

Urinary concentrations of aminoglycosides reach levels about 25–100 times peak plasma aminoglycoside concentrations within an hour after dosing and remain well above therapeutic levels for several days after even a single dose (85–88). After termination of a multiple dosing regimen, urinary aminoglycoside concentrations remain above therapeutic levels for many days, with a terminal half-life of about 48–200 hours (86–89).

Metabolism. Aminoglycosides are not metabolized by humans.

Excretion. Aminoglycosides are eliminated entirely as unchanged drugs and almost entirely from the kidneys. Less than 1 percent of a parenterally administered dose appears in the feces and none in saliva (90,91).

Aminoglycosides are filtered by the glomerulus. Although they are negligibly protein bound, their filtration is not completely free since their polycationic nature appears to impede filtration at the positively charged glomerular capillary surface (92). After entering the luminal fluid of the proximal renal tubule, a small but toxicologically important portion of the total filtered aminoglycoside is reabsorbed exclusively into the proximal renal tubular cells (67,93,94). This reabsorption appears to involve binding of the aminoglycosides to negatively charged phospholipids in the renal tubular brush border membranes with subsequent internalization by pinocytosis (95–99). There is no conclusive evidence for secretion of aminoglycosides into the urine. Quantitatively, most of the filtered aminoglycoside is excreted into the urine.

OVERALL PHARMACOKINETICS

The overall pharmacokinetics of aminoglycosides can be quite accurately described as a composite of contributions from absorption and three phases of elimination (100,101). Since absorption is predictably complete and rapid after either intramuscular or intermittent intravenous administration, it is the three phases of elimination that deserve emphasis.

The three phases of aminoglycoside elimination can be considered to be related to three connected compartments in the commonly used model of the pharmacokinetic behavior of drugs or simply as mathematical components of a triexponential equation that has been found to fit the experimentally derived decay curve of plasma aminoglycoside levels versus time. Although neither of the above approaches allows the designation of anatomic or physiologic spaces for the compartments or for the components of the equation, it is clearly of practical value to consider the disposition of aminoglycosides in physiologic terms.

The first (or alpha or distributive) phase of aminoglycoside elimination is made up predominantly of the process of drug distribution from the vascular space to some extravascular space. Since aminoglycosides enter most cells poorly, the extravascular space may be considered to be similar to the extracellular fluid volume. The time course of this phase can be described as having a half-life of about 15–30 minutes (100–102). Measurement of plasma aminoglycoside levels after the end of this phase provides levels that approach the levels in interstitial fluid and avoid the rapidly changing plasma levels that occur earlier. For this reason it has been suggested that "peak" aminoglycoside levels should be drawn 30 minutes–1 hour after the end of an intravenous infusion (103).

The second (or beta) phase of aminoglycoside elimination involves the excretion of the drug from the plasma and simultaneously from most of the extravascular space. The time course of this beta phase is determined nearly exclusively by the glomular filtration rate, and it is this phase that is most important in terms of clinical dosing. It is also this phase that is altered by a number of clinically important factors as discussed below. In the young healthy adult with normal renal function this phase can be reasonably described by a small number of pharmacokinetic parameters. The volume of distribution is about 25–30 percent of body weight (104–106), the half-life is 1.5–3.5 hours (104–107), and the plasma clearance is about 1 ml/min/kg (108). Each of these pharmacokinetic parameters can be altered, however, by a number of clinically important conditions, and rational dosing of the aminoglycosides must take cognizance of these alterations, which are described below.

The third (or gamma) phase of aminoglycoside elimination involves the prolonged and slow excretion of the drug from the plasma and simultaneously from a relatively small portion of an extravascular space either through the plasma space or directly into the urine. This portion of the extravascular space has been termed a *deep compartment* to distinguish it from the portion of the extravascular space that readily equilibrates with the vascular space. It has also been considered to represent primarily the kidneys since aminoglycosides accumulate in kidney parenchymal tissue and leave very slowly. The importance of this third phase of aminoglycoside elimination has been clearly demonstrated in terms of rigorously describing the overall pharmacokinetics of aminoglycoside elimination (100,109–111). However, the importance of this phase in terms of rational aminoglycoside dosing remains unclear. The third phase can be described in pharmacokinetic terms as having a large volume of distribution (the volume of distribution at steady state) of 45–100 percent of the body weight, a very long half-life of 35–200 hours, and a clearance of about 1 ml/min/kg (100, 101,109–111). The influence of various clinical conditions on the pharmacokinetics of the third phase have not been defined, although individual aminoglycosides appear to vary with respect to their volumes of distribution at steady state (100,101,109–111).

Alterations with Age. The pharmacokinetics of aminoglycosides in both children and the elderly differ significantly from those in young healthy adults. The differences are attributable to known differences in glomerular function in newborns, children, and the elderly and are seen primarily as deviations during the second phase of elimination.

In the newborn the volume of distribution is considerably larger as a percentage of body weight (34–78 percent), and the half-life of the second phase is significantly prolonged (3–14 hours). Both the volume of distribution and the half-life of the second phase are inversely correlated with either gestational age or postnatal age (112–120).

After the newborn period, infants and children have volumes of distribution that are close to those of young adults and half-lives that are shorter (0.4–3 hours) than those of young adults (112,120–130).

In the elderly the volumes of distribution are similar to those of young adults, but the half-lives are considerably longer due to decreased glomerular function with age (131). Since the diminution in glomerular function in the elderly is not necessarily reflected in a higher serum creatinine (due to a decrease in creatinine production in the elderly), it is important to use a calculated creatinine clearance (C_{cr}) in order to estimate the half-life or clearance of an aminoglycoside in the elderly (132). The equation of Cockcroft and Gault is as follows:

$$C_{cr}(\text{ml/min}) = \frac{(140 - \text{age}) \times \text{weight}}{\text{Cr} \times 72}$$

Its modification by Spyker and Guerrant is as follows:

$$C_{cr}(\text{ml/min}) = \frac{(140 - \text{age}) \times (1.03 - 0.053 \times \text{Cr})}{\text{Cr}}$$

The nomogram of Siersbaek-Nielson et al. is useful in calculating the creatinine clearance (132–134). In the above equations weight is in kilograms, creatinine in milligrams per deciliter, and age in years.

Alterations with Disease States. Kidney disease with glomerular dysfunction is the most common disease state associated with altered aminoglycoside pharmcokinetics. The clearance of an aminoglycoside is linearly related to the clearance of creatinine since aminoglycosides are nearly entirely eliminated renally and their elimination rate is highly dependent on the glomerular filtration rate. A useful estimation of aminoglycoside clearance (135) is given by the following equation:

$$\text{Aminoglycoside clearance} = (C_{cr})(0.6) + 10$$

Since the creatinine clearance, as a measure of glomerular filtration rate, can also be calculated reasonably accurately using the equation of Cockcroft and Gault (given above), we can easily estimate the clearance of an aminoglycoside in a patient with renal disease. The volume of distribution as a percent of body weight of an aminoglycoside may be increased in patients with marked renal dysfunction (135–137). The half-life, which is a function of the ratio of the volume of distribution to clearance, is prolonged in patients with renal disease and may in fact be somewhat longer than would be predicted on the basis of the creatinine clearance alone due to the somewhat larger volume of distribution.

In obese patients, the volume of distribution of aminoglycosides as a fraction of the total body weight is about 75 percent of that seen in nonobese patients or about 20 percent of total body weight. The rates of elimination and half-lives, however, are similar in obese and nonobese patients (138,139).

Conversely, in protein–calorie malnutrition (marasmus) the volume of distribution of aminoglycosides as a fraction of the total body weight is about 120 percent of that seen in well-nourished patients (140).

Fever appears to alter aminoglycoside pharmacokinetics. Lower plasma aminoglycoside levels are found in febrile patients (141).

In severe burns the glomerular filtration rate and consequently the rate of elimination of aminoglycosides may be markedly enhanced (142,143).

Alterations with Other Drugs. The aminoglycosides can be inactivated by many of the β-lactam antibiotics in vitro and to a lesser extent in vivo. The inactivation occurs as a result of a covalent bond being formed between the carboxyl group of a broken β-lactam ring and an amino group on the aminoglycoside. The reaction occurs at high molar ratios of β-lactam to aminoglycoside and is thus especially important when carbenicillin or ticarcillin is used with an aminoglycoside since large doses of these β-lactams provide the requisite high molar ratios. Since 1 mol of β-lactam is inactivated at the same time that 1 mol of aminoglycoside is being inactivated, theoretically there should be a loss of both activities. The disproportionate number of β-lactam molecules, however, is not significantly diminished by having lost a few molecules through these interactions. The reaction occurs more readily in a protein free setting and, therefore, the reaction is more relevant to the situation in an intravenous bottle containing both drugs than to the patient containing both drugs. The rapid elimination of most β-lactams also tends to minimize the ability of the β-lactam to inactivate the aminoglycoside since the required molar ratios of the two antibiotics exist for only a brief period in patients with normal renal function. The shortening of the half-life of the aminoglycoside in patients with renal failure may be clinically significant.

Aminoglycoside Dosing

The existence of extensive pharmacokinetic data on aminoglycosides provides information that permits the construction of dosage regimens that will achieve and maintain plasma aminoglycoside levels within practically any desired range. Numerous dosage regimens have been proposed, and extensive and rigorous clinical trials have been conducted with a few of the proposed regimens. However, studies comparing one regimen to another with respect to both effectiveness and safety are virtually nonexistent. A dosage regimen that has been used extensively and rigorously and that has been carefully assessed with respect to both effectiveness and toxicity is presented as one approach (103). Although other regimens may be equally or even more effective and equally or even less toxic, there is currently no comparative information to verify such differences.

Initiation of therapy should involve the administration of a loading dose of aminoglycoside in order to achieve therapeutic aminoglycoside plasma levels quickly. This principle is especially relevant in situations in which the elimination of the aminoglycoside is delayed since in these situations it will take many hours to achieve a plateau level unless a loading dose is given. The loading dose will be determined exclusively by the volume of distribution of the aminoglycoside and the desired maximum plasma aminoglycoside level. Considerable evidence suggests that a reasonable goal in terms of the maximal plasma aminoglycoside level is between 5 and 10 μg/ml for gentamicin, tobramycin, and netilmicin and between 20 and 40 μg/ml for kanamycin and amikacin (144–148). Based on an average volume of distribution of 25 percent of the body weight, a loading dose of 1.5–2 mg/kg for gentamicin, tobramycin, or netilmicin or 7.5–8 mg/kg for kanamycin or amikacin will provide plasma levels of 6–8 and 30–32 μg/ml, respectively.

Several aspects of the loading dose deserve emphasis. First, the loading dose should be the same whether or not there is reason to believe that elimination will be impaired. Thus, no matter what the degree of renal dysfunction, the same loading dose should be given. Second, in calculating a loading dose, we should aim at the maximal plasma level desired since some drug will be eliminated before the first maintenance dose and we would not choose to provide suboptimal levels during the critical initiation of aminoglycoside therapy. Third, the loading dose should be given intravenously over 20–30 minutes or intramuscularly rather than as a rapid intravenous bolus in order to minimize the risk of transient neuromuscular paralysis.

The next step is to calculate a maintenance dosage regimen, including the size of individual doses and the dosing intervals. In adult patients with normal renal function, a dose of 1.5–2 mg/kg of gentamicin, tobramycin, or netilmicin given every 8 hours or 7.5–8 mg/kg of kanamycin or amikacin given every 12 hours will provide levels that oscillate between peaks of about 8 or 32 μg/ml, respectively, and troughs of about 1 or 4 μg/ml, respectively.

In patients with diminished renal glomerular function, the total daily dose of aminoglycosides must be reduced. A convenient method of calculating the appropriate daily dose of an aminoglycoside in the presence of renal glomerular dysfunction is to multiply the usual daily dose for a patient with normal renal function by the ratio of the clearance of the drug in renal insufficiency to the clearance of the drug with normal renal function. Since the clearance of aminoglycosides is linearly related to the endogenous creatinine clearance, the ratio of the patient's creatinine clearance to normal creatinine clearance will closely approximate the ratio of aminoglycoside clearances. Thus, if the calculated creatinine clearance, taking into account the patient's age, sex, weight, and serum creatinine, is 40 ml/min/1.73 m^2, the appropriate ratio is (40 ml/min/1.73 m^2)/ (100 ml/min/1.73 m^2) = 0.4, and the total daily aminoglycoside dose should be 0.4 times or 40 percent of the usual daily aminoglycoside dose. Instead of 4.5–6 mg/kg/day, the reduced dose should be 1.8–2.4 mg/kg/day.

Having derived a reduced daily maintenance dose, there are two commonly advocated methods of giving the reduced dose. One can either reduce the individual dose given at the usual dosage interval or give the usual individual dose at less frequent intervals. There is currently no evidence to support one method over the other.

It must be emphasized that any calculation of dosage reduction will be approximate and should only be used to provide an estimate of the appropriate maintenance dose. As soon as convenient (usually within 24–48 hours), plasma aminoglycoside levels should be measured and the maintenance doses adjusted to provide selected plasma levels. Plasma levels of 5–10 μg/ml 30 minutes–1 hour after the end of an intravenous infusion over 20–30 minutes or after an intramuscular injection of gentamicin, tobramycin, or netilmicin have been associated with effectiveness and acceptibly low toxicity as have plasma levels of 20–40 μg/ml for amikacin (and presumably kanamycin)(103,149).

Aminoglycoside Toxicity

All aminoglycosides share three principal toxicities, although there are quantitative differences among individual aminoglycosides for each of the three. The principal toxicities are neuromuscular paralysis, ototoxicity, and nephrotoxicity. Although the detailed mechanisms involved in these toxicities remain to be defined, an intriguing thread that appears to run through each involves the interactions of the polycationic aminoglycosides, polyamines, calcium, and magnesium with the polyanionic phosphatidylinositol, phosphatidylinositol diphosphate, and phosphatidylinositol triphosphate.

Neuromuscular Paralysis. The aminoglycosides are all capable of producing clinically significant neuromuscular paralysis. Whereas this phenomenon is rare, it is potentially quite serious.

The mechanism responsible for aminoglycoside-induced neuromuscular paralysis appears to involve both an inhibition of the presynaptic release of acetylcholine and a blockade of the postsynaptic receptor sites for acetylcholine. The presynaptic site of inhibition is dependent on the ability of an aminoglycoside to inhibit the internalization of calcium into the presynaptic region of the neuronal axon, thus preventing an event that necessarily precedes the release of acetylcholine (150). This presynaptic effect is manifest more by neomycin or tobramycin than by streptomycin and is prevented or reversed by the provision of additional local calcium (150–152). The postsynaptic site of blockade involves an effect on the postsynaptic receptor for acetylcholine such that the response to acetylcholine is blunted. The postsynaptic effect is produced more potently by streptomycin or netilmicin than by neomycin (151,152).

The neuromuscular paralysis associated with aminoglycosides is enhanced by the presence of curarelike drugs, succinylcholine, magnesium, by the simultaneous presence of botulinus toxin in patients with botulism, and in patients with myasthenia gravis (153–158).

The neuromuscular paralysis of aminoglycosides is clearly associated with the presence of very high concentrations of drug at the neuromuscular junctions. Sufficiently high concentrations are achieved only by the very rapid intravenous administration of a bolus of aminoglycoside or as a result of absorption of the drug from the pleural or peritoneal space after instillation of a highly concentrated solution.

The neuromuscular paralysis of aminoglycosides can be prevented by administering intravenous doses over 20–30 minutes, by the intramuscular administration of the drugs, and by the instillation of less concentrated solutions into the pleural or peritoneal spaces.

Once manifest, the neuromuscular paralysis of aminoglycosides can be treated by the prompt administration of calcium. Neostigmine has also been advocated, but neostigmine may be less rational if it is the presynaptic release of acetylcholine that is inhibited by aminoglycosides.

Aminoglycosides are capable of inhibiting both myocardial and vascular smooth muscle contractility in experimental situations but the clinical relevance is uncertain (159–161).

Ototoxicity. All aminoglycosides are capable of causing ototoxicity. Although individual aminoglycosides preferentially produce either auditory toxicity or vestibular toxicity in experimental animals, all aminoglycosides are capable of producing both in humans. Although relatively uncommon, ototoxicity is especially worrisome because of its frequent irreversibility, its occurrence even after discontinuation of the drug, and its cumulative nature with repeated courses of the drug (162).

The mechanism of auditory toxicity of aminoglycosides involves the selective destruction of the outer hair cells of the organ of Corti, especially those located in the basal turn (162–165). Subsequently, retrograde degeneration of the auditory nerve occurs (166). Inner hair cells and cells of the stria vascularis are affected with more extensive damage. The vestibular system is affected primarily by damage to type I hair cells of the summit of the ampullar cristae (167). Neither cochlear nor ampullar cells can regenerate once they have been destroyed, thus accounting for irreversibility.

The cellular damage may be related to the concentrations of aminoglycosides in the perilymph and endolymph that bathe the relevant cells. Aminoglycosides enter and leave the perilymph slowly when compared to their pharmacokinetics in plasma (168). Endolymph levels rise and disappear even more slowly (168). Thus cells bathed by these fluids may be exposed to aminoglycosides for prolonged periods of time even after discontinuation of the drug.

The biochemical events associated with aminoglycoside ototoxicity appear to be biphasic with an immediate effect that is reversible by calcium and a subsequent irreversible event that may involve binding of the aminoglycoside by phosphatidylinositol biphosphate (169,170). An inhibition of a sodium–potassium ATPase has also been found (171). This inhibition might lead to alterations in endolymph or perilymph ion gradients with subsequent effects on the integrity of cochlear cells.

The incidence of aminoglycoside-induced auditory and vestibular toxicity in humans is quite low if clinically detectable hearing loss or vestibular dysfunction is required, but it is clearly higher if more sensitive measures of auditory or vestibular function, such as audiometry or electronystagmography, are used. Large prospective comparative clinical trials of aminoglycosides, usually using rigorous dosing regimens, have delineated relative incidences of aminoglycoside ototoxicity and have also contributed significantly to an understanding of the clinical course of the ototoxicity and risk factors involved with the development of ototoxicity.

Clinically detectable toxicity has been reported to occur in 3–5 percent of patients receiving gentamicin, tobramycin, or amikacin and in whom audiometric testing could be performed (172,173). In other extensive clinical trials of gentamicin, tobramycin, and amikacin, only 3 patients with clinically detectable hearing loss were seen out of a total of 674 patients receiving an aminoglycoside. Thus another estimate of the incidence of clinically detectable hearing loss is less than 0.5 percent of those receiving an aminoglycoside (103,149).

Using audiometric testing, the incidence of auditory toxicity in patients receiving gentamicin, tobramycin, or amikacin has not been shown to differ significantly when individual aminoglycosides are directly compared (103,149,172,173). Netilmicin, however, has been shown to produce auditory toxicity less frequently than tobramycin in one multicenter study (174).

Vestibular dysfunction has been reported as clinically significant in 0.4 percent of patients receiving gentamicin, tobramycin, or amikacin (172,173) and present by electronystagmography in 4 percent of patients receiving gentamicin and 6 percent of patients receiving amikacin (172). In a prospective but unblinded study tobramycin produced vestibular dysfunction significantly less frequently than did gentamicin (173).

Auditory toxicity associated with aminoglycosides is seen clinically as hearing loss. Although tinnitus and a feeling of fullness in the ears have been said to precede hearing loss, these are clearly unreliable premonitors of auditory toxicity since they often occur without subsequent hearing loss and hearing loss often occurs without these symptoms. The hearing loss is usually bilateral, although unilateral hearing loss has been reported and usually involves the loss of high-tone hearing before the loss of low-tone hearing. The occurrence and severity of the hearing loss are dose related, as well as related to the duration of aminoglycoside therapy (174,175). There is, however, a somewhat less clear relationship between plasma aminoglycoside levels and auditory toxicity. In prospective clinical trials in which aminoglycoside levels have been carefully monitored and adjusted there has been no correlation of auditory toxicity and plasma aminoglycoside levels within the narrow range of levels seen. However, if plasma aminoglycoside levels are not carefully adjusted, high plasma levels would surely be associated with greater auditory toxicity. Transient aminoglycoside levels above the usual limits of 10 μg/ml for gentamicin, tobramycin, and netilmicin or 40 μg/ml for amikacin (and presumably kanamycin) are unlikely to be ototoxic.

Even when plasma aminoglycoside levels are carefully monitored, some patients will suffer hearing loss by audiometry and even clinical hearing loss. Risk factors for the development of auditory toxicity include the duration of aminoglycoside use, the presence of bacteremia, fever, liver dysfunction, and the ratio of serum urea nitrogen to serum creatinine as a measure of hypovolemia (176).

Another important risk factor for auditory aminoglycoside toxicity is the concurrent use of ethacrynic acid (177–179). Fortunately, furosemide at clinically used doses and with proper attention to hydration does not appear to be associated with enhanced aminoglycoside auditory toxicity (179).

Several other potential risk factors that have been identified in experimental animals but that have not yet been proven in humans include noise and age with increased susceptibility in the very young and elderly (180–183).

It bears emphasis that auditory toxicity is cumulative. Thus with repeated aminoglycoside courses, hearing loss may become detectable as a result of cumulative damage even during a carefully monitored course of therapy (173–176). This is surely related to the inability of damaged or destroyed cochlear hair cells to regenerate.

Vestibular dysfunction is manifest clinically by nausea, vomiting, vertigo, dizziness, and an unsteady gait with nystagmus. These symptoms and signs are difficult to evaluate in ill patients. More sophisticated laboratory tests are too cumbersome for use in most ill patients (175).

As with auditory toxicity, vestibular toxicity is dose related, duration related, and probably related to plasma levels outside the therapeutic range. However, because of the difficulties of evaluating vestibular function, it has been less well defined than has been auditory toxicity.

Nephrotoxicity. All aminoglycosides are capable of causing nephrotoxicity, although individual differences exist among members of the family with respect to nephrotoxic potential.

The mechanisms involved in aminoglycoside nephrotoxicity include the rapid transport, extensive accumulation, and avid retention of aminoglycosides for prolonged periods of time. In addition the aminoglycosides are assumed to produce biochemical effects on proximal tubular metabolism that lead to pathophysiologic effects linking proximal tubular damage to diminished glomerular function. The transport of aminoglycosides is primarily across the luminal brush border of the proximal renal tubular cells and involves an initial binding of the positively charged aminoglycoside to the negatively charged phosphatidylinositol within the membrane (93, 95,96,99). Internalization is believed to occur by pinocytosis into vesicles that eventually coalesce with lysosomes whose highly negative interior effectively traps the aminoglycoside (94,184). The extensive accumulation of aminoglycosides is confined to the renal cortex where concentrations 5–50-fold higher than plasma concentrations are found (185). Within the renal cortex the aminoglycosides are further localized exclusively to the proximal renal tubular cells (67,94).

It remains unclear whether the proximal tubular cell damage that is characteristic of the aminoglycosides is attributable to lysosomal or extralysosomal effects. Lysosomes may be a primary site of aminoglycoside toxicity or may be salvage organelles responsible for keeping the intracellular aminoglycoside in a nontoxic site. Morphologically, aminoglycosides cause an accumulation of multilamellar structures within lysosomes called myeloid bodies (184,186,187). Biochemically, aminoglycosides inhibit lysosomal phospholipases A_1, A_2, and C_1 and are also associated with a loss of sphingomyelinase activity (188,189). Extralysosomal effects of aminoglycosides include both structural and functional effects on mitochondria (190–192), the inhibition of a sodium–potassium adenosine triphosphatase localized on the basolateral portion of the plasma membrane (193), and the inhibition of a cytosolic phosphatidylinositol specific phospholipase C (194). The inhibition of this cytosolic phospholipase may be particularly important since this enzyme may be responsible for an early and pivotal step in the biosynthesis of prostaglandins and prostacyclin. Such an effect might be quite relevant to the reduction of glomerular filtration that is produced by the aminoglycosides subsequent to proximal tubular damage since an inhibition of the production of vasodilatory prostaglandins would allow the unopposed vasoconstrictor action of angiotensin II leading to arteriolar vasoconstriction and a decrease in glomerular filtration (195). Structural and functional alterations of glomeruli have also been identified and may be directly related to amingoglycosides or secondary to effects on prostaglandin or angiotensin systems (196–199).

Clinical nephrotoxicity, as defined by a reduced glomerular filtration rate (GFR), occurs in between 5 and 25 percent of aminoglycoside recipients (103,149). The earliest manifestation of an effect of aminoglycosides on the kidney is an increase in the urinary excretion of several renal tubular enzymes, including alanine aminopeptidase, β-D-glucosaminidase, and alkaline phosphatase (200). In addition, the reabsorption of β-2-microglobulin is competitively inhibited and its excretion is enhanced (201). These early indicators of renal effects are too sensitive and too nonspecific to be of clinical value since every patient receiving an aminoglycoside will exhibit these effects (200). It appears to be more useful to define aminoglycoside nephrotoxicity in terms of a reduction in GFR as reflected by a rise in serum creatinine, and the serum creatinine is an adequate and convenient parameter to follow when monitoring for aminoglycoside nephrotoxicity.

The onset of glomerular dysfunction usually occurs several days after the initiation of therapy, although a more rapid onset is possible. The glomerular dysfunction in humans increases in severity over a few days, although in experimental animals a cyclic phenomenon of damage and repair occurs even with continuing administration of the aminoglycoside (202). Whether the same phenomenon occurs in humans remains unknown.

The extent of human kidney damage associated with aminoglycosides is most often mild, occasionally moderate, and rarely severe (203). It appears that severe nephrotoxicity does not occur if the aminoglycoside dosage is carefully adjusted for changing glomerular function.

The degree of reversibility of renal dysfunction associated with aminoglycosides is remarkable since the potential of the proximal renal tubule for regeneration is extensive and no or very little irreversible renal damage is associated with aminoglycosides. The type of renal dysfunction is nonoliguric.

Although individual functions served by the proximal renal tubule such as glucose reabsorption or amino acid reabsorption have been abnormal in experimental animals, these individual proximal tubular functions are usually remarkably well preserved in humans. A syndrome of hypokalemia, hypocalcemia, and hypomagnesemia has been reported in a very few patients (204–208).

Recently, considerable attention has centered on risk factors in an effort to identify patients who are likely to develop renal dysfunction while receiving an aminoglycoside. Risk factors include older age, female sex, concomitant liver disease, and concomitant hypotension at the onset of aminoglycoside therapy (209). Concomitant cephalothin administration has been reported to be associated with an increased incidence of renal dysfunction (210). Other nephrotoxic drugs including *cis*-platinum, amphotericin B, and cyclosporin also contribute to the renal dysfunction associated with aminoglycosides.

In addition different aminoglycosides possess differing degrees of inherent nephrotoxic potential. Of the currently available aminoglycosides, gentamicin is more nephrotoxic than tobramycin (149). Amikacin is also less nephrotoxic than gentamicin on a weight basis in animals. At a clinical level, however, higher doses of amikacin are allowed because of this lesser nephrotoxicity, and at least some of the difference may be abolished. Netilmicin is also less nephrotoxic than gentamicin in animal studies, but the evidence in humans is currently unconvincing.

Since aminoglycoside nephrotoxicity is usually mild and reversible, we should not err on the side of undertreatment as a result of excessive fear of this adverse effect.

INDIVIDUAL DRUGS

Streptomycin

Streptomycin is available as streptomycin sulfate for parenteral administration in vials either premixed or to be reconstituted to concentrations of 400 or 500 mg/ml.

Streptomycin is primarily considered as an antituberculous drug with good activity against both *M. tuberculosis* and *Mycobacterium bovis* and less activity against atypical mycobacteria. Streptomycin also is considered the drug of choice for *Francisella tularensis* (tularemia) and *Y. pestis* (plague) and is often used for infections caused by *Brucella.* In addition, streptomycin is frequently used, in combination with penicillin or vancomycin, for infections caused by *Streptococcus faecalis* or *Streptococci viridans* especially endocarditis, and in prophylactic regimens designed to prevent endocarditis. Enterococcal resistance to streptomycin in some areas, however, may preclude the use of streptomycin and favor gentamicin (46).

The dosage of streptomycin for tuberculosis is generally 1 g/day followed in a few weeks by 1 g three times a week. For tularemia an accepted dosage is 2 g/day in divided doses (12 hourly), for plague 2 g/day in divided doses (12 hourly), and for brucellosis 1 g/day in divided doses (12 hourly) along with tetracycline. For the treatment of enterococcal endocarditis a recommended dosage regimen is 1 g/day in divided doses (12 hourly) for 4–6 weeks. Enterococci may be highly resistant to streptomycin, and gentamicin is usually recommended for treatment of endocarditis caused by streptomycin-resistant organisms. For the prevention of endocarditis, a recommended dosage regimen of streptomycin is 1 g given ½–1 hour before dental or surgical intervention and for genitourinary (GU) or gastrointestinal (GI) surgery an additional 1 g at 12 hours and again at 24 hours postoperatively.

As with other aminoglycosides, the dosage should be reduced in the elderly, in newborns, and in patients with diminished glomerular function.

Neomycin

Neomycin is available as neomycin sulfate for oral administration in tablets containing 500 mg each. In addition neomycin sulfate is available either alone or in combination with other agents in numerous ophthalmologic, otic, and dermatologic formulations for topical application.

For preoperative suppression of intestinal bacteria a dosage regimen of 6 g/day (divided four hourly) for 2–3 days has been recommended. In hepatic coma a dosage regimen of 4–12 g/day (divided four or six hourly) has been recommended. It is imperative to recognize that a small percentage of the oral dose of neomycin will be absorbed and that this may provide toxic systemic levels in a patient with renal dysfunction.

Kanamycin

Kanamycin is available as kanamycin sulfate in both parenteral and oral formulations. For parenteral use kanamycin sulfate is available at concentrations of 250, 333, or 37.5 mg/ml. All parenteral formulations contain sodium bisulfite as a preservative. For oral use kanamycin sulfate is available in capsules of 500 mg each.

The place for kanamycin for systemic infections is debatable. Its widespread usage during the 1960s was sharply curtailed in the 1970s as a result of the relatively common emergence of resistance in common gram-negative bacillary organisms in conjunction with the usual resistance of *Pseudomonas* species. With its disuse, however, the level of resistance has decreased in many areas, and it has again enjoyed some increase in use in infections unlikely to be associated with *Pseudomonas* species. In general, however, its place has been taken by gentamicin, tobramycin, and amikacin.

The dosage of kanamycin (either intramuscularly or intravenously) for systemic infections has been 15 mg/kg/day in divided doses (usually 12 hourly) with a maximal dose of 1.5 g/day. If given intravenously, the dose should be administered over at least 30 minutes.

The parenteral formulation of kanamycin sulfate may be diluted with sterile distilled water to provide solutions for intraperitoneal instillation or for the irrigation of abscess cavities, pleural or peritoneal spaces, the bladder, or wounds. Although concentrations of 25 mg/ml for intraperitoneal instillation and 2.5 mg/ml for irrigating solutions have been recommended, it is important to recognize that absorption can occur, especially from the peritoneum, pleura, or open wounds, and that very large daily systemic doses can be achieved inadvertently with these concentrated solutions. It would seem more prudent to use solutions of 25 μg/ml since this is the peak level achieved in plasma with systemic dosing and since this level is unlikely to produce toxicity in the absence of renal dysfunction.

The oral dose of kanamycin for the suppression of intestinal bacteria preoperatively or in hepatic coma is 8–12 g/day in divided doses (four or six hourly). As with neomycin, some kanamycin will be absorbed, and toxic systemic levels may result in patients with renal dysfunction.

As with all aminoglycosides, the systemic dosing of kanamycin must be adjusted for renal glomerular dysfunction, including that seen in the elderly and the newborn.

Gentamicin

Gentamicin is available as gentamicin sulfate for parenteral and topical use. For parenteral use gentamicin sulfate is available in concentrations of 2 mg/ml (without methyl and propylparabens, ethylenediaminetetraacetic acid (EDTA), and sodium bisulfite as preservatives) for intrathecal or intraventricular use, 10 mg/ml (pediatric), 40 mg/ml (intravenous or intramuscular), or 1 mg/

ml (intravenous piggyback without preservative) in various sized vials, prefilled syringes, or piggyback units.

Gentamicin sulfate is also available in several topical formulations for ophthalmologic or dermatologic use.

Gentamicin remains a mainstay in the treatment of gram-negative bacillary infections, in part because of its relatively low cost after the expiration of its patent.

Gentamicin dosing is discussed above.

Tobramycin

Tobramycin is available as tobramycin sulfate for parenteral or topical use. For parenteral use tobramycin sulfate is available in concentrations of 10 mg/ml (pediatric) and 40 mg/ml (intravenous or intramuscular) in vials or prefilled syringes. Each of these formulations contains phenol, EDTA, and sodium bisulfite as preservatives. In addition a powder for injection is available, which can be reconstituted with sterile water to a concentration of 40 mg/ml. This formulation contains no preservatives and may be a more reasonable choice for intrathecal or intraventricular injections.

Tobramycin sulfate is also available as ophthalmic drops containing 3 mg/ml.

Tobramycin is widely used in the treatment of gram-negative bacillary infections. At a clinical level there is no evidence for its superiority or inferiority when compared to gentamicin, amikacin, or netilmicin with respect to effectiveness in infections caused by susceptible organisms. Its in vitro activity is somewhat greater than gentamicin for *P. aeruginosa* and somewhat less for *Serratia,* but this has not led to demonstrable differences in clinical effectiveness. A few organisms are resistant to gentamicin and yet sensitive to tobramycin, but the resistance profiles of the two are very similar. Tobramycin is somewhat less nephrotoxic than gentamicin and may be somewhat less ototoxic as well, but the lesser ototoxicity that exists in animals has been supported only with respect to vestibular dysfunction in humans.

Tobramycin dosing is discussed above and is identical to gentamicin dosing.

Amikacin

Amikacin is available as amikacin sulfate for parenteral use in solutions containing 50 or 250 mg/ml. Only one formulation of amikacin sulfate contains no preservatives (sodium bisulfite and sulfuric acid), and this is probably the preferred formulation for intrathecal or intraventricular use.

Amikacin is widely used in the treatment of gram-negative bacillary infections. At a clinical level there is no evidence for its superiority or inferiority when compared to gentamicin, tobramycin, or netilmicin with respect to effectiveness in infections caused by susceptible organisms. Although its in vitro potency is somewhat less, on a weight basis, than that of gentamicin, tobramycin, or netilmicin, the larger dosages used compensate for this lesser potency. A clear advantage of amikacin lies in its resistance profile. Many of the aminoglycoside-inactivating enzymes that inactivate other aminoglycosides cannot inactivate amikacin and consequently many organisms that are resistant to gentamicin, tobramycin, or netilmicin remain sensitive to amikacin. Thus amikacin has clearcut advantages in treating infections caused by organisms known to be resistant to other aminoglycosides and in nosocomial infections in which the likelihood of resistant organisms is increased. The use of amikacin in other and more general settings currently presents a dilemma for the clinician. On the one hand, the restriction of amikacin usage is often believed to be wise in order to delay the emergence of resistance to this valuable drug. On the other hand, there is no evidence that the restriction of amikacin usage will delay the emergence of resistance, and there is a theoretical reason that resistance may not be delayed. This is based on the fact that each of the relatively few aminoglycoside-inactivating enzymes that can inactivate amikacin can also inactivate other aminoglycosides. Thus the continued use of other aminoglycosides may provide ecologic pressure for the development of those enzymes capable of inactivating amikacin even though amikacin use is restricted.

With respect to toxicity, amikacin is probably less nephrotoxic and less ototoxic than gentamicin on a weight basis. However, since larger doses of amikacin are used, the differences on a weight basis may be at least partially lost. At a clinical level there have been no direct prospective and blinded comparisons between amikacin and either tobramycin or netilmicin with respect to toxicity. Therefore, the precise placement of amikacin with respect to its relative toxicity remains unclear.

Netilmicin

Netilmicin is available as netilmicin sulfate for parenteral use, in formulations containing 10 mg/ml (neonatal; with sodium metabisulfite and sodium sulfite as preservatives), 25 mg/ml (pediatric; with methyl and propyl parabens, EDTA, sodium metabisulfite, and sodium sulfite as preservatives) and 100 mg/ml (with benzyl alcohol, EDTA, sodium metabisulfite, and sodium sulfite as preservatives) in vials or prefilled syringes.

Netilmicin has only recently been marketed, and its place in therapy is yet to be established. Its clinical effectiveness is probably similar to gentamicin, tobramycin, and amikacin. In vitro its resistance profile resembles gentamicin and tobramycin, with only a few strains of bacteria being resistant to gentamicin or tobramycin and sensitive to netilmicin. From a toxicologic point of view, netilmicin is less nephrotoxic than gentamicin in experimental animals, but this has not been confirmed in humans. Subclinical auditory toxicity, as detected by audiometry, is less with netilmicin than with tobramycin (174). Clinically detectable auditory toxicity is very rare with any of the commonly used aminoglycosides if dosing is appropriately controlled.

Spectinomycin

Spectinomycin is isolated from *Streptomyces spectabilis* and is classified as an aminocyclitol antibiotic but is not an aminoglycoside since it contains neither an aminosugar nor a glycosidic bond (Fig. 2) (211,212).

The site of action of spectinomycin may be similar to the aminoglycosides since spectinomycin binds to the smaller (30s) ribosomal subunits and protein synthesis is inhibited (213). However, misreading of the genetic code does not occur, and a membrane effect does appear to exist by electron microscopy (214).

Resistance to spectinomycin is rarely seen in *Neisseria gonorrhoea,* and there is no cross resistance with penicillins (211).

Although the spectrum of activity of spectinomycin is broader, spectinomycin is used only as an agent for infections caused by *N. gonorrhoea.* Significantly, it is not effective against *Treponema pallidum* or *Chlamydia trachomatis,* but it may be somewhat effective against *Ureaplasma urealyticum* and *Gardnerella vaginalis* (211,212,215).

Spectinomycin is rapidly and completely absorbed after intramuscular administration. Its volume of distribution is about 0.33 liter/kg and its half-life about 1 hour (216). It is not metabolized and is excreted completely into the urine as unchanged drug. Spectinomycin does not enter saliva and is not predictably effective in eliminating pharyngeal *Neisseria* (212).

Toxicologically, spectinomycin differs considerably from the aminoglycosides in that it is neither ototoxic nor nephrotoxic, and, in fact, few side effects exist with the usual dosing of the drug. Urticaria, chills, fever, dizziness, nausea, and insomnia have been reported.

Therapeutically spectinomycin is clearly highly effective in the treatment of uncomplicated gonorrhea and disseminated gonoccal infection. It is unpredictable in the treatment of pharyngeal gonorrhea. Spectinomycin is the drug of choice in the treatment of penicillinase-producing gonococcal infections and in the treatment of patients who fail to respond to treatment.

Spectinomycin is available as spectinomycin hydrochloride in a powder form that is reconstituted with 0.9 percent benzyl alcohol as a diluent to a concentration of 400 mg/ml. It can be given only intramuscularly.

For uncomplicated gonorrheal infections 2 g as a single intramuscular dose is recommended. For disseminated gonococcal infections the recommended dose is 4 g/day in divided doses (12 hourly) for 3 days.

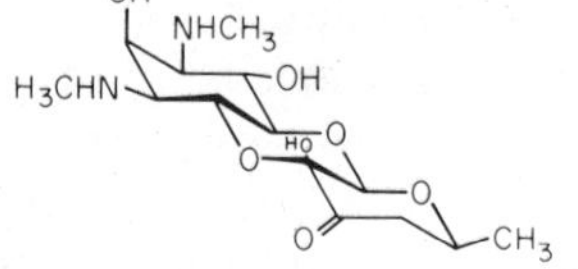

SPECTINOMYCIN

FIGURE 2. Structure of spectinomycin—an aminocyclitol.

REFERENCES

1. Rinehart KL: Comparative chemistry of the aminoglycoside and aminocyclitol antibiotics. *J Infect Dis* 119:345, 1969.
2. Daniels PJL: Antibiotics (aminoglycosides), in Grayson M (ed): *Kirk-Othmer: Encyclopedia of Chemical Technology*, ed 3. New York, John Wiley and Sons, 1978, vol 2 p 819.
3. Hooper, IR: The naturally occurring aminoglycoside antibiotics, in Umezawa H, Hooper IR (eds): *Aminoglycoside Antibiotics.* Springer-Verlag, New York, 1982, p 1.
4. Umezawa S, Tsuchiya T: Total synthesis and chemical modification of the aminoglycoside antibiotics, in Umezawa H, Hooper IR (eds): *Aminoglycoside Antibiotics.* Springer-Verlag, New York, 1982, p 37.
5. Price KE, Godfrey JC, Kawaguchi H: Effect of structural modifications on the biological properties of aminoglycoside antibiotics containing 2-deoxystreptamine. *Adv Appl Microbiol* 18:191, 1974.
6. Hancock REW: Aminoglycoside uptake and mode of action: With special reference to streptomycin and gentamicin. I. Antagonists and mutants. *J Antimicrob Chemother* 8:249, 1981.
7. Hancock REW: Aminoglycoside uptake and mode of action: With special reference to streptomycin and gentamicin. II. Effects of aminoglycosides on cells. *J Antimicrob Chemother* 8:429, 1981.
8. Pestka S: Inhibitors of protein synthesis, in Weissbach H, Pestka S (eds): *Molecular Mechanisms of Protein Synthesis.* New York, Academic Press, 1977, p 467.
9. Stoffler G, Wittmann HG: Primary structure and three-dimensional arrangement of proteins within the *Escherichia coli* ribosome, in Weissbach H, Pestka S (eds): *Molecular Mechanisms of Protein Synthesis.* New York, Academic Press, 1977, p 117.
10. Hummel H, Piepersberg W, Bock A: 30s subunit mutations relieving restriction of ribosomal misreading caused by L6 mutations. *Mol Gen Genet* 179:147, 1980.
11. Kuhberger R, Piepersberg W, Petzet A, et al: Alteration of ribosomal protein L6 in gentamicin-resistant strains of *Escherichia coli.* Effects on fidelity of protein synthesis. *Biochemistry* 18:187, 1979.
12. Tai P-C, Davis BD: Triphasic concentration effects of gentamicin on activity and misreading in protein synthesis. *Biochemistry* 18:193, 1979.
13. Chang FN, Flaks JG: Binding of dihydrostreptomycin to *Escherichia coli* ribosomes: Characteristics and equilibrium of the reaction. *Antimicrob Agents Chemother* 2:294, 1972.
14. Chang FN, Flaks JG: Binding of dihydrostreptomycin to *Escherichia coli* ribosomes: Kinetics of the reaction. *Antimicrob Agents Chemother* 2:308, 1972.
15. Ozaki M, Mizushima S, Nomura M: Identification and functional characterization of the protein controlled by the streptomycin-resistant locus in *E. coli. Nature* 222:333, 1969.
16. Schreiner G, Nierhaus KH: Protein involved in the binding of dihydrostreptomycin to ribosomes of *Escherichia coli. J Mol Biol* 81:71, 1973.
17. Wallace BJ, Davis BD: Cyclic blockade of initiation sites by streptomycin-damaged ribosomes in *Escherichia coli:* An explanation for dominance of sensitivity. *J Mol Biol* 75:377, 1973.
18. Wallace BJ, Tai P-C, Davis BD: Effect of streptomycin on the response of *Escherichia coli* ribosomes to the dissociation factor. *J Mol Biol* 75:391, 1973.
19. Luzzatto L, Apirion D, Schlessinger D: Mechanism of action of streptomycin in *E. coli:* Interruption of the ribosome cycle of the initiation of protein synthesis. *Proc Natl Acad Sci USA* 60:873, 1968.
20. Luzzatto L, Apirion D, Schlessinger D: Polyribosome depletion and blockage of the ribosome cycle by streptomycin in *Escherichia coli. J Mol Biol* 42:315, 1969.
21. Bryan LE, van den Elzen HM: Effects of membrane-energy mutations and cations on streptomycin and gentamicin accumulation by bacteria: A model for entry of streptomycin and gentamicin in susceptible and resistant bacteria. *Antimicrob Agents Chemother* 12:163, 1977.
22. Mak L, Lietman PS: Aminoglycoside transport by bacteria, in Fillastre J-P (ed): *Néphrotoxicité, Ototoxicité Médicamenteuses.* Rouen, Editions INSERM, 1981, p 55.

23. Damper PD, Epstein W: Role of the membrane potential in bacterial resistance to aminoglycoside antibiotics. *Antimicrob Agents Chemother* 20:803, 1981.
24. Mates SM, Patel L, Kaback HR, et al: Membrane potential in anaerobically growing *Staphylococcus aureus* and its relationship to gentamicin uptake. *Antimicrob Agents Chemother* 23:526, 1983.
25. Holtje J-V: Regulation of polyamine and streptomycin transport during stringent and relaxed control in *Escherichia coli. J Bacteriol* 137:661, 1979.
26. Hurwitz C, Rosano CL: Chloramphenicol-sensitive and -insensitive phases of the lethal action of streptomycin. *J Bacteriol* 83:1202, 1962.
27. Mitsuhashi S, Kawabe H: Aminoglycoside antibiotic resistance in bacteria, in Whelton A, Neu HC (eds): *The Aminoglycosides.* New York, Marcel Dekker, Inc, 1983, p 97.
28. Davies JE: Resistance to aminoglycosides: Mechanism and frequency. *Rev Infect Dis* 5(suppl):3261, 1983.
29. Sanders CC, Sanders WE Jr, Goering RV: *In vitro* studies with Sch 21420 and Sch 22591: Activity in comparison with six other aminoglycosides and synergy with penicillin against enterococci. *Antimicrob Agents Chemother* 14:178, 1978.
30. Moellering RC Jr: Clinical microbiology and the *in vitro* activity of aminoglycosides, in Whelton A, Neu HC (eds): *The Aminoglycosides: Microbiology, Clinical Use, and Toxicology.* New York, Marcel Dekker, Inc, 1982, p 65.
31. Kabins SA, Nathan C, Cohen S: *In vitro* comparison of netilmicin, a semisynthetic derivative of sisomicin, and four other aminoglycoside antibiotics. *Antimicrob Agents Chemother* 10:139, 1976.
32. Fu K, Neu HC: *In vitro* study of netilmicin compared with other aminoglycosides. *Antimicrob Agents Chemother* 10:526, 1976.
33. National Committee for Clinical Laboratory Standards: Performance standards for antimicrobial disc susceptibility tests. Approved Standard: ASM-2, Villanova, Pa, 1979.
34. Thornsberry C, Gavan TL, Gerlach EH, et al: New developments in antimicrobial agent susceptibility testing, in Sherris JC (ed): *Cumitech 6.* Washington, DC, American Society of Microbiology, 1977, p 1.
35. McDonald PJ, Craig WA, Konin CM: Persistent effect of antibiotics on Staphylococcus aureus after exposure for limited periods of time. *J Infect Dis* 135:217, 1977.
36. Grasso S, Meinardi G, DeCarneri J, et al: New *in vitro* model to study the effect of antibiotic concentration and rate of elimination on antibacterial activity. *Antimicrob Agents Chemother* 13:570, 1978.
37. Nishida M, Marakawa T, Kamimura T, et al: Bactericidal activity of cephalosporins in an *in vitro* model simulating serum levels. *Antimicrob Agents Chemother* 14:6, 1978.
38. Al-Asadi MJS, Greenwood D, O'Grady F: *In vitro* model simulating the form of exposure of bacteria to antimicrobial drugs encountered in infection. *Antimicrob Agents Chemother* 16:77, 1979.
39. Murakawa T, Sakamoto H, Hinrose T, et al: New *in vitro* kinetic model for evaluating bactericidal efficacy of antibiotics. *Antimicrob Agents Chemother* 18:77, 1980.
40. Bergan T, Carlsen IB, Fuglesang JE: An *in vitro* model for monitoring bacterial responses to antibiotic agents under simulated *in vivo* conditions. *Infection* 8(suppl 1): S96, 1980.
41. Longstreth JA: Interaction of aminoglycoside pharmacokinetics and bacterial population kinetics in a chemostat. PhD dissertation. Johns Hopkins University, 1982.
42. Hammond BJ, Kogot M, Lightbown JW: Analogue computer studies of the growth characteristics of *Escherichia coli* following dihydrostreptomycin treatment. *J Gen Microbiol* 48:189, 1967.
43. Kogut M, Lightbown JW, Isaacson P: Effects of dihydrostreptomycin treatment on the growth of *Escherichia coli* after removal of extracellular antibiotic. *J Gen Microbiol* 39:165, 1965.
44. Bundtzen RW, Gerber AU, Cohn DL, et al: Postantibiotic suppression of bacterial growth. *Rev Infect Dis* 3:28, 1981.
45. Klastersky J, Cappel R, Danpau D: Clinical significance of *in vitro* synergism between antibiotics in gram-negative infections. *Antimicrob Agents Chemother* 2:470, 1972.

46. Moellering RC Jr, Wennerstein C, Weinberg AN: Studies on antibiotic synergism against enterocooci: I. Bacteriologic studies. *J Lab Clin Med* 77:821, 1971.
47. Kunin CM, Chalmers TC, Leevy CM: Absorption of orally administered neomycin and kanamycin. *N Engl J Med* 262:380, 1960.
48. Last PM, Sherlock S: Systemic absorption of orally administered neomycin in liver disease. *N Engl J Med* 262:385, 1960.
49. Kunin CM: Absorption, distribution, excretion and fate of kanamycin. *Ann NY Acad Sci* 132:811, 1966.
50. Breen KF, Bryant RE, Levinson JD, et al: Neomycin absorption in man. *Ann Intern Med* 76:211, 1972.
51. Mitch WE, Lietman PS, Walser M: Effects of oral neomycin and kanamycin in chronic uremic patients: I. Urea metabolism. *Kidney Int* 11:116, 1977.
52. King JT: Severe deafness in an infant following oral administration of neomycin. *J Med Assoc Ga* 51:530, 1962.
53. Ruben RJ, Daly JF: Neomycin ototoxicity and nephrotoxicity. *Laryngoscope* 78:1734, 1968.
54. Kalbian VV: Deafness following oral use of neomycin. *South Med J* 65:499, 1972.
55. Ward KM, Rounthwaite FJ: Neomycin ototoxicity. *Ann Otol* 87:211, 1978.
56. Doluisio JT, Dittert LW, LaPiana JC: Pharmacokinetics of kanamycin following intramuscular administration. *J Pharmacokinet Biopharm* 1:253, 1973.
57. Barza M, Lauermann M: Why monitor serum levels of gentamicin. *Clin Pharmacokinet* 3:202, 1978.
58. Little PJ, Lynn KL: Neomycin toxicity. *NZ Med J* 81:445, 1975.
59. Bamford MFM, Jones LF: Deafness and biochemical imbalance after burns treatment with topical antibiotics in young children. *Arch Dis Child* 53:326, 1978.
60. Somani P, Shapiro RS, Stockard H, et al: Unidirectional absorption of gentamicin from the peritoneum during continuous ambulatory peritoneal dialysis. *Clin Pharmacol Ther* 32:113, 1982.
61. DePaepe M, Lameire N, Belpaire F, et al: Peritoneal pharmacokinetics of gentamicin in man. *Clin Nephrol* 19:107, 1983.
62. Chamberlain G, Needham P: The absorption of antibiotics from the bladder. *J Urol* 116:172, 1976.
63. Lifschitz MI, Denning CR: Safety of kanamycin aerosol. *Clin Pharmacol Ther* 12:91, 1971.
64. Odio W, VanLeier E, Klastersky J: Concentrations of gentamicin in bronchial secretions after intramuscular and endotracheal administration. *J Clin Pharmacol* 15:518, 1975.
65. Rahal JJ Jr, Hyams PJ, Simberkoff MS, et al: Combined intrathecal and intramuscular gentamicin for gram-negative meningitis. *N Engl J Med* 290:1394, 1974.
66. Van Etta LL, Kravitz GR, Russ TE, et al: Effect of method of administration on extravascular penetration of four antibiotics. *Antimicrob Agents Chemother* 21:873, 1982.
67. Kuhar MJ, MaK LL, Lietman PS: Localization of ^{3}H-gentamicin in the proximal renal tubule of the mouse. *Antimicrob Agents Chemother* 15:131, 1979.
68. Thys JP, Klastersky J, Mombelli G: Peak or sustained antibiotic levels for optimal tissue penetration. *J Antimicrob Chemother* 8(suppl C):29, 1981.
69. Klastersky J, Meunier-Carpentier F, Kahan-Coppens L, et al: Endotracheally administered antibiotics for gram negative bronchopneumonia. *Chest* 75:586, 1979.
70. Kaiser AB, McGee ZA: Aminoglycoside therapy of gram-negative bacillary meningitis. *N Engl J Med* 293:1215, 1975.
71. Wirt TC, McGee ZA, Oldfield EH, et al: Intraventricular administration of amikacin for complicated gram-negative meningitis and ventriculitis. *J Neurosurg* 50:95, 1979.
72. McCracken GH Jr, Mize S, Threlkeld N: Intraventricular gentamicin therapy in gram-negative bacillary meningitis of infancy. *Lancet* i:787, 1980.
73. Barza M, Kane A, Baum J: Comparison of the effects of continuous and intermittent systemic administration on the penetration of gentamicin into infected rabbit eyes. *J Infect Dis* 147:144, 1983.

74. Gorden TB, Cunningham RD: Tobramycin levels in aqueous humor after subconjunctival injection in humans. *Am J Ophthalmol* 93:107, 1982.
75. Rubenstein E, Goldfarb J, Keren G, et al: The penetration of gentamicin into the vitreous humor in man. *Invest Ophthalmol Vis Sci* 24:637, 1983.
76. Marsh DC Jr, Matthew EB, Perselin RA: Transport of gentamicin into synovial fluid. *JAMA* 228:607, 1974.
77. Dee TH, Koein F: Gentamicin and tobramycin penetration into synovial fluid. *Antimicrob Agents Chemother* 12:548, 1977.
78. Chow A, Hecht R, Winters R: Gentamicin and carbenicillin penetration into the septic joint. *N Engl J Med* 285:178, 1971.
79. Baciocco EA, Iles RI: Ampicillin and kanamycin concentration in joint fluid. *Clin Pharmacol Ther* 12:858, 1971.
80. Schurman DJ, Wheeler R: Bone and joint gram-negative infection and amikacin treatment. *Am J Med* 62(suppl):160, 1977.
81. Alftan O, Renkonen OV, Sironen A: Concentration of gentamicin in serum, urine and urogenital tissue in man. *Acta Pathol Microbiol Scand* [B] 81(suppl 241):92, 1973.
82. Mahmod S, Al-Hakiem MHH, Landon J, et al: Aminoglycoside antibiotics do not appear in saliva. *Clin Chem* 29:988, 1983.
83. Pitt HA, Roberts RB, Johnson WD Jr: Gentamicin levels in the human biliary tract. *J Infect Dis* 127:299, 1973.
84. Mendelson J, Portnoy J, Sigman H: Pharmacology of gentamicin in the biliary tract of humans. *Antimicrob Agents Chemother* 4:538, 1973.
85. Wood MJ, Farrell W: Comparison of urinary excretion of tobramycin and gentamicin in adults. *J Infect Dis* 134(suppl):S133, 1976.
86. Kahlmeter G, Kamme C: Prolonged excretion of gentamicin in a patient with unimpaired renal function. *Lancet* i:286, 1975.
87. Kahlmeter G, Jonsson S, Kamme C: Multiple-compartment pharmacokinetics of tobramycin. *J Antimicrob Chemother* 4(suppl A):5, 1978.
88. Kahlmeter G: Netilmicin: Clinical pharmacokinetics and aspects on dosage schedules. An overview. *Scand J Infect Dis* 23:74, 1980.
89. Laskin OL, Longstsreth JA, Smith CR, et al: Netilmicin and gentamicin multidose kinetics in normal subjects. *Clin Pharmacol Ther* 34:644, 1983.
90. Wilson TW, Mahon WA, Inaba T, et al: Elimination of tritiated gentamicin in normal human subjects and in patients with severely impaired renal function. *Clin Pharmacol Ther* 14:815, 1973.
91. Kahlmeter G: Gentamicin and tobramycin: Clinical pharmacokinetics and nephrotoxicity: Aspects on assay techniques. Thesis, Department of Medical Microbiology, University of Lund, Sweden, 1979.
92. Pastoriza-Munoz E, Timmerman D, Feldman S, et al: Ultrafiltration of gentamicin and netilmicin *in vivo*. *J Pharmacol Exp Ther* 220:604, 1982.
93. Collier VU, Lietman PS, Mitch WE: Evidence for luminal uptake of gentamicin in perfused rat kidney. *J Pharmacol Exp Ther* 210:247, 1979.
94. Silverblatt FJ, Kuehn C: Autoradiography of gentamicin uptake by the rat proximal tubular cell. *Kidney Int* 15:335, 1979.
95. Lipsky JJ, Cheng L, Saktor B, et al: Gentamicin uptake by renal tubule brush border membrane vesicles. *J Pharmacol Exp Ther* 215:390, 1980.
96. Sastrasinh M, Knauss TC, Weinberg JM, et al: Identification of the aminoglycoside binding site in rat renal brush border membranes. *J Pharmacol Exp Ther* 222:350, 1982.
97. Senekjian HO, Knight TF, Weinman EJ: Micropuncture study of the handling of gentamicin by the rat kidney. *Kidney Int* 19:416, 1981.
98. Pastoriza-Munoz E, Bowman RL, Kaloyanides GJ: Renal tubular transport of gentamicin in the rat. *Kidney Int* 16:440, 1979.
99. Frommer JP, Senekjian HO, Babino H, et al: Intratubular microinjection study of gentamicin transport in the rat. *Mineral Electrolyte Metab* 9:108, 1983.

100. Wenk M, Spring P, Vozeh S, et al: Multicompartment pharmacokinetics of netilmicin. *Eur J Clin Pharmacol* 16:331, 1979.
101. Laskin OL, Longstsreth JA, Smith CR, et al: Netilmicin and gentamicin multidose kinetics in normal subjects. *Clin Pharmacol Ther* 34:644, 1983.
102. Lanao JM, Dominguez-Gil A, Tabernero JM, et al: Pharmacokinetics of amikacin (BB-K8) in patients with normal or impaired renal function. *Int J Clin Pharmacol Biopharm* 17:171, 1979.
103. Smith CR, Baughman KL, Edwards CQ, et al: Controlled comparison of amikacin and gentamicin. *N Engl J Med* 296:349, 1977.
104. Gyselynck A-M, Forrey A, Cutler R: Pharmacokinetics of gentamicin: Distribution and plasma and renal clearance. *J Infect Dis* 124(suppl):S70, 1971.
105. Plantier J, Forrey AW, O'Neill MA, et al: Pharmacokinetics of amikacin in patients with normal or impaired renal function: Radioenzymatic acetylation assay. *J Infect Dis* 134(suppl):S323, 1976.
106. Barza M, Brown RB, Shen D, et al: Predictability of blood levels of gentamicin in man. *J Infect Dis* 132:165, 1975.
107. Clarke JT, Libke RD, Regamey C, et al: Comparative pharmacokinetics of amikacin and kanamycin. *Clin Pharmacol Ther* 15:610, 1974.
108. Walker JM, Wise R, Mitchard M: The pharmacokinetics of amikacin and gentamicin in volunteers: A comparison of individual differences. *J Antimicrob Chemother* 5:95, 1979.
109. Kahlmeter G, Jonsson S, Kamme C: Multiple-compartment pharmacokinetics of tobramycin. *J Antimicrob Chemother* 4(suppl A):5, 1978.
110. Kahlmeter G: Gentamicin and tobramycin: Clinical pharmacokinetics and nephrotoxicity: Aspects on assay techniques. Berlings, Lund, 1979.
111. Adelman M, Evans E, Schentag JJ: Two-compartment comparison of gentamicin and tobramycin in normal volunteers. *Antimicrob Agents Chemother* 22:800, 1982.
112. Assael BM, Cavanna G, Jusko WJ, et al: Multiexponential elimination of gentamicin. A kinetic study during development. *Dev Pharmacol Ther* 1:171, 1980.
113. Driessen OMJ, Sorgedrager N, Michel MF, et al: Pharmacokinetic aspects of therapy with ampicillin and kanamycin in new-born infants. *Eur J Clin Pharmacol* 13:449, 1978.
114. Haughey DB, Hilligoss DM, Grassi A, et al: Two compartment gentamicin pharmacokinetics in premature neonates. A comparison to adults with decreased glomerular filtration rate. *J Pediatr* 96:325, 1980.
115. Herngren L, Boreus LO, Jalling B, et al: Pharmacokinetic aspects of streptomycin treatment of neonatal septicemia. *Scand J Infect Dis* 9:301, 1977.
116. Howard JB, McCracken GH: Reappraisal of kanamycin usage in neonates. *J Pediatr* 86:949, 1975.
117. Howard JB, McCracken GH, Trujillo H, et al: Amikacin in newborn infants: Comparative pharmacology with kanamycin and clinical efficacy in 45 neonates with bacterial diseases. *Antimicrob Agents Chemother* 10:205, 1976.
118. McCracken GH Jr, Gay Jones L: Gentamicin in the neonatal period. *Am J Dis Child* 120:524, 1970.
119. McCracken GH Jr, Nelson JD: Antimicrobial therapy for newborns: *Practical Application of Pharmacology to Clinical Use.* New York, Grune and Stratton, 1977.
120. Yoshioka H, Takimoto M, Matsudi I, et al: Dosage schedule of gentamicin for chronic renal insufficiency in children. *Arch Dis Child* 53:334, 1978.
121. Echeverria P, Siber GR, Paisley J, et al: Age dependent dose response to gentamicin. *J Pediatr* 87:805, 1975.
122. Evans WE, Feldman S, Barker LF, et al: Use of gentamicin serum levels to individualize therapy in children. *J Pediatr* 93:133, 1978.
123. Evans WE, Huntley Taylor R, Feldman S, et al: A model for dosing gentamicin in children and adolescents that adjusts for tissue accumulation with continuous dosing. *Clin Pharmacokinet* 5:295, 1980.

124. Hoecker JL, Pickering LK, Swaney J, et al: Clinical pharmacology of tobramycin in children. *J Infect Dis* 137:592, 1978.
125. Karetzis DA, Sinaniotis CA, Papadatos CJ, et al: Pharmacokintics of amikacin in infants and preschool children. *Acta Paediat Scand* 68:419, 1979.
126. Kramer WG, Cleary T, Frankel LS, et al: Multiple-dose amikacin kinetics in pediatric oncology patients. *Clin Pharmacol Ther* 26:635, 1979.
127. Marks MI, Vose A, Hammerberg S, et al: Clinico-pharmacological studies of sisomicin in ill children. *Antimicrob Agents Chemother* 13:753, 1978.
128. McCracken GH Jr: Clinical pharmacology of gentamicin in infants 2 to 24 months of age. *Am J Dis Child* 124:884, 1972.
129. Siber GR, Echeverria P, Smith AL, et al: Pharmacokinetics of gentamicin in children and adults. *J Infect Dis* 132:637, 1975.
130. Vogelstein B, Kowarski AA, Lietman PS: The pharmacokinetics of amikacin in children. *J Pediatr* 91:333, 1977.
131. Welling PG, Baumueller A, Lau CC, et al: Netilmicin pharmacokinetics after single intravenous doses to elderly male patients. *Antimicrob Agents Chemother* 12:328, 1977.
132. Spyker DA, Guerrant RL: Dosage nomograms for aminoglycoside antibiotics. *Hosp Formulary* 16:132, 1981.
133. Cockcroft DW, Gault MH: Prediction of creatinine clearance from serum creatinine. *Nephron* 16:31, 1976.
134. Siersbaek-Nielsen K, Molholm-Hansen J, Kampmann J: Rapid evaluation of creatinine clearance. *Lancet* i:1133, 1971.
135. Plantier J, Forrey AW, O'Neill MA, et al: Pharmacokinetics of amikacin in patients with normal or impaired renal function: Radioenzymatic acetylation assay. *J Infect Dis* 134(suppl):5323, 1976.
136. Gyselynck A-M, Forrey A, Cutler R: Pharmacokinetics of gentamicin: Distribution and plasma and renal clearance. *J Infect Dis* 124(suppl):570, 1971.
137. Lanao JM, Dominguez-Gil A, Tabernero JM, et al: Pharmacokinetics of amikacin (BB-K8) in patients with normal or impaired renal function. *Int J Clin Pharmacol Biopharm* 17:171, 1979.
138. Schwartz SN, Pazin GJ, Lyon JA, et al: A controlled investigation of the pharmacokinetics of gentamicin and tobramycin in obese subjects. *J Infect Dis* 138:499, 1978.
139. Blouin RA, Mann HJ, Griffen WO Jr, et al: Tobramycin pharmacokinetics in morbidly obese patients. *Clin Pharmacol Ther* 26:508, 1979.
140. Bravo ME, Arancibia A, Jarpa S, et al: Pharmacokinetics of gentamicin in malnourished infants. *Eur J Clin Pharmacol* 21:499, 1982.
141. Pennington JE, Dale DC, Reynolds HY, et al: Gentamicin sulfate pharmacokinetics: Lower levels of gentamicin in blood during fever. *J Infect Dis* 132:270, 1975.
142. Sawchuk RJ, Zaske DE: Pharmacokinetics of dosing regimens which utilize multiple intravenous infusions: Gentamicin in burn patients. *J Pharmacokinet Biopharm* 4:183, 1976.
143. Loirat P, Rohan J, Baillet A, et al: Increased glomerular filtration rate in patients with major burns and its effect on the pharmacokinetics of tobramycin. *N Engl J Med* 299:915, 1978.
144. Noone P, Parsons TMC, Pattison JR, et al: Experience in monitoring gentamicin therapy during treatment of series gram-negative sepsis. *Br Med J* 1:477, 1974.
145. Tally FP, Louie TJ, Weinstein WM, et al: Amikacin therapy for severe gram-negative sepsis. *Ann Intern Med* 83:484, 1975.
146. Anderson ET, Young LS, Hewitt WL: Simultaneous antibiotic levels in "breakthrough" gram-negative and bacteremia. *Am J Med* 61:493, 1976.
147. Klastersky J, Meunier-Copenter F, Prevase J: Significance of antimicrobial synergism for the outcome of gram-negative sepsis. *Am J Med Sci* 273:157, 1977.
148. Moore RD, Smith CR, Lietman PS: The association of aminoglycoside plasma levels with mortality in patients with gram-negative bacteremia. *J Infect Dis* 149:443, 1984.
149. Smith CR, Lipsky JJ, Laskin OL, et al: Double-blind comparison of the nephrotoxicity and auditory toxicity of gentamicin and tobramycin. *N Engl J Med* 302:106, 1980.

150. Wright JM, Collier B: The effects of neomycin upon transmitter release and action. *J Pharmacol Exp Ther* 200:576, 1977.
151. Lee C, DeSilva JC: Acute and subchronic neuromuscular blocking characteristics of streptomycin: A comparison with neomycin. *Br J Anaesth* 51:431, 1979.
152. Caputy AJ, Kim YI, Sanders DB: The neuromuscular blocking effects of therapeutic concentrations of various antibiotics on normal rat skeletal muscle: A quantitative comparison. *J Pharmacol Exp Ther* 217:369, 1981.
153. Chinyanga HM, Stoyka WW: The effect of colymycin M, gentamycin and kanamycin on depression of neuromuscular transmission induced by pancuronium bromide. *Can Anaesth Soc J* 21:569, 1974.
154. L'Hommedieu CS, Huber PA, Rasch DK: Potentiation of magnesium-induced neuromuscular weakness by gentamicin. *Crit Care Med* 11:55, 1983.
155. L'Hommedieu C, Stough R, Brown L, et al: Potentiation of neuromuscular weakness in infant botulism by aminoglycosides. *J Pediatr* 95:1065, 1979.
156. Hokkanen E: The aggravating effect of some antibiotics on the neuromuscular blockade in myasthenia gravis. *Acta Neurol Scand* 40:346, 1964.
157. Sanders DB, Kim YI, Howard JF, et al: Intercostal muscle biopsy studies in myasthenia gravis: Clinical correlations and the direct effects of drugs and myasthenic serum. *Ann NY Acad Sci* 377:544, 1981.
158. Pittinger CB, Adamson R: Antibiotic blockade of neuromuscular function. *Ann Rev Pharmacol* 12:169, 1972.
159. Adams HR: Direct myocardial depressant effects of gentamicin. *Eur J Pharmacol* 30:272, 1975.
160. Descotes J, Evreux JC: Cardiac depressant effects of some recent aminoglycoside antibiotics. *J Antimicrob Chemother* 7:197, 1981.
161. Adams HR, Goodman FR, Wass GB: Alteration of contractile function and calcium ion movements in vascular smooth muscle by gentamicin and other aminoglycoside antibiotics. *Antimicrob Agents Chemother* 5:640, 1974.
162. Lerner SA, Matz GJ, Hawkins JE (eds): *Aminoglycoside Ototoxicity.* Boston, Little, Brown and Company, 1981.
163. Brummett RE, Meikle MM, Vernon JA: Ototoxicity of tobramycin in guinea pigs. *Arch Otolaryngol* 94:59, 1971.
164. Theopold HM: Comparative surface studies of ototoxic effects of various aminoglycoside antibiotics on the organ of Corti in the guinea pig. *Acta Otolaryngol* 84:57, 1977.
165. Johnsson L-G, Hawkins JE Jr, Kinesley TC, et al: Aminoglycoside-induced cochlear pathology in man. *Acta Otolaryngol (Suppl) (Stockh)* 383:1, 1981.
166. Koitchev K, Guilhaume A, Cazals Y, et al: Spiral ganglion changes after massive aminoglycoside treatment in the guinea pig. *Acta Otolaryngol* (*Stockh*) 94:431, 1982.
167. Igarashi M: Vestibular ototoxicity in primates. *Audiology* 12:337, 1973.
168. Tran Ba Hay P, Muelemans A, Wassef M, et al: Gentamicin persistence in rat endolymph and perilymph after a two-day constant infusion. *Antimicrob Agents Chemother* 23:344, 1983.
169. Takada A, Schacht J: Calcium antagonism and reversibility of gentamicin-induced loss of cochlear microphonics in the guinea pig. *Hear Res* 8:179, 1982.
170. Schacht J: Biochemistry of neomycin ototoxicity. *J Acoust Soc Am* 59:940, 1978.
171. Iinuma T, Mizukoshi O, Daly JF: Possible effects of various ototoxic drugs upon the ATP-hydrolyzing system in the stria vascularis and spiral ligament of the guinea pig. *Laryngoscope* 77:159, 1967.
172. Matz GJ, Lerner SA: Prospective studies of aminoglycoside ototoxicity in adults, in Lerner SA, Matz GJ, Hawkins JE (eds): *Aminoglycoside Ototoxicity.* Boston, Little, Brown and Company, 1981, p 327.
173. Fee WE Jr: Aminoglycoside ototoxicity in the human. *Laryngoscope* 90(suppl 24):1, 1980.
174. Lerner AM, Reyes MP, Cone LA, et al: Randomized, controlled trial of the comparative efficacy, auditory toxicity, and nephrotoxicity of tobramycin and netilmicin. *Lancet* i:1123, 1983.

175. Bendush CL: Ototoxicity: Clinical considerations and comparative information, in Whelton A, Neu HC (eds): *The Aminoglycosides.* New York, Marcel Dekker Inc, 1982, p 453.
176. Moore RD, Smith CR, Lietman PS: Risk factors for the development of auditory toxicity in patients receiving aminoglycosides. *J Infect Dis* 149:23, 1984.
177. Mathog RH, Klein WJ, Jr: Ototoxicity of ethacrynic acid and aminoglycoside antibiotics in uremia. *N Engl J Med* 280:1223, 1969.
178. Brummett RE, Brown RT, Himes DL: Quantitative relationships of the ototoxic interaction of kanamycin and ethacrynic acid. *Arch Otolaryngol* 105:240, 1979.
179. Smith CR, Lietman PS: Effect of furosemide on aminoglycoside-induced nephrotoxicity and auditory toxicity in humans. *Antimicrob Agents Chemother* 23:133, 1983.
180. Dodson HC, Bannister LH, Dovek EE: The effects of combined gentamicin and white noise on the spiral organ of young guinea pigs. *Acta Otolaryngol* (Stockh) 94:193, 1982.
181. Ryan AF, Bone RC: Non-simultaneous interaction of exposure to noise and kanamycin intoxication in the chinchilla. *Am J Otolaryngol* 3:264, 1982.
182. Henry KR, Chole RA, McGinn MD, et al: Increased ototoxicity in both young and old mice. *Arch Otolaryngol* 107:92, 1981.
183. Dumas G, Charachon R: Ototoxicity of kanamycin in developing guinea pigs: An electrophysiological study. *Acta Otolaryngol* (Stockh) 94:203, 1982.
184. Silverblatt F: Pathogenesis of nephrotoxicity of cephalosporins and aminoglycosides: A Review of current concepts. *Rev Infect Dis* 4(suppl):S360, 1982.
185. Edwards CQ, Smith CR, Baughman KL, et al: Concentrations of gentamicin and amikacin in human kidneys. *Antimicrob Agents Chemother* 9:925, 1976.
186. Luft FC, Yun MN, Walker PD, et al: Gentamicin gradient patterns and morphological changes in human kidneys. *Nephron* 18:167, 1977.
187. Houghton DC, Campbell-Boswell MV, Bennett WM, et al: Myeloid bodies in the renal tubules of humans: relationship to gentamicin therapy. *Clin Nephrol* 10:140, 1978.
188. Aubert-Tulkens G, Van Hoof F, Tulkens P: Gentamicin-induced lysosomal phospholipidosis in cultured rat fibroblasts. Quantitative ultrastructural and biochemical study. *Lab Invest* 40:481, 1979.
189. Carlier MB, Laurent G, Claes PJ, et al: Inhibition of lysosomal phospholipases by aminoglycoside antibiotics: In vitro comparative studies. *Antimicrob Agents Chemother* 23:440, 1983.
190. Bennett WM, Gilbert DN, Houghton D, et al: Gentamicin nephrotoxicitymorphologic and pharmacologic features. *West J Med* 126:65, 1977.
191. Wellwood JM, Simpson PM, Tighe JR, et al: Evidence of gentamicin nephrotoxicity in patients with renal allographs. *Br Med J* 3:278, 1975.
192. Simmons CF, Bogusky RT, Humes HD: Inhibitory effects of gentamicin on renal mitochondrial oxidative phosphorylation. *J Pharmacol Exp Ther* 214:709, 1980.
193. Lipsky JJ, Lietman PS: Neomycin inhibition of adenosine triphosphatase: Evidence for a neomycin-phospholipid interaction. *Antimicrob Agents Chemother* 18:532, 1980.
194. Lipsky JJ, Lietman PS: Aminoglycoside inhibition of a renal phosphatidylinositol phospholipase C. *J Pharmacol Exp Ther* 220:287, 1981.
195. McNeil JS, Jackson B, Nelson L, et al: The role of prostaglandins in gentamicin-induced nephrotoxicity in the dog. *Nephron* 33:202, 1983.
196. Baylis C, Rennke HR, Brenner BM: Mechanism of the defect in glomerular ultrafiltration associated with aminoglycoside administration. *Kidney Int* 12:344, 1977.
197. Cojocel C, Hook JB: Differential effect of aminoglycoside treatment on glomerular filtration and renal reabsorption of lysozyme in rats. *Toxicology* 22:261, 1981.
198. Luft FC, Aronoff GR, Evan AP, et al: The effect of aminoglycosides on glomerular endothelium: A comparative study. *Res Commun Chem Pathol Pharmacol* 34:89, 1981.
199. Cojocel C, Dociu N, Maita K, et al: Effects of aminoglycosides on glomerular permeability, tubular reabsorption, and intracellular catabolism of the cationic low-molecular-weight protein lysozyme. *Toxicol Appl Pharmacol* 68:96, 1983.
200. Carlier B, Ninane G: Effects of aminoglycosides on enzymuria and beta 2 microglobulinuria. *Acta Clin Belg* 37:23, 1982.

201. Walenkamp GHIM, Vree TB, Guelen PJM, et al: Interaction between the renal excretion rates of Beta-2-microglobulin and gentamicin in man. *Clin Chim Acta* 127:229, 1983.

202. Elliott WC, Houghton DC, Gilbert DN, et al: Gentamicin nephrotoxicity: 1. Degree and permanence of acquired insensitivity. *J Lab Clin Med* 100:501, 1982.

203. Lietman PS, Smith CR: Aminoglycoside nephrotoxicity in humans. *J Infect Dis* 5(suppl 2):S284, 1983.

204. Holmes AM, Hesling CM, Wilson TM: Drug-induced secondary hyperaldosteronism in patients with pulmonary tuberculosis. *Q J Med* 39:299, 1970.

205. Bar RS, Wilson HE, Mazzaferri EL: Hypomagnesemic hypocalcemia secondary to renal magnesium wasting: A possible consequence of high-dose gentamicin therapy. *Ann Intern Med* 82:646, 1975.

206. Roediger WEW, Ludwin D, Hinder RA: Hypocalcaemic response to streptomycin in malignant hypercalcaemia. *Postgrad Med J* 51:399, 1975.

207. Keating MJ, Seth MR, Bodey GP, et al: Hypocalcemia with hypoparathyroidism and renal tubular dysfunction associated with aminoglycoside therapy. *Cancer* 39:1410, 1977.

208. Patel R, Savage A: Symptomatic hypomagnesemia associated with gentamicin therapy. *Nephron* 23:50, 1979.

209. Moore RD, Smith CR, Lipsky JJ, et al: Risk Factors for renal dysfunction in patients treated with aminoglycosides. *Ann Intern Med* 100:352, 1984.

210. Wade JC, Petty BG, Conrad G, et al: Cephalothin plus an aminoglycoside is more nephrotoxic than methicillin plus an aminoglycoside. *Lancet* ii:604, 1978.

211. Davies J, Anderson P, Davis BD: Inhibition of protein synthesis by spectinomycin. *Science* 149:1096, 1965.

212. Ward ME: The bactericidal action of spectinomycin on *Neisseria gonorrhoeae*. *J Antimicrob Chemother* 3:323, 1977.

213. Holloway WJ: Spectinomycin. *Med Clin North Am* 66:169, 1982.

214. McCormack WM, Finland M: Spectinomycin. *Ann Intern Med* 84:712, 1976.

215. Virtanen S: Sensitivity of *Haemophilus vaginalis* (*Carynebacterium* vaginale) to oleandomycin and spectinomycin. *Pathol Microbiol* 42:36, 1975.

216. Wagner JG, Novak E, Leslie LG: Absorption, distribution and elimination of spectinomycin dihydrochloride in man. *Int J Clin Pharmacol Biopharm* 14:261, 1967.

7

TETRACYCLINES AND CHLORAMPHENICOL

HAROLD C. STANDIFORD

THE TETRACYCLINES

All the tetracyclines are primarily bacteriostatic and have a broad spectrum, which includes gram-positive, gram-negative, aerobic, and anaerobic bacteria, spirochetes, mycoplasmas, rickettsia, chlamydiae, and some protozoa. The analogues can be divided into three groups based on differences in their pharmacology: (*1*) the short-acting compounds—chlortetracycline, oxytetracycline, and tetracycline; (*2*) an intermediate group consisting of demeclocycline and methacycline; and (*3*) the more recently discovered, longer-acting compounds, doxycycline and minocycline.

Structure, Derivation, Nomenclature, and Brand Names

Unlike the fortuitous discovery of penicillin by Flemming, the first tetracycline, chlortetracycline, was discovered by screening organisms obtained from the soil for their antimicrobial properties. Benjamin M. Duggar, a meticulous mycologist in his 70s, noted unusual antimicrobial activity from organisms that formed a golden-yellow colony (1). He designated the organism *Streptomyces aureofaciens* (L. *aurum,* golden) and named the product aureomycin. Oxytetracycline was derived from *Streptomyces rimosus* in 1950, and tetracycline was produced by the catalytic dehalogenation of chlortetracyline in 1953. The two long-acting compounds were derived semisynthetically: doxycycline in 1966 and minocycline in 1967. The compounds currently available in the United States, their major brand names, doses, and costs are listed in Table 1. Chlortetracycline (aureomycin), the first member of the family, is no longer available except for topical use. The low cost of tetracycline compared to the other agents is frequently an important consideration in selecting an agent from this family of related antibiotics. The generic names of the analogues are determined by the substitu-

TABLE 1. The Names, Preparations, Usual Adult Oral Dose, and Costs for the Tetracyclines Currently Available in the United States

Generic Name (Major Brand Name[a])	*Oral Preparations*	*Usual Adult Oral Dose*	*Cost for 10 Days[d]*
Short acting[b]			
Oxytetracycline (Terramycin, Pfizer)	Capsules: 125, 250 mg	500 mg q6h	$27.00
Tetracycline (Achromycin, Lederle)	Capsules: 100, 250, 500 mg Syrup: 125 mg/5 ml	500 mg q6h	5.10
Intermediate			
Methacycline (Rondomycin, Wallace)	Capsules: 150, 300 mg Capsules: 150 mg	300 mg q12h	24.60
Demeclocycline (Declomycine, Lederle)	Tablets: 150 mg	300 mg q12h	31.00
Long acting[c]			
Doxycycline (Vibramycin, Pfizer)	Capsules (hyclate): 50 mg, 100 mg Syrup (calcium): 50 mg/5 ml Suspension (monohydrate): 25 mg/5 ml	200 mg (or 100 mg q12h for first day), then 100 mg q24h	17.55 13.00[e]
Minocycline (Minocin, Lederle)	Capsules: 50, 100 mg Suspension: 50 mg/5 ml	200 mg, then 100 mg q12h	16.60

[a] Many other brands are available for some of the analogues.
[b] The short-acting tetracyclines are also available for intravenous administration at usual doses of 500 mg every 6–12 hours not to exceed 2 g daily. However, most prefer doxycycline for this route of administration. Preparations combined with a local anesthetic agent can be given intramuscularly, but these are not recommended.
[c] The longer-acting agents can be given intravenously in the same doses that are recommended for oral therapy. Doxycycline is available in 100 or 200 mg/vial; minocycline in 100 mg/vial.
[d] The costs are those for a 10-day adult treatment regimen when the antibiotics are purchased by the patient at a community pharmacy. Courtesy of Robert Plummer, Dell's Pharmacy, Aberdeen, Md.
[e] Cost for generic form.

tions on the basic structure of tetracycline, which consists of a hydronaphthacene nucleus containing four fused rings (Fig. 1).

Mechanism of Action

The mechanism of action of the tetracyclines has been reviewed in detail by Pratt (2). The antibiotics enter bacteria by an energy-dependent process. Once within the cell, they reversibly bind primarily to the 30S ribosomal subunit at a position that blocks the binding of the aminoacyl-tRNA to the accepter site on the mRNA-ribosome complex (3). This prevents the addition of new amino acids into the growing peptide chain. The tetracyclines also inhibit protein synthesis in mammalian cells but do not accumulate within these cells by an active process. This may partially explain the difference in the degree of protein inhibition produced in the host and in the microorganism.

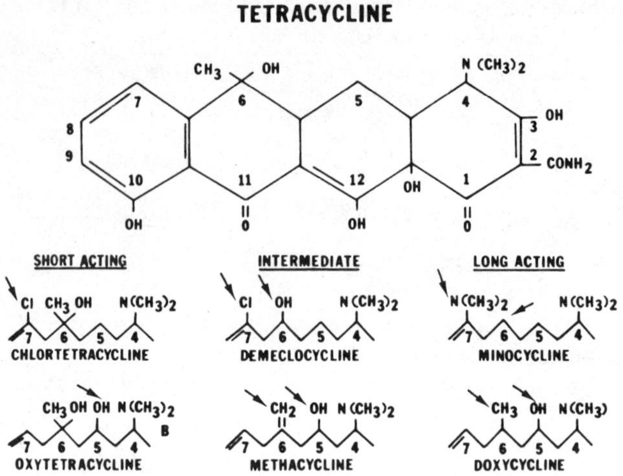

FIGURE 1. The chemical structure of the tetracyclines. The analogues differ from tetracycline at the fifth, sixth, or seventh position, as indicated by the arrows.

In Vitro Activity

The antimicrobial spectra of all the tetracyclines are almost identical. Some differences, however, in the degree of activity against these organisms do exist among the analogues. In general, minocycline is the most active of the analogues, closely followed by doxycycline. The minimum inhibitory concentration (MIC) of oxytetracycline and tetracycline are two- to fourfold higher against many bacteria and are the least-active analogues (4). To save space on crowded sensitivity plates, the tetracycline disk is used to evaluate susceptibility for all the analogues. Minimum inhibitory concentrations of tetracycline and doxycycline for many aerobic bacteria are given in Table 2. For the activity of the other analogues, the reader is referred to the extensive work from the laboratory of Finland et al. (4–6).

Although many of the aerobic and facultative anaerobic organisms are within the spectrum of the tetracyclines, more effective agents are available for the treatment of infections caused by most of these bacteria. The pneumonococci and many *Hemophilus influenzae* can be inhibited by concentrations of tetracyclines achieved in the serum, and this provides rationale for their use in sinusitis and acute exacerbations of chronic bronchitis (7). Gonococci and meningococci are extremely susceptible; unfortunately, gonococci resistant to penicillin G also tend to be resistant to tetracycline (8). Most *Escherichia coli* acquired outside the hospital setting can be inhibited by concentrations achieved in the serum or urine. Tetracyclines, therefore, are useful agents for the treatment of acute, uncomplicated, urinary tract infections. *Pseudomonas pseudomallei* are generally sensitive, and this has therapeutic importance, as does the high degree of susceptibility of *Brucella* sp. (9,10). Although *Campylobacter* sp. are generally susceptible, a high percentage of resistant isolates has been noted in some countries (11–13). Therefore, it is not the drug of choice for infections caused by these bacteria. *Shigella* have become increasingly resistant to these agents (14). *Mycobacterium marinum* is susceptible and appears to respond clinically (15).

The tetracyclines have activity against many anaerobic organisms (16) (Table 3). Their activity against *Actinomyces* is particularly relevant clinically. Doxycycline is more active against *Bacteroides fragilis* than tetracycline, but clindamycin or metronidazole are the preferred agents for infections caused by this organism. The activity of the tetracyclines against anaerobic bacteria, however, may be partially responsible for the effectiveness of the neomycin–tetracycline combination and doxycycline alone as oral presurgical bowel preperations (17,18). Other organisms generally inhibited by this group of antibiotics include rickettsia, chlamydiae, mycoplasmas, and to a limited degree, *Entamoeba histolytica.*

Bacteria develop resistance to the tetracyclines predominantly by preventing the accumulation of tetracycline within the cell. This is accomplished by decreasing the influx transport system and/or increasing the ability of the cell to export the antibiotic. Rarely, if ever, are the tetracyclines inactivated biologically or altered chemically by resistant bacteria (19,20). Resistance to one tetracycline usually implies resistance to all, except for *S. aureus* for minocycline and *B. fragilis* for doxycycline. The resistance among enteric organisms can be mediated by R factors, a mechanism particularly important for *Shigella.* The tetracyclines have been widely used in feeds to promote growth in animals. This may be a major factor in providing selective antibiotic pressure for the spread of R-factor-mediated resistance to these and other antibiotics (21,22).

Pharmacology

Serum levels achieved by usual oral doses in adults are seen in Figure 2. Absorption occurs primarily in the proximal small bowel, producing peak serum concentration 1–3 hours after administration. The commonly used 500-mg therapeutic dose of tetracycline gives a serum level of 4 μg/ml, highest of all the short-acting analogues (23). Doxycycline and minocycline (200 mg) achieve serum levels of about 2.5 μg/ml, slightly higher than levels attained by the larger therapeutic doses of the intermediate agents (24–28).

After intravenous administration of 500 mg, serum levels of the short-acting agents (not shown) are approximately 8 μg/ml at 30 minutes and decrease to 2–3 μg/ml by 5 hours (29). Intravenous injection of the usual 200-mg loading dose of the long-acting agents, doxycycline and minocycline, produce serum levels of approximately 4 μg/ml at 30 minutes. Once tissue distribution occurs for the long-acting analogues, levels are almost identical to concentrations achieved orally (25,30). Thrombophlebitis is a frequent complication of the intravenous preparations. Intramuscular preparations are available for the short-acting compounds but are not recommended because of the severe pain produced on injection, even when they are mixed with local anesthetics.

TABLE 2. Minimum Inhibitory Concentration (MIC) of Tetracycline and Doxycycline for Common Aerobic and Facultative Anaerobic Bacteria

	Number of		*Cumulative % Inhibited by Indicated Concentrations (μg/ml)*						
Organism	*Strains*	*Antibiotic*	*0.4*	*0.8*	*1.6*	*3.1*	*6.3*	*12.5*	*25*
Gram positive									
S. aureus	56	Tetracycline	0	2	20	65	67	67	67
		Doxycycline	2	25	63	65	68	80	87
S. pyogenes[a]	63	Tetracycline	10	50	80	87	90	92	98
		Doxycycline	56	90	90	95	95	98	100
S. pneumoniae[b]	35	Tetracycline	70	96	96	100			
		Doxycycline	100						
Streptococcus (Group B)	12	Tetracycline	0	0	50	50	50	50	75
		Doxycycline	0	50	50	50	50	58	100
Streptococcus (Group D)	36	Tetracycline	0	0	0	0	10	15	15
		Doxycycline	0	0	0	0	10	18	22

Gram negative[c]									
N. gonorrhoeae	25	Tetracycline	5	60	85	88	100		
		Doxycycline	60	75	80	92	100		
N. meningitidis[d]	10	Tetracycline	0	50		100			
		Doxycycline	0		50		100		
H. influenzae	15	Tetracycline	0	0	0	33	87	100	
		Doxycycline	0	0	60	93	100		
E. coli	48	Tetracycline	0	0	0	5	35	60	65
		Doxycycline	0	0	0	5	35	60	70
K. pneumoniae	17	Tetracycline	0	0	0	0	5	30	40
		Doxycycline	0	0	0	0	12	35	40
Enterobacter sp.	10	Tetracycline	0	10	30	50	70	80	90
		Doxycycline	0	0	0	0	10	30	60
Pseudomonas pseudomallei	10	Tetracycline	0	0	60	100			
Campylobacter	172	Tetracycline	44	62	74	81	84	85	88
jejuni	107	Doxycycline	68	74	79	80	86	98	100
Shigella sp.	213	Tetracycline	0	10	12	50	50	55	62

SOURCE: Adapted from Steigbigel et al. (14), Finland (5), Sabath et al. (6), Eickhoff et al. (9), Karmali et al. (12), and Gordon et al. (14). Organisms should be considered susceptible if the MICs are 4 μg/ml or less. An intermediate susceptibility range up to 12.5 μg/ml is useful for the treatment of urinary tract infections.

[a] More recent series indicate that 20–40 percent of *S. pyogenes* have become resistant to the tetracyclines.

[b] Tetracycline-resistant *S. pneumoniae* are more common in some areas.

[c] *P. mirabilis,* indole-positive *Proteus* sp., and *P. aeruginosa* are generally resistant to 25 μg/ml.

[d] The medium inhibitory concentration of minocycline for meningococci is 1.6 μg/ml (range: 0.8–1.6 μg/ml).

TABLE 3. Minimum Inhibitory Concentrations (MIC) of Tetracycline and Doxycycline for Common Anaerobic Bacteria[a]

Organism	Number of Strains	Antibiotic	Cumulative % Susceptible to Indicated Concentration (μg/ml)						
			0.5	*1.0*	*2.0*	*4.0*	*8.0*	*16.0*	*32.0*
Gram positive									
Peptococcus and *Gaffkya*	59	Tetracycline	25	29	36	36	37	61	92
		Doxycycline	28	35	40	70	93	98	100
Peptostreptococcus	29	Tetracycline	38	41	48	52	72	86	97
		Doxycycline	45	45	66	79	97	100	
Streptococci anaerobic and microaerophilic	10	Tetracycline	50	60	70	90	90	90	100
		Doxycycline	70	90	90	90	100		
Eubacterium	17	Tetracycline	24	59	65	65	77	82	94
		Doxycycline	59	65	77	82	88	100	
Propioni bacterium	12	Tetracycline	58	75	83	83	83	83	100
		Doxycycline	75	83	83	92	92	92	100
Clostridium perfringens	9	Tetracycline	22	22	56	67	67	78	78
		Doxycycline	67	67	67	78	89	100	
Other clostridia	33	Tetracycline	36	46	49	52	61	67	76
		Doxycycline	49	52	61	68	82	97	97
Actinomyces	16	Tetracycline	56	69	94	94	94	100	
		Doxycycline	63	69	94	100			
Gram negative									
Gram-negative cocci	26	Tetracycline	54	69	73	73	73	85	92
		Doxycycline	58	69	73	81	96	100	
Fusobacterium	34	Tetracycline	94	97	97	97	97	100	
		Doxycycline	94	94	94	94	100		
Bacteroides fragilis	76	Tetracycline	25	40	40	42	46	68	63
		Doxycycline	41	42	50	75	88	97	100
Bacteroides melaninogenicus	67	Tetracycline	75	76	79	87	94	96	99
		Doxycycline	75	78	90	96	97	99	99
Other *Bacteroides Selenomonas*	72	Tetracycline	33	35	43	50	60	75	93
		Doxycycline	40	43	53	68	79	85	96

SOURCE: Adapted from Sutter and Finegold (16).

[a] An organism with a MIC of 4 μg/ml or less should be considered susceptible.

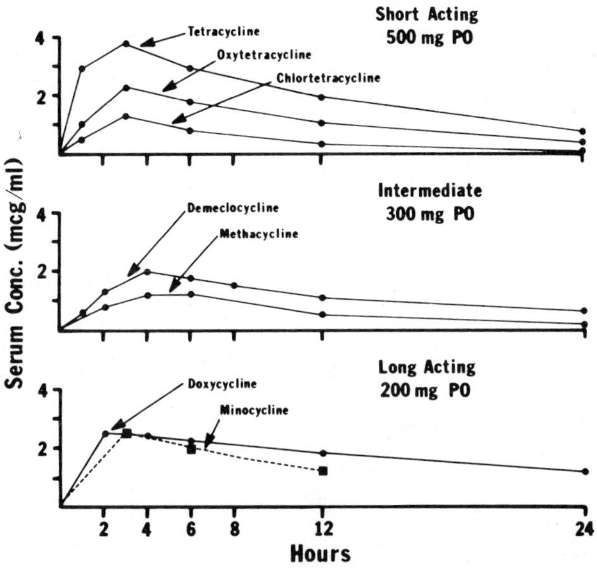

FIGURE 2. Serum levels achieved with the usually recommended oral doses of the tetracyclines. Chlortetracycline is no longer available for oral or parenteral administration. [Adapted from Finland and Garrod (23), Fabre et al. (25), Lederle Laboratories (26), Rosenblatt et al. (27), and Kirby et al. (28).]

Some of the pharmacokinetic properties of the tetracyclines are compared in Table 4. The high levels obtained orally with tetracycline compared with other short-acting agents are due primarily to better absorption from the gastrointestinal tract. The long-acting analogues, doxycycline and minocycline, are absorbed almost completely: Thus, high serum levels are achieved with relatively small doses (25,26). The tetracyclines can be differentiated into three groups on the basis of their different half-lives. Doxycycline has the longest of all, allowing therapeutic levels to be maintained with a single daily dose (25). The 8-hour half-life of tetracycline (29) suggests that the dosage interval could be 8 hours for this antibiotic when it is used to treat minor infections. The half-lives of the compounds are determined mainly by the rate of excretion by the kidneys. Chlortetracycline is an exception, having a short half-life despite a slow rate of clearance as a result of the marked instability of the compound in vitro as well as in vivo (29). With the possible exception of chlortetracycline and minocycline, adequate therapeutic concentrations of all the tetracyclines are achieved in the urine for treatment of urinary tract infections caused by sensitive organisms. The degree of protein binding of the analogues is variable, depending on the methods used for the determination, but it tends to be greater for the intermediate and long-acting compounds (30–32). This may be one of the factors that determines their slow rate of renal excretion. The apparent

TABLE 4. Pharmacokinetic Features of the Tetracyclines[a]

Antibiotic	*GI Absorption (%)*	*Half-Life (hours)*	*Renal Clearance*[b] *(ml/min/1.73m²)*	*Urinary Recovery (%)*	*Apparent Volume of Distribution*[b] *(liters)*	*Protein Binding*[c] *(%)*
Short acting						
Chlortetracycline	30	6	32	18	100	47
Oxytetracycline	58	9	99	70	128	35
Tetracycline	77	8	74	60	108	65
Intermediate						
Demeclocycline	66	12	35	39	121	91
Methacycline	58	14	31	60	79	90
Long acting						
Doxycycline	93	18	20	42	50	93
Minocycline	95	16	9	6	60	76

SOURCE: Adapted from Fabre et al. (25), Lederle Laboratories (26), Rosenblatt et al. (27), Kunin et al. (29), MacDonald et al. (30), Kunin (31), and Bennett et al. (32).

[a] The pharmacokinetic values vary considerably from laboratory to laboratory. These values were selected in most instances because comparative data were available from reliable investigators.

[b] Following single dose intravenous administration.

[c] Ultrafiltration technique.

volume of distribution for most of the tetracyclines is greater than that of extracellular body water, indicating sequestration in tissues, presumably the liver (29). Minocycline and doxycycline have the smallest volume of distribution, another factor that tends to enhance their serum levels (30).

Tissue Distribution. The tetracyclines can be found in small amounts in many tissues and fluids, including lung, liver, kidney, brain, sputum, and mucosal fluid. For tetracycline, the levels in the cerebral spinal fluid are approximately 10–20 percent of the serum levels (33), whereas concentrations in synovial fluid and the maxillary sinus mucosa approach serum levels (34,35). All the tetracyclines are concentrated in the bile and produce levels in this fluid 5–20 times those obtained in the serum. It has been suggested that lipid solubility is a primary determinant for the diffusion in many tissues. Minocycline, followed by doxycycline, is more lipophilic at a physiologic pH than are the other drugs. This may explain why minocycline reaches sufficient concentrations in saliva and tears to eradicate the meningococcal carrier state, whereas the other tetracyclines do not (36,37). The tetracyclines cross the placenta, accumulate in fetal bone and teeth, and, therefore, should not be given during pregnancy (38). Because they are excreted in breast milk, caution is advised in the postpartum period.

Renal Insufficiency. The tetracyclines should not be used in patients with renal failure. Doxycycline, the only exception, is excreted in the gastrointestinal tract under these circumstances. Neither the half-life nor therapeutic dose of this antibiotic varies with alterations of renal function (39).

Assay

The tetracyclines generally are measured by bioassay using *Bacillis cereus* as the test organism (40). A spectrofluorometric assay is available for some of the analogues (41), but monitoring of serum levels during therapy is rarely indicated.

Toxicity

Skin and Allergy. Hypersensitivity reactions including anaphylaxis, urticuria, periorbital edema, fixed drug eruptions, and morbilliform rashes occur with tetracyclines but are not common (42–44). When a patient is allergic to one analogue, he or she should be considered to be allergic to all. Photosensitivity reactions consisting of a red rash on areas exposed to sunlight frequently associated with onycholysis are most common in patients receiving demeclocycline but occur with all analogues. They appear to be a toxic, rather than an allergic, reaction (45,46).

Teeth and Bones. A gray-brown to yellow discoloration of the teeth has been noted in 80 percent of the children taking tetracyclines in some communities

(47). This side effect is permanent and may be associated with hypoplasia of the enamel (45,48) and depression of skeletal growth in premature infants (49). The darkening effect of tetracyclines on permanent teeth appears to be related to the total dose of the antibiotic administered. In a retrospective study, cosmetically noticeable, but mild, darkening of the permanent teeth occurred in 3 out of 14 children receiving five courses of tetracycline whereas 4 out of 6 children receiving eight courses had moderate darkening of the enamel (50). Primary teeth generally show more darkening than the larger, thicker, and more opaque permanent teeth. Since there is some variability in staining with similar tetracycline exposure, it is prudent not to administer these agents to pregnant women and to children up to age 8, the period when tooth enamel is being formed. For this reason, the Food and Drug Administration (FDA) has withdrawn from the market the concentrated liquid dosage forms (drops) specifically intended for pediatric use (51). It is not unreasonable, however, to administer a single course of tetracycline therapy to young children for specifically defined indications where the alternative regime may produce more severe toxicity. Thus, the tetracyclines are indicated for children suspected of having Rocky Mountain spotted fever who can tolerate oral medications. Doxycycline binds less with calcium than do other tetracyclines and may cause dental changes less frequently in children (52).

Gastrointestinal. The tetracyclines are irritative substances and frequently produce gastrointestinal symptoms following oral administration. Esophageal ulcerations that manifest as retrosternal pain exacerbated by swallowing have been clearly documented following tetracycline and doxycycline administration. In most cases, the patients were taking the capsules with little or no fluid just before going to bed. A word of caution to the patient is indicated in order to prevent this toxicity. The complication may also occur in patients with esophageal obstruction or motility disorders (53,54). Nausea, vomiting, and epigastric distress are dose related and limit the dose of most the analogues. Administration of food with doxycycline, minocycline, or oxytetracycline may ameliorate some of these symptoms, but food seriously decreases the absorption of the other tetracyclines. Diarrhea is most often associated with analogues that are poorly absorbed and appears to be related to alterations in the enteric flora. Doxycycline produces less of an effect on bowel flora than does tetracycline (55). The diarrhea usually subsides when the antibiotic is stopped, but prolonged symptoms due to pseudomembranous colitis have been reported (56). Tetracycline also has been noted, rarely, to cause pancreatitis with or without overt liver disease (57).

Superinfection. Colonization by tetracycline-resistant organisms is a frequent occurrence during tetracycline therapy and is generally of little clinical significance. Rarely, a fulminating diarrhea resulting from staphlococcal enteritis may occur after oral or parenteral therapy (58,59). More often and less serious, oral or vaginal monaliasis complicates therapy, a complication that may require specific therapy.

Liver. The hepatoxicity of the tetracyclines, first described in patients receiving intravenous chlortetracycline but now described with other analogues, appears pathologically as a fine droplet fatty metamorphosis and results in a high mortality (60,61). Administration of less than 2 g/day intravenously is not associated with liver dysfunction or injury except in pregnant women who are particularly at risk (62) and in patients with an excessive serum level due to renal failure (63).

Renal Function. Tetracycline aggravates preexisting renal failure by inhibiting protein synthesis, which increases the azotemia from amino acid metabolism (64). Nephrogenic diabetes insipidus is produced by demeclocycline, a side effect that has been used therapeutically to reverse chronic inappropriate antidiuretic hormone secretion (65); renal failure has complicated its use for this purpose in patients with cirrhosis (66). Out-dated tetracycline has produced a reversible Fanconilike syndrome with renal tubular acidosis, but tetracycline formulations producing this syndrome have been modified. It is unlikely that this complication will recur (39).

Nervous and Sensory Systems. Vertigo is a side effect unique to minocycline. Symptoms of light headedness, loss of balance, dizziness, and tinnitus usually begin on the second and third day of therapy and have been noted more frequently in women (70 percent) than in men (28 percent). The symptoms are reversible within several days after discontinuation of the antibiotic, but this side effect has seriously limited the use of minocycline (67). Benign intracranial hypertension (pseudotumor cerebri) has been described in infants and adults with many of the analogues (68,69).

Significant Drug Interactions

Food adversely affects the absorption of tetracycline, chlortetracycline, methacycline, and demeclocycline. All the tetracyclines form complexes with divalent or tivalent cations. Therefore, absorption is markedly decreased when these drugs are administered simultaneously with calcium, magnesium, and aluminum in antacids, milk, or iron and iron-containing tonics (70). Sodium bicarbonate also has an adverse effect on absorption and should not be administered simultaneously (71). Cimetidine has been shown to decrease the absorption of tetracycline, but this is unlikely to be significant in the clinical situation (72). Carbamazepine (Tegretol), diphenylhydantoin, and barbiturates decrease the normal half-life of doxycycline to almost one-half by increasing the hepatic metabolism of the antibiotic (73,74). Methyoxyflurane anesthesia may cause nephrotoxicity when administered with tetracyclines (75). The use of these antibiotics concurrently with diuretics produces an elevated blood urea nitrogen (BUN), although the exact mechanism has not been determined (76).

Indications

The tetracyclines are the drugs of choice or very effective alternative therapy for a wide variety of infections (Table 5). Their role in the therapy for many of the sexually transmitted diseases, including infections caused by the gonococci and chlamydia, and for the treatment of the syndromes of acute pelvic inflammatory disease, nonspecific urethritis, and sexually transmitted epididymoorchitis in young adults is particularly noteworthy (77). The reader is referred to the specific chapter for details. They have no role in the treatment of viral or fungal diseases. Tetracycline, the least expensive of the analogues, is generally preferred for oral administration. Doxycycline, however, appears equally effective and is preferred by most when intravenous administration is required.

CHLORAMPHENICOL

Soon after chloramphenicol was released in the United States in 1949, reports linked this highly effective agent with aplastic anemia, and it quickly fell into disfavor. The increased awareness of the pathogenicity of anaerobic organisms and the development of ampicillin resistant *H. influenzae* accounted for an increase in the use of the compound. However, the availability of both clindamycin and metronidazole for anaerobic infections has reduced the need for chloramphenicol for this indication, and its use for ampicillin-resistant *H. influenzae* is currently being challenged by the newer cephalosporins. Chloramphenicol remains a useful antibiotic but only for well-defined indications in seriously ill patients.

Structure, Derivation, Brand Names, and Preparations

Like the early tetracyclines, chloramphenicol was discovered by screening organisms for their antimicrobial activity. Isolated independently by Burkholder from a mulched field near Caracas, Venezuela (78) and by workers at the University of Illinois from compost (79), the organism producing the active compound was named *Streptomyces venezuelae* (80). The structure of chloramphenicol is shown in Figure 3. It was the first antibiotic whose chemical synthesis was economically and technically practical for large-scale production (81). Preparations currently available and the usual doses are given in Table 6.

Mechanism of Action

Chloramphenicol inhibits protein synthesis. This is accomplished by reversibily binding to the larger 50S ribosomal subunit at a locus that prevents the attach-

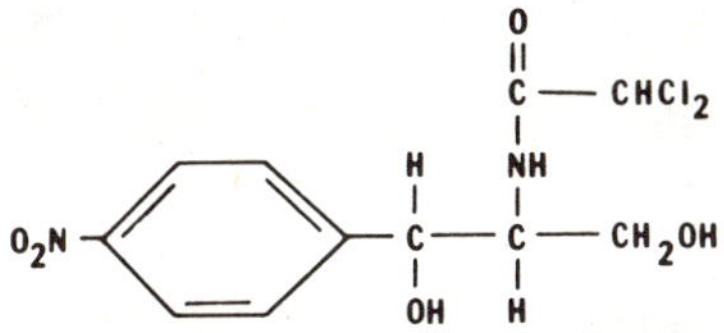

FIGURE 3. The chemical structure of chloramphenicol.

TABLE 5. Major Therapeutic Indications for the Tetracyclines[a]

Therapy of Choice	*Effective Alternative Therapy*
Brucellosis (with streptomycin in seriously ill patients)	Acne, severe Actinomycosis
Chlamydial infections	Anthrax
Ornithosis	*Campylobacter fetus, jejuni*
Trachoma	
Urethral, endocervical, or rectal infections in adults	
Lymphogranuloma venereum	
Cholera	Chronic bronchitis (acute exacerbations)
Epididymitis, acute (sexually transmitted form)	
Gonococcal infections (uncomplicated in adults: penicillin or amoxicillin equally effective)	
Granuloma inguinale	
Leptospirosis	*Pasteurella multocida*
Lyme disease (adults)	Rat-bite fever (Spirillum minus, *Streptobacillus moniliformis*)
Melioidosis (with chloramphenicol in seriously ill patients)	
Mycobacterium fortuitum (amikacin plus doxycycline)	
Mycoplasma pneumoniae (some prefer erythromycin)	Syphilis Tularemia
Pelvic inflammatory disease (acute)	Vincent's infection
Plague (uncomplicated bubonic)	
Prostatitis	
Relapsing fever (*Borrelia* recurrentis)	Whipple's disease
Rickettsial infections (some prefer chloramphenicol for severe infections)	Yaws, nasopalatal *Yersinia enterocolitica*
Rocky Mountain spotted fever	
Typhus fever	
Q fever	
Rickettsial pox	
Urethritis, nonspecific	
Urethral syndrome (dysuria-frequency syndrome)	
Prophylaxis of Choice	*Effective Alternative Prophylaxis*
None	Oral bowel prep for intestinal surgery (tetracycline in combination with neomycin or doxycycline alone) Meningococcal disease (only minocycline) Traveler's diarrhea (doxycycline)

[a] Unless otherwise specified, tetracycline hydrochloride is the preferred analogue for oral administration.

TABLE 6. Systemic Chloramphenicol Preparations Currently Available in the United States

Preparation	*How Supplied*	*Usual dose*
Oral		
Capsules		
Chloromycetin (Parke-Davis)	50, 100, 250 mg	25 mg/kg/day for neonates less than 1 week old; 25 mg/kg q 12 h for infants 1–4 weeks; 50 mg/kg/day in 6-hour intervals for older children and adults; 100 mg/kg/day for older children and adults with meningitis
Mychel (Rachelle)	250 mg	
Suspension		
Chloromycetin Palmitate (Parke-Davis)	150 mg/5 ml	Same as above
Parenteral (intravenous)		
Chloromycetin Sodium Succinate (Parke-Davis)	1 g (powder)	Same as above

ment of the amino-acid-containing end of the aminoacyl-tRNA to its binding region. Without this attachment, the association of the amino acid substrate with peptidyl transferase does not occur, and peptide bond formation is prevented (2). This block in protein synthesis produces a static effect against most sensitive microorganisms. However, in vitro evidence indicates that chloramphenicol is bactericidal against some meningeal pathogens such as *H. influenzae, Streptococcus pneumoniae* and *Neisseria meningitidus* but not group B streptococci at concentrations that can be achieved therapeutically (82–84).

In Vitro Activity

Chloramphenicol is extremely active against a variety of organisms, including bacteria, spirochetes, richettsia, chlamydiae, and mycoplasmas. The minimum inhibitory concentrations required for bacteria are listed in Table 7. Most of the gram-positive and gram-negative aerobic bacteria are inhibited by concentrations easily achieved in the serum of patients, but more active or less toxic therapeutic agents are available for most of these pathogens (5,6, 9,16,81,85–89). Salmonellae, including *Salmonella typhosa,* are generally susceptible (87). In the United States, resistant strains seldom occur (90) but imported strains may be highly resistant. The three most common organisms causing meningitis in childhood (*H. influenzae, S. pneumoniae,* and *N. meningitidis*) are highly susceptible (6) although rare resistant strains of each species have been reported (91,92). Indeed, strains of *H. influenzae* causing clinical infections have been shown to be resistant to both chloramphenicol and ampicillin (93–95). Chloramphenicol is one of the most active antibiotics against anaerobic bacteria including

B. fragilis, but clindamycin and metronidazole have become more important clinically to treat infections caused by these bacteria (16,96).

Bacteria develop resistance to chloramphenicol by becoming impermeable to the drug or by producing an enzyme, acetyltransferase, that acetylates the antibiotic to an inactive diacetyl derivative (97,98). This latter mechanism has been R-factor mediated and has been responsible for widespread epidemics of chloramphenicol-resistant typhoid fever and *Shigella* dysentery in Central and South America, Vietnam, and other countries (99,100,101). It has been suggested that the unrestricted over-the-counter sale of chloramphenicol in the countries involved may be an important factor that provides antibiotic pressure for the development of these resistant strains (101,102).

Pharmacology

Chloramphenicol serum levels achieved by different routes of administration and with different product forms are listed in Figure 4. Chloramphenicol in the encapsulated form is well absorbed from the gastrointestinal tract, resulting in peak serum levels of 12 μg/ml of active antibiotic after a 1-g dose (103,104). Since it is a very bitter substance, aqueous solutions may not be accepted by children. A tasteless suspension in the form of chloramphenicol palmitate is available. This preparation must be hydrolized in the intestine to produce active chloramphenicol. Although earlier formulations sometimes produced erratic serum levels, the bioavailability of chloramphenicol palmitate in the current formulation is the same as in the capsules (A.J. Glazko, Warner-Lambert/Parke-Davis Pharmaceutical Research Division, Ann Arbor, Michigan, personal communication, 105).

The intravenous preparation of the drug is the soluble but inactive chloramphenicol succinate ester that is rapidly hydrolized within the body to biologically active chloramphenicol (106). This preparation produces predictable active chloramphenicol levels in the serum that are 70 percent of those obtained after oral administration due to incomplete hydrolysis (104). Peak serum concentrations after intramuscular administration of this preparation are only one-half to two-thirds of those obtained by the intravenous route, and this has been associated with a delayed therapeutic response and increased relapse rate of typhoid fever (107). Since 30 percent of the unhydrolyzed inactive succinate ester is found in the urine, regardless of which parenteral route is used, the lower serum levels produced by intramuscular injection appear to be due to delayed absorption of the ester from the site of injection rather than to decreased hydrolysis (104). The intramuscular route of administration is currently not recommended.

Chloramphenicol is metabolized primarily by the liver where it is conjugated with glucuronic acid and is excreted in this inactive form by the kidneys. Only about 5–10 percent of the administered dose is recovered in the urine as biologically active choramphenicol. Nevertheless, in the absence of renal disease, con-

TABLE 7. Activity of Chloramphenicol Against Bacteria[a]

Bacteria	Number of Strains	Cumulative % Inhibited at Indicated Concentration (μg/ml)						
		0.4	*0.8*	*1.6*	*3.1*	*6.3*	*12.5*	*25*
Aerobic bacteria								
Gram positive								
S. aureus	291	0	0	0	5	55	95	96
S. aureus (methicillin-resistant)	22	0	0	0	0	20	20	20
S. pyogenes	303	0	0	20	92	99	100	
Streptococci, group B	146	0	0	0	85	99	100	
S. viridans	193	0	0	0	60	90	100	
Streptococci, group D	382	0	0	0	0	0	12	48
S. pneumoniae	78				50	100		
Gram negative								
H. influenzae	17			50	100			
N. meningitidis	7		50		100			
N. gonorrhoeae	106	5	52	97	100			
E. coli	71	0	0	5	30	75	95	95
K. pneumoniae	35	0	0	6	70	75	75	75
Enterobacter	10	0	0	0	10	20	50	80
Serratia marcescens	111	0	0	0	0	5	33	60
P. mirabilis	209	0	0	0	20	60	90	95
Proteus (indole-positive)	32	0	0	0	10	40	50	65

Salmonella typhosa	81	0	0	0	50	95	100	
S. paratyphi A	31				28	97	97	97
Shigella sp.	44		20	30	75	90	90	95
Vibrio cholera	64					84		89
Brucella sp.	25	0	0	28	92	100		
P. aeruginosa	11	0	0	0	0	0	0	0
P. pseudomallei	10	0	0	0	0	50	100	
Bordetella pertussia	31	20	45	85	97	99		
Anaerobic bacteria								
Gram positive								
Peptococcus sp.	145	8	25	67	97	98	98	99
Peptostreptococcus sp.	72	11	37	63	96	100		
Propionibacterium acnes	16	12	31	94	100			
Eubacterium lentum	14	14	14	28	71	100		
Clostridium perfringens	34	0	0	15	100			
Clostridium sp.	17	12	12	53	88	100		
Gram negative								
Veillonella sp.	13	23	46	85	100			
B. fragilis	195	0	1	2	23	98	100	
B. melaninogenicus	29	14	31	93	96	100		
Fusobacterium fusiforme	18	39	44	56	89	100		

SOURCE: Data adapted from Finland (5), Sabath et al. (6), Eickhoff et al. (9), Gordon et al. (14), Sutter and Finegold (16), Woodward and Wisseman (81), McGowan et al. (85), Yow and Spink (86), Robertson et al. (87), Rubinstein and Shainberg (88), Wells et al. (89), and Martin et al. (96).

[a] An organism with a MIC of 12.5 μg/ml or less can be considered susceptible.

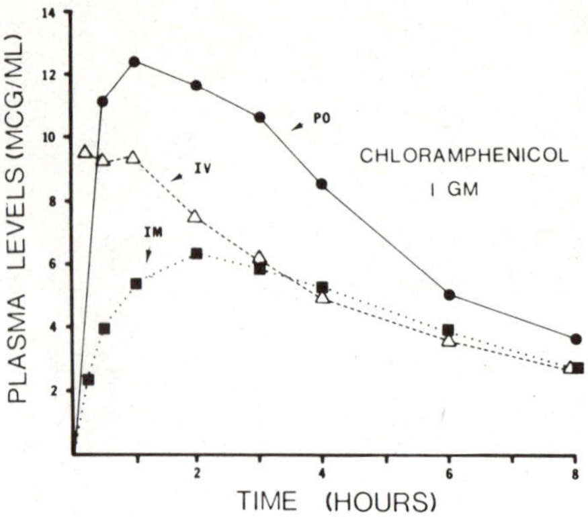

FIGURE 4. Plasma levels of active chloramphenicol achieved with 1 g of chloramphenicol administered orally (Chloromycetin Kapseals) and with chloramphenicol sodium succinate intravenously (IV) and intramuscularly (IM). [Adapted with permission from presentation at the 78th Annual Meeting, American Society for Clinical Pharmacology and Therapeutics (104).]

centrations of 150–200 μg/ml of active drug are achieved, sufficient to treat urinary tract infections, if necessary. Urinary concentrations are markedly diminished, however, in patients with renal failure (108).

The increased use of chloramphenicol in children has led to a better understanding of the pharmacokinetics. It is clear that there is a wide variation in the metabolism and excretion in that age group. Dosage requirements may vary threefold in children of the same age, with even greater variation noted in newborn and young infants. Because they metabolize the antibiotic at a slow rate, the initial dose for newborns less than 1 week old should be 25 mg/kg every 24 hours and for infants from 1–4 weeks, 25 mg/kg every 12 hours instead of the usual 50 mg/kg/day divided into 6 hour dosing intervals for older children and adults. However, the wide variation makes monitoring serum levels imperative (109,110).

Chloramphenicol has a half-life in adults of 4.1 hours after single intravenous injections, is not highly bound to protein (25–50 percent), and has an apparent volume of distribution of 100 liters (81,104,111). The antibiotic diffuses well into many tissues and body fluids. Kramer et al. (112) have shown levels in the brain to be 36 μg/ml, whereas corresponding serum levels were 4 μg/ml. These high levels may reflect the antibiotic's high degree of lipid solubility in conjunction with low protein binding and small molecular size (113). Levels in the cerebral spinal fluid even without inflamed meninges are generally 30–50 percent of serum concentrations, much higher than those of most other antibiotics (81). Therapeutic levels are obtained in pleural, ascitic, and synovial fluid (81,114). In the aqueous humor levels are approximately 50 percent of those in the serum (115), but studies in rabbits and humans suggest that topical administration may be more efficient in providing high aqueous concentrations (116,117). Subconjuctival injections are not satisfactory (118). The antibiotic crosses the placenta to the fetal circulation but produces negligible amounts in the amniotic fluid. Only small amounts of active chloramphenicol are recovered in the bile (0.14 percent of a 1-g dose) (81).

Renal and Hepatic Insufficiency. The half-life of biologically active chloramphenicol in patients with renal disease differs only slightly from healthy subjects, whereas its metabolites increase markedly. The dose, however, should not be modified if therapeutic levels of the active drug are to be maintained. Fortunately, the metabolites do not appear to be as toxic as the active compound. Neither peritoneal nor hemodialysis alters serum levels sufficiently to require dose alternations (111,119).

Patients with hepatic failure, as evidenced by jaundice or ascites, conjugate chloramphenicol at a slower rate. Serum levels of active chloramphenicol increase to levels capable of bone marrow suppression (120). The regime suggested for adults with hepatic insufficiency is an initial 1-g loading dose, followed by 500 mg every 6 hours. The course of therapy should be limited where possible to 10–14 days.

Assay

Because of the narrow therapeutic-to-toxic ratio, it is important to monitor serum levels of this antibiotic, particularly in newborn and premature infants, in patients with hepatic disease, and in those patients taking interacting drugs. There are a number of very effective assays that can be used, including bioassays, radioenzymatic assays, and high-performance chromotography (121–126). Serum levels in most cases should be maintained between 10 and 25 μg/ml.

Toxicity

Hematologic. The most important toxic effects of chloramphenicol occurs in the bone marrow. The effects can be divided into two types. The first is a reversible bone marrow depression due to a direct pharmacologic effect of the antibiotic as a result of inhibition of mitochondrial protein synthesis. It is manifested by reticulocytopenia, anemia, leukopenia, thrombocytopenia, or any combination thereof. There is an increase in serum iron in association with a reduced uptake of radioactive iron by the red blood cells, indicating diminished hemoglobin synthesis. The bone marrow reveals vacuolization of the erythyroid and myeloid precursors, but these changes are not specific for chloramphenicol. This type of toxicity is extremely common, occurs during the course of therapy, and is dose related (127). It is more likely to occur in patients receiving 4 g or more per day or in patients in whom serum levels are above 25 μg/ml, a level that may occur in patients with severe liver disease who are receiving usual doses. It is reversible when the antibiotic is discontinued (128).

The second type of toxicity is a rare but generally fatal "idiosyncratic" response that is most frequently manifested as aplastic anemia (129). Indeed, chloramphenicol is the most common cause of this syndrome. According to the best epidemiologic studies in the United States, aplastic anemia occurs once in 24,500–40,800 patients who receive the antibiotic, a risk about 13 times greater than that for aplastic anemia in the general population (130). The aplastic anemia most commonly occurs weeks to months following completion of therapy and is not necessarily dose related. It appears that this toxic effect is caused by a different mechanism than the direct bone marrow suppression previously described. Although the pathogenesis of this idiosyncratic response is not known, there have been several observations and theories that deserve comment. The type of toxicity has occurred in identical twins suggesting a genetic predisposition (131). Morley et al. (132) have observed that mice given chloramphenicol after treatment with busulfan had a progressive fall in pluripotential stem cells, whereas control mice did not. Since most of the animals had entirely normal hemograms before receiving chloramphenicol, they suggest that the aplastic anemia might result in patients with unrecognized preexisting residual marrow damage either genetic or acquired. In 1967, Holt observed that the aplastic anemia only occurred after oral administration of the antibiotic (133). He postulates that the fatal reaction may be caused by the absorption of toxic products produced by enzymatic degradation of chloramphenicol, perhaps as a result of specific types of bacteria colonizing the gut of affected people. Since that time, a number of cases of aplastic anemia from parenteral chloramphenicol and following administration of eye drops have been reported. Although the number of cases reported is greater after oral therapy, the parenteral form of the antibiotic should also be considered to be potentially toxic (134–136). It has been speculated that the nitrobenzene moiety of chloramphenicol may be the culprit responsible for the aplastic anemia. Thiamphenicol, an analogue of chloramphenicol that is currently used in Europe and Japan, has the nitro group on the benzene ring replaced by methysulfone. This analogue produces the reversible bone marrow suppression as readily as chloramphenicol but has not been associated with the aplastic anemia (137). Although most cases of aplastic anemia from chloramphenicol become apparent after completion of therapy, it should be emphasized that 22 percent of the cases occur concurrently with antibiotic administration (129,136). Whether some of these episodes can be prevented by checking the blood counts of patients is not known. Until the pathogenesis of the toxicity is clearly understood, it is recommended that a complete blood count be obtained on all patients receiving chloramphenicol on a twice-a-week basis. If the white blood cell count decreases below 2500/mm^3, it is desirable to discontinue the antibiotic if the clinical condition allows. It should be recognized, however, that low numbers of white blood cells may occur in illnesses such as typhoid fever for which chloramphenicol is used.

Chloramphenicol may also produce a hemolytic anemia in patients with the Mediterranean form of glucose-6-phosphate dehydrogenase (G6PD) deficiency. This apparently does not occur with the milder A type G6PD deficiency, which is the most common form in blacks (138).

Gray Syndrome. The gray syndrome of neonates is characterized by abdominal distention, vomiting, flacidity, cynosis, circulatory collapse, and death. The side effect results from a diminished ability of neonates to conjugate chloramphenicol and to excrete the active form in the urine (139). If chloramphenicol is necessary in premature infants and neonates, the dose should be reduced to 25 mg/kg/day and the antibiotic levels should be monitored. This syndrome has also been recognized in toddlers and after accidental overdoses in adults (140,141).

Optic Neuritis. Optic neuritis resulting in decreased visual acuity has been described in patients receiving prolonged chloramphenicol therapy (142). The symptoms are generally reversible, but loss of vision has occurred. Other neurologic sequelae such as peripheral neuritis, headache, depression, opthalmoplegia, and mental confusion have also been described.

Other Types. Hypersensitivity reactions including rashes and drug fevers and anaphylaxis are rare. Herxheimerlike responses during therapy for syphilis, brucellosis, and typhoid fever have been observed. Symptoms involving the gastrointestinal tract, including nausea, vomiting and diarrhea, glossitis, and stomatitis, occur but have not been a major problem. Bleeding due to decreased vitamin K synthesis has resulted from prolonged administration.

Significant Drug Interactions

Chloramphenicol prolongs the half-life of tolbutamide, chlorpropamide, phenytoin, and warfarin (Coumadin), apparently by inhibiting hepatic microsomal enzymes (143–145). Severe toxicity and death have occurred. Phenytoin and phenobarbital have been observed to decrease the serum concentration and increase the total body clearance of chloramphenicol, perhaps by inducing hepatic microsomal enzymes. Serum concentrations should be monitored when these drugs are administered concurrently (147). The physician should be on the alert for toxicity from other agents that are metabolized by the liver when administering this agent, and should monitor serum levels when these drugs are administered concurrently. Chloramphenicol may delay the response of anemias to iron, folic acid, and vitamin B_{12} (146).

Chloramphenicol is primarily a bacteriostatic agent and will antagonize in vitro the bactericidal activity of the penicillins, cephalosporins, and the aminoglycoside antibiotics. This has doubtful clinical significance in most instances. However, care should be exercised in the use of such combinations for infections that require bactericidal activity for efficacy, such as for infections in the granulocytopenic host or in the treatment of endocarditis (148). In the treatment of

TABLE 8. Indications for Chloramphenicol

Indication	*Usual Adult Dose*	*Comment*
Therapy of choice		
Brain abscess	100 mg/kg/day	Used with a penicillin; some prefer metronidazole
Meningitis		
H. influenzae	100 mg/kg/day	Use for this indication currently challenged by newer cephalosporins
Typhoid fever and salmonellosis (invasive)	50 mg/kg/day	Strains in some areas may be chloramphenicol resistant; not used for gastroenteritis or carrier state
Acute melioidosis		Used with tetracycline
Effective alternative therapy		
Meningitis	100 mg/kg/day	For penicillin-allergic patients
S. pneumoniae		
N. meningitidis		
Rickettsial infections	50 mg/kg/day	Preferred drug when patients require parenteral therapy
Rocky Mountain spotted fever		
Typhus		

meningitis, the bacteriostatic activity of chloramphenicol against group B streptococci and its in vitro antagonism with ampicillin against this organism is of concern and should be considered in selecting therapy when this organism is likely to be a pathogen (84).

Indications

The clinical indications for the use of chloramphenicol are listed in Table 8. In most cases, these indications are clearly defined. Occasionally, the antibiotic is useful when the differential diagnosis includes both meningococcemia and Rocky Mountain spotted fever, diseases that may be difficult to distinguish on clinical characteristics. It also may be useful in the place of a nephrotoxic agent for the treatment of severe infections due to sensitive organisms in patients with decreased renal function.

Chloramphenicol is a valuable antimicrobial agent. Like many other agents, it is toxic and can cause death. When the clinical indications are present, however, the antibiotic should not be avoided because of its possible toxicity.

REFERENCES

1. Finland M: Twenty-fifth anniversary of the discovery of Aureomycin: The place of the tetracyclines in antimicrobial therapy. *Clin Pharmacol Ther* 15:3, 1974.
2. Pratt WB: *Chemotherapy of Infection.* New York, Oxford University Press, 1977, pp 128.
3. Craven GR, Gavin R, Fanning T: The transfer RNA binding site of the 30 s ribosome and the site of tetracycline inhibition. *Symp Quant Biol* 34:129, 1969.

4. Steigbigel NH, Reed CR, Finland M: Susceptibility of common pathogenic bacteria to seven tetracycline antibiotics in vitro. *Am J Med Sci* 255:179, 1968.
5. Finland M: Changing patterns of susceptibility of common bacterial pathogens to antimicrobial agents. *Ann Intern Med* 76:1009, 1972.
6. Sabath LD, Stumpf LL, Wallace SJ, et al: Susceptibility of *Diplococcus pneumoniae, Haemophilus influenzae,* and *Neisseria meningitidis* to 23 antibiotics. *Antimicrob Agents Chemother 1970,* 1971, p 53.
7. Neu HC: A symposium on the tetracyclines: A major appraisal. Introduction. *Bull NY Acad Med* 54:141, 1978.
8. Sparling PF: Antibiotic resistance in *Neisseria gonorrhoeae. Med Clin North Am* 56:1133, 1972.
9. Eickhoff TC, Bennett JV, Hayes PS, et al: *Psudomonas pseudomallei* susceptibility to chemotherapeutic agents. *J Infect Dis* 121:95, 1970.
10. Farrell ID, Hinchliffe PM, Robertson L: Susceptibility of *Brucella* spp. to tetramycline and its analogues. *J Clin Pathol* 29:1097, 1976.
11. Chow AW, Patten V, Dominick B: Susceptibility of *Campylobacter fetus* to twenty-two. *Antimicrob Agents Chomether* 13:416, 1978.
12. Karmali MA, DeGrandis S, Fleming PC: Antimicrobial susceptibility of *Campylobacter jejuni* with special reference to resistance patterns of Canadian isolates. *Antimicrob Agents Chemother* 19:593, 1981.
13. Michel J, Rogol M, Dickman D: Susceptibility of clinical isolates of *Campylobacter jejuni* to sixteen. *Antimicrob Agents Chemother* 23:796, 1983.
14. Gordon RC, Thompson TR, Carlson W, et al: Antimicrobial resistance of shigellae isolated in Michigan. *JAMA* 231:1159, 1975.
15. Wallace RJ, Wiss K: Susceptibility of *Mycobacterium marinum* to tetracyclines and aminoglycosides. *Antimicrob Agents Chemother* 20:610, 1981.
16. Sutter VL, Finegold SM: Susceptibility of anaerobic bacteria to 23 antimicrobial agents. *Antimicrob Agents Chemother* 10:736, 1976.
17. Washington JA, Dearing WH, Judd ES, et al: Effect of preoperative antibiotic regimen on development of infection after intestinal surgery: Prospective, randomized, double-blind study. *Ann Surg* 180:567, 1974.
18. Hojer H, Wetterfors J: Systemic prophylaxis with doxycycline in surgery of the colon and rectum. *Ann Surg* 187:362, 1978.
19. Benveniste R, Davies J: Mechanisms of antibiotic resistance in bacteria. *Ann Rev Biochem* 42:471, 1973.
20. Sompolinsky D, Zemira S: Plasmid-determined resistance to tetracycline. *Microbios* 30:109, 1981.
21. Rapoport MI, Calia FM: The use of antibiotics in animal feeds. *JAMA* 229:1212, 1974.
22. VanLeeuwen WJ, VanEmbden J, Guinee PAM, et al: Decrease in drug resistance in salmonella in the Netherlands. *Antimicrob Agents Chemother* 16:237, 1979.
23. Finland M, Garrod LP: Demethylchlortetracycline. *Br Med J* 2:959, 1960.
24. Fabre J, Pitton JS, Junz JP, et al: Distribution and excretion of doxycycline in man. *Chemotherapia* 11:73, 1966.
25. Fabre J, Milek E, Kalfopoulos P, et al: The kinetics of tetracyclines in man: Digestive absorption and serum concentrations, in: *Doxycycline (Vibramycin), A Compendium of Clinical Evaluation.* New York, Pfizer Laboratories Division, Pfizer, Inc, 1973, p 13.
26. Lederle Laboratories: *Minocin: Minocycline.* Pearl River, NY, Lederle Laboratories, American Cyanamid Co, 1975.
27. Rosenblatt JE, Barrett JE, Brodie JL, et al: Comparison of in vitro activity and clinical pharmacology of doxycycline with other tetracyclines. *Antimicrob Agents Chemother 1966,* 1967, p 134.
28. Kirby WMM, Roberts CE, Burdick RE: Comparison of two new tetracyclines with tetracycline and demethylchlortetracycline. *Antimicrob Agents Chemother 1961,* 1962, p 286.

29. Kunin CM, Dornbush AC, Finland M: Distribution and excretion of four tetracycline analogues in normal young men. *J Clin Invest* 38:1950, 1959.
30. MacDonald H, Kelley RG, Allen ES, et al: Pharmacokinetic studies on minocycline in man. *Clin Pharmacol Ther* 14:852, 1973.
31. Kunin CM: Comparative serum binding distribution and excretion of tetracycline and a new analogue methacycline. *Proc Soc Exp Biol Med* 110:311, 1962.
32. Bennett JV, Mickewait JS, Barrett JE, et al: Comparative serum binding of four tetracyclines under simulated in vivo conditions. *Antimicrob Agents Chemother 1965,* 1966, p 180.
33. Wood WS, Kipnis GR: The concentrations of tetracycline, chlortetracycline and oxytetracycline in the cerebrospinal fluid after intravenous administration. *Antibiotics Annual 1953–1954,* 1953, p 98.
34. Parker RH, Schmid F: Antimicrobial activity of synovial fluid during therapy of septic arthritis. *Arthritis Rheum* 14:96, 1971.
35. Lundberg C, Malmburg A, Ivemark BI: Antibiotic concentrations in relation to structural changes in maxillary sinus mucosa following intramuscular or peroral treatment. *Scand J Infect Dis* 6:187, 1974.
36. Fabre J, Milek E, Kalopoulos P, et al: The kinetics of tetracyclines in man II. Excretion, penetration in normal and inflammatory tissues, behavior in renal insufficiency and hemodialysis, in: *Doxycycline (Vibramycin): A Compendium of Clinical Evaluations.* New York, Pfizer Laboratories Division, Pfizer, Inc, 1973, p 19.
37. Hoeprich PD, Warshauer DM: Entry of four tetracyclines into saliva and tears. *Antimicrob Agents Chemother* 5:330, 1974.
38. LeBlanc AL, Perry JE: Transfer of tetracycline across the human placenta. *Tex Rep Biol Med* 25:541, 1967.
39. Whelton A: Tetracyclines in renal insufficiency: Resolution of a therapeutic dilemma. *Bull NY Acad Med* 54:223, 1978.
40. Bennett JV, Brodie JL, Benner EJ, et al: Simplified accurate method for antibiotic assay of clinical specimens. *Appl Microbiol* 14:170, 1966.
41. Kohn KW: Determination of tetracyclines by extraction of fluorescent complexes: Application to biological materials. *Anal Chem* 33:862, 1961.
42. Csonka GW, Rosedale N, Walkden L: Balanitis due to fixed drug eruption associated with tetracycline therapy. *Br J Vener Dis* 47:42, 1970.
43. Fellner MJ, Baer RL: Anaphylactic reaction to tetracycline in a penicillin-allergic patient: Immunologic Studies. *JAMA* 192:997, 1965.
44. Furey WW, Tan C: Anaphylactic shock due to oral demethylchlortetracycline. *Ann Intern Med* 70:357, 1969.
45. Carey BW: Photodynamic response of a new tetracycline. *JAMA* 172:1196, 1960.
46. Frost P, Weinstein GD, Gomez EC: Phototoxic potential of minocycline and doxycycline. *Arch Dermatol* 105:681, 1972.
47. Brearley LJ, Storey E: Tetracycline-induced tooth changes: Part 2. Prevalence localization and nature of staining in extracted deciduous teeth. *Med J Aust* 2:714, 1968.
48. Witkop CJ, Wolf RO: Hypoplasia and intrinsic staining of enamel following tetracycline therapy. *JAMA* 185:1008, 1963.
49. Cohan S, Bevelander G, Tiamsic T: Growth inhibition of prematures receiving tetracycline. *Am J Dis Child* 105:453, 1963.
50. Grossman ER, Walcheck A, Freedman H: Tetracycline and permanent teeth: The relationship between doses and tooth color. *Pediatrics* 47:567, 1971.
51. Department of Health Education and Welfare: Tetracycline pediatric drops to be withdrawn from the market. *FDA Drug Bull* 8:23, 1978.
52. Forti G, Benincori C: Doxycycline and the teeth. *Lancet* 1:782, 1969.
53. Schneider R: Doxycycline esophageal ulcers. *Am J Dig Dis* 22:805, 1977.
54. Winckler K: Tetracycline ulcers of the oesophagus: Endoscopy, histology, and roentgenology in two cases, and review of the literature. *Endoscopy* 13:225, 1981.
55. Hinton NA: The effect of oral tetracycline HCl and doxycycline on the intestinal flora. *Curr Therap Res* 12:341, 1970.

56. Gorbach SL, Bartlett JG: Anaerobic infections. *N Engl J Med* 290:1289, 1974.
57. Elmore MF, Rogge JD: Tetracycline induced pancreatitis. *Gastroenterology* 81:1134, 1981.
58. Jackson GG, Haight TH, Kass EH, et al: Terramycin therapy of pneumonia: Clinical and bacteriologic studies in 91 cases. *Ann Intern Med* 35:1175, 1951.
59. Lundsgaard-Hansen P, Senn A, Roos B, et al: Staphylococcal enteritis: Report of six cases with two fatalities after intravenous administration of *N*-(Pyrrolidinomethyl) tetracycline. *JAMA* 173:1008, 1960.
60. Lepper MH, Wolfe CK, Zimmerman HJ, et al: Effect of large doses of Aureomycin on human liver. *Arch Intern Med* 88:271, 1951.
61. Schultz JC, Adamson JS Jr, Workman WW, et al: Fatal liver disease after intravenous administration of tetracycline in high doses. *N Engl J Med* 269:999, 1963.
62. Whalley PJ, Adams RH, Combes B: Tetracycline toxicity in pregnancy: Liver and pancreatic dysfunction. *JAMA* 189:357, 1964.
63. Damjanov I, Arnold R, Faour M: Tetracycline toxicity in a non-pregnant woman. *JAMA* 204:934, 1968.
64. Shils ME: Renal disease and the metabolic effects of tetracycline. *Ann Intern Med* 58:389, 1963.
65. Forrest JN, Cox M, Hong C, et al: Superiority of demeclocycline over lithium in the treatment of chronic syndrome of inappropriate secretion of antidiuretic hormone. *N Engl J Med* 298:173, 1978.
66. Carrilho F, Bosch J, Arroyo V, et al: Renal failure associated with demeclocycline in cirrhosis. *Ann Intern Med* 87:195, 1977.
67. Fanning WL, Gump DW, Sofferman RA: Side effects of minocycline: A double blind study. *Antimicrob Agents Chemother* 11:712, 1977.
68. Koch-Weser J, Gilmore EB: Benign intracranial hypertension in an adult after tetracycline therapy. *JAMA* 200:345, 1967.
69. Walters BNJ, Gubbay SS: Tetracycline and benign intracranial hypertension: Report of five cases. *Br Med J* 282:19, 1981.
70. Neuvonen PJ, Gothoni G, Hackman R, et al: Interference of iron with the absorption of tetracyclines in man. *Br Med J* 4:532, 1970.
71. Bar WH, Adir J, Garrettson L: Decrease of tetracycline in man by sodium bicarbonate. *Clin Pharmacol Ther* 12:779, 1971.
72. Fisher P, House F, Inns P, et al: Effect of cimetidine on the absorption of orally administered tetracycline. *Br J Clin Pharmacol* 9:153, 1980.
73. Neuvonem PJ, Penttila O: Interaction between doxycycline and barbiturates. *Br Med J* 1:535, 1974.
74. Penttila O, Neuvonen PJ, Lehtovaara R: Interaction between doxycycline and some antiepileptic drugs. *Br Med J* 2:470, 1974.
75. Kuzucu EY: Methoxyflurane, tetracycline and renal failure. *JAMA* 211:1162, 1970.
76. Boston collaborative drug surveillance program: Tetracycline and drug-attributed rises in blood urea nitrogen. *JAMA* 220:377, 1972.
77. U.S. Department of Health and Human Services: Sexually transmitted diseases treatment guidelines, 1982, *Morbidity and Mortality Weekly Report* 31(suppl):35S, 1982.
78. Ehrlich J, Bartz QR, Smith RM, et al: Chloromycetin, a new antibiotic from a soil actinomycete. *Science* 106:417, 1947.
79. Carter HE, Gottlieb D, Anderson HW: Comments and communications. *Science* 107:113, 1947.
80. Ehrlich J, Gottlieb D, Burkholder PR, et al: *Streptomyces venezuelae,* N. sp., the source of Chloromycetin. *J Bacteriol* 56:467, 1948.
81. Woodward TE, Wisseman CL: *Chloromycetin* (*Chloramphenicol*). New York, Medical Encyclopedia, 1958.
82. Turk DC: A comparison of chloramphenicol and ampicillin as bactericidal agents for *Haemophilus influenzae* type B. *J Med Microbiol* 10:127, 1977.
83. Rahal JJ, Simberkoff MS: Bactericidal and bacteriostatic action of chloramphenicol against meningeal pathogens. *Antimicrob Agents Chemother* 16:13, 1979.

84. Weeks JL, Mason EO Jr, Baker CJ: Antagonism of ampicillin and chloramphenicol for meningeal isolates of group B Streptococci. *Antimicrob Agents Chemother* 20:281, 1981.
85. McGowan JE, Garner C, Wilcox C, et al: Antibiotic suceptibility of gram negative bacilli isolated from blood cultures: Results of tests with 35 agents and strains from 169 patients at Boston City Hospital during 1972. *Am J Med* 57:225, 1974.
86. Yow EM, Spink WW: Experimental studies on the action of streptomycin, Aureomycin and Chloromycetin on *Brucella. J Clin Invest* 28:871, 1949.
87. Robertson RP, Wahab MFA, Raasch FO: Evaluation of chloramphenicol and ampicillin in *Salmonella* enteric fever. *N Engl J Med* 278:171, 1968.
88. Rubinstein E, Shainberg B: In vitro activity of cinoxacin, ampicillin, and chloramphenicol against *Shigella* and non-typhoid *Salmonella. Antimicrob Agents Chemother* 11:577, 1977.
89. Wells EB, Chang SM, Jackson GG, et al: Antibiotic spectrum of *Hemophilus pertussis. J Pediatr* 36:752, 1950.
90. Cherubin CE, Neu HC, Rahal JJ, et al: Emergence of resistance to chloramphenicol in *Salmonella. J Infect Dis* 135:807, 1977.
91. Long SS, Phillips SE: Chloramphenicol-resistant *Hemophilus influenzae. J Pediatr* 90:1030, 1976.
92. Mathies AW Jr: Penicillins in the treatment of bacterial meningitis. *J R Coll Physicians Lond* 6:139, 1972.
93. MacMahon P, Sills J, Hall E, et al: Haemophilus influenzae type b resistant to both chloramphenicol and ampicillin in Britain. *Br Med J* 24:1229, 1982.
94. Bergeron MC, Claveau S, Simard P: Limited in vitro activity of cefamandole against 100 beta-lactamase- and non-beta-lactamase-producing haemophilus influenzae strains: Comparison of moxalactam, chloramphenicol and ampicillin *Antimicrob Agents Chemother* 19:101, 1981.
95. Kenny JF, Isburg CD, Michaels RH: Meningitis due to haemophilus influenzae type b resistant to both ampicillin and chloramphenicol. *Pediatrics* 66:14, 1980.
96. Martin WJ, Gardner M, Washington JA II: In vitro antimicrobial susceptibility of anaerobic bacteria isolated from clinical specimens. *Antimicrob Agents Chemother* 1:148, 1972.
97. Okamoto S, Mizuno D: Mechanism of chloramphenicol and tetracycline resistance in *Escherichia coli. J Gen Microbiol* 35:125, 1964.
98. Okamoto S, Suzuki Y: Chloramphenicol-, dihydrostreptomycin-, and kanamycin-inactivating enzymes from multiple drug-resistant *Escherichia coli* carrying episome "R." *Nature* 208:1301, 1965.
99. Gangarosa EJ, Bennett JV, Wyatt C, et al: An epidemic-associated episome? *J Infect Dis* 126:215, 1972.
100. Butler T, Linh NN, Arnold K, et al: Chloramphenicol-resistant typhoid fever in Vietnam associated with R-factor. *Lancet* 2:983, 1973.
101. Editorial: Drug resistance in salmonellas. *Lancet* 1:1391, 1982.
102. Anderson ES, Smith HR: Chloramphenicol resistance in the typhoid bacillus. *Br Med J* 3:329, 1972.
103. Bartelloni PJ, Calia FM, Minchew BH, et al: Absorption and excretion of two chloramphenicol products in humans after oral administration. *Am J Med Sci* 258:203, 1969.
104. Glazko AJ, Dill WA, Kinkel AW, et al: Absorption and excretion of parenteral doses of chloramphenicol sodium succinate in comparison with peroral doses of chloramphenicol, abstract. *Clin Pharmacol Ther* 21:104, 1977.
105. Pickering LK, Hoecker JL, Kramer WG, et al: Clinical pharmacology of two chloramphenicol preparations in children: Sodium succinate (IV) and palmitate (oral) esters. *J Pediatr* 96:757, 1980.
106. McCrumb FR, Snyder MJ, Hicken WJ: The use of chloramphenicol acid succinate in the treatment of acute infections. *Antibiotics Annual 1957–1958.* New York, Medical Encyclopedia, 1958, p 837.
107. DuPont HL, Hornick RB, Weiss CF, et al: Evaluation of chloramphenicol acid succinate therapy of induced typhoid fever and Rocky Mountain spotted fever. *N Engl J Med* 282:53, 1970.

108. Lindberg AA, Nilsson LH, Bucht H, et al: Concentration of chloramphenicol in the urine and blood in relation to renal function. *Br Med J* 2:724, 1966.
109. Kauffman RE, Miceti JN, Strebel L, et al: Pharmacokinetics of chloamphenicol and chloramphenicol succinate in infants and children. *J Pediatr* 98:315, 1981.
110. Kauffman RE, Thirumoorthi MC, Buckley JA, et al: Relative bioavailability of intravenous chloramphenicol succinate and oral chloramphenicol palmitate in infants and children. *J Pediatr* 99:363, 1981.
111. Kunin CM: A guide to use of antibiotics in patients with renal disease. *Ann Intern Med* 67:151, 1967.
112. Kramer PW, Griffith RS, Campbell RL, et al: Antibiotic penetration of the brain: A comparative study. *J. Neurosurg* 31:295, 1969.
113. Braude AI: *Antimicrobial Drug Therapy.* Philadelphia, WB Saunders, 1976, p 82.
114. Rapp GF, Griffith RS, Hebble WM: The permeability of traumatically inflamed synovial membrane to commonly used antibiotics. *J Bone Joint Surg* 48-A:1534, 1966.
115. Abraham RK, Burnett HH: Tetracycline and chloramphenicol studies on rabbit and human eyes. *Arch Ophthalmol* 54:641, 1955.
116. Beasley H, Boltralik JJ, Baldwin HA: Chloramphenicol in aqueous humor after topical application. *Arch Ophthalmol* 93:184, 1975.
117. George FJ, Hanna C: Ocular penetration of chloramphenicol. *Arch Ophthalmol* 95:879, 1977.
118. McPherson SD Jr, Presley GD, Crawford JR: Aqueous humor assays of subconjunctival antibiotics. *Am J Ophthalmol* 66:430, 1968.
119. Kunin CM, Glazko AJ, Finland M: Persistence of antibiotics in blood of patients with acute renal failure. II. Chloramphenicol and its metabolic products in the blood of patients with severe renal disease or hepatic cirrhosis. *J Clin Invest* 38:1498, 1959.
120. Suhrland LG, Weisberger AS: Chloramphenicol toxicity in liver and renal disease. *Arch Intern Med* 112:161, 1963.
121. Louie TJ, Tally FP, Bartlett JG, et al: Rapid microbiological assay for chloramphenicol and tetracyclines. *Antimicrob Agents Chemother* 9:874, 1976.
122. Jorgensen JH, Alexander GA: Rapid bioassay for chloramphenicol in the presence of other antibiotics. *Am J Clin Pathol* 76:474, 1981.
123. Lietman PS, White TJ, Shaw WV: Chloramphenicol: An enzymological microassay. *Antimicrob Agents Chemother* 10:347, 1976.
124. Smith AL, Smith DH: Improved enzymatic analysis of chloramphenicol. *Clin Chem* 24:1452, 1978.
125. Aravind MK, Miceli JN, Kauffman RE, et al: Simultaneous measurements of chloramphenicol and chloramphenicol succinate in body fluids utilizing HPLC. *J Chromatogr* 221:176, 1980.
126. Nahata MC, Powell DA: Simultaneous determination of chloramphenicol and its succinate ester by high-performance liquid chromatography. *J Chromatogr* 223:247, 1981.
127. Yunis AA: Chloramphenicol-induced bone marrow suppression. *Semin Hematol* 10:225, 1973.
128. Scott JL, Finegold SM, Belkin GA, et al: A controlled double-blind study of the hematologic toxicity of chloramphenicol. *N Engl J Med* 272:1137, 1965.
129. Best WR: Choramphenicol-associated blood dyscrasias. A review of cases submitted to the American Medical Association Registry. *JAMA* 201:181, 1967.
130. Wallerstein RO, Condit PK, Kasper CK, et al: Statewide study of chloramphenicol therapy and fatal aplastic anemia. *JAMA* 208:2045, 1969.
131. Nagao T, Mauer AM: Concordance for drug-induced aplastic anemia in identical twins. *N Engl J Med* 281:7, 1969.
132. Morley A, Trainor K, Remes J: Residual marrow damage: Possible explanation for idiosyncrasy to chloramphenicol. *Br J Haematol* 32:525, 1976.
133. Holt R: The bacterial degradation of chloramphenicol. *Lancet* 1:1259, 1967.
134. Polin HB, Plaut ME. Chloramphenicol. *NY State J Med* 77:378, 1977.
135. Plaut ME, Best WR: Aplastic anemia after parenteral chloramphenicol: Warning renewal, letter. *N Engl J Med* 306:1486, 1982.

136. Daum RS, Cohen DL, Smith AL: Fatal aplastic anemia following apparent "dose-related" chloramphenicol toxicity. *J Pediatr* 94:403, 1979.
137. Keiser G: Introduction: Symposium on thiampenicol. *Postgrad Med J* 50(suppl 5):13, 1974.
138. Beutler E: Glucose 6-phosphate dehydrogenase deficiency, in Williams WJ, Beutler E, Erslev AJ, et al (eds): *Hematology.* New York, McGraw Hill, 1977, p 466.
139. Burns LE, Hodgman JE, Cass AB: Fatal circulatory collapse in premature infants receiving chloramphenicol. *N Engl J Med* 261:1318, 1959.
140. Craft AW, Brocklebank JT, Hey EN, et al: The "grey toddler": Chloramphenicol toxicity. *Arch Dis Child* 49:235, 1974.
141. Thompson WL, Anderson SE, Lipsky JJ, et al: Overdoses of chloramphenicol. *JAMA* 234:149, 1975.
142. Chloramphenicol blindness, editorial. *Br Med J* 1:1511, 1965.
143. Christensen LK, Skovsted L: Inhibition of drug metabolism by chloramphenicol. *Lancet* 2:1397, 1969.
144. Petitpierre B, Fabre J: Chlorpropamide and chloramphenicol. *Lancet* 1:789, 1970.
145. Rose JQ, Choi HK, Schentag JJ: Intoxication caused by interaction of chloramphenicol and phenytoin. *JAMA* 237:2630, 1977.
146. JiJi RM, Gangarosa EJ, de la Macorra F: Chloramphenicol and its sulfamoyl analogue. Report of reversible erythropoietic toxicity in healthy volunteers. *Arch Intern Med* 11:70, 1963.
147. Powell DA, Nahata MC, Durrell DC, et al: Interactions among chloramphenicol, phenytoin and phenobarbital in a pediatric patient. *J Pediatr* 98:1001, 1981.
148. Sande MA, Overton JW: In vivo antagonism between gentamicin and chloramphenicol in neutropenic mice. *J Infect Dis* 128:247, 1973.

8

RIFAMPIN

BARRY FARR
GERALD L. MANDELL

Rifampin is a semisynthetic derivative of rifamycin B, a macrocyclic antibiotic compound produced by the mold *Streptomyces mediterranei.* First isolated from fermentation culture of a soil isolate in 1957, rifamycins were named for a then current Italian movie, *Le Riffi.* Rifampin, which is the 3-4-methyl-piperazinyl-iminomethyl derivative of rifamycin SV, is more soluble and active in vitro than is its parent compound (1). Rifampin is a zwitterion (inner salt) that is soluble in acidic aqueous solution, is even more soluble in organic solvents, and displays remarkable diffusion through lipids (2).

MECHANISM OF ACTION

The rifamycins exert a bactericidal effect by inhibition of DNA- dependent RNA polymerase at the β-subunit, preventing chain initiation but not elongation (3). Mammalian mitochondrial RNA synthesis is not impaired at clinically achievable concentrations.

PHARMACOLOGY

Rifampin is available in the United States as a capsule of orange-red powder that is almost completely absorbed from the gastrointestinal tract yielding peak plasma concentrations of approximately 7 μg/ml (range, 4–32) within 1–4 hours after ingestion of 600 mg in adults or 10 mg/kg of body weight in children. The drug is 75 percent protein bound in serum and distributes into a volume calculated to be 160 percent of body weight. Plasma clearance is through hepatic uptake, desacetylation to an active metabolite, and biliary excretion. Desacetylation diminishes reabsorption and increases fecal excretion, but there is significant enterohepatic circulation. The half-life is initially 2–5 hours, but it decreases by 40 percent during the first 2 weeks of therapy due to enhanced biliary excretion. From 6 to 30 percent of a dose is excreted in the urine. An intravenous preparation available in several countries (not licensed in the United States) yields similar pharmacokinetics. Dosage adjustment is unnecessary in renal failure, but rifampin should be avoided or used with caution (perhaps at a lower dosage) in patients with hepatic dysfunction.

Food interferes with absorption, lowering and delaying peak blood levels. Para-amino salicylic acid also interferes with absorption. Probenecid does not consistently affect rifampin serum levels. Slow acetylators of isoniazid have an accelerated clearance of rifampin.

Rifampin penetrates well into almost all body tissues. It achieves concentrations in lung, liver, bile, cholecystic wall, and urine that exceed peak blood levels (4). The concentration in tears is similar to that in serum, and salivary concentrations are about 20 percent of those in serum. It achieves therapeutic levels in pleural exudate, ascites, cavity fluid, milk, urinary bladder wall, and soft tissues. It penetrates bone, with higher levels being reached in the presence of osteomyelitis (4). Levels in cerebrospinal fluid (CSF) of 0–0.5 μg/ml have been achieved in healthy people, and higher levels (up to 1.3 μg/ml) have been observed during meningitis after a standard oral dosage of 600 mg/day. Rifampin has also been shown to penetrate and sterilize abscess fluid more readily than other antibiotics with similar antibacterial activity (5,6). This may relate both to the drug's high lipid solubility and to its unusual ability to enter living phagocytes and kill living intracellular bacteria (2).

ANTIMICROBIAL ACTIVITY

Rifampin exhibits bactericidal activity against a wide range of organisms (Table 1) (7). It is extremely active against staphylococci (both coagulase-positive and coagulase-negative strains) and is also effective against other gram-positive cocci, although somewhat less so than penicillin. *Neisseria meningitidis, Neisseria gonorrhoeae,* and *Hemophilus influenzae* are the most sensitive gram-negative species. Rifampin has less activity than tetracycline, chloramphenicol, or aminoglycosides against most gram-negative aerobic bacilli.

Rifampin is the most active agent known against *Legionella pneumophila,* being 200 times as active as erythromycin in plaque reduction in cell culture monolayers. It is also effective in a whole embryo model against *Legionella micdadei,* the Pittsburgh pneumonia agent. It is as active as vancomycin in vitro against *Clostridium difficile,* the organism associated with pseudomembranous colitis.

Mycobacterium tuberculosis has remained quite sensitive to rifampin, with most epidemiologic surveys finding less than 1 percent initial resistance to the drug (8). *Mycobacterium ulcerans* is equally sensitive. A new spiro-piperidyl-rifamycin called ansamycin (LM427) appears to have remarkable in vitro activity against many mycobacteria, including the *Mycobacterium avium/intracellulare* complex and *Mycobacterium fortuitum* (9).

TABLE 1. Minimal Inhibitory Concentrations of Rifampin

Organism	*MIC* (μg/*ml*)
Clostridium difficile	<1
Enterobacter sp.	5–50
Enterococcus sp.	0.01–0.5
Escherichia coli	5–50
Hemophilus influenzae	0.02–0.63
Klebsiella sp.	5–50
Legionella pneumophila	<0.01
Mycobacterium avium/intracellulare	2–>20
Mycobacterium fortuitum	>20
Mycobacterium kansasii	0.1–1.0
Mycobacterium marinum	0.64–2.5
Mycobacterium tuberculosis	0.005–0.2
Mycobacterium ulcerans	0.005–0.2
Neisseria gonorrhoeae	0.02
Neisseria meningitidis	0.1–0.8
Proteus sp.	5–50
Pseudomonas sp.	5–50
Staphylococcus aureus	0.005–0.01
Staphylococcus epidermidis	0.003–0.005
Streptococcus pneumoniae	0.01
Streptococcus pyogenes	0.01–0.5

The rifamycins possess antiviral and possible antitumor activity, which have not proved clinically useful at usual therapeutic levels. There is also activity against some *Chlamydia,* including *Chlamydia trachomatis* (lymphogranuloma venereum—LGV and non-LGV strains) and *Chlamydia psittaci. Ureaplasma urealyticum* and *Treponema pallidum* are usually resistant.

Bacteria rapidly develop resistance to rifampin in vitro or in vivo due to a mutation altering DNA-dependent RNA polymerase. Approximately one out of every 10^{10} tubercle bacilli is a resistant mutant. There is a low incidence of rifampin resistance among previously untreated tuberculous patients. The mutation rate to rifampin resistance among other bacteria is higher than that for *M. tuberculosis* (e.g., *Staphylococcus aureus,* 10^{-7}; *Streptococcus* sp., 10^{-7}; *H. influenzae* type B 10^{-7}; meningococcus, 10^{-7}; and *Escherichia coli,* 10^{-8}) (7,10). Except for short-term meningitis prophylaxis, rifampin should not be used alone because of this rapid development of resistance during monotherapy.

ADVERSE EFFECTS

Short-term meningitis prophylaxis is usually associated with very few side effects except for red discoloration of urine and permanent staining of soft contact lenses.

Chronic daily therapy is associated with a mild, usually self-limited rash in up to 5 percent of patients, gastrointestinal complaints in 1–2 percent of patients, asymptomatic elevation of serum enzymes in up to 14 percent of patients, and overt hepatitis in less than 1 percent of patients (7). At least seven cases of acute renal failure have been reported during daily therapy with three of these requiring dialysis (11). A vast majority of patients receiving rifampin develop light-chain proteinuria without apparent ill effect.

Intermittent administration (less than twice per week) and high individual dosage (greater than or equal to 1200 mg) have been associated with an increased incidence of side effects. A flulike syndrome with fever, chills, and myalgias may develop in up to 20 percent of patients, beginning after several months of intermittent therapy and correlating with the presence of antirifampin antibodies. These patients may develop eosinophila, interstitial nephritis, acute tubular necrosis, thrombocytopenia, hemolytic anemia, and even shock (12).

Various effects of rifampin on the central nervous system have been reported, including rare cases of organic brain syndrome. Pseudomembranous colitis has been reported during rifampin administration although clear causality has not been proven. Pancreatitis has also been reported in rare cases. Patients have survived overdoses of up to 12 g, turning "lobster red" for several days.

Rifampin causes an increase in serum bile acids and may cause slight elevation of serum bilirubin concentrations that return to normal during the first week of therapy in the absence of hepatitis. Rifampin causes a reduction in 25-hydroxycholecalciferol levels without changing levels of 1,25-dihydroxycholecalciferol or parathyroid hormone, and osteomalacia has been mentioned as a possible side effect with long-term treatment. It causes increased deiodination and biliary clearance of thyroxine and lowers the serum concentration of thryoxine. The serum concentration of triiodothyronine remains normal.

Immunosuppression has been an alleged side effect of rifampin therapy. Contradictory studies have found diminished or normal antibody responses to various antigens such as sheep red blood cells, pneumococcal vaccine, and tetanus toxoid. Some workers have suggested blunted cell-mediated immunity with diminished response to phytohemagglutinin in vitro, whereas others have shown no change in response to phytohemagglutin, concanavalin A, pokeweed mitogen, or purified protein derivative (PPD). Skin tests with PPD have not been altered by rifampin therapy, and no ill effect from this possible immunosuppression in the form of opportunistic infection or inability to heal tuberculosis has been reported (13).

Rifampin readily crosses the placenta and has caused teratogenic effects in rodents treated with high doses; such effects have not been observed in humans, except in patients with severe tuberculosis, but rifampin should only be used for severe tuberculosis infections during pregnancy (14).

DRUG INTERACTIONS

Rifampin competitively inhibits the hepatic uptake of several compounds such as cholecystografin and sulfobromophthalein. Addition of isoniazid to rifampin increases the risk of hepatitis slightly, but the combination is usually safe in the absence of prior liver disease (15). Rifampin is one of the most potent inducing agents for hepatic microsomal enzymes (16), leading to a decreased half-life for a number of compounds including prednisone, norethisterone, digitoxin, quinidine, ketoconazole, and the sulfonylureas (17,18). These effects have been reported to cause decreased efficacy of oral contraceptive agents, relapse of arrhythmias during quinidine therapy, decompensation of heart failure during digitoxin therapy, and exacerbation of diabetes during oral hypoglycemic therapy. Rifampin also reduces the efficacy of warfarin, causing a reduction in prothrombin time in patients anticoagulated with this drug.

THERAPEUTIC USES

Mycobacterial Infections

The unique pharmacology and bactericidal activity of rifampin have revolutionized chemotherapy for pulmonary tuberculosis with rifampin-containing treatment courses of 6–9 months yielding cure rates equal to those achieved with 18 months of nonrifampin- containing regimens (19). It should be emphasized that rifampin monotherapy is contraindicated in mycobacterial disease, as illustrated by one study in which 5 out of 11 tuberculous patients developed rifampin-resistant isolates within 3 months on rifampin alone (20). Rifampin-containing regimens have also proven useful in the therapy of *M. avium/intracellulare* (21), *Mycobacterium kansasii* (22), *Mycobacterium xenopi* (23), and bacille Calmette-Guérin (BCG) infections (24,25).

Rifampin seems to kill *Mycobacterium leprae* faster than do the sulfones. If used in patients with lepromatous leprosy, however, it should be combined with dapsone to prevent the development of resistance. It has been used successfully with monthly rifampin doses being added to daily dapsone therapy without producing the flu-like side effects usually seen with intermittent rifampin administration (26).

Meningitis Prophylaxis

Rifampin has been recommended as prophylaxis for close contacts of patients with meningococcal meningitis at a daily dose of 600 mg for 4 days in adults or 20 mg/kg for 4 days in children. Although prevention of secondary disease with this therapy has never been rigorously demonstrated, rifampin has been shown to eradicate meningococci from the nasopharynx in approximately 90 percent of carriers. Sulfadiazine was formerly recommended for meningococcal prophylaxis, but up to 70 percent of meningococcal isolates are resistant to sulfa. Minocycline is also an effective prophylactic agent, but it is associated with a much higher incidence of side effects, especially vestibular symptoms.

Recent epidemiologic studies of *H. influenzae* type B meningitis have shown a high incidence of secondary disease among preschool contacts. Secondary disease attack rates for this group have been approximately 2 percent, yielding a relative risk approximately 800 times that of the general population. Rifampin at a single daily dose of 20 mg/kg (up to a maximum dose of 600 mg) for 4 days has been shown to eradicate *H. influenzae* from the nasopharynx in over 90 percent of carriers. It has been recommended that families with children under 4 years old and day-care classmates under 4 years old exposed within a week of diagnosis to a patient with invasive *H. influenzae* type B disease (meningitis, epiglottitis, or pneumonia) take rifampin prophylaxis (27). The risk of secondary disease declines after the first week, obviating the need for prophylaxis if more than a week has passed since exposure to the index patient. Index cases with invasive *H. influenzae* diseases should also be given the same rifampin regimen before hospital discharge. Attempts to eradicate nasopharyngeal carriage with other drugs active against *H. influenzae* including ampicillin and trimethoprim-sulfamethoxazole have been less successful.

Endocarditis

The use of rifampin in therapy for endocarditis remains an unsettled and controversial issue (27a). No prospective, comparative trials are available in human infection. One retrospective series of 75 cases of prosthetic valve endocarditis due to *Staphylococcus epidermidis,* the most common cause of prosthetic valve endocarditis, suggested a trend toward higher survival ($p = 0.10$) in patients receiving rifampin (900–1200 mg/day) or an aminoglycoside plus vancomycin, as opposed to vancomycin alone (28). Enhancement of serum bactericidal activity was noted in 8 of these patients after addition of rifampin to vancomycin, but this test was not performed in all patients nor were in vitro synergy studies reported. A multicenter prospective study is now examining the role of rifampin in prosthetic valve endocarditis due to *S. epidermidis.*

Several patients with endocarditis due to *S. aureus* have been reported to respond only after addition of rifampin to nafcillin or vancomycin (7). Studies have been published, however, showing antagonism between nafcillin or vancomycin and rifampin against many *S. aureus* isolates in vitro (29–31). In these studies some isolates have shown synergy, whereas others have shown indifference or antagonism with the rifampin combination, and one study revealed that the concentrations of the individual drugs were important, with synergy being obtained at one ratio and antagonism at another (31). These data suggest that both synergy and antagonism may occur in vivo depending upon dose and timing of administration of the two drugs.

Experimental endocarditis due to *S. aureus* in rabbits has been examined by Sande et al. (5); combination of rifampin with penicillin was antagonistic in vitro against a strain of *S. aureus,* and there was a trend toward slower sterilization of vegetations with the rifampin combination than with penicillin alone. Sterilization of renal abscesses, however, occurred faster in the rifampin combination group than in the group taking penicillin alone despite in vitro antagonism. It was suggested that this was due to rifampin's unique ability to penetrate and sterilize abscess fluid and living polymorphonuclear neutrophil (PMN) leukocytes.

Rifampin may be a useful addition to the antibiotic regimen in *S. aureus* endocarditis complicated by renal, myocardial, splenic, or cerebral abscess for the reasons cited above, but clinical studies are needed to confirm this impression. In the absence of such complications, rifampin (or an aminoglycoside) could be considered for addition to the regimen if therapy with a β-lactam or vancomycin were failing. Serum bactericidal levels should be compared before and after addition of rifampin.

Rifampin (300 mg po bid) has also been recommended in combination with vancomycin and gentamicin for therapy for endocarditis due to *Corynebacterium* spp. (32). One case of endocarditis due to psittacosis was refractory to several other antibiotics but subsequently responsive to rifampin (33).

Tolerant Staphylococci

Staphylococci with an antibiotic minimal bactericidal concentration (MBC) much greater than the minimal inhibitory concentration (MIC) (MBC equal to or greater than 32 × MIC) are said to be tolerant to the antibiotic in question. Tolerance to nafcillin and/or vancomycin has been described in several cases with persistent staphylococcal infection. Addition of rifampin has led to improved serum bactericidal levels and the successful treatment of such infections (34,35).

Staphylococcal Carriage and Furunculosis

Rifampin has been shown to reduce the rate of staphylococcal nasal colonization markedly (36), whereas systemic penicillinase-resistant penicillins or intranasal gentamicin cream have not eradicated nasal carriage (37). Mandell and Sande (unpublished data) have used cloxacillin plus rifampin to eradicate nasal carriage and interrupt the course of recurrent furunculosis. Methicillin-resistant staphylococcal nasal carriage in nosocomial epidemics has been successfully eradicated using a combination of rifampin plus either vancomycin or trimethoprim-sulfamethoxazole (37,38).

Methicillin-Resistant Staphylococcal Infection

Methicillin-resistant infections should be treated with vancomycin to which they are uniformly sensitive. There are no data to support the routine addition of rifampin to vancomycin, but if there is inadequate response to vancomycin alone then addition of gentamicin or rifampin should be considered.

Osteomyelitis and Septic Arthritis

Experimental animal data suggest that rifampin combined with another antistaphylococcal drug such as nafcillin or vancomycin provides better results than single drug therapy for chronic staphylococcal osteomyelitis even when the drug combination is antagonistic in vitro (39). Controlled trials are necessary to confirm these data in human infection, however, and a multicenter study is currently evaluating a rifampin-containing regimen in chronic staphylococcal osteomyelitis. Rifampin is not part of the usual regimen for staphylococcal arthritis, but it has been added with success in occasional cases initially refractory to nafcillin alone (40).

Legionella

Both *L. pneumophila* and *L. micdadei* are sensitive to rifampin. It has been suggested that rifampin be added to erythromycin for patients with legionnaires' disease when the illness does not respond to erythromycin alone.

Brucellosis

Rifampin has been shown to be superior to tetracycline in the therapy for experimental brucellosis in rodents and there have been several case reports of successful therapy for human infections, but controlled clinical trials are lacking. In one uncontrolled study, relapses occurred after rifampin monotherapy, suggesting the need for combination therapy if rifampin is used (41).

Infection Occurring in Patients with Chronic Granulomatous Disease of Childhood

Rifampin has been shown to kill living intracellular staphylococci in neutrophils from healthy people and from patients with chronic granulomatous disease (42). One patient with an axillary staphylococcal abscess responded dramatically to the addition of rifampin after unsuccessful months of therapy with vancomycin, nafcillin, and gentamicin (43).

Infected Cerebrospinal Fluid Shunts

Cerebrospinal fluid shunt infections have responded to the addition of rifampin in several cases after initial failure with multiple-drug therapy excluding rifampin (44–46).

Cutaneous Leishmaniasis

When a patient with *Leishmania mexicana amazonensis* refractory to previous antileishmanial therapy was treated with rifampin and isoniazid for intercurrent mycobacterial infection, the cutaneous leishmaniasis improved (47). A small uncontrolled series has also suggested that rifampin may be efficacious for this disease (48).

REFERENCES

1. Sensi P, Maggi N, Furesz S, et al: Chemical modifications and biological properties of rifamycins. *Antimicrob Agents Chemother* 6:699, 1966.
2. Mandell GL: Interaction of intraleukocytic bacteria and antibiotics. *J Clin Invest* 52:1673, 1973.
3. Wehrli W, Knusel F, Schmid K, et al: Interaction of rifamycn with bacterial RNA polymerase. *Proc Natl Acad Sci USA* 61:667, 1968.
4. Furesz S: Chemical and biological properties of rifampicin. *Antibiot Chemother* 16:316, 1970.
5. Sande MA, Johnson ML: Antimicrobial therapy of experimental endocarditis caused by *Staphylococcus aureus. J Infect Dis* 131:367, 1975.
6. Mandell GL, Vest TK: Killing of intraleukocytic *Staphylococcus aureus* by rifampin: In vitro and in vivo studies. *J Infect Dis* 125:486, 1972.
7. Farr B, Mandell GL: Rifampin. *Med Clin North Am* 66:157, 1982.
8. Collins CH, Yates MD: Low incidence of rifampin resistant tubercle bacilli. *Thorax* 37:526, 1982.
9. Woodley CL, Kilburn JO: In vitro susceptibility of *Mycobacterium avium* complex and *Mycobacterium tuberculosis* strains to a spiro-piperidyl rifamycin. *Am Rev Respir Dis* 126:586, 1982.
10. Yogev R, Melick C, Glogowski W: In vitro development of rifampin resistance in clinical isolates of *Haemophilus influenzae* type B. *Antimicrob Agents Chemother* 21:387, 1982.
11. Qunibi WY, Godwin J, Eknoyan G: Toxic nephropathy during continuous rifampin therapy. *South Med J* 73:791, 1980.
12. Girling DJ, Hitze HL: Adverse reactions to rifampicin. *Bull WHO* 57:45, 1979.
13. Humber DP, Nsanzumuhire H, Aluoch JA, et al: Controlled double-blind study of the effect of rifampin on humoral and cellular immune responses in patients with pulmonary tuberculosis and in tuberculosis contacts. *Am Rev Respir Dis* 122:425, 1980.
14. Snider DE Jr, Layde PM, Johnson MW, et al: Treatment of tuberculosis during pregnancy. *Am Rev Respir Dis* 122:65, 1980.
15. Mandell GL, Sande MA: Drugs used in the chemotherapy of tuberculosis and leprosy, in Goodman AG, Goodman LS, Gilman A (eds): *The Pharmacological Basis of Therapeutics,* 6th ed. New York. Macmillian, 1980, pp 1203–1206.
16. Ohnhaus EE, Kirchhof B, Peheim E: Effect of enzyme induction on plasma lipids using antipyrine, phenobarbital, and rifampicin. *Clin Pharmacol Ther* 25:591, 1979.
17. Twum-Barima Y, Carruthers SG: Quinidine-rifampin interaction. *New Engl J Med* 304:1466, 1981.
18. Brass C, Galgiani JN, Blaschke TF, et al: Disposition of ketoconazole, an oral antifungal, in humans. *Antimicrob Agents Chemother* 21:151, 1982.
19. British Thoracic Association: A controlled trial of six months chemotherapy in pulmonary tuberculosis. Second report: Results during the 24 months after the end of chemotherapy. *Am Rev Respir Dis* 126:460, 1982.
20. Baronti A, Lukinovich N: A pilot trial of rifampicin in tuberculosis. *Tubercle* 49:180, 1968.
21. Hunter AM, Campbell IA, Jenkins PA, et al: Treatment of pulmonary infections caused by mycobacteria of the *Mycobacterium avium-intracellulare* complex. *Thorax* 36:326, 1981.
22. Ahn CH, Lowell JR, Ahn SS, et al: Chemotherapy for pulmonary disease due to *Mycobaterium kansasii:* Efficacies of some individual drugs. *Rev Infect Dis* 3:1028, 1981.
23. Bogaerts Y, Elinck W, van Renterghem D, et al: Pulmonary disease due to *Mycobacterium xenopi:* Report of two cases. *Eur J Respir Dis* 63:298, 1982.
24. Kallenius G, Moller E, Ringden O, et al: The first infant to survive a generalized BCG infection. *Acta Paediatr Scand* 71:161, 1982.
25. Izumi AK, Matsunaga J: BCG vaccine-induced lupus vulgaris. *Arch Dermatol* 118:171, 1982.
26. Yawalkar SJ, McDougall AC, Longuillon J, et al: Once monthly rifampicin plus daily dapsone in initial treatment of lepromatous leprosy. *Lancet* 1:1119, 1982.
27. Respiratory and Special Pathogens Epidemiology Branch (CDC): Prevention of secondary cases of *Haemophilus influenzae* type B disease. *MMWR* 31:672, 1982.

27a. Sande MA (ed): The use of rifampin in treatment of nontuberculous infections. *Rev Infect Dis* 5:S399, 1983.
28. Karchmer AW, Archer GL, Dismukes WE: *Staphylococcus epidermidis* causing prosthetic valve endocarditis: Microbiologic and clinical observations as guides to therapy. *Ann Intern Med* 48:447, 1983.
29. Traczewski MM, Goldmann DA, Murphy P: In vitro activity of rifampin in combination with oxacillin against *Staphylococcus aureus. Antimicrob Agents Chemother* 23:571, 1983.
30. Watanakunakorn C, Guerriero JC: Interaction between vancomycin and rifampin against *Staphylococcus aureus. Antimicrob Agents Chemother* 19:1089, 1981.
31. Zinner SH, Lagast H, Klastersky J: Antistaphylococcal activity of rifampin with other antibiotics. *J Infect Dis* 144:365, 1981.
32. Sande MA, Scheld WM: Combination antibiotic therapy of bacterial endocarditis. *Ann Intern Med* 92:390, 1980.
33. Jariwalla AG, Davies BH, White J: Infective endocarditis complicating psittacosis: response to rifampicin. *Br Med J* 280:155, 1980.
34. Faville RJ, Zaske DE, Kaplan EL, et al: *Staphylococcus aureus* endocarditis: Combined therapy with vancomycin and rifampin. *JAMA* 240:1963, 1978.
35. Simmons NA: Synergy and rifampicin. *J Antimicrob Chemother* 3:109, 1977.
36. Wheat LJ, Kohler RB, White AL, et al: Effect of rifampin on nasal carriers of coagulase-positive staphylococci. *J Infect Dis* 144:177, 1981.
37. Locksley RM, Cohen ML, Quinn TC, et al: Multiply antibiotic-resistant *Staphylococcus aureus:* Introduction, transmission, and evolution of nosocomial infection. *Ann Intern Med* 97:317, 1982.
38. Ward TT, Winn RE, Hartstein AI, et al: Observations relating to an interhospital outbreak of methicillin resistant *Staphylococcus aureus:* Role of anticrobial therapy in infection control. *Infect Control* 2:453, 1981.
39. Norden CW, Shaffer M: Treatment of experimental chronic osteomyelitis due to *Staphylococcus aureus* with vancomycin and rifampin. *J Infect Dis* 147:352, 1983.
40. Beam TR: Sequestration of *Staphylococcus aureus* at an inaccessible focus. *Lancet* 2:227, 1979.
41. Llorens-Terol J, Busquets RM: Brucellosis treated with rifampicin. *Arch Dis Child* 55:486, 1980.
42. Ezer G, Soothill JF: Intracellular bactericidal effect of rifampicin in both normal and chronic granulomatous disease polymorphs. *Arch Dis Child* 49:463, 1974.
43. Lorber B: Rifampin in chronic granulomatous disease. *N Engl J Med* 303:111, 1980.
44. Archer G, Tenenbaum MJ, Haywood HB: Rifampin therapy of *S. epidermidis:* Use in infections from indwelling artificial devices. *JAMA* 240:751, 1978.
45. Bolton WK, Sande MA, Normansell DE, et al: Ventriculojugular shunt nephritis with *Corynebacterium bovis. Am J Med* 59:417, 1975.
46. Ring JC, Cates KL, Belani KK, et al: Rifampin for CSF shunt infections caused by coagulase-negative staphylococci. *J Pediatr* 95:317, 1979.
47. Peters W, Shaw JJ, Lainson R, et al: Potentiating action of rifampicin and isoniazid against *Leishmania mexicana amazonensis. Lancet* 1:1122, 1981.
48. Even-Paz Z, Weinrauch L, Livshin R, et al: Rifampicin treatment of cutaneous leishmaniasis. *Int J Dermatol* 21:110, 1982.

9

METRONIDAZOLE

SYDNEY M. FINEGOLD

DESCRIPTION

Metronidazole was introduced in 1959 for treatment of *Trichomonas vaginalis* infections. It is now known to be effective against most infections involving anaerobic bacteria and against certain other parasitic infections. Metronidazole diffuses well into all tissues, including the central nervous system. It is well tolerated. It has the best bactericidal activity of all drugs active against anaerobic bacteria.

Metronidazole is a nitroimidazole drug with the chemical formula, 1-(2-hydroxyethyl)-2-methyl-5-nitroimidazole. It has a low molecular weight, 171.

SPECTRUM OF ACTIVITY, RESISTANCE

Table 1 from Sutter (1) summarizes the activity of metronidazole against 793 strains of anaerobic and microaerophilic bacteria. Note that virtually all of the organisms tested were inhibited by 16 μg/ml or less except for one-third of gram-positive nonspore-forming bacilli and 7 percent of *Capnocytophaga* sp. Metabolites are found in serum and urine, and Sutter found that the hydroxy metabolite of metronidazole was slightly less active than the parent compound against many anaerobes but had equivalent or better activity against some. The acid metabolite has poor activity against anaerobes. In general, studies by other workers have given comparable results in terms of in vitro activity of metronidazole. Wüst (2) found that seven strains of *Propionibacterium acnes* required 100 μg/ml for inhibition. Werner et al. (3) also noted that the hydroxy metabolite of metronidazole was roughly comparable in activity to the parent compound. We found that only about 25 percent of strains of *Actinomyces* and *Arachnia* are susceptible to metronidazole at achievable levels. In a recent study, Rosenblatt and Edson (4) noted somewhat less activity against anaerobic gram-positive cocci (MIC_{70} of 6.25 and MIC_{90} of >25 μg/ml). *Propionibacterium acnes* was highly resistant. The study by Chow et al. (5) found significantly more resistance

TABLE 1. Activity of Metronidazole Against Anaerobic and Microaerophilic Bacteria

		Cumulative Percent Susceptible to Indicated Concentration (μg/ml)			
Bacteria	*No. Strains*	*4*	*8*	*16*	*32*
Bacteroides fragilis[a]	161	90	99	100	—
B. melaninogenicus[b]	60	98	100	—	—
Other bacteroides and *Selenomonas* sp.	154	95	98	100	—
Fusobacterium sp.	65	100	—	—	—
Anaerobic gram-negative cocci	24	92	96	100	—
Anaerobic gram-positive cocci	124	98	—	—	—
Clostridium perfringens	18	94	100	—	—
Other *Clostridium* sp.	73	97	99	—	100
Gram-positive nonsporulating bacilli	87	57	60	62	66
Capnocytophaga sp.	27	52	70	93	—

SOURCE: Sutter VL (1).

[a] Includes all species of the *B. fragilis* group.

[b] Includes *B. melaninogenicus* and *B. asaccharolyticus* ssp.

among anaerobes to metronidazole than was indicated by the studies previously cited.

Also sensitive to metronidazole are *Treponema pallidum,* oral spirochetes, *Campylobacter fetus,* and *Gardnerella vaginalis.* In certain animal models, *Escherichia coli* may be inhibited by metronidazole when it is present together in a mixture with *Bacteroides fragilis.* However, in another animal model (6), there was no activity against *E. coli.* We have noted decreased counts of *E. coli* initially present together with anaerobes in the bypassed loop of patients with ileal bypass for obesity who were treated with metronidazole for "bypass enteropathy."

Development of resistance to metronidazole is rare. Resistant strains identified include one strain each of *Bacteroides fragilis, Bacteroides distasonis, Bacteroides melaninogenicus* ss *melaninogenicus* and *Bacteroides bivius.* Phillips et al. (7) note that they have seen occasional marginally resistant isolates of *B. bivius, Bacteroides ureolyticus* and perhaps *B. melaninogenicus.* Tally et al. (8) studied a metronidazole-resistant strain of *B. fragilis.* They found uptake of metronidazole by cells was slower than in a sensitive strain. Also, the rate of reduction of metronidazole was four times less than with a sensitive control strain, possibly due to decreased nitro-reductase activity.

MODE OF ACTION

Mechanism of Action

It is convenient to think of the action as occurring in four successive steps (9): (*1*) entry of the drug into the bacterial cell, (*2*) reductive activation, (*3*) toxic effect of the reduced intermediate product(s), and (*4*) release of inactive end products. A key feature is reduction of the nitro group of the drug; the drug acts as a preferential electron acceptor, being reduced by low redox potential electron-transport proteins (ferredoxinlike and flavodoxinlike). Reduction of the drug decreases the intracellular concentration of unchanged drug, thus maintaining a gradient that drives the uptake and generates compounds that are toxic to the cell. The toxicity is due to short-lived intermediate compounds or free radicals that produce damage by interaction with DNA and possibly other macromolecules. The cytotoxic intermediates decompose into nontoxic and inactive end products, including acetamide and 2-hydroxethyl oxamic acid.

Metabolic Products

As noted above, the hydroxy derivative of metronidazole has significant antianaerobic activity; it is more active than metronidazole on *G. vaginalis.* The acid derivative of metronidazole has relatively little activity, less than one-tenth as much as metronidazole versus *B. fragilis* and *Trichomonas* (9). The drug is also conjugated; the glucuronide has no activity on *Trichomonas* and is not taken up (9).

Bactericidal Activity

Metronidazole is a potent bactericidal agent. It typically kills organisms at the same concentration as, or within one twofold dilution of, that required for inhibition (10). Under reduced conditions, metronidazole has a rapid onset of bactericidal activity. Killing rates are not affected by inoculum size, nutritional requirements, or growth rate (11,12).

Bartlett et al. (13) found metronidazole to be the most effective drug in a *B. fragilis* subcutaneous abscess model in mice even when treatment was delayed for 8–120 hours after challenge.

PHARMACOLOGY

When given orally, metronidazole is absorbed rapidly and almost completely. Serum levels are similar during the elimination phase after equivalent doses by the intravenous and oral routes. Blood levels are proportional to the administered dose. The standard intravenous dosage regimen that has been used in the United States consists of a loading dose of 15 mg/kg of body weight followed by 7.5 mg/kg every 6 hours. This results in peak and trough steady-state plasma levels averaging 25 μg/ml and 18 μg/ml, respectively. There is very little protein binding of metronidazole. The half-life is 8 hours. Absorption of metronidazole is not affected by ingestion of food, but peak levels may be markedly delayed. Metronidazole is absorbed relatively well, though slowly, when given rectally or vaginally.

There is a large apparent volume of distribution of metronidazole, equivalent to about 80 percent of body weight; it reaches all tissues and fluids. Therapeutic levels are achieved in amniotic fluid, the unobstructed biliary tract, alveolar bone, cerebrospinal fluid and brain abscess contents, cord blood, pleural empyema fluid, hepatic abscesses, middle ear discharge, middle ear mucosa, breast milk, pelvic tissues (concentrations attained in the myometrium and fallopian tubes are nearly the same as concomitant serum levels), saliva, seminal fluid, and vaginal secretions. Levels achieved in the aqueous humor were between one-third and one-half those attained in the serum (14).

During metabolization of metronidazole, five major products are formed. The most important one is the hydroxy derivative. In addition, there is an acid metabolite, acetylmetronidazole, metronidazole glucuronide, and the glucuronide conjugate of hydroxy metronidazole. A sulfate conjugate may also be found on occasion. Metronidazole and its metabolites are eliminated primarily in the urine (60–80 percent of the dose). From 6 to 15 percent is excreted in the feces.

The elimination half-life of metronidazole in patients with no renal function is the same as in healthy people. However, the hydroxy metabolite may accumulate in patients with absent renal function, and although dosage adjustment is usually not considered necessary in the absence of hepatic disease, consideration might be given to dosage adjustment in patients initially receiving large doses. Metronidazole and its metabolites are rapidly removed by hemodialysis; the elimination half-life of metronidazole is reduced to 2.6 hours. In patients with impaired hepatic function, even without concomitant renal functional impairment, the plasma clearance of metronidazole is delayed. Therefore, dosage adjustment will likely be necessary. Unfortunately, there are no good guidelines to follow and we must monitor serum levels and make adjustments as indicated.

ADMINISTRATION AND DOSAGE

Table 2 gives dosage recommendations and routes of administration for the major indications for metronidazole therapy. The intravenous (IV) route is recommended initially for seriously ill patients. Since oral therapy gives blood levels comparable to those achieved by the intravenous route, we may switch when conditions warrant.

As noted, the standard regimen in the United States for intravenous administration has been a loading dose of 15 mg/kg of body weight, followed by a maintenance schedule of 7.5 mg/kg every 6 hours. Clearly, the half-life of the drug would warrant administration at longer intervals such as every 8 or even every 12 hours. The manufacturer recommends that intravenous infusions be administered over a period of 1 hour. However, a number of foreign investigators have administered the drug in as little as 20 minutes without any apparent adverse effects. The maximum daily dose recommended is 4 g.

After reconstitution, metronidazole hydrochloride should be diluted with in-

TABLE 2. Major Indications for Metronidazole: Administration and Dosage

Indication	*Route of Administration*	*Dosage*
Susceptible anaerobic infections	Intravenous	Loading dose of 15 mg/kg, then 7.5 mg/kg q6h
	Oral	1–2 g/day in 2–4 doses q6–12h
Nonspecific vaginitis	Oral	500 mg bid for 7 days
Trichomonas vaginitis	Oral	250 mg tid for 7 days *or* 500 mg bid for 5 days *or* 2 g in single dose
Amebiasis (intestinal or extraintestinal)	Intravenous or oral	750 mg tid for 10 days
Giardiasis	Oral	250 mg bid or tid for 5–7 days *or* 2 g/day for 3 days

travenous fluid to a concentration not exceeding 8 mg/ml and should be neutralized to pH 6.0–7.0 with sodium bicarbonate before administration. There is also a metronidazole intravenous solution (Flagyl IV RTU), a ready-to-use isotonic solution that does not require dilution or buffering before infusion.

Duration of therapy will vary according to the entity being treated. Certain recommendations are made in Table 2. For serious infections, however, we may often need to treat the patient for 2–4 weeks or longer.

Comments regarding dosage in patients with impaired renal and/or hepatic function have been noted in the section above on pharmacology.

ADVERSE REACTIONS, PRECAUTIONS

In general, metronidazole is well tolerated. The more commonly encountered major and minor adverse reactions are listed in Table 3. There may also be furring of the tongue, glossitis, stomatitis, dry mouth, headache, fever, dizziness, syncope, and occasionally overgrowth of *Candida* in the oral cavity or vagina. Thrombophlebitis has been reported with intravenous infusion but is seldom seen now with proper buffering of the preparation. Gastrointestinal side effects include nausea, epigastric distress, anorexia, and, less commonly, vomiting or diarrhea. Although pseudomembranous colitis has been reported rarely with metronidazole therapy, the drug has proved effective therapeutically for this condition and is probably comparable to vancomycin in effectiveness. The most serious adverse effects are those involving the central nervous system. These are rare unless large doses and/or prolonged therapy are used. If abnormal neurologic symptoms are observed, the drug must be discontinued immediately. Metronidazole should be used with caution in people with a history of seizures

TABLE 3. Adverse Effects Related to Metronidazole Therapy

Major adverse reactions (rare)
Seizures, encephalopathy
Cerebellar dysfunction, ataxia
Peripheral neuropathy
Disulfiram reaction with alcohol
Potentiation of effects of warfarin
Pseudomembranous colitis
Minor adverse reactions
Minor gastrointestinal disturbances
Reversible neutropenia
Metallic taste
Dark or red-brown urine
Maculopapular rash, urticaria
Urethral, vaginal burning

or other central nervous system disorders. The peripheral neuropathy may take a considerable period of time to resolve.

There has been concern about mutagenicity in the Ames *Salmonella* mutant system and carcinogenicity of metronidazole. Reduction of the nitro group of the compound is necessary for both antibacterial activity and mutagenic activity. Mutagenic activity has been detected in urine of patients receiving 750 mg/day of metronidazole. When a mutant *Salmonella* that did not possess nitro reductase was used in the mutagenic testing system, metronidazole could not be demonstrated to be a mutagen. Thus, the drug itself is not mutagenic, but rather it is one or more reduction products of it. Some protozoa, bacteria (including facultative anaerobes), and fungi possess nitro-reductase activity. Eukaryotic tissues have very little nitro-reductase activity. It has been suggested that during metronidazole therapy some reduction products of the drug might escape from the bacterial cells and serve as mutagens to the host's mammalian tissue. However, these active derivatives are very short-lived and either promptly bind to macromolecules within the bacterial cell or are promptly reduced to compounds that are not mutagenic or carcinogenic. The drug has been studied specifically for mutagenic potential in eukaryotic test systems (human lymphocytes in vitro and lymphocytes of patients receiving metronidazole therapy). No chromosomal aberrations or sister chromatid exchanges could be detected in vitro with metronidazole or its metabolites in concentrations of 1000–10,000 μg/ml. No lymphocyte abnormalities were noted in patients receiving a short course of metronidazole therapy (15,16). Metronidazole has shown tumorigenic activity in several studies in mice involving lifetime (or almost lifetime) oral administration. Female rats given metronidazole over long periods (sometimes for life) had a significant increase in neoplasms, especially mammary tumors, compared to controls. Interestingly, in one study drug-fed rats lived longer than controls. Two lifetime studies in hamsters were negative (above studies are summarized in Ref. 17).

It should be noted that acetamide has been found in the urine of patients receiving metronidazole, and prolonged feeding of high doses of this compound to rats has produced hepatocarcinomas (18). A recent study in rats (19) using the dimethylhydrazine (DMH) model for colon neoplasia noted that addition of metronidazole on a long-term basis had an apparent cocarcinogenic effect. As Condon notes in the discussion of this paper, the DMH tumor model is relatively specific and may not readily be extrapolated to humans.

One follow-up study of women treated with metronidazole up to 10 years earlier for trichomoniasis and another shorter follow-up study failed to show an increased incidence of malignancy (cited in Ref. 17). Clearly, more studies are needed in patients receiving high dose metronidazole therapy for long periods of time and with a follow-up period of 20 years or longer.

There has been no evidence of teratogenicity in animals or in humans, but more data are needed to rule out this possibility. Metronidazole does cross the placental barrier and enters the fetal circulation. It should be used during pregnancy only if clearly needed, and it should be avoided during the first trimester.

Because metronidazole is excreted into breast milk, nursing should be discontinued during and for 2 days after therapy with metronidazole.

Drug Interactions, Interference with Laboratory Tests

In patients ingesting alcohol, metronidazole may cause reactions similar to those produced by disulfiram. Patients should be advised not to drink alcohol when taking this drug. Metronidazole inhibits the metabolism of warfarin and other oral coumarin-type anticoagulants. Therefore, if concomitant use must be carried out, the dosage of the anticoagulant should be reduced to maintain the desired prothrombin time.

Metronidazole interferes with certain chemical analyses for the serum enzyme, glutamic oxaloacetic transaminase, resulting in falsely low or negative values.

EFFECT ON NORMAL FECAL FLORA

In subjects who have a normal gastrointestinal tract and are not receiving other drugs, metronidazole has very little effect on the fecal flora (20). This is thought to be due to the drug being rapidly reduced by the bowel flora under the usual anaerobic conditions in the colon. Why this would not have an impact on the organisms carrying out the reduction, as it does in the course of treating infections, is not at all clear. In patients on high dosage regimens, in patients with diarrhea, and in patients receiving certain other antimicrobial agents concurrently, there may be a significant impact of metronidazole on the fecal flora. For example, when oral neomycin or kanamycin (active primarily versus nonanaerobes) are given with metronidazole there is a significant impact on both the anaerobic and aerobic flora. Thus, it has been feasible to use metronidazole for therapy in certain conditions such as ileal bypass enteropathy and for preoperative "bowel preparation" along with an oral aminoglycoside.

CLINICAL USES

Parasitic Infections

Metronidazole has been used successfully for therapy of *Trichomonas* vaginitis for many years. It is also an effective agent for therapy for amoebic liver abscess and has been used with generally good results in intestinal amebiasis. The drug is also effective against giardiasis, being at least as active as quinacrine for this purpose.

Some workers have felt that metronidazole has been effective in *Balantidium coli* infection and in infection due to *Dracunculus medinensis,* but these indications are certainly not well established.

Anaerobic Infections

As is suggested by the spectrum of activity of metronidazole, this drug is useful for the vast majority of anaerobic infections. Certainly actinomycosis is one notable exception, and infections with *P. acnes,* which are quite rare, would be another. There is one other setting in which metronidazole may represent less than optimum therapy—anaerobic infections of the lower respiratory tract. Data from Sanders et al. (21) show a relatively high rate of suboptimal response. Most treatment failures had mixed infections with aerobic bacteria as well as anaerobes. Addition of penicillin G or ampicillin for mixed infections involving streptococci, pneumococci or *Hemophilus influenzae* or addition of erythromycin in the case of a penicillin-allergic patient would likely provide an excellent regimen. In the case of aspiration pneumonia involving aerobic and/or facultative gram-negative bacilli and/or *Staphylococcus aureus,* other appropriate therapy to cover these agents would be needed along with metronidazole. Many anaerobic infections are mixed with aerobic or facultative bacteria, of course, and particularly in sicker patients, therapy aimed at both categories of organisms is desirable.

The excellent distribution of metronidazole throughout the body, including the central nervous system, and the impressive bactericidal activity of this compound, even against organisms that are not actively multiplying, make it an excellent choice for a number of serious infections, including brain abscess and other central nervous system infections involving anaerobes, endocarditis due to anaerobic bacteria, and, perhaps, any anaerobic infection of serious nature in patients who are immunocompromised.

The *B. fragilis* group of organisms is the one most commonly encountered in anaerobic infections overall. Until recently, there were only three drugs that were consistently active against this group—metronidazole, chloramphenicol, and clindamycin. Recently, a number of centers are encountering varying degrees of resistance of the *B. fragilis* group to clindamycin. Thus, metronidazole may become an even more important part of our armamentarium for management of anaerobic infections. It should be noted, however, that in intra-abdominal infections, in which *B. fragilis* is almost always involved, comparative studies (cited in Ref. 11) failed to show any significant difference among metronidazole, clindamycin, chloramphenicol, ticarcillin, or cefoxitin; most of these used together with an aminoglycoside.

The resistance of a number of clostridia, other than *Clostridium perfringens,* to cefoxitin and clindamycin again suggests that metronidazole might have an advantage in selected intra-abdominal and obstetric and gynecologic infections. However, there are no specific data to back up this point.

Metronidazole has been useful against other types of anaerobic infections, including bacteremia, infections of bones and joints, soft tissue infections, oral and dental infections, and head and neck infections. Metronidazole has also provided good results in the therapy for nonspecific vaginitis, a condition in which various anaerobes or *G. vaginalis* or both may be important. As noted elsewhere, it has been effective in the management of pseudomembranous colitis due to *Clostridium difficile.* Metronidazole is not a suitable alternative to penicillin for syphilis.

Other Therapeutic Uses

Metronidazole has been used experimentally in very high doses as a hypoxic cell sensitizer in radiotherapy of malignancy.

Metronidazole has been useful in a number of types of bowel bacterial overgrowth syndromes such as complications of jejunoileal bypass for obesity (22), dysfunction of the continent ileostomy (23), and for prevention of intrahepatic cholestasis associated with total parenteral nutrition (24). Although not everyone agrees, it appears that metronidazole has had a beneficial effect in Crohn's disease, producing a lessening of diarrhea (in patients with colonic involvement) and promoting the healing of perianal lesions and erythema nodosum (25). There is concern about using the drug for very extended periods as might be necessary in this disease.

Metronidazole is said to be beneficial in the treatment of acne rosacea whether used orally or topically (26).

An intriguing report (27) notes striking decreases in serum cholesterol and triglyceride levels in patients receiving metronidazole for other indications. Only short courses of therapy were used. There is no information as to the mechanism of this effect.

Prophylactic Use

Several groups have carried out prospective controlled studies of metronidazole, alone or in combination with other agents, for prophylaxis in patients undergoing elective colonic surgery, gynecologic surgery, or emergency appendectomy. In the case of appendectomy, a perforated appendix is an indication for therapy rather than prophylaxis, and in uncomplicated appendicitis, the frequency of postoperative infection is quite low. In general, however, in these studies metronidazole has appeared to be as effective as other effective prophylactic agents. It should be kept in mind, however, that the prophylactic use of metronidazole is not an approved indication for the drug in the United States at present. Finally, it should be appreciated that not all of the prophylactic trials have found metronidazole effective. Metronidazole was not effective prophylactically in one study of hysterectomy (28) and in one study of appendectomy for nonperforated appendicitis (29).

REFERENCES

1. Sutter VL: In vitro susceptibility of anaerobic and microaerophilic bacteria to metronidazole and its hydroxy metabolite, in: Finegold SM, George WL, Rolfe RD (eds): *First United States Metronidazole Conference.* Proc Symp, Tarpon Springs, Fla, February 1982. New York, Biomedical Information Corp, 1982, p 61.
2. Wüst J: Susceptibility of anaerobic bacteria to metronidazole, ornidazole, and tinidazole and routine susceptibility testing by standardized methods. *Antimicrob Agents Chemother* 11:631, 1977.
3. Werner H, Schädler G, Krasemann C: In vitro activity of azlocillin, metronidazole and its hydroxy metabolite against anaerobes. *Arzneimittel-Forschung Drug Res* 33:574, 1983.
4. Rosenblatt JE, Edson RS: Metronidazole. *Mayo Clin Proc* 58:154, 1983.
5. Chow AW, Bednorz D, Guze LB: Susceptibility of obligate anaerobes to metronidazole: an extended study of 1,054 clinical isolates, in: Finegold SM, McFadzean JA, Roe FJC (eds): *Metronidazole.* Proc Internat Metronidazole Conf, Montreal, May 1976. Princeton, NJ, Excerpta Medica, 1977, p 286.
6. Reznikov M, McDonald PJ: Effect of metronidazole on *Escherichia coli* in the presence of *Bacteroides fragilis:* An investigation in mice. *Chemotherapy* 29:225, 1983.
7. Phillips I, Warren C, Taylor E, et al: The antimicrobial susceptibility of anaerobic bacteria in a London teaching hospital. *J Antimicrob Chemother* 8:17, 1981.
8. Tally FP, Snydman DR, Shimell MJ et al: Mechanisms of antimicrobial resistance of *Bacteroides fragilis,* in: Phillips I, Collier J (eds): *Metronidazole.* Proc 2nd Internat Symp Anaerobic Infections, Geneva, April 1979. London, The Royal Society of Medicine and Academic Press and New York, Grune & Stratton, 1979, p 19.
9. Müller Rhône M: Mode of action of metronidazole on anaerobic bacteria and protozoa, in: Rhône-Poulenc Pharma Inc, Montreal, Proc North American Metronidazole Symp, Anaerobic Infections, Scottsdale, Ariz, October 1981. *Surgery* 93:165, 1983.
10. Nastro LJ, Finegold SM: Bactericidal activity of five antimicrobial agents against *Bacteroides fragilis. J Infect Dis* 126:104, 1972.
11. Tally FP, Sullivan CE: Metronidazole: In vitro activity, pharmacology and efficacy in anaerobic bacterial infections. *Pharmacotherapy* 1:28, 1981.
12. Corrodi P, Busch DF, Sutter VL, et al: Factors affecting the *in vitro* antibacterial activity of metronidazole, in: Finegold SM, McFadzean JA, Roe FJC (eds): *Metronidazole.* Proc Internat Metronidazole Conf, Montreal, May 1976. Princeton, NJ, Excerpta Medica, 1977, p 299.
13. Bartlett JG, Dezfulian M, Joiner K: Relative efficacy and critical interval of antimicrobial agents in experimental infections involving *Bacteroides fragilis. Arch Surg* 118:181, 1983.
14. Mattila J, Nerdrum K, Rouhiainen H, et al: Penetration of metronidazole and tinidazole into the aqueous humor in man. *Chemotherapy* 29:188, 1983.
15. Lambert B, Lindblad A, Lindsten J, et al: Genotoxic effects of metronidazole in human lympho-

cytes in vitro and in vivo, in: Phillips I and Collier J (eds): *Metronidazole.* Proc 2nd Internat Symp Anaerobic Infections, Geneva, April 1979. London, The Royal Society of Medicine and Academic Press and New York, Grune & Stratton, 1979, p 229.

16. Hartley-Asp B: Chromosomal studies on human lymphocytes exposed to metronidazole in vivo and in vitro, in: Phillips I, Collier J, (eds): *Metronidazole.* Proc 2nd Internat Symp Anaerobic Infections, Geneva, April 1979. London, The Royal Society of Medicine and Academic Press and New York, Grune & Stratton, 1979, p 237.
17. Finegold SM: Metronidazole. *Ann Intern Med* 93:585, 1980.
18. Koch RL, Chrystal EJT, Beaulieu BB, et al: Acetamide—a metabolite of metronidazole formed by the intestinal flora. *Biochem Pharmacol* 28:3611, 1979.
19. Sloan DA, Fleiszer DM, Richards GK, et al: Increased incidence of experimental colon cancer associated with long-term metronidazole therapy. *Am J Surg* 145:66, 1983.
20. Lewis RP, Wideman P, Sutter VL, et al: The effect of metronidazole on human fecal flora, in: Finegold SM, McFadzean JA, Roe FJC (eds): *Metronidazole.* Proc Internat Metronidazole Conf, Montreal, May 1976. Princeton, NJ, Excerpta Medica, 1977, p 307.
21. Sanders CV, Hanna BJ, Lewis AC, et al: The use of metronidazole in the treatment of anaerobic pleuropulmonary infections, in: Phillips I, Collier J (eds): *Metronidazole.* Proc 2nd Internat Symp Anaerobic Infections, Geneva, April 1979. London, The Royal Society of Medicine and Academic Press and New York, Grune & Stratton, 1979, p 83.
22. Drenick EJ: Extraintestinal complications of jejunoileal bypass for obesity, in: Finegold SM, George WL, Rolfe RD (eds): *First United States Metronidazole Conference,* Proc Symp, Tarpon Springs, Fla, February 1982. New York, Biomedical Information Corp, 1982, p 371.
23. Kelly DG, Phillips SF, Kelly KA, et al: Dysfunction of the continent ileostomy: Clinical features and bacteriology. *Gut* 24:193, 1983.
24. Capron J-P, Herve M-A, Gineston J-L, et al: Metronidazole in prevention of cholestasis associated with total parenteral nutrition. *Lancet* i:446, 1983.
25. Gilat T: Metronidazole in Crohn's disease (editorial). *Gastroenterology* 83:702, 1982.
26. Nielsen PG: Treatment of rosacea with 1% metronidazole cream. A double-blind study. *Br J Dermatol* 108:327, 1983.
27. Davis JL, Schultz TA, Mosley CA: Metronidazole lowers serum lipids. *Ann Intern Med* 99:43, 1983.
28. Vincelette J, Finkelstein F, Aoki FY, et al: Double-blind trial of perioperative intravenous metronidazole prophylaxis for abdominal and vaginal hysterectomy, in: Rhône-Poulenc Pharma Inc, Montreal: Proc North American Metronidazole Symp, Anaerobic Infections, Scottsdale, Ariz, October 1981. *Surgery* 93:185, 1983.
29. Keiser TA, MacKenzie RL, Feld R, et al: Prophylactic metronidazole in appendectomy: A double-blind controlled trial, in: Rhône-Poulenc Pharma Inc, Montreal: Proc North American Metronidazole Symp, Anaerobic Infections, Scottsdale, Ariz, October 1981. *Surgery* 93:201, 1983.

BIBLIOGRAPHY

Finegold SM, McFadzean JA, Roe FJC, eds: *Metronidazole.* Proc Internat Metronidazole Conf, Montreal, May 1976. Princeton, NJ, Excerpta Medica, 1977.

Finegold SM: Metronidazole. *Ann Intern Med* 93:585, 1980.

Finegold SM, George WL, Rolfe RD, eds: *First United States Metronidazole Conference.* Proc Symp, Tarpon Springs, Fla, February 1982. New York, Biomedical Information Corp, 1982.

May & Baker, Ltd: *"Flagyl" (Metronidazole) in anaerobic infections.* Essex, England, May & Baker, Ltd, 1979.

Phillips I, Collier J, eds: *Metronidazole.* Proc 2nd Internat Symp Anaerobic Infections, Geneva, April 1979. London, The Royal Society of Medicine and Academic Press and New York, Grune & Stratton, 1979.

Rhône-Poulenc Pharma Inc., Montreal: Proc North American Metronidazole Symp, Anaerobic Infections, Scottsdale, Ariz, October 1981. *Surgery* 93:123, 1983.
Rosenblatt JE, Edson RS: Metronidazole. *Mayo Clin Proc* 58:154, 1983.
Stranz MH, Bradley WE: Metronidazole (Flagyl IV, Searle). *Drug Intelligence Clin Pharm* 15:838, 1981.

10

ERYTHROMYCIN, LINCOMYCIN, AND CLINDAMYCIN

NEAL H. STEIGBIGEL

Erythromycin and the lincosamide antibiotics, lincomycin and clindamycin, are chemically unrelated but possess similar biologic properties in terms of mechanisms of action and resistance, antimicrobial activity, and clinical pharmacology. Erythromycin, currently the most important of the macrolide antibiotics, has a few primary indications in therapy and is often useful as an alternative to penicillin G. It is one of the safest antibiotics in clinical use. Clindamycin has been restricted in use by its potential gastrointestinal toxicity but remains particularly important in the treatment of certain anaerobic infections. Lincomycin is now mainly of historic interest.

ERYTHROMYCIN

Derivation, Chemistry, and Preparations

Erythromycin was derived in 1952 from a strain of *Streptomyces erythreus* obtained from soil from the Philippines. The structure (Fig. 1) consists of a macrocyclic lactone ring, therefore the class name macrolide, attached to two sugar moities. Erythromycin base is poorly soluble in water, has a pK of 8.8, is rapidly inactivated by gastric acid, and is often inconsistently absorbed after oral administration. Pharmaceutical preparations for oral use have been made with an aim to diminish destruction by gastric acid and to promote better absorption. Six preparations for oral use are available: enteric-coated tablets (Ilotycin, E-mycin, Ery-Tab, Robimycin, and generics), enteric-coated pellets in capsules (Eryc), and "film"-coated (Filmtab, Abbott) tablets of the base; stearate salt (formed in association with the amino group on desosamine) and available as "film"-coated tablets (Erythrocin, Bristamycin, other brand names, and generics); ethyl-

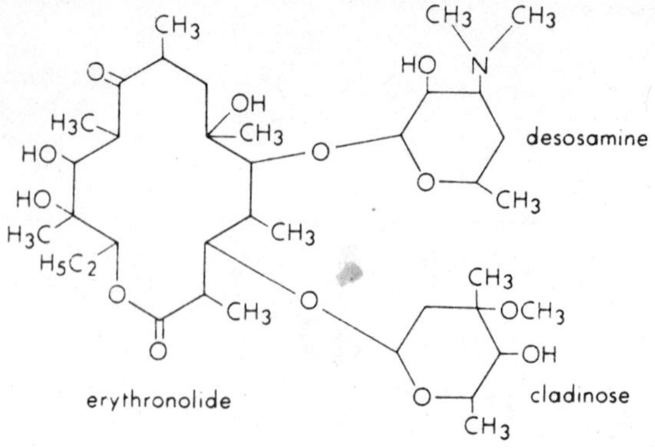

FIGURE 1. Erythromycin base.

succinate ester (formed with the hydroxyl group on desosamine) available in tablet, chewable and liquid forms (Erythrocin, Eryped, EES, Pediamycin); lauryl sulfate salt of the propionyl ester (the estolate) available in tablet, capsule, or liquid forms (Ilosone). There are two water-soluble salts of erythromycin prepared for intravenous use, erythromycin gluceptate (Ilotycin gluceptate) and erythromycin lactobionate (Erythrocin lactobionate). The drug is not given intramuscularly because of pain on injection. Erythromycin base is also available in 1.5 and 2 percent topical solutions used for the treatment of acne vulgaris and in an ophthalmic ointment for treatment of bacterial conjunctivitis and prevention of neonatal gonococcal and chlamydial conjunctivitis.

Mechanisms of Action

Erythromycin inhibits RNA-dependent protein synthesis at the step of chain elongation in susceptible prokaryotic organisms. A single molecule of the antibiotic reversibly binds to the 50S ribosomal subunit resulting in blockage of the transpeptidation and/or translocation reactions (1–3). In some bacteria erythromycin interferes with the ribosomal binding of other macrolides, lincomycin, and chloramphenicol, suggesting common or overlapping binding sites for these antibiotics.

Antimicrobial Activity and Mechanisms of Resistance

The antimicrobial activity of erythromycin is broad in spectrum being exhibited against gram-positive and gram-negative bacteria, including actinomycetes and mycobacteria, as well as against treponemes, mycoplasmas, *Chlamydia,* and rickettsia. Depending on drug concentration, bacterial species, phase of growth, and density of the inoculum, erythromycin may be primarily bacteriostatic or bactericidal. Bacterial killing is favored by higher antibiotic concentrations, lower bacterial density, and rapid growth (4). The activity of erythromycin, which is a weak base, increases markedly with increasing pH over the range 5.5–8.5, for both gram-positive and gram-negative bacteria (5,6), possibly reflecting increased entry into the bacterial cell of the un-ionized drug that is more plentiful at the higher pH.

The in vitro susceptibilities of potential pathogens to erythromycin are listed in Table 1 (7–12). Erythromycin shows high activity against pneumococci and group A streptococci, although occasional resistant clinical isolates have been encountered, especially from patient populations recently exposed to erythromycin or lincomycin (13,14). Of 200 strains of *Streptococcus pneumoniae* isolated from patients with pneumococcal disease, in a survey conducted recently in Spain, 5 were found to be highly resistant to erythromycin and clindamycin (15). In a recent study in Japan, 60 percent of strains of group A streptococci isolated from infected children were highly resistant to erythromycin and lincomycin (16). Almost all of these resistant strains were of type 12, and erythromycin had been widely used to treat respiratory infections in Japan in the several years before the study. A survey of 474 group A streptococcal strains isolated from patients in Oklahoma in 1980 indicated that 5 percent had minimal inhibitory concentrations (MIC) to erythromycin by microtiter broth dilution ≥ 1 μg/ml (17). The emergence of resistance to erythromycin encountered in clinical isolates of these organisms from patient populations treated with this antibiotic is consistent with in vitro studies with pneumococci and streptococci subcultured sequentially in the presence of erythromycin demonstrating the selection of

TABLE 1. In Vitro Susceptibilities to Erythromycin

	Minimum Inhibitory Concentration (μ*g/ml*)	
Organism	*Range*	*Median*
S. pneumoniae	0.001–0.2[a]	0.05
S. pyogenes	0.005–0.2[a]	0.04
S. "viridans"	0.02–3.1[a]	0.06
Enterococcus	0.1–>100	1.5
S. aureus	0.005–>100	0.4
S. epidermidis	0.2–>100	0.6
C. diptheriae	0.006–3.1[a]	0.02
C. perfringens	0.1–6[a]	0.8
L. monocytogenes	0.1–0.3	0.2
B. pertussis	0.02–1.6	0.3
N. gonorrhoeae	0.005–0.4[a]	0.1
N. meningitidis	0.1–1.6	0.4
H. influenzae	0.1–6	3.1
C. jejuni	0.05–>50	0.2
B. fragilis	0.1–>100	≤0.25
L. pneumophila	0.06–0.5	0.1
M. pneumoniae	0.001–0.02	0.005
C. trachomatis	0.1–0.5	0.1

[a] Occasional clinical isolates are more resistant.

erythromycin resistance and often cross-resistance to other macrolides and lincomycin. Similar in vitro results are obtained with staphylococci (18). Although resistance to erythromycin by *Staphlococcus aureus* may be selected by its use in hospitals (19), most clinical isolates are presently sensitive to this agent. However, there always exits a potential for the emergence, during treatment in an individual patient, of erythromycin resistance by *S. aureus* (7,18,20,21). These strains may demonstrate the emergence of one-step high-level resistance to erythromycin alone or may show cross resistance to other macrolides and to lincomycin and clindamycin. In addition, staphylococci isolated from patients treated with erythromycin may exhibit a phenomenon called *dissociated resistance* by Garrod (22). Only a small proportion of the population of such staphylococcal isolates exhibit resistance when grown in large concentrations of erythromycin; however, in the presence of lower concentrations of erythromycin almost the entire population demonstrates resistance to erythromycin, other macrolides, and to the lincosamide antibiotics. In the absence of erythromycin these organisms appear sensitive to these antibiotics.

The majority of strains of the "viridans" group of streptococci, *Listeria monocytogenes,* and *Corynebacterium diphtheriae* show appreciable susceptibility to erthromycin. Many strains of *Clostridium perfringens* may be only moderately sensitive (23). Appreciable in vitro activity has been demonstrated against *Actinomyces israelii, Mycobacterium scrofulaceum,* and *Mycobacterium kansasii* (24), and against *Nocardia asteroides* when combined with ampicillin (25).

With gram-negative bacteria erythromycin displays consistent and useful activity against *Neisseria meningitidis, Neisseria gonorrhoeae,* and *Bordetella pertussis* (8) and somewhat lower activity against *Hemophilus influenzae* (26). High bacteriostatic and bactericidal activity is demonstrated against over 90 percent of strains of *Campylobacter jejuni* (10). Erythromycin has activity against some species of gram-negative anaerobes, but *Bacteroides fragilis* strains are usually resistant (27). The Enterobacteriaceae are usually resistant, except as the pH rises to 8.5 (6).

The extensive spectrum of activity of erythromycin is also demonstrated by its clinically useful activity against such diverse organisms as *Treponema pallidium, Legionella pneumophila* (9), *Mycoplasma pneumoniae, Ureaplasma urealyticum,* some strains of *Rickettsia,* and *Chlamydia trachomatis.* Erythromycin is about 50 times more potent against *M. pneumoniae* than tetracycline (28). Erythromycin-resistant variants of *M. pneumoniae* have been isolated in the laboratory and from a patient (29).

Resistance to erythromycin may be the result of the following: (*1*) Decreased permeability of the cell envelope to the drug is exhibited by the Enterobacteriaceae; cell-free systems and protoplasts of these organisms are susceptible to the drug (30,31). (*2*) Alteration in a single 50S ribosomal protein of the receptor site confers resistance to erythromycin and often to other macrolides, lincomycin, and clindamycin; in some but not all strains this is associated with a decreased binding affinity for erythromycin (2). This one-step high-level resistance is the result of chromosomal mutation, has been demonstrated in some strains of

Bacillus subtilis, Streptococcus pyogenes, Escherichia coli, and probably occurs in *S. aureus.* (*3*) Alteration in the 23S ribosomal RNA of the 50S ribosomal subunit by methylation of adenine (32–35). This is associated with resistance to erythromycin and often to other macrolides, lincomycin, and clindamycin and is due to decreased binding of the antibiotics to their targets on the ribosome. This resistance is mediated by a plasmid and can be exhibited by strains of *S. aureus, Streptomyces* sp., and probably *S. pyogenes* and *Streptococcus faecalis.* The phenomenon may be constituitive or inducible by subinhibitory concentrations of erythromycin that brings about induction of a methylating enzyme. The inducible mechanism seems to explain the phenomenon of "dissociated resistance" already described.

Clinical Pharmacology

The peak serum levels obtained after single doses of various erythromycin preparations are given in Table 2 (7,8,27,36,37). Erythromycin base is subject to destruction by gastric acid, and preparations of the base have been made with an acid-resistant coating to delay drug dissolution until it reaches the small bowel. The esters and ester salts of erythromycin are more acid stabile, form a stable suspension in water, and are tasteless. These characteristics are utilized in the liquid suspensions for children. Erythromycin base (absorbed intact), stearate (absorbed as the base), and ethylsuccinate (absorbed both as the intact

TABLE 2. Serum Levels of Erythromycin in Adults

			Peak Serum Level	
Preparation	*Dose (mg)*	*Route*	*Hours After Dose*	*μg/ml*
Base	250	Oral	4	0.3–1.0[a]
	500			0.3–1.9
Stearate	250 (fasting)	Oral	3	0.2–1.3
	500 (fasting)		3	0.4–1.8
	500 (after food)		3	0.1–0.4[b]
Ethylsuccinate	500	Oral	0.5–2.5	1.5[c] (0.6[d])
Estolate	250	Oral	2–4	1.4–1.7
	500		3.5–4	4.2[c] (1.1[d])
Lactobionate	200	Intravenous	Immediately	3–4
	500		1	9.9
Gluceptate	250	Intravenous	Immediately	3.5–10.7
	1000		1	9.9

[a] Somewhat higher levels reported with some enteric-coated preparations after repeated doses (38,39).
[b] Recent studies note higher levels (to 2.8 μg/ml) with dose taken during a meal (37).
[c] Total drug (inactive ester and free base).
[d] Free base.

ester and the free base after hydrolysis in the intestine) are usually absorbed more completely in the fasting state, although recent studies demonstrate increased absorption of a stearate preparation when taken with a meal (37). After absorption, about 45 percent of the ethylsuccinate preparation is present in the serum as the inactive ester and about 55 percent as the active base. Average serum levels achieved under fasting conditions with these preparations are similar; however, results with the base may be erratic. Erythromycin base has recently become available in a capsule containing enteric-coated granules; this preparation is promoted as giving more uniform absorption (38), but some enteric-coated tablets may provide similar blood levels (39). The absorption of the estolate is not effected by food, and the resulting peak serum level consists of both free base (20–30 percent) (active form) and estolate (70–80 percent) (much less active); the level of base thus achieved is similar to that achieved by the other oral preparations taken in comparable doses in the fasting state. The clinical significance of the much less active esterified form of the drug that is present in serum in appreciable concentration is controversial. It would seem in treatment of infections of only moderate severity by organisms highly sensitive to erythromycin (*S. pneumoniae, S. pyogenes, M. pneumoniae*) that differences in therapeutic results using the various oral preparations will be insignificant. Limited clinical comparisons confirm that suspicion (40). Intravenous preparations of erythromycin achieve appreciably higher serum levels and should be used to treat serious infections requiring erythromycin.

Erythromycin is distributed through total body water. Values given for protein binding vary from 40 to 90 percent; however, the significance of such binding is speculative (41,42). The drug persists in tissues longer than in the blood. The ratios of tissue or body fluid concentrations to simultaneous serum concentrations (usually at peak) are for aqueous humor, 0.3; ascites, 0.4; bile, 28; middle ear exudate in otitis media, 0.3–0.7; pleural fluid, 0.7; prostatic fluid, 0.4; cerebrospinal fluid without meningitis, 0–0.02, with meningitis, 0.05–0.1; infected maxillary paranasal sinus, 0.4–0.8; tonsil, 0.3. Concentrations achieved in the middle ear in otitis media are adequate to treat pneumococcal and group A streptococcal infections but are not adequate to consistently eradicate *H. influenzae* (43,44).

There are very limited data on concentrations of erythromycin achieved in the cerebrospinal fluid of patients with meningitis, which suggest that large parenteral doses may be effective against meningeal infection by highly susceptible organisms such as the pneumococci (45). Limited data from patients with septic arthritis suggest poor penetration of synovial fluid. Erythromycin is transferred across the placenta; fetal serum concentrations are about 2 percent of those in maternal serum, but higher concentrations accumulate in fetal tissue and amniotic fluid (46). The drug is excreted in breast milk.

Up to 4.5 percent of an oral dose and 15 percent of a parenteral dose of erythromycin are recoverable in the urine (7,8). Urine concentrations after oral doses are often high, but quite variable. Erythromycin is concentrated by the liver and excreted into the bile in high concentrations; however, only about

1.5 percent of the dose of the base and 0.2 percent of the ester can be recovered in bile in the first 8 hours, and some of this is reabsorbed from the intestine (47). The higher serum levels achieved by the estolate have been attributed to both better absorption and lower biliary excretion. After an oral dose, large concentrations of the antibiotic are found in feces, probably representing ingested drug that was never absorbed as well as some that was excreted in bile. A large proportion of absorbed drug cannot be accounted for by urinary or biliary excretion or by tissue binding and may be inactivated in the liver by demethylation (48).

The normal serum half-life of erythromycin is 1.4 hours, and appreciable serum levels are maintained for 6 hours. In anuric patients, half-life is only prolonged to about 5 hours, and dosage reduction in patients with renal failure is generally therefore not necessary (49). Erythromycin is not removed by peritoneal dialysis or hemodialysis.

ADVERSE REACTIONS

Erythromycin is one of the safest antibiotics in clinical use. Untoward reactions except for pseudomembranous colitis are not life threatening and, with the exception of the irritative reactions, are rare.

1. Irritative reactions are as follows: dose-related epigastric distress, nausea, vomiting, and diarrhea; thrombophlebitis with intravenous use can be decreased by appropriate dilution of the dose in at least 250 ml of solution and by avoiding rapid "bolus" infusions (infuse over about 45–60 minutes).
2. Allergic reactions include skin rash, fever, and eosinophilia.
3. Cholestatic hepatitis occurs only with the estolate preparation and chiefly in adults (50). The syndrome typically begins after 10 days of therapy, but more rapidly in those previously treated, and consists of nausea, vomiting, and abdominal pain followed by jaundice, fever, and abnormal liver function tests consistent with cholestatic hepatitis. These findings are sometimes accompanied by rash, leukocytosis, and eosinophilia. The abnormalities generally clear within days to a few weeks after stopping the drug but may return rapidly on rechallenge. The syndrome appears to represent a hypersensitivity reaction to the specific structure of the estolate compound (51). Milder forms of the syndrome occur with the estolate and may be more common in pregnant women (52). It must be distinguished from false-positive serum glutamic-oxaloacetic transaminase (SGOT) elevations that occur in patients taking the estolate (53). The latter may be found when SGOT is determined by colorimetric procedures rather than by an enzymatic method and seems to result from an interfering substance present in the blood in association with estolate administration. Reversible hepatotoxicity has occurred with the ethysuccinate ester of erythromycin and possibly with other preparations of erythromycin (54).

4. Transient hearing loss has been reported very rarely in association with the use of large intravenous doses of erythromycin lactobionate or large doses of oral erythromycin (55,56). This may occur more commonly in elderly patients with renal insufficiency (57,58).
5. Hypertrophic pyloric stenosis developed in five infants during administration of erythromycin estolate (59).
6. Superinfection, especially of the gastrointestinal tract or vagina, with *Candida* species or gram-negative bacilli may occur as with other antibiotics.
7. Pseudomembrabous colitis caused by overgrowth of toxin-producing *Clostridium difficile* occurs rarely with the use of erythromycin (60,61).

Drug Interactions

Incompatibility during administration between intravenous preparations of erythromycin and other drugs has been reported; the latter include vitamin B complex and vitamin C, cephalothin, tetracycline, chloramphenicol, colistin, heparin, metraminol, and diphenylhydantoin. When oral theophylline and oral erythromycin are used concurrently, increased blood levels of theophylline and potential theophylline toxicity may result (62). False elevations during erythromycin therapy have been reported for urinary catecholamines and 17-hydroxycorticosteroids (8), as well as in the colorimetrically determined transaminase levels discussed above. Erythromycin may inhibit the assay organism used in some determinations of serum folic acid. Sequential use of erythromycin and clindamycin should be avoided when possible because of the potential for the development of cross or "dissociated" resistance.

Uses of Erythromycin

Erythromycin has a few indications for use as the drug of choice and a larger number of important applications as an alternative drug to penicillin G (Table 3) (63). When used in adults by the oral route, preparations other than the estolate are generally preferable because they give less risk of cholestatic hepatitis. Absorption, particularly with the enteric-coated base, stearate, or ethylsuccinate preparations taken in the fasting state, or before meals is usually adequate. The estolate preparation should be particularly avoided during pregnancy when hepatotoxicity may be more common (52). When higher serum levels are needed in more severe infections requiring erythromycin therapy, the drug should be given intravenously.

Treatment of *M. pneumoniae* infection with erythromycin, as with tetracycline, shortens the clinical course of the infection; radiologic clearing of pulmonary lesions occurs earlier with erythromycin (64). Clinical experience and studies in vitro and in guinea pigs suggest that erythromycin is the most active available agent in treating pneumonia caused by *L. pneumophila* or *L. micdadei* (9,65–67). Erythromycin treatment of patients with gastroenteritis caused by *C. jejuni* hastens the eradication of the organism from the feces, but it does

TABLE 3. Major Uses of Erythromycin

Indication	*Doses of Erythromycin for Adults*	*Alternative Drug*
Infection in which erythromycin is the drug of first choice		
M. pneumoniae infections	0.5 g tid–qid po[a]	Tetracycline
Legionella pneumonia	0.5–1.0 g qid po[a]	Rifampin + erythromycin
Diphtheria[b]	carrier state: 500 mg qid po for 10 days disease:[a] followed by oral for 10 days	Penicillin G Penicillin G
Pertussis	0.5 g qid po	Ampicillin
Chlamydia trachomatis pneumonia or conjunctivitis	10 mg/kg qid po[a]	Sulfisoxazole
Chlamydial pelvic infection in pregnancy	0.5–1.0 g qid po[a,c]	Sulfisoxazole
Campylobacter jejuni gastroenteritis	250 mg qid po	Tetracycline
Prevention of infection after colorectal surgery	1 g po each of neomycin and erythromycin base at 1, 2, and 11 P.M. on the day before surgery combined with vigorous purgation over the 2 days before surgery	Parenteral cephalosporin

TABLE 3. (Continued)

Indication	*Doses of Erythromycin for Adults*	*Alternative Drug*
Infections in which erythromycin is an important alternative drug		*Drug of First Choice*
Groups A, B, C, G streptococcal infection	250–500 mg qid po[a,d]	Penicillin G
Streptococcus pneumoniae infection	250–500 mg qid po[a]	Penicillin G
Rheumatic fever prophylaxis	250 mg bid po	Penicillin G
Prevention of bacterial endocarditis (in dental procedures)	1.0 g po 1–2 hr before procedure; then 500 mg 6 hr later	Penicillin G
Gonorrhea: disseminated	500 mg q6h IV (3 days) or po (5 days)	Penicillin G
Nongonococcal urethritis	500 mg qid po for 7 days	Tetracycline
Syphilis 1°, 2°, latent (< 1 yr) in pregnancy	500 mg qid po for 15 days[e]	Penicillin G
latent (> 1 yr) in pregnancy	500 mg qid po for 30 days[e]	Penicillin G
Bronchopulmonary anaerobic infections	0.5 gm qid po	Penicillin G; clindamycin
Acne vulgaris	250 mg qid po or topical preparation	Tetracycline po and a number of topical drugs
Urinary tract infection	500 mg qid po[f]	Many agents

[a] Intravenous therapy (2–4 g/day) should be used in serious illness or when oral therapy is not possible or reliable.
[b] Antitoxin is essential primary therapy for disease.
[c] Severe pelvic inflammatory disease is often polymicrobial in origin; treatment of such cases should include other agents more active against likely facultative and anaerobic enteric bacteria and/or *N. gonorrhoeae.*
[d] Treatment should be continued for 10 days for Group A.
[e] Careful follow-up needed when used in pregnancy. Effectiveness uncertain.
[f] Urine pH must be raised to greater than 8 with sodium bicarbonate.

not appear to alter the clinical course of uncomplicated infection when therapy begins 4 days or more after the onset of symptoms (68). Treatment is particularly recommended for people who may transmit the organism (68) or for those with prolonged or severe illness (69). Treatment of infants with erythromycin for pneumonia due to *C. trachomatis* appears to speed recovery and eradication of the shedding of organisms (70). Erythromycin is preferable to tetracycline in treating chlamydial pelvic infection during pregnancy (27). Erythromycin base given orally together with neomycin on the day before colorectal surgery and combined with vigorous purgation is about as effective as parenteral cephalosporin administration just before surgery in decreasing the incidence of septic complications (71). The oral regimen is generally less expensive; however, in the presence of bowel obstruction or when there is need for emergency surgery, the parenteral antibiotic regimen should be used (63). The results of treating syphilis with erythromycin during pregnancy must be considered uncertain at best; fetal syphilis may not be eradicated, and therefore convincing evidence of potentially dangerous penicillin allergy should be obtained before this type of therapy is used (72). Erythromycin may occasionally be useful in treating urinary tract infections due to gram-negative bacilli that might otherwise require the use of more toxic agents (73). Urine pH must generally be raised to 8.0 or above to achieve effective activity at urinary concentrations against the gram-negative bacilli. Erythromycin may be used as an alternative antibiotic in the treatment of anthrax and in infections by *L. monocytogenes.* Erythromycin is not consistently effective in treatment of infections due to *H. influenzae* (43,44), and *in vitro* studies suggest resistance by some strains of *C. perfringens* (23). In view of the availability of more effective alternative drugs, erythromycin should not be used alone in the treatment of deep-seated staphylococcal infections because of the potential for the emergence of resistant strains during therapy (18,20,21). Experimental studies and limited clinical data suggest that erythromycin combined with a penicillin may demonstrate synergy (20,74) against *S. aureus;* further studies are needed to exploit the potential in therapy.

Other Macrolides

Troleandomycin, an ester of the macrolide, oleandomycin, has no advantages over erythromycin and may occasionally cause cholestatic hepatitis.

LINCOMYCIN AND CLINDAMYCIN

Derivation, Chemistry, and Preparations

Lincomycin was isolated in 1962 from an organism, *Streptomyces lincolnensis,* obtained from soil near Lincoln, Nebraska. Its biologic properties are similar to erythromycin, but it is chemically unrelated, consisting of an amino acid linked to an amino sugar (Fig. 2). Chemical modification provided clindamycin

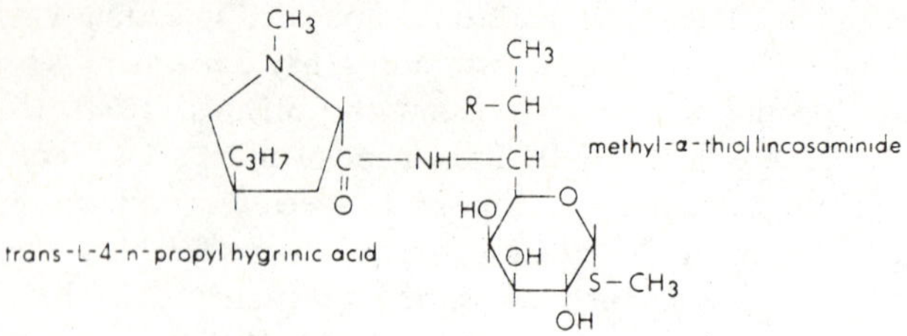

FIGURE 2. The lincosamide antibiotics: lincomycin, R = OH; clindamycin, R = Cl.

(7-chloro-7-deoxylincomycin) (Fig. 2) with increased antibacterial potency and absorption after oral administration (75). Since there are no therapeutic advantages for lincomycin over clindamycin, the discussion will concentrate on the latter, although both are still marketed as pharmaceuticals. Both are weak bases that are readily water soluble when provided as salts.

Lincomycin (Lincocin) is available as the hydrochloride salt in 250- and 500-mg capsules and syrup for oral administration and in solution (300 mg/ml) for parenteral use. Clindamycin (Cleocin) is prepared as the hydrochloride salt of the base in 75- and 150-mg capsules and of the palmitate ester for pediatric suspension. It is supplied as the phosphate ester for intramuscular or intravenous use (150 mg/ml). It is also available in a topical solution for the treatment of acne vulgaris.

Mechanisms of Action

The lincosamide antibiotics have, in susceptible organisms, the same or overlapping 50S ribosomal binding sites as those for the macrolides and chloramphenicol, and they may compete with these drugs for binding (2,3). Protein synthesis is inhibited primarily in early chain elongation by interference with the transpeptidation reaction (1,3).

Antimicrobial Activity and Mechanisms of Resistance

In vitro susceptibilities to clindamycin are given in Table 4 (7, 12,75,76). Clindamycin is more potent than lincomycin but similar in degree of activity to erythromycin against staphylococci, pneumococci, *S. pyogenes,* and streptococci of the "viridans" group. However, while erythromycin demonstrates at least moderate activity against the enterococcus, *H. influenzae,* and *N. meningitidis,* clindamycin is generally inactive against these organisms at clinically achievable concentrations. In contrast, clindamycin shows significantly greater activity than erythromycin against most clinically significant anaerobic bacteria, particularly *B. fragilis* (76,77) and some erythromycin-resistant strains of *S. aureus* (78). Clindamycin is one of the most active antibiotics available against *B. fragilis.* In a survey of nine hospitals in the United States that provided 750 strains of the

TABLE 4. In Vitro Susceptibilities to Clindamycin

Organism	*Minimum Inhibitory Concentration (μg/ml)* Range	Median
S. pneumoniae	0.002–0.04[a]	0.01
S. pyogenes	0.02–0.1[a]	0.04
S. "viridans"	0.005–0.04[a]	0.02
Enterococcus	12.5–>100	100
S. aureus	0.04–>100	0.1
S. epidermidis	0.1–>100	0.1
C. perfringens	<0.1–8	0.8
N. gonorrhoeae	0.01–6.3	3.1
N. meningitidis	6.3–25	12.5
H. influenzae	0.4–50	12.5
B. fragilis group	≤0.25–>32	≤0.25
B. melaninogenicus	≤0.1–1	≤0.1
Fusobacterium sp.	≤0.5[a]	≤0.5
Peptococcus sp.	≤0.1–>100	≤0.5
Peptostreptococcus sp.	≤0.1–0.8	≤0.5
M. pneumoniae	1.6–3.1	3.1

[a] Occasional clinical isolates are more resistant.

B. fragilis group in 1981, 6 percent of isolates were resistant to clindamycin (MIC > 4 μg/ml by an agar dilution method); this represented 0–13 percent of strains in individual institutions (12). Of the species belonging to the *B. fragilis* group, clindamycin resistance was found in 5 percent of *B. fragilis,* 17 percent of *Bacteroides thetaiotaomicron,* and 12 percent of *Bacteroides vulgatus* strains. Resistance to clindamycin by anaerobes also includes 10–20 percent of clostridial species other than *C. perfringens,* about 10 percent of peptococci, and most *Fusobacterium varium* strains (76,77). All the Enterobacteriaceae are resistant to clindamycin.

There have been occasional reports of clinical isolates of lincosamide-resistant *S. pneumoniae* (14,15), *S. pyogenes* (13,16), and "viridans" group streptococci; these strains are usually also resistant to erythromycin. In most hospitals at present, the vast majority of isolates of *S. aureus* are sensitive to lincomycin or clindamycin (77); however, there are a few reports of resistance in 15–20 percent of strains (79). Lincomycin resistance has been reported in 20 percent of methicillin-resistant strains (80) and in 50 percent of erythromycin-resistant strains (81) of *S. aureus.* Cross resistance of *S. aureus* between lincomycin and clindamycin is complete. The minimal inhibitory concentrations of clindamycin and erythromycin in vitro are generally similar for *S. aureus* strains that are sensitive to both agents; however resistance can be selected in vitro by serial subculture in the presence of subinhibitory concentrations of either, and it occurs slowly for clindamycin and more rapidly for erythromycin (78,82). In contrast, strains that are sensitive to clindamycin and resistant to erythromycin can be rapidly selected for clindamycin resistance by serial subculture on clindamycin. Consistent with these in vitro observations, the emergence of clindamycin-resistant *S. aureus* has been noted in clindamycin-treated patients, in particular when the organisms had demonstrated erythromycin resistance at the onset of treatment (78). Clindamycin resistance, often crossing to erythromycin, has also emerged from treated patients infected with *S. aureus* that were initially sensitive to erythromycin (83). Resistance of the "dissociated" type may also emerge during treatment of patients (82).

The antibacterial activity of lincomycin and clindamycin has been shown, in limited in vitro studies, to be bactericidal for *S. pneumoniae, S. pyogenes,* and *S. aureus.* Its killing activity is similar to erythromycin and therefore probably varies with concentration, bacterial species, and inoculum. It is more slowly bactericidal for *S. aureus* than the penicillins (84) and is inconsistently bactericidal for *B. fragilis* (85).

The known mechanisms of resistance to the lincosamide antibiotics have been discussed and relate to alteration in the ribosomal binding site that overlaps with that for the macrolide antibiotics (2,32–35). Plasmid-mediated resistance involving both erythromycin and clindamycin has been described recently for *B. fragilis* (12,86). It is likely that this resistance is brought about by methylation of the 23S ribosomal RNA of the 50S ribosomal subunit; however, the mechanism has not yet been elucidated for the bacteroides group.

Clinical Pharmacology

Peak serum levels achieved after oral administration of clindamycin occur earlier and are at least twice as high as those of lincomycin. Absorption of clindamycin is about 90 percent and is slightly delayed, but not decreased, by ingestion of food, whereas that of lincomycin is markedly decreased (75). Mean peak serum concentrations of clindamycin in adults after single oral doses of 150 and 300 mg occur at 1 hour and are 2.5 and 3.6 μg/ml, respectively; at 6 hours they are 0.7 and 1.1 μg/ml, respectively. The esters, clindamycin palmitate in suspension for oral use and clindamycin phosphate for parenteral use, are absorbed as the inactive ester and rapidly hydrolyzed in the blood to the active base. After intramuscular administration, which causes little pain, mean peak serum levels are reached in 3 hours and are about 6 μg/ml after a 300 mg dose and 9 μg/ml after a 600 mg dose; at 12 hours they are 0.7 and 0.9 μg/ml, respectively (87). In adult healthy volunteers, immediately following 20–45-minute intravenous infusions of 600, 900, or 1200 mg of clindamycin phosphate, serum levels of base are 10, 11, and 14 μg/ml, respectively. Higher levels after intravenous infusion have been reported in infected patients under treatment (88).

Limited studies have demonstrated good penetration of most tissues by the lincosamides excepting clinically insignificant entry of clindamycin into the cerebrospinal fluid, even with meningitis (7,89). Concentration in bone in relationship to serum levels is particularly high (90). Clindamycin administered to pregnant women readily passes the placental barrier and enters fetal blood and tissues (46). Clindamycin is actively transported into polymorphonuclear leukocytes and macrophages (91) and is present in relatively high concentrations, compared to peak serum levels, in experimental abscesses (92).

The normal half-life of clindamycin is 2.4 hours. Most of the absorbed drug is metabolized, probably by the liver, to products with variable antibacterial activity, including *N*-demethyl-clindamycin (more active than the parent compound) and clindamycin sulfoxide (less active), which have been detected in bile and urine but not in serum (87). High bioactivity is found in bile, mostly as the *N*-demethyl metabolite; this represents a minor route of excretion and accounts for the activity assayed in feces after parenteral administration (87,93). Clindamycin activity in feces persists for at least 5 days after 48 hours of parenteral administration and is associated with a major reduction in the population of sensitive bacteria in the colon lasting up to 14 days (94). Clindamycin concentration in bile is markedly diminished or absent when the common bile duct is obstructed (95). High clindamycin bioactivity, also mostly in the *N*-demethyl form, is found in the urine and persists for up to 4 days after a single dose, suggesting slow release from tissues (87). Accurate data on the proportion of absorbed clindamycin that is excreted in the urine are not available because of the variable activity of the metabolites and their unknown proportions in urine.

Half-life of clindamycin is increased from 2.4 to about 6 hours in patients with severe renal failure, and peak blood levels after parenteral administration are about twice those in healthy people (96). If modified at all, parenteral doses should be halved in such patients. Some prolongation of clindamycin activity in serum is noted in patients with severe liver disease (97). Appreciable dose modification should be made when there is concomitant severe renal and hepatic disease in the same patient. Neither hemodialysis nor peritoneal dialysis removes significant amounts of clindamycin.

Adverse Reactions

1. Allergic reactions include a variety of rashes, fever, and rare cases of erythema multiforme and anaphylaxis.
2. Diarrhea occurs in up to 20 percent of patients and is more common with oral administration. However, the major toxicity of lincomycin and clindamycin that now appreciably limits their use is the occurrence of pseudomembranous colitis caused by a toxin secreted by *C. difficile* that overgrows in the presence of these antibiotics (98–100). This has been reported in 0.01–10 percent of clindamycin-treated patients (77,101). The syndrome may occur in association with administration of other antibiotics but does so less frequently; it is not related to dose and may occur after oral or parenteral therapy. The variable incidence of colitis in different reports has been ascribed to different diagnostic methods and the variable epidemiology of *C. difficile* (77,101). It may begin during or as long as several weeks after a course of lincomycin or clindamycin therapy and is characterized by diarrhea, some-

times bloody, with fever and cramps and the appearance of yellow-white plaques on the colonic mucosa, seen by proctoscopy. The toxin of *C. difficile* can be detected in the stool of nearly all patients with antibiotic-associated pseudomembranous colitis and in about 20 percent of patients with antibiotic-associated diarrhea by a cytotoxicity assay using tissue culture cells (61,100). The cytotoxic effect can be prevented by neutralization of the toxin in the stool extract with *Clostridium sordelli* antitoxin. The syndrome can be protracted and may end fatally. Prompt cessation of the antibiotic is essential. Use of antiperistaltic drugs should be avoided since they may worsen the condition. Vancomycin given by mouth in doses of 125–500 mg qid is the drug of choice for treatment of this type of pseudomembranous colitis, although oral bacitracin and oral metronidazole may be effective as well (102). Relapse after treatment may occur.

3. Hepatotoxicity: Minor reversible elevation of transaminase levels, unassociated with other evidence of liver abnormality, has been commonly observed in patients receiving clindamycin, especially by the parenteral route. Some of these may have been false-positive reactions associated with colorimetric rather than specific enzymatic measurements (75). However, rare cases of frank hepatotoxicity, including jaundice associated with hepatocellular damage, have been observed (103).
4. Isolated cases of reversible neutropenia, thrombocytopenia, and agranulocytosis associated with lincomycin or clindamycin therapy have been reported; their relationship to the antibiotic administration was uncertain.
5. Occasional reports of hypotension, ECG changes, and rarely cardiopulmonary arrest have been reported when large intravenous doses of lincomycin were given rapidly. This has not been reported with clindamycin.
6. Local irritative reactions are rare with these drugs. Intramuscular and intravenous administration is generally well tolerated.

Drug Interactions

Clindamycin may block neuromuscular transmission and may enhance the action of other blocking agents (104). Clindamycin phosphate in solution is physically incompatible with ampicillin, diphenylhydantoin, barbituates, aminophylline, calcium gluconate, and magnesium sulfate.

Uses of Clindamycin

The higher activity and absorption properties of clindamycin along with no greater potential for toxicity, compared with lincomycin, favors the former in all indications for use of these antibiotics. The lincosamides have been used in a variety of infections, often with good effect; however, the appreciation of the potential for serious or even fatal toxicity with pseudomembranous colitis and the availability of safer alternative antibiotics should now generally limit the use of clindamycin to a few indications (63):

1. Infections that are outside of the central nervous system and are likely to involve *B. fragilis* or other penicillin-resistant anaerobic bacteria. These particularly involve polymicrobial intra-abdominal or gynecologic pelvic infections (77). Clindamycin is likely to be beneficial where there is spillage of fecal flora associated with tissue damage, as in cases involving bowel damage or perforation. In these situations studies of experimental animal models and patients with infection suggest that clindamycin decreases the likelihood of abscess formation involving fecal organisms, especially *B. fragilis* (105,106). In these conditions clindamycin is administered together with an aminoglycoside, because additional activity is required against Enterobacteriaceae. The beneficial effect of clindamycin in preventing or ameliorating morbidity from fecal abscess formation or other infection appears to be superior to that of penicillin, cephalothin, or aminoglycosides (105,107). However, in comparative trials of therapy for intra-abdominal or pelvic sepsis, clindamycin, cefoxitin, metronidazole, and chloramphenicol have shown similar effectiveness (77).

   Until recently clindamycin appeared to offer no advantage over penicillin G in the treatment of anaerobic bronchopulmonary infections (108) except that it served as an alternative in patients allergic to penicillin. However, in a recent prospective randomized study of 39 patients with community-acquired putrid lung abscess, clindamycin was more effective than penicillin in terms of time until eradication of fever and fetid sputum and "overall response" to treatment (109). The study involved small numbers of patients and had some flaws in the analysis (110); however, the superiority of clindamycin for some patients was demonstrated and may relate to recent observations that 15–25 percent of anaerobic pulmonary infections involve β-lactamase-producing strains of *B. fragilis, Bacteroides melaninogenicus, Bacteroides ruminicola,* and *Bacteroides ureolyticus,* which are resistant to penicillin (77, 110). Clindamycin may therefore be preferable for the treatment of this condition, particularly in seriously ill patients or in those who have responded poorly to penicillin.
2. Clindamycin is useful as an alternative to penicillin in treatment of *C. perfringens* infections.
3. Clindamycin may sometimes be useful as an alternative to a penicillin in the treatment of staphylococcal infections. However, its more limited bactericidal rate for staphylococci compared with the penicillins and particularly the real potential for the emergence of clindamycin-resistant strains in treated patients are disadvantages. The latter problem, noted especially, but not only, with erythromycin-resistant strains, appreciably limits its effectiveness in therapy of deep-seated staphylococcal infections, particularly endocarditis (83,90). Vancomycin or the cephalosporins are usually better alternatives to the penicillins for the latter. Although high concentrations of clindamycin are achieved in bone, an advantage of clindamycin for the treatment of osteomyelitis in patients has not been established.
4. The topical solution of clindamycin may be used to treat acne vulgaris (111).

Doses of clindamycin, for adults depend on the site, severity of the infection, and condition of the patient. Oral doses are usually 150–300 mg every 6 hours and parenteral doses, given every 8–12 hours, usually total 600–2700 mg/day, occasionally higher.

REFERENCES

1. Pestka S: Inhibitors of protein synthesis, in Weissbach H, Pestka S (eds): *Molecular Mechanisms of Protein Biosynthesis.* New York, Academic Press, 1977, p 467.
2. Oleinick NL: The erythromycins, in Corcoran JW, Hahn FE (eds): *Mechanism of Action of Antimicrobial and Antitumor Agents.* New York, Springer-Verlag, 1975, p 396.
3. Franklin TJ, Snow GA: *Biochemistry of Antimicrobial Action,* ed 3. London, Chapman and Hall, 1981 p 128.
4. Haight TH, Finland M: Observations on mode of action of erythromycin. *Proc Soc Exp Biol Med* 81:188, 1952.
5. Haight TH, Finland M: The antibacterial action of erythromycin. *Proc Soc Exp Biol Med* 81:175, 1952.
6. Sabath LD, Gerstein DA, Loder PB, et al: Excretion of erythromycin and its enhanced activity in urine against gram-negative bacilli with alkalinization. *J Lab Clin Med* 72:916, 1968.
7. Garrod LP, Lambert HP, O'Grady F: *Antibiotic and Chemotherapy,* ed 5. Edinburgh, Churchill Livingstone, 1981, p 183.
8. Nicholas P: Erythromycin: Clinical review I. Clinical pharmacology. *NY State J Med* 77:2088, 1977.
9. Edelstein PM, Meyer RD: Susceptibility of *Legionella pneumophila* to twenty antimicrobial agents. *Antimicrob Agents Chemother* 18:403, 1980.
10. Vanhoof R, Gordts B, Dierickx R, et al: Bacteriostatic and bactericidal activities of 24 antimicrobial agents against *Campylobacter fetus* subsp. *jejuni. Antimicrob Agents Chemother* 18:118, 1980.
11. Kuo C, Wang S, Grayston T: Antimicrobial activity of several antibiotics and a sulfonamide against *Chlamydia trachomitis* organisms in cell culture. *Antimicrob Agents Chemother* 12:80, 1977.
12. Tally FP, Cuchural GJ, Jacobus NV, et al: Susceptibility of the *Bacteriodes fragilis* group in the United States in 1981. *Antimicrob Agents Chemother* 23:536, 1983.
13. Sanders E, Foster MT, Scott D: Group A beta-haemolytic streptococci resistant to erythromycin and lincomycin. *New Engl J Med* 278:538, 1968.
14. Dixon JM: Pneumococcus resistant to erythromycin and lincomycin. *Lancet* 1:573, 1967.
15. Linares J, Garau J, Dominquez C, et al: Antibiotic resistance and serotypes of *Streptococcus pneumoniae* from patients with community acquired pneumococcal disease. *Antimicrob Agents Chemother* 23:545, 1983.
16. Maruyama S, Yoshioka H, Fujita K, et al: Sensitivity of Group A streptococci to antibiotics. *Am J Dis Child* 133:1143, 1979.
17. Istre GR, Welch DF, Marks MI, et al: Susceptibility of Group A beta-hemolytic *Streptococcus* isolates to penicillin and erythromycin. *Antimicrob Agents Chemother* 20:244, 1981.
18. Haight TH, Finland M: Resistance of bacteria to erythromycin. *Proc Soc Exp Biol Med* 81:183, 1952.
19. Lepper MH, Dowling HF, Jackson GG, et al: Effect of antibiotic usage in the hospital on the incidence of antibiotic-resistant strains among personnel carrying staphylococci. *J Lab Clin Med* 42:832, 1953.
20. Griffith RS, Black HR: Erythromycin. *Med Clin North Am* 54:1199, 1970.
21. Haight TH, Finland M: Laboratory and clinical studies on erythromycin. *New Engl J Med* 247:227, 1952.

22. Garrod LP: The erythromycin group of antibiotics. *Br Med J* 2:57, 1957.
23. Sapcio FL, Kwok Y, Sutter V, et al: Standardized antimicrobial disc susceptibility testing of anaerobic bacteria: *In vitro* susceptibility of *Clostridium perfringens* to nine antibiotics. *Antimicrob Agents Chemother* 2:320, 1972.
24. Molavi A, Weinstein L: *In vitro* activity of erythromycin against atypical mycobacteria. *J Infect Dis* 123:216, 1971.
25. Finland M, Bach MC, Garner C, et al: Synergistic action of ampicillin against *Nocardia asteroides:* Effect of time of incubation. *Antimicrob Agents Chemother* 5:344, 1974.
26. McLinn SE, Nelson JD, Haltalin KC: Antimicrobial susceptibility of *Hemophilus influenzae. Pediatrics* 45:827, 1970.
27. Kucers A: Chloramphenicol, erythromycin, vancomycin, tetracyclines. *Lancet* ii:425, 1982.
28. Jao RL, Finland M: Susceptibility of *Mycoplasma pneumoniae* to 21 antibiotics *in vitro. Am J Med Sci* 253:639, 1967.
29. Niitu Y, Hasegawa S, Kubota H: *In vitro* development of resistance to erythromycin, other macrolide antibiotics, and lincomycin in *Mycoplasma pneumoniae. Antimicrob Agents Chemother* 5:513, 1974.
30. Mao JC-H, Putterman M: Accumulation in gram-positive and gram-negative bacteria as a mechanism of resistance to erythromycin. *J Bacteriol* 95:1111, 1968.
31. Taubeneck U: Susceptibility of *Proteus mirabilis* and its stable L-forms to erythromycin and other macrolides. *Nature* 196:195, 1962.
32. Weisblum B, Siddhikol C, Lai CJ, et al: Erythromycin inducible resistance in *Staphylococcus aureus:* requirements for induction. *J Bacteriol* 106:835, 1971.
33. Lai CJ, Weissblum B, Fahnestock SR, et al: Alteration of 23S ribosomal RNA and erythromycin-induced resistance to lincomycin and spiramycin in *Staphylococcus aureus. J Mol Biol* 74:67, 1973.
34. Levy SB: Microbial resistance to antibiotics: An evolving and persistant problem. *Lancet* ii:83, 1982.
35. Fujisawa Y, Weisblum B: A family of r-determinants in Streptomyces spp. that specifies inducible resistance to macrolide, lincosamide, and streptogramin type B antibiotics. *J Bacteriol* 146:621, 1981.
36. Bechtol LD, Stephen VC, Pugh CT, et al: Erythromycin esters: Comparative in-vivo hydrolysis and bioavailability. *Curr Therap Res* 20:610, 1976.
37. Malmborg A: Effect of food on absorption of erythromycin. A study of two derivatives, the stearate and the base. *J Antimicrob Chemother* 5:591, 1979.
38. McDonald PJ, Mather LE, Story MJ: Studies on absorption of a newly developed enteric-coated erythromycin base. *J Clin Pharmacol* 17:601, 1977.
39. DiSanto AR, Chodos DJ: Influence of study design in assessing food effects on absorption of erythromycin base and erythromycin stearate. *Antimicrob Agents Chemother* 20:190, 1981.
40. Janicki RS, Garnham JC, Worland MC, et al: Comparison of erythromycin ethyl succinate, stearate and estolate treatments of group A streptococcus infections of the upper respiratory tract. *Clin Pediatr* (*Phila*) 14:1098, 1975.
41. Braude Al: *Antimicrobial Drug Therapy.* Philadelphia, WB Saunders Co, 1976.
42. Welling PG: The esters of erythromycin. *J Antimicrob Chemother* 5:633, 1979.
43. Bass JW, Steele RW, Wiebe RA, et al: Erythromycin concentrations in middle ear exudates. *Pediatrics* 48:417, 1971.
44. Howard JE, Nelson JD, Clahsen J, et al: Otitis media of infancy and early childhood. *Am J Dis Child* 130:965, 1976.
45. Romansky MJ, Nasou JP, Davis DS, et al: The treatment of 171 patients with erythromycin, including 132 with bacterial pneumonia. *Antibiotics Annual,* New York, Medical Encyclopedia, Inc, 1956, 1955–1956, p 48.
46. Philipson A, Sabath LD, Charles D: Transplacental passage of erythromycin and clindamycin. *New Engl J Med* 288:1219, 1973.
47. Hammond JB, Griffith RS: Factors affecting the absorption and biliary excretion of erythromycin and two of its derivatives in humans. *Clin Pharmacol Ther* 2:308, 1961.

48. Mao JC-H, Tardrew PL: Demethylation of erythromycin by rabbit tissues *in vitro. Biochem Pharm* 14:1049, 1965.
49. Kunin CM: A guide to use of antibiotics in patients with renal disease. *Ann Intern Med* 67:151, 1967.
50. Braun P: Hepatotoxicity of erythromycin. *J Infect Dis* 119:300, 1969.
51. Tolman KG, Sannella JJ, Freston JW: Chemical structure of erythromycin and hepatotoxicity. *Ann Intern Med* 81:58, 1974.
52. McCormack WM, George H, Donner A, et al: Hepatotoxicity of erythromycin estolate during pregnancy. *Antimicrob Agents Chemother* 12:630, 1977.
53. Sabath LD, Gerstein DA, Finland M: Serum glutamic oxalacetic transaminase: False elevation during administration of erythromycin. *New Engl J Med* 279:1137, 1968.
54. Sullivan D, Csuka ME, Blanchard B: Erythromycin ethylsuccinate hepatotoxicity. *JAMA* 243:1074, 1980.
55. Karmody CS, Weinstein L: Reversible sensorineural hearing loss with intravenous erythromycin lactobionate. *Ann Otol Rhinol Laryngol* 86:9, 1977.
56. Eckman MR, Johnson T, Riess R: Letter: Partial deafness after erythromycin. *New Engl J Med* 292:649, 1975.
57. Mery JP, Kanfer A: Ototoxicity of erythromycin in patients with renal insufficiency, letter. *New Engl J Med* 301:944, 1979.
58. Taylor R, Schofield IS, Ramos JM, et al: Ototoxicity of erythromycin in peritoneal dialysis patients, letter. *Lancet* ii:935, 1981.
59. Filippo JA: Infantile hypertrophic pyloric stenosis related to ingestions of erythromycin estolate: A report of five cases. *J Pediatr Surg* 11:177, 1976.
60. Gantz NM, Zawacki JK, Dickerson J, et al: Pseudomembranous colitis associated with erythromycin. *Ann Intern Med* 91:866, 1979.
61. Bartlett JG: Antimicrobial agents implicated in *Clostridium difficile* toxin-associated diarrhea or colitis. *Johns Hopkins Med J* 149:6, 1981.
62. Kozak Jr PP, Cummins LH, Gillman SA: Administration of erythromycin to patients on theophylline. *J Allergy Clin Immunol* 60:149, 1977.
63. *Handbook of Antimicrobial Therapy,* The Medical Letter on Drugs and Therapeutics, New Rochelle, NY, The Medical Letter, Inc. 1984.
64. Rasch JR, Mogabgab WJ: Therapeutic effect of erythromycin on *Mycoplasma pneumoniae* pneumonia. *Antimicrob Agents Chemother* 5:693, 1965.
65. Kirby BD, Snyder KM, Myer RD, et al: Legionnaires' Disease: Report of sixty-five nosocomially acquired cases and review of the literature. *Medicine* 59:188, 1980.
66. Broome CV: Pneumonia due to Legionella species, in Weinstein L, Fields BN (eds): *Seminars in Infectious Disease,* vol V, Pneumonias. New York, Thieme-Stratton, 1983, p 16.
67. Muder RF, Yu VL, Zuravleff MS: Pneumonia due to the Pittsburgh pneumonia agent: New clinical perspective with a review of the literature. *Medicine* 62:120, 1983.
68. Anders BJ, Lauer BA, Paisley JW, et al: Double-blind placebo controlled trial of erythromycin for treatment of Campylobacter enteritis. *Lancet* i:131, 1982.
69. Blaser MJ, Reller LB: Campylobacter enteritis. *New Engl J Med* 305:1444, 1981.
70. Beem MD, Saxon E, Tipple MA: Treatment of chlamydial pneumonia of infancy. *Pediatrics* 63:198, 1979.
71. Clarke JS, Condon RE, Fenton LJ, et al: Preoperative oral antibiotics reduce septic complications of colon operations: Results of prospective, randomized, double-blind clinical study. *Ann Surg* 186:251, 1977.
72. Fenton LJ, Light IJ: Congenital syphilis after maternal treatment with erythromycin. *Obstet Gynecol* 47:492, 1976.
73. Zinner SK, Sabath LD, Casey JI, et al: Erythromycin and alkalinization of the urine in treatment of urinary tract infections due to gram-negative bacilli. *Lancet* 1:1267, 1971.
74. Steigbigel RT, Greenman RL, Remington JS: Antibiotic combinations in the treatment of experimental *Staphylococcus aureus* infection. *J Infect Dis* 131:245, 1975.
75. McGehee RF Jr, Smith CB, Wilcox C, et al: Comparative studies of antibacterial activity *in*

vitro and absorption and excretion of lincomycin and clindamycin. *Am J Med Sci* 256:279, 1968.
76. Sutter VL: *In vitro* susceptibility of anaerobes: Comparison of clindamycin and other antimicrobial agents. *J Infect Dis* 135(suppl):S7, 1977.
77. Bartlett JG: Anti-anaerobic antibacterial agents. *Lancet* ii:478, 1982.
78. McGehee RF, Barrett FF, Finland M: Resistance of *Staphylococcus aureus* to lincomycin, clindamycin and erythromycin. *Antimicrob Agents Chemother–1968:*392, 1969.
79. Nunnery AW, Riley HD: Clinical and laboratory studies of lincomycin in children. *Antimicrob Agents Chemother–1964:*142, 1965.
80. Barrett FF, McGehee RF Jr, Finland M: Methicillin-resistant *Staphylococcus aureus* at Boston City Hospital. *New Engl J Med* 279:441, 1968.
81. Desmyter J, Reybrouck G: Lincomycin sensitivity of erythromycin-resistant staphylococci. *Chemotherapia* 9:183, 1964.
82. Duncan IBR: Development of lincomycin resistance by staphylococci. *Antimicrob Agents Chemother*–1967:723, 1968.
83. Watanakunakorn C: Clindamycin therapy of *Staphylococcus aureus* endocarditis. Clinical relapse and development of resistance to clindamycin, lincomycin and erythromycin. *Am J Med* 60:419, 1976.
84. Sande MA, Johnson ML: Antimicrobial therapy of experimental endocarditis caused by *Staphylococcus aureus. J Infect Dis* 131:367, 1975.
85. Nastro LJ, Finegold SM: Bactericidal activity of five antimicrobial agents against *Bacteroides fragilis. J Infect Dis* 126:104, 1972.
86. Tally F, Snydman DR, Gorbach SL, et al: Plasmid mediated transferable resistance to clindamycin and erythromycin in *Bacteriodes fragilis. J Infect Dis* 139:83, 1979.
87. DeHaan RM, Metzler CM, Schellenberg D, et al: Pharmacokinetic studies of clindamycin phosphate. *J Clin Pharmacol* 13:190, 1973.
88. Fass RJ, Saslow S: Clindamycin: Clinical and laboratory evaluations of parenteral therapy. *Am J Med Sc* 263:369, 1972.
89. Panzer JD, Brown DC, Epstein WL, et al: Clindamycin levels in various body tissues and fluids. *J Clin Pharmacol* 12:259, 1972.
90. Nicholas P, Meyers BR, Levy RN: Concentration of clindamycin in human bone. *Antimicrob Agents Chemother* 8:220, 1975.
91. Prokesch RC, Hand WL: Antibiotic entry into human polymorphonuclear leukocytes. *Antimicrob Agents Chemother* 23:373, 1982.
92. Joiner KA, Lowe BR, Dzink JL, et al: Antibiotic levels in infected and sterile subcutaneous abscesses in mice. *J Infect Dis* 143:487, 1981.
93. McCall CE, Steigbigel NH, Finland M: Lincomycin: Activity *in vitro* and absorption and excretion in normal young men. *Am J Med Sci* 254:144, 1967.
94. Kager L, Liljeqvist L, Malmborg AS, et al: Effect of clindamycin prophylaxis on the colonic microflora in patients undergoing colorectal surgery. *Antimicrob Agents Chemother* 20:736, 1981.
95. Brown RB, Martyak SN, Barza M, et al: Penetration of clindamycin phosphate into the abnormal human biliary tract. *Ann Intern Med* 84:168, 1976.
96. Joshi A, Stein R: Altered serum clearance of intravenously administered clindamycin phosphate in patients with uremia. *J Clin Pharmacol* 14:140, 1974.
97. Williams DN, Crossley K, Hoffman C, et al: Parenteral clindamycin phosphate: pharmacology with normal and abnormal liver function and effect on nasal staphylococci. *Antimicrob Agents Chemother* 7:153, 1975.
98. Rifkin GD, Fekety FR, Silva J Jr, et al: Antibiotic-induced colitis: Implication of a toxin neutralized by *Clostridium sordellii* antitoxin. *Lancet* 11:1103, 1977.
99. Bartlett JG, Chang TW, Gurwith M, et al: Antibiotic-associated pseudomembranous colitis due to toxin-producing clostridia. *New Engl J Med* 298:531, 1978.
100. Bartlett JG: Antibiotic-associated pseudomembranous colitis *Rev Infect Dis* 1:530, 1979.
101. Tedesco FJ: Clindamycin and colitis: A review. *J Infect Dis* 135(suppl):S95, 1977.

102. George WL, Rolfe RD, Finegold SM: Treatment and prevention of antimicrobial agent-induced colitis and diarrhea. *Gastroenterology* 79:366, 1980.

103. Elmore M, Rissing JP, Rink L, et al: Clindamycin-associated hepatotoxicity. *Am J Med* 57:627, 1974.

104. Fogdall RP, Miller RD: Prolongation of a pancuronium-induced neuromuscular blockade by clindamycin. *Anesthesiology* 41:407, 1974.

105. Thadepalli H, Gorbach SL, Broido PW, et al: Abdominal trauma, anaerobes, and antibiotics. *Surg Gynecol Obstet* 137:270, 1973.

106. Weinstein WM, Onderdonk AB, Bartlett JG, et al: Antimicrobial therapy of experimental intra-abdominal sepsis. *J Infect Dis* 132:282, 1975.

107. diZerega G, Yonekura L, Roy S, et al: A comparison of clindamycin-gentamicin and penicillin-gentamicin in the treatment of post-cesarean section endometritis. *Am J Obstet Gynecol* 134:238, 1979.

108. Bartlett JG, Gorbach SL: Treatment of aspiration pneumonia and primary lung abscess: penicillin G vs clindamycin. *JAMA* 234:935, 1975.

109. Levison ME, Mangura CT, Lorber B, et al: Clindamycin compared with penicillin for the treatment of anaerobic lung abscess. *Ann Intern Med* 98:466, 1983.

110. Bartlett JG, Gorbach SL: Penicillin or clindamycin for primary lung abscess? An editorial. *Ann Intern Med* 98:546, 1983.

111. Mills Jr, OH, Kligman AM: Therapeutic options in the management of acne and its variants. *Semin Dermatol* 1:233, 1982.

11

VANCOMYCIN

ROBERT FEKETY

STRUCTURE

Vancomycin is a complex soluble glycopolypeptide that has a molecular weight of approximately 1450. While similar to teichomycin, it is unrelated to all other antibiotics. When first introduced, commercial preparations of vancomycin contained as much as 20 percent of another substance of unknown nature that probably contributed to its side effects (1). Current preparations are much purer and less toxic.

DERIVATION AND NOMENCLATURE

Vancomycin (Vancocin, Lilly) is a narrow spectrum bactericidal antibiotic obtained from *Streptomyces orientales.* Introduced in 1956 because of its effectiveness against penicillin-resistant staphylococci, it was relegated, because of its toxicity, to the role of alternate therapy when methicillin became available. With spread of methicillin-resistant staphylococci in the United States in recent years, vancomycin is now being used frequently, since it is the drug of choice for treating infections with such organisms. It is also the drug of choice for oral treatment of antibiotic-associated colitis caused by *Clostridium difficile.*

MECHANISM OF ACTION

Vancomycin inhibits synthesis and assembly of the second stage of cell wall peptidoglycan polymers and also injures protoplasts by altering the permeability of their cytoplasmic membrane (2). Rapidly and tightly bound to organisms, vancomycin exerts its bactericidal effect without a lag period, but only on multiplying organisms.

ANTIMICROBIAL ACTIVITY

Both *Staphylococcus aureus* and *Staphylococcus epidermidis* are susceptible to vancomycin. Increasing resistance of these organisms has not been observed. Concentrations of 1–5 μg/ml or less are almost invariably inhibitory, even with isolates resistant to methicillin, and most organisms are killed at about the same concentrations. A small proportion of strains require 10–20 μg/ml for inhibition, and about 20 percent of organisms are deficient in autolysins and relatively tolerant to the bactericidal action of vancomycin (3,4). *Streptococcus pyogenes,* group B streptococci, J.K. bacillus, and *Streptococcus pneumoniae* are highly susceptible. *Listeria monocytogenes* is often susceptible. Anaerobic or microaerophilic streptococci, clostridia, including *Clostridium perfringens* and *C. difficile, Bacillus anthracis,* actinomyces, lactobacilli, diphtheroids, *Clostridium diphtheriae,* and *Neisseria gonorrhoeae* are usually susceptible (5,6). Viridans streptococci *Streptococcus agalactiae, Streptococcus bovis,* and *Streptococcus faecalis* are usually inhibited at concentrations attainable in serum, but some isolates are not killed at these concentrations (4). *S. faecalis* isolates usually require concentrations greater than 100 μg/ml for killing. Forty to 70 percent of *S. faecalis* isolates show a synergistic bactericidal effect when vancomycin is combined with streptomycin, but the combination of vancomycin plus gentamicin is almost always bactericidal at attainable concentrations (7,8). There is no cross-resistance between vancomycin and other unrelated antibiotics, and significant resistance rarely develops during therapy. Antibacterial activity varies little between pH 6.5 and 8. *Flavobacterium meningosepticum* is susceptible at concentrations between 16 and 25 μg/ml, but other gram-negative bacilli, mycobacteria, fungi, and bacteroides are not susceptible.

PHARMACOLOGY

Administration

After being dissolved in sterile water, vancomycin should be given intravenously in 100–250 ml of 5% dextrose or 0.9% NaCl over 30–60 minutes (1). It can also be given by continuous intravenous drip, but intermittent infusion is preferred. Rapid or bolus administration is dangerous, and can cause flushing and anaphylactoid reactions. Hydrocortisone (20 mg) can be added to the infusion to reduce side effects, but this mixture may precipitate when mixed with high concentrations of vancomycin. Heparin and vancomycin also can precipitate at high concentrations, so they should not be infused simultaneously through the same intravenous line (9). Because of pain on injection, no satisfactory intramuscular preparation is available. Vancomycin is absorbed poorly from the gastrointestinal tract and is used orally only in the treatment of enterocolitis (1,10–12) and for prevention of infection in cancer patients (13).

Distribution, Excretion, and Protein Binding

Vancomycin is eliminated from the body almost exclusively by glomerular filtration. Eighty to 90 percent of an administered dose appears in the urine within 24 hours. A small amount may be eliminated via the liver and biliary tract. The half-life of vancomycin in serum is approximately 6 hours in people with normal renal function. In anuria, it may be prolonged to about 9 days, and the drug may be detected in serum for as long as 21 days after a single 1 g dose (14,15). From 10 to 55 percent is protein bound in serum.

Concentrations in Body Fluids and Tissues

Serum levels 1 to 2 hours after intravenous administration of a 500 mg dose to adults range from 6–10 μg/ml, with an average of 8 μg/ml after repeated dosing. Peak levels of up to 50 μg/ml may be seen. When 1 g is given slowly intravenously, peak and trough levels of 20–50 μg/ml and 5–10 μg/ml respectively can be achieved. Urinary concentrations range from 100–300 μg/ml. When vancomycin (0.5 g q 6 h) is given orally, levels of 1000–9000 μg/ml are found in the stool, but only trace amounts are usually found in serum (5,6,11). Higher and potentially toxic serum concentrations have been reported in an anuric patient given oral vancomycin for treatment of colitis (15a). When 125 mg is given, stool concentrations range from 100–800 μg/ml. When vancomycin is given intravenously, levels of up to 100 μg/ml may be found in stools, but the drug is undetectable in stools of many patients (6). Vancomycin is not found in normal cerebrospinal fluid (CSF), but bactericidal levels have been found in the CSF of some patients with meningitis (<1–7 g/ml). Small amounts (3–5 mg) may be given intrathecally in meningitis if there is no response after 48 hours of intravenous therapy (16). A larger intrathecal dose may be needed for less susceptible organisms, such as flavobacteria. Vancomycin is irritating when infected into serous or synovial cavities. Adequate concentrations are reached in pleural, pericardial, synovial, and ascitic fluids, but low levels are found in bile (5).

Since the kidney is the only significant organ of elimination of vancomycin, high and potentially toxic serum levels can be attained in patients with renal insufficiency unless dosage is reduced appropriately (14,15,17). A loading dose of 15 mg/kg can be given to all adults. To achieve a mean therapeutic concentration of 20 μg/ml in serum of adults with renal impairment, a simple formula can be used to estimate maintenance dosage: the daily parenteral dose of vancomycin in milligrams is 150 plus 15 times the creatinine clearance in ml/min (17). Another scheme is to give 1 g every 36 hours when the serum creatinine concentration is 1.5–5 mg/100 ml, and 1 g every 10 to 14 days when the creatinine level is greater than 5 mg/100 ml. As little as 1 g may yield effective serum concentrations for 7 to 14 days in anuric patients (15). A nomogram (Fig. 1) that may be useful for dosing patients with renal failure is designed to provide

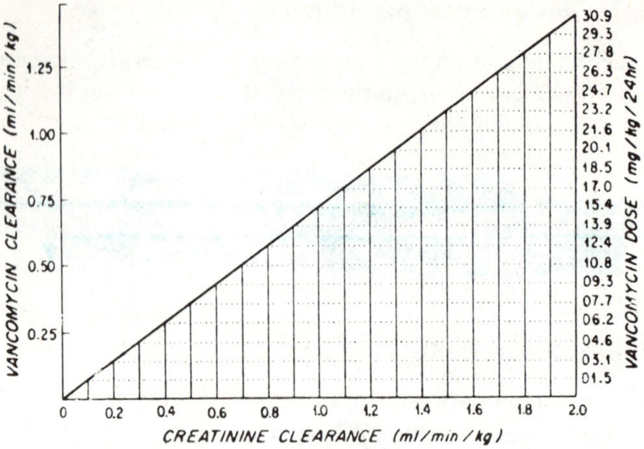

FIGURE 1. Dosage nomogram for vancomycin in patients with impaired renal function. The nomogram is not valid for functionally anephric patients on dialysis. For such patients, the dosage is 1.9 mg/kg · 24 hr. (From *Ann Intern Med* 94:343, 1981.)

a steady state concentration of 15 μg/ml (18). Hemodialysis does not remove significant amounts of vancomycin, but peritoneal dialysis may (14,15,19). It is best to monitor serum levels in dialyzed, uremic, or seriously ill patients to ascertain that safe yet adequate concentrations are present. Cardiopulmonary bypass is associated with a fall in serum levels because of dilution. A preoperative dose of 15 mg/kg is needed before bypass surgery and 10 mg/kg should be given postoperatively if renal function is normal.

TOXICITY AND ADVERSE REACTIONS

With the purified preparations now available, adverse reactions are less frequent than when vancomycin was first introduced. The most frequent side effects consist of fever, chills, and phlebitis at the site of the infusion. These are less frequent if the drug is infused slowly in a large volume of fluid. Tingling and flushing of the face, neck, and thorax (the "red-neck syndrome") are occasionally experienced if the drug is infused very rapidly (20). Shock has occurred after rapid intravenous infusion of the drug. Leukopenia or eosinophilia have been seen in a few patients. Rashes occur in 4 to 5 percent of patients, and may persist for weeks despite discontinuation of vancomycin in patients with marked renal failure.

The most important adverse reaction to vancomycin is neurotoxicity, which is manifested by auditory nerve damage and hearing loss. This is infrequent if serum concentrations are maintained below 30 μg/ml and is common with concentrations of 80 μg/ml or more. Tinnitus and high tone hearing loss are frequently an antecedent to deafness. Hearing occasionally improves when the drug is discontinued, but often continues to deteriorate (21,22). Nephrotoxicity was relatively common with early impure preparations of vancomycin, especially when given in high doses, and was usually transient or reversible. With appropriate doses (judged by quantitative susceptibility tests and by monitoring renal function and serum concentrations), nephrotoxicity is now uncommon (22–24). Though vancomycin is no longer appreciably nephrotoxic, high doses should be avoided by the parenteral route and serum levels should be carefully monitored when other nephrotoxic drugs are being given. When vancomycin and an aminoglycoside are both administered, a high instance of nephrotoxicity has been reported (24a).

Drug Interactions

Vancomycin is incompatible with many other drugs in intravenous solutions, especially chloramphenicol, adrenal corticosteroids, methicillin, and heparin (9).

MAJOR USES AND DOSES

The usual intravenous dose of vancomycin for adults with normal renal function is 1 g every 12 hours (15 mg/kg), or 500 mg (6.5–8 mg/kg) every 6 hours. In severely ill patients with normal renal function, such as those with meningitis, 1 g may be given every 8 hours for 2 or 3 days until the infection is under control. Morbidly obese patients may require high doses which should be based upon total body weight (25) and serum levels. Various dosage regimens have been proposed for pediatric usage. For newborn infants, 15 mg/kg doses should be given slowly intravenously every 12 hours during the first week of life, or every 8 hours in those 8 to 30 days of age; 10 mg/kg every 6 hours to older infants and children; and 15 mg/kg every 6 hours to infants and children with staphylococcal central nervous system infections. A continuous drip can be used (26,27). In infants and children with *C. difficile* colitis, an oral dose of 500 mg/1.73 m^2 every 6 hours has been recommended (28).

Dosage must be reduced in patients with renal impairment, and monitored to achieve peak serum concentrations no higher than 30–40 μg/ml, and troughs ranging from 5–10 μg/ml; if a continuous infusion is used, a steady state concentration of 15 μg/ml seems desirable (17,18,22,23,29). Recent evidence indicates that impaired liver function may also delay elimination of vancomycin and require dosage modification (30). It is most important that dosage be reduced and serum levels be monitored in patients with renal impairment (see above).

Vancomycin should be used only for serious infections. Intravenous vancomycin is the therapy of choice for serious staphylococcal infections in patients with methicillin-oxacillin-nafcillin- or cephalothin-resistant organisms, or in patients who cannot be given these primary drugs (5,23,31–35).

All strains of methicillin-resistant staphylococci have been susceptible to low concentrations of vancomycin, but some isolates show tolerance to its bactericidal action (4,31,34,36). When treatment of serious infections with vancomycin alone has failed, gentamicin, rifampin, or trimethoprim/sulfamethoxazole may be added. Since antagonism can occur with these combinations of antimicrobials (31), serum bacteriostatic and bactericidal levels should be monitored as a guide to therapy. When vancomycin is used for adults in conjunction with an aminoglycoside, its dosage should not exceed 0.5 g every 8 hours (23). Methicillin-resistant *S. epidermidis* endocarditis of prosthetic valves is best treated with vancomycin, usually in combination with rifampin and/or an aminoglycoside (35).

Vancomycin has a very rapid bactericidal effect, and were it not for its toxicity, it might be the preferred drug for treating serious staphylococcal infections. Survival rates of 60–75 percent have been achieved with vancomycin in patients with staphylococcal endocarditis or bacteremia (1,5). Survival in patients aged 70 or above is about 50 percent. The usual duration of therapy is 4 to 6 weeks. Success rates of 75 percent or greater have been reported in patients with pneumonia, parotitis, or meningitis.

While vancomycin penetrates into the central nervous system in most patients in amounts adequate to treat meningitis and shunt infections, this is not always the case (16), and removal of foreign bodies or supplemental intraventricular or intrathecal instillation of vancomycin may be required in patients with a poor prognosis and response (36,37).

Vancomycin is the treatment of choice in patients with *S. faecalis* (enterococcal) endocarditis who are allergic to penicillin. In this case, it is best given along with an aminoglycoside, since vancomycin alone is not dependably bactericidal against these streptococci (7,8,38,39). Since bactericidal synergism between gentamicin and vancomycin has been demonstrated with essentially all enterococci, gentamicin may be preferable to streptomycin, which is not synergistic with as many as 40 percent of these organisms. Laboratory studies of synergism with the patient's organism or Schlichter tests on their serum may be helpful in determining the best regimen. A vancomycin dose of 0.5 g every 8 hours IV plus streptomycin (0.5 g every 12 hours IM) or gentamicin (60–80 mg every 8 hours IV) for 4 to 6 weeks is recommended for adults with normal renal function. Patients should be monitored closely for signs of ototoxicity or nephrotoxicity, and drug dosages should be carefully adjusted in renal failure. Viridans streptococcal or *S. bovis* endocarditis may be treated with vancomycin alone if the minimum bactericidal concentration for the isolate is no more than 10 μg/ml; otherwise it should be combined with streptomycin or another aminoglycoside (5,23).

Other serious infections with resistant organisms that have been responsive to vancomycin include *Corynebacterium* endocarditis in patients with prosthetic valves, and *Flavobacterium meningosepticum* meningitis (5,16,37).

Vancomycin has been considered the drug of choice for treating acute staphylococcal pseudomembranous enterocolitis, which is now a rare disease. In two series of cases, 67 of 72 patients were cured (93 percent) (10,40). It is usually given orally, 500 mg diluted in water every 6 hours.

Orally administered vancomycin is the drug of choice for treating seriously ill patients with antibiotic-associated *C. difficile* (pseudomembranous) colitis. This organism is always susceptible (11, 12,41,42). A dose of 125–500 mg four times daily has been effective. Vancomycin is useful in treating relapses (42). Intravenous vancomycin is not as reliable. When nasogastric tubes are needed for administering the drug, they can be clamped for 1 hour after giving vancomycin.

Staphylococcal peritonitis occurring during peritoneal dialysis can be treated with parenteral vancomycin alone. One gram given intravenously will yield peritoneal fluid concentrations greater than 5 μg/ml for a week or more (19). Others have noted peritoneal dialysis may remove vancomycin from blood, and have recommended instilling vancomycin into the peritoneal cavity at a concentration of 25 μg/ml, in addition to parenteral vancomycin, to insure good levels in peritoneal fluid (43). In fact, it may be possible to treat staphylococcal peritonitis in chronic peritoneal dialysis patients solely by the intraperitoneal administration of vancomycin at a concentration of 50 μg/ml in the dialysate (43).

According to an American Heart Association Advisory Committee, vancomycin is useful in the prevention of bacterial endocarditis in patients who are allergic to penicillin and undergoing certain dental or surgical procedures. The mechanism of prevention may be either by the bactericidal action of vancomycin, or by its interference with the ability of the organism to adhere to the endocardium. One gram is given intravenously over the 30 to 60 minutes before the procedure, in combination with erythromycin (dental or upper respiratory surgery) or streptomycin (genitourinary or gastrointestinal surgery or instrumentation) (44). Vancomycin can be used safely IV at a dose of 15 mg/ml given over 1 hour starting just before surgery for prophylaxis in patients undergoing open heart surgery (45).

Vancomycin has been useful in prophylactic oral nonabsorbable antibiotic regimens designed to prevent endogenous infections in patients with cancer or leukemia (13). These regimens are probably of no value unless protective environments and leukocyte transfusions are available and used.

It is obvious that there has been a resurgence of vancomycin use. Many new indications for its use have been established, and much new information about it has accumulated. An excellent review of newer knowledge about vancomycin has been published (46).

REFERENCES

1. Alexander MR: Review of vancomycin after 15 years of use. *Drug Intell Clin Pharm* 8:520, 1974.
2. Perkins HR, Nieto M: The chemical basis for the action of the vancomycin group of antibiotics. *Ann NY Acad Sci* 235:348, 1974.

3. Gopal V, Bisno AL, Silverblatt FJ: Failure of vancomycin treatment in *Staphylococcus aureus* endocarditis. In vivo and in vitro observations. *JAMA* 236:1604, 1976.
4. Sabath L, Wheeler N, Laverdiere M, et al: A new type of penicillin resistance of *Staphylococcus aureus. Lancet* 1:443, 1977.
5. Geraci JE: Vancomycin. *Mayo Clin Proc* 52:631, 1977.
6. Geraci JE, Heilman FR, Nichols DR, et al: Some laboratory and clinical experiences with a new antibiotic, vancomycin. *Proc Staff Meet Mayo Clin* 31:564, 1956.
7. Watanakunakorn C, Bakie C: Synergism of vancomycin-gentamicin and vancomycin-streptomycin against enterococci. *Antimicrob Agents Chemother* 4:120, 1973.
8. Harwick HJ, Kalmanson GM, Guze LB: In vitro activity of ampicillin or vancomycin combined with gentamicin or streptomycin against enterococci. *Antimicrob Agents Chemother* 4:383, 1973.
9. Barg N, Fekety R, Supena R: Unpublished observations.
10. Khan MY, Hall WH: Staphylococcal enterocolitis treatment with oral vancomycin. *Ann Intern Med* 65:1, 1966.
11. Tedesco F, Markham R, Gurwith M, et al: Oral vancomycin for antibiotic-associated pseudomembranous colitis. *Lancet* 2:226–228, 1978.
12. Silva J, Batts DH, Fekety R, et al: Treatment of *Clostridium difficile* colitis and diarrhea with vancomycin. *Am J Med* 71:815–222, 1981.
13. Bodey G: Oral antibiotic prophylaxis in protected environment units: effect of nonabsorbable and absorbable antibiotics on the fecal flora. *Antimicrob Agents Chemother* 1:343, 1972.
14. Lindholm DD, Murray JS: Persistence of vancomycin in the blood during renal failure and its treatment by hemodialysis. *N Engl J Med* 274:1047, 1966.
15. Eykyn S, Phillip I, Evans J: Vancomycin for staphylococcal shunt infections in patients on regular hemodialysis. Br Med J 3:80, 1970.
15a. Spitzer PG, Eliopoulos GM: Systemic absorption of enteral vancomycin in a patient with pseudomembranous colitis. *Ann Intern Med* 100:533–534, 1984.
16. Hawley HB, Gump DW: Vancomycin therapy of bacterial meningitis. *Am J Dis Child* 126:261, 1973.
17. Nielsen HE, Hansen HE, Korsager B, et al: Renal excretion of vancomycin in kidney disease. *Acta Med Scand* 197:261, 1975.
18. Moellering RC, Krogstad DJ, Greenblatt DJ: Vancomycin therapy in patients with impaired renal function. A nomogram for dosage. *Ann Intern Med* 94:343–346, 1981.
19. Ayus JC, Enkas JF, Tong TG, et al: Peritoneal clearance and total body elimination of vancomycin during chronic intermittent peritoneal dialysis. *Clin Nephrol* 11:129–132, 1979.
20. Newfield P, Roizen MF: Hazards of rapid administration of vancomycin. *Ann Intern Med* 91:581, 1979.
21. Traber PG, Levine DP: Vancomycin ototoxicity in a patient with normal renal function. *Ann Intern Med* 95:458–460, 1981.
22. McHenry MC, Gavan TL: Vancomycin. *Pediatr Clin North Am* 30:31–47, 1983.
23. Geraci JE, Hermans PE: Vancomycin. *Mayo Clin Proc* 58:88–91, 1983.
24. Appel GB, Neu HC: The nephrotoxicity of antimicrobial agents. *N Engl J Med* 296:722, 1977.
24a. Farber BF, Moellering RC: Retrospective study of the toxicity of preparations of vancomycin for 1974 to 1981. *Antimicrob Agents Chemother* 23:138–141, 1983.
25. Blovin RA, Bauer LA, Miller DD, Record KL, Griffin WO: Vancomycin pharmacokinetics in normal and morbidly obese subjects. *Antimicrob Agents Chemother* 21:575–580, 1982.
26. Riley HD: Vancomycin and novobiocin. *Med Clin North Am* 54:1277, 1970.
27. Schaad VB, McCracken GH, Nelson JD: Clinical pharmacology and efficacy of vancomycin in pediatric patients. *J Pediatr* 96:119–126, 1980.
28. Batts DH, Martin D, Holmes R, et al: Treatment of antibiotic-associated *Clostridium difficile* diarrhea with oral vancomycin. *J Pediatr* 97:151–153, 1980.
29. Rotschafer JC, Crossley K, Zaski DE, et al: Pharmacokinetics of vancomycin. Observations in 28 patients and dosage recommendations. *Antimicrob Agents Chemother* 22:391–394, 1982.
30. Brown N, Ho DHW, Fong KL, et al: Effects of hepatic function on vancomycin clinical pharmacology. *Antimicrob Agents Chemother* 23:603–609, 1983.

31. Watanakunakorn C: Treatment of infections due to methicillin-resistant *Staphylococcus aureus. Ann Intern Med* 97:376–378, 1982.
32. Myers JP, Linnemann CC: Bacteremia due to methicillin-resistant *Staphylococcus aureus. J Infect Dis* 4:532–536, 1982.
33. Sorrell TC, Packham DR, Shanker S, et al: Vancomycin therapy for methicillin-resistant *Staphylococcus aureus. Ann Intern Med* 97:344–350, 1982.
34. Levine DP, Cushing R, Jim J, et al: Community-acquired methicillin-resistant *Staphylococcus aureus* endocarditis in the Detroit Medical Center. *Ann Intern Med* 97:330–338, 1982.
35. Karchmer AW, Archer GL, Dismukes WE: *Staphylococcus epidermidis* causing prosthetic-valve endocarditis: microbiologic and clinical observations as guides to therapy. *Ann Intern Med* 98:447–455, 1983.
36. Sutherland GE, Palitang EG, Marr JJ, et al: Sterilization of Ommaya reservoir by instillation of vancomycin. *Am J Med* 71:1068–1070, 1981.
37. Gump DW: Vancomycin for treatment of bacterial meningitis. *Rev Infect Dis* 3:S289–S292, 1981.
38. Westenfelder GO, Paterson PY, Reisberg BE, et al: Vancomycin-streptomycin synergism in enterococcal endocarditis. *JAMA* 223:37, 1973.
39. Harwick HJ, Kalmanson GM, Guze LB: Pyelonephritis. XVII. Comparison of combinations of vancomycin, ampicillin, streptomycin, and gentamicin in the treatment of enterococcal infection in the rat. *J Infect Dis* 129:358, 1974.
40. Esposito AL, Gleckman RA: Vancomycin, a second look. *JAMA* 238:1756, 1977.
41. Fekety R, Silva J, Armstrong J, et al: Treatment of antibiotic-associated enterocolitis with vancomycin. *Rev Infect Dis* 3:S273–S281, 1981.
42. Tedesco FJ: Treatment of recurrent antibiotic-associated pseudomembranous colitis. *Am J Gastroenterol* 77:220–221, 1982.
43. Nielsen HE, Sorensen I, Hansen HE: Peritoneal transport of vancomycin during peritoneal dialysis. *Nephron* 24:274–277, 1979.
44. Kaplan EL, Anthony BF, Bisno A, et al: Prevention of bacterial endocarditis. *Circulation* 56:139A–143A, 1977.
45. Austin TW, Leake J, Coles JC, et al: Vancomycin blood levels during cardiac surgery. *Can Card J Surg* 24:423–425, 1981.
46. Wise RI, Kory M (ed): Reassessments of vancomycin—a potentially useful antibiotic. *Rev Infect Dis* 3:S199–S300, 1981.

12

POLYMYXINS

ROBERT FEKETY

STRUCTURE

Polymyxin A, B, C, D, and E are related cyclic basic polypeptides characterized by poor diffusibility, a molecular weight of about 1100, a limited antimicrobial spectrum, and significant toxicity. All but polymyxin B and E are too toxic for therapeutic use in man (1). Colistin is identical to polymyxin E, and differs from polymyxin B in only 1 of its 10 amino acids (2).

DERIVATION AND NOMENCLATURE

Polymyxins are derived from *Bacillus polymyxa.* Polymyxin B sulfate was introduced for clinical use in 1947. As marketed, it is only 65 to 75 percent pure; 1 unit of polymyxin B sulfate is equivalent to 0.1 μg of pure polymyxin base. Colistin (polymyxin E, Coly-Mycin) was introduced clinically in 1961 as the methanesulfonate (colistimethate) derivative, which is less painful than polymyxin B sulfate on intramuscular injection (3). Methanesulfonation of the free amino groups of polymyxins has a definitely negative effect on their antibacterial action, and colistimethate is essentially inactive until hydrolyzed within the body to the colistin base (4). Thus, colistimethate may be thought of as a repository form of intramuscular polymyxin.

MECHANISM OF ACTION

The polymyxins act like cationic detergents or surfactants. They disrupt the osmotic integrity of the cell's membrane by interacting with its phospholipids and increasing cell permeability. This damage allows important intracellular constituents such as nucleic acids and proteins to leak out, with subsequent breakdown and death of the cell. It may also interfere with some of the actions of endotoxin. The polymyxins are bactericidal and kill resting cells without necessarily lysing them. Susceptibility may be related to the phospholipid content of the cell wall-membrane complex (3). Resistant organisms have cell walls that prevent access of the drug to the membrane. Calcium reduces the antibacterial action of polymyxins by interfering with their attachment to the membrane.

ANTIMICROBIAL ACTIVITY

Polymyxin B and colistin (polymyxin E) have identical antibacterial spectra and show complete cross resistance (1,3,5). On a weight basis, polymyxin B sulfate is slightly more antibacterially active and toxic than colistin sulfate and much more so than colistin methanesulfonate (6). The polymyxins are active against gram-negative bacilli almost exclusively. Their primary clinical usefulness is for *Pseudomonas aeruginosa* isolates, which are almost always inhibited by concentrations lower than 8 μg/ml. *E. coli, Klebsiella pneumoniae, Enterobacter, Salmonella, Shigella, Vibrios, Hemophilus, Pasteurella,* and *Bordetella* isolates are usually susceptible. *Proteus, Providencia, Serratia,* and *Neisseria* isolates are usually resistant, as are gram-positive organisms and obligate anaerobes (1,5). There is no cross resistance with other antibiotics, and resistance rarely develops during therapy. Polymyxins have slight activity against various fungi, but this has had no clinical significance. Rifampin and polymyxin B may be synergistic against multiply-resistant *Serratia* isolates. Synergism against *Pseudomonas* has been demonstrated in vitro between polymyxins and tetracycline, chloramphenicol, and carbenicillin, and trimethoprim/sulfamethoxazole, but the clinical significance of this enhancement is not known (1,3,6).

PHARMACOLOGY

Administration and Absorption

The polymyxins are not absorbed when given orally. Polymyxin B sulfate is the only derivative of polymyxin B available for treatment. It can be given intravenously, intramuscularly, intrathecally, orally, topically, endobronchially, or by aerosol. Polymyxins are quite painful when given intramuscularly, and the pain may persist for several hours. However, when the drugs are given intravenously, local effects are minimal. Colistin is available as the sulfate for oral use and as the sodium salt of the colistimethate derivative for parenteral use. Colistimethate can be given by slow intravenous infusion, but this may result in inadequate serum and tissue antibacterial activity if colistimethate is eliminated from the body by the kidneys before hydrolysis to the active base can take place (4).*

* Bioassay of colistimethate in serum following intravenous or intramuscular administration encounters a related problem in that unhydrolyzed drug may become hydrolyzed and therefore may become more active during the assay.

When a total daily dose of parenteral polymyxin B of 2.5 mg (25,000 units)/kg is infused in 300–500 ml of D5W, peak serum concentrations of approximately 5 μg/ml are obtained. Ninety-five percent of *P. aeruginosa* isolates are susceptible at this concentration. These organisms are also susceptible at the serum levels of 5–8 μg/ml achieved with intramuscular colistin (2.5–5.0 mg/kg/day). By virtue of renal excretion, urinary concentrations of 10–160 μg/ml are achieved with colistimethate. The half-life in serum of colistin is 2 to 4.5 hours, and of polymyxin B, 6 to 7 hours. With intramuscular injection, there may be a delay of several hours before effective urinary levels are achieved with both drugs, but colistimethate being less bound to kidney tissues is excreted more rapidly than polymyxin B (4). These drugs may be found in the urine for 2 to 3 days after they have been discontinued. Polymyxins do not pass into the cerebrospinal fluid well, even in the presence of inflammation, and in the treatment of meningitis they must be given intrathecally (3). Neither do they pass readily into pleural, synovial, or brain tissues. Furthermore, they may combine with tissue cell membranes and exudate constituents (such as polyphosphates), which may explain why they seem to be relatively ineffective in infections of pleura, synovium, or brain (3). Polymyxins do cross the placental barrier, and concentrations of 1 μg/ml may be found in the fetus.

The excretion of the polymyxins is mostly via the kidneys. They are excreted primarily by glomerular filtration; there is no tubular secretion or reabsorption. Renal insufficiency results in decreased renal excretion of polymyxins, increased serum levels, and a greater likelihood of toxicity. The half-life in serum of polymyxin B or E in anuric patients is 48 to 72 hours. Doses must be reduced appropriately and renal function monitored carefully to avoid toxicity (Table 1). Urinary concentrations are reduced in the presence of renal failure (5). Hemodialysis has no appreciable effect on serum concentrations, but peritoneal dialysis removes small amounts (1 mg/hr) and may be useful in overdosage (7).

While orally administered polymyxins are poorly absorbed from the intact gastrointestinal tract of adults, they may be absorbed from the gastrointestinal tract of premature or newborn infants, and their oral use is thus hazardous and contraindicated in this group (5). After being given orally, polymyxins are not found in the tissues of the bowel wall in significant amounts, which may be responsible for their ineffectiveness in treatment of shigellosis.

Polymyxin is often used topically, usually in concentrations of 0.1% polymyxin (1 mg/ml or g), in combination with other antibiotics such as bacitracin or neomycin for the treatment of skin, mucous membrane, eye, and ear infections. Polymyxins are poorly absorbed from these surfaces. Polymyxin B is sometimes used for irrigation of various sites of infection. This can be dangerous, since polymyxin B is absorbed well from serous cavities such as the peritoneum, and the resultant high serum concentrations may result in the induction of apnea.

The protein binding of polymyxins has not been studied extensively, but may be as high as 75 percent. These drugs lose much of their activity in the presence of serum (1).

TABLE 1. Reduction in Polymyxin Dosage to Avoid Drug-Induced Renal Injury

	Parenteral Dose (mg/kg Body Weight)			
	When Creatinine Clearance Is			
	Normal, or ≥ 80% of Normal	*80%–≥30% of Normal*	*<30% of Normal*	*With Anuria*
Polymyxin B, sulfate	2.5–3.0 mg/day	1st day: 2.5 mg Daily thereafter: 1.0–1.5 mg	1st day: 2.5 mg Every 2–3 days thereafter: 1.0–1.5 mg	1st day: 2.5 mg Every 5–7 days thereafter: 1.0 mg
Colistimethate (polymyxin E)	3.0–5.0 mg/day	1st day: 3.0 mg Daily thereafter: 1.5–2.5 mg	1st day: 3.0 mg Every 2–3 days thereafter: 1.5–2.5 mg	1st day: 2.5 mg Every 5–7 days thereafter: 1.5 mg

TOXICITY AND ADVERSE REACTIONS

The two most important side effects of polymyxins are neurotoxicity and nephrotoxicity. Allergic reactions (including fever and skin rashes) are rare after polymyxin administration, but they are histamine-releasers, and some patients have developed urticaria or shock after rapid intravenous infusion. Pain at the site of injection is common. This can be reduced by mixing with a local anesthetic. For example, 50 mg polymyxin B may be mixed with 2 ml of 2% procaine in saline; colistimethate formerly was supplied mixed with dibucaine. When a serum concentration of 1–2 μg/ml or more of polymyxins is achieved, most patients will experience circumoral or stocking-glove paresthesias, sometimes with flushing, dizziness, vertigo, ataxia, slurred speech, drowsiness, or confusion. These are less frequent with lower doses and in children and when injections are given no more frequently than every 8 hours. These neurotoxic side effects disappear soon after the drugs have been discontinued. Polymyxins also have a curarelike action on striated muscles and block neuromuscular transmission. High serum concentrations may result in apnea, which can be treated with intravenous calcium chloride.

Dose-related nephrotoxicity is the most important side effect of polymyxins. In general, the more antibacterially active derivative, polymyxin B, is more toxic than colistin. At therapeutically equivalent doses, they are frequently and equally nephrotoxic (3,6), and renal function should be carefully monitored during therapy. Renal toxicity probably follows attachment of the antibiotics to the membrane of the renal convoluted tubular epithelium. This may be accentuated or potentiated by cephaloridine, aminoglycosides, or other nephrotoxic drugs which should therefore be avoided. At appropriate therapeutic dosages, approximately 20 percent of the patients experience nephrotoxity manifested by a rising serum creatinine level and an abnormal urinary sediment, and 1 to 2 percent develop acute tubular necrosis. Nitrogen retention, probably related to a reduction in glomerular filtration rate, frequently increases for a week or so after these drugs have been discontinued but is usually reversible (8). Anuria and tubular necrosis with serious renal failure are particularly common in patients who have received excessive doses or in whom the drug is continued in usual doses in the face of impaired renal function. In renal failure, polymyxins should be used only with great care and in reduced doses (Table 1) (3,5,8,9). Patients receiving no more than 2.2 mg/kg daily usually tolerate polymyxin B well even for long periods.

Little diarrhea or disturbance of the gastrointestinal flora results when these drugs are used. Dyspnea may occur after use of polymyxin by aerosol, and respiratory arrest has been reported.

MAJOR USES AND DOSES

The polymyxins are used parenterally infrequently and almost exclusively for serious, life-threatening *Pseudomonas* or gram-negative bacillary infections caused by organisms resistant to other drugs, or in patients with these infections who are intolerant or allergic to the preferred drugs. The usual dose of polymyxin B for adults with normal renal function is 1.5–2.5 mg (15,000–25,000 units)/kg/day given by continuous intravenous infusion. The intramuscular dosage is 2.5–3.0 mg/kg/day, given at 4- or 6-hour intervals. Septic infants may receive up to 40,000–45,000 units/kg/day. Adults with normal renal function may be given 2.5–5.0 mg/kg colistimethate/day in two or three divided doses (IV or IM). Polymyxin B is preferred to colistimethate for intravenous use, for it does not require hydrolysis for activation (5).

Polymyxins are second-line or alternate drugs, since they are relatively ineffective in patients with bacteremia and involvement of deep tissues, and they are especially ineffective in compromised hosts with granulocytopenia (10). Endocarditis usually cannot be cured with the polymyxins without the aid of surgery or other drugs. When bacteremia is associated with a removable or treatable focus, these drugs may be useful. Best results have been obtained with urinary tract infections or septicemias arising from the urinary tract (3,7).

Patients with meningitis requiring polymyxins should be treated intrathecally. The usual intrathecal dose of polymyxin B is 5–10 mg/day in adults; in children less than 2 years of age, a dose of 2 mg/day is used. Amounts greater than 10 mg (100,000 units) should never be used intrathecally. Nothing is gained by adding intravenous therapy when patients are treated intrathecally. Daily intrathecal therapy should be given for 3 to 5 days and then every other day for 3 weeks or for 2 weeks after cultures are negative and the CSF glucose level is normal.

Urinary tract infections can be treated with relatively low and well tolerated doses of intramuscular colistimethate (2.5 mg/kg/day in divided dosage for 7 to 10 days). Results are better with acute than with chronic urinary infections, in which relapses are frequent within a few months.

Prevention of urinary tract infections in patients requiring indwelling (Foley) catheters for periods up to 2 weeks may be achieved by using triple-lumen catheters and continuous irrigation of the bladder with a solution of neomycin (40 mg/liter) and polymyxin B (20 mg/liter). Usually, no more than 1 liter of irrigant is used per day unless urine flow rates are very high (11).

Aerosolized polymyxins have been used in the treatment of respiratory infections due to *Pseudomonas* in patients with cystic fibrosis or bronchiectasis and in the prevention of *Pseudomonas* infections in respiratory intensive care units during periods of high risk (12). Usually, the solution contains 2–10 mg/ml, and 2 ml is aerosolized six to eight times per day. Ultimately, the development of resistant organisms has limited the efficacy of this measure; to delay this, intermittent use of the regimens has been tried.

In creams, sprays, and solutions containing 0.5–3 mg/ml, polymyxins are useful in prevention and treatment of skin infections and in the treatment of external otitis or corneal ulcers. When given topically, it is often combined with neomycin and bacitracin. Subconjunctival injection of up to 100,000 units polymyxin B/day may be used in treatment of *Pseudomonas* infections of the cornea and conjunctivae. A total dose of 200 mg/day should not be exceeded.

Polymyxins may be useful when given orally to small children with localized gastroenteritis due to enteropathogenic *E. coli* but are relatively useless in patients with *Salmonella* or invasive *Shigella* enteritis. An oral dose of colistin sulfate of 15–20 mg/kg/day in three divided doses for 5 to 20 days has been used with *E. coli* outbreaks, but 3–5 mg/kg/day is the usual oral dose. These drugs should not be used orally in neonates and premature infants.

When polymyxins are combined with sulfamethoxazole and trimethoprim, they are often synergistic and can be useful in the treatment of serious infections with multiply drug-resistant *Serratia* and *Pseudomonas cepacia, P. maltophilia,* or *P. aeruginosa* isolates (13–15). A combination of polymyxin B and rifampin has also been used successfully in seriously ill patients with drug-resistant nosocomial *Serratia* infections (16).

REFERENCES

1. Jawetz E: Polymyxin, colistin and bacitracin. *Pediatr Clin North Am* 8:1057, 1961.
2. Wilkinson S: Identity of colistin and polymyxin E. *Lancet* 1:922, 1963.
3. Goodwin NJ: Colistin and sodium colistimethate. *Med Clin North Am* 54:1267, 1970.
4. Barnett M, Bushby SRM, Wilkinson S: Sodium sulphomethyl derivatives of polymyxins. *Bri J Pharmacol* 23:552, 1964.
5. Hoeprich PD: The polymyxins. *Med Clin North Am* 54:1257, 1970.
6. Nord NM, Hoeprich PD: Polymyxin B and colistin. A critical comparison. *N Engl J Med* 270:1030, 1964.
7. Goodwin N, Friedman E: The effects of renal impairment, peritoneal dialysis, and hemodialysis on serum sodium colistimethate levels. *Ann Intern Med* 68:984, 1968.
8. Fekety FR, Norman PS, Cluff LE: The treatment of gram-negative bacillary infections. The toxicity and efficacy of large doses in forty-eight patients. *Ann Intern Med* 57:214, 1962.
9. Appel GB, Neu HC: The neprotoxicity of antimicrobial agents. *N Engl J Med* 296:663, 1977.
10. Whitecar JP, Luna M, Bodey GP: Pseudomonas bacteremia in patients with malignant diseases. *Am J Med Sci* 260:216, 1970.
11. Marten CM, Bookrajian EN: Bacteriuria prevention after indwelling urinary catheterization. *Arch Int Med* 110:703, 1962.
12. Feeley TW, duMoulin GC, Hedley-Whyte J, et al: Aerosol polymyxin and pneumonia in seriously ill patients. *N Engl J Med* 293:471, 1975.
13. Thomas FE, Leonard JM, Alford RH: Sulfamethoxazole-trimethoprim polymyxin therapy of serious multiply drug-resistant *Serratia* infections. *Antimicrob Agents Chemother* 9:201, 1976.
14. Rosenblatt JE, Stewart PR: Combined activity of sulfamethoxazole, trimethoprim, and polymyxin B against gram-negative bacilli. *Antimicrob Agents Chemother* 6:84, 1974.
15. Nord C, Wadstrom T, Wretlind B: Synergistic effects of combinations of sulfamethoxazole, trimethoprim and colistin against *Pseudomonas maltophilia* and *P. cepacia. Antimicrob Agents Chemother* 6:521, 1974.
16. Ostenson RC, Fields BT, Nolan CM: Polymyxin B and rifampin: new regimen for multiresistant *Serratia marcescens* infections. *Antimicrob Agents Chemother* 12:655, 1977.

13

SULFONAMIDES AND TRIMETHOPRIM

STEPHEN H. ZINNER
KENNETH H. MAYER

The modern era of antimicrobial chemotherapy began in 1932 with the first reports by Gerhard Domagk of the protective activity of prontosil against murine streptococcal infections. This drug was an outgrowth of the German dye industry and had been available in this industry since the early twentieth century. Prontosil (sulfachrysoidine) exerted its antibacterial activity due to the release in vivo of para-aminobenzenesulfonamide or sulfanilamide. This agent was the first antibacterial used in the United States in an unsuccessful attempt, in July 1935, to treat a 10-year-old girl late in the course of meningitis and sepsis due to *Hemophilus influenzae* (1). During the late 1930s, the basic sulfanilamide compound was modified to remove unpleasant side effects while expanding its spectrum of activity. More recent modifications have resulted in compounds of specific usefulness, for example, in urinary infections (those compounds that are highly soluble), or those nonabsorbable sulfonamides that act only within the gastrointestinal tract.

Trimethoprim is a 2,4-diamino-pyrimidine and, as such, inhibits the enzyme dihydrofolate reductase resulting in interference in folic acid and subsequent pyrimidine synthesis in the bacterial cell. Trimethoprim is one of several such compounds synthesized and studied by Hitchings and coworkers in the 1950s and 1960s. The use of trimethoprim as a potentiator of sulfonamide activity was introduced by Bushby and Hitchings in 1968 (2). In the subsequent decade the combination of trimethoprim-sulfamethoxazole has been introduced clinically and has found a place in the chemotherapy of many infectious diseases. These agents, available in a fixed drug combination, show true antibacterial synergism against a wide variety of organisms.

SULFONAMIDES

Structure

The clinically useful sulfonamides are derived from sulfanilamide (para-aminobenzenesulfonamide) that is similar in structure to para-aminobenzoic acid (PABA), a factor required by bacteria for folic acid synthesis (Fig. 1).

A free amino group at the 4 position is associated with enhanced activity. Increased activity due to increased PABA inhibition is associated with substitutions at the sulfonyl radical (SO_2)—attached to the 1 carbon as seen with sulfadiazine, sulfisoxazole, and sulfamethoxazole, all of which are more active than the parent compound, sulfanilamide. The nature of these substitutions determines other pharmacologic properties of the drug such as absorption, solubility, and gastrointestinal tolerance. Substitutions at the 4-amino group result in decreased absorption from the gastrointestinal tract (e.g., phthalylsulfathiazole).

Derivation and Nomenclature

Since the introduction of sulfonamides into clinical medicine, dozens of compounds have been used. However, relatively few survive today, and they can be classified as (*1*) short- or medium-acting sulfonamides, (*2*) long-acting sulfonamides, (*3*) sulfonamides limited to the gastrointestinal tract, and (*4*) topical sulfonamides.

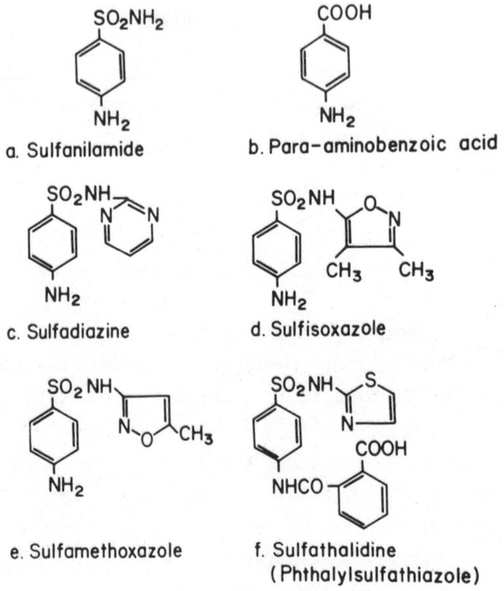

FIGURE 1. Structural formulas of selected sulfonamides.

Short- or Medium-Acting Sulfonamides. Sulfisoxazole *United States Pharmacopeia* (USP) (sulphafurazole *British Pharmacopeia*—BP, 3,4-dimethyl-5-sulfanilamidoisoxazole, Gantrisin, SK-Soxazole) is a highly soluble drug especially useful in urinary tract infections. Sulfamethoxazole USP (5-methyl-3-sulfanilamido-isoxazole; Gantanol) is somewhat less soluble than sulfisoxazole and yields higher blood levels. It is the sulfonamide presently most frequently combined with trimethoprim. Sulfadiazine USP (2-sulfanilamidopyridine) is highly active and attains high blood and cerebrospinal fluid levels and is associated with low protein binding and lower solubility than the above drugs. Sulfamethizole USP (2-sulfanilamide-5-methyl-1:3:4-thiazole; Microsul, Thiosulfil) is used for urinary tract infections. Sulfadimidine and sulfacarbamide are available in the United Kingdom.

Short-acting sulfonamides are also available in several combinations. Sulfisoxazole, sulfamethoxazole, and sulfamethizole are each combined with phenazopyridine, a urinary analgesic, as Azo Gantrisin, Azo Gantanol, Microsul-A, Sul-Azo, and Thiosulfil-A Forte. Phenazopyridine is also present with sulfamethazole and sulfadiazine in Suladyne. Sulfamethizole is also combined with tetracycline and phenazopyridine in Urobiotic and Azotrex, but these two preparations have been classified by the Food and Drug Administration (FDA) as lacking evidence of effectiveness as a fixed drug combination.

Long-Acting Sulfonamides. Sulfamethoxypyridazine (3-sulfanilamido-6-methoxy-pyridazine) and sulfameter [4-amino-*N*-(5-methoxy-2-pyrimidinyl)] benzene-sulfonamide are no longer available for single daily dose therapy, as they were associated with hypersensitivity reactions such as Stevens-Johnson syndrome. Neither sulfadimethoxine (Madribon) nor any other long-acting sulfonamides other than sulfadoxine are currently available in the United States.

Sulfadoxine, originally known as sulformethoxine [*N*'-(5,6-dimethoxy-4-pyrimidyl) sulfanilamide] is a very long-acting sulfonamide that, combined with pyrimethamine, is available as Fansidar. Sulfadoxine has a half-life of 100–230 hours and reaches a peak serum level of 51–76 μg/ml 2.5–6 hours after an oral dose of 500 mg. Fansidar is active in the treatment and prophylaxis of malaria due to chloroquine resistant *Plasmodium falciparum* (3). Due to the unknown teratogenic potential of pyrimethamine, Fansidar should not be recommended for prophylaxis of pregnant women, and its use has been associated with Stevens-Johnson syndrome. Also, some strains of *P. falciparum* from Southeast Asia and South America may be resistant.

Sulfonamides Limited to the Gastrointestinal Tract. Sulfaguanidine (*N*'amidinosulfanilamide), sulfasuxidine (2-(para-succinylsulfanilamido)-thiazole, succinylsulfathiazole), and sulfathalidine [2(para-phthalyl-sulfanilamido)-thiazole] are relatively poorly absorbed from the gastrointestinal tract. They have been used to suppress the susceptible bowel flora before surgery.

Salicylazosulfapyridine (sulfasalazine, Azulfidine) is a sulfonamide derivative used in the treatment of ulcerative colitis. This drug is absorbed in its parent form as sulfapyridine, and significant blood levels of this compound are measurable.

Topical Sulfonamides. Mafenide acetate (para-aminomethylbenzene sulfonamide, Sulfamylon cream) is available for use in the topical therapy of burns. However, its use has been limited by metabolic acidosis due to carbonic anhydrase inhibition. Silver sulfadiazine has fewer side effects and is used extensively for burns (4). Here the sulfonamide acts primarily as a vehicle for release of silver ions that exert an antibacterial effect. Recent reports of outbreaks of silver-resistant infections in burn units may ultimately limit its usefulness (5,6). Various combinations of other sulfonamides are available as vaginal creams or suppositories (e.g., Sultrin vaginal cream and tablets, AVC cream and suppositories, Sulfamel, Vagitrol).

There are a variety of ophthalmic ointments and solutions of sulfacetamide sodium USP available for use in treating conjunctivitis due to susceptible bacteria and as adjunctive therapy of trachoma (e.g., Bleph, Cetamide, Isoph, Sulamyd).

Mechanisms of Action

Although a wide variety of chemical modifications of the sulfonamides has been synthesized, all basically share the same mechanism of action. The sulfonamides are bacteriostatic in that they inhibit bacterial growth via interference with microbial folic acid synthesis. More specifically, sulfonamides inhibit competitively the incorporation of PABA into tetrahydropteroic acid (7–9), and they in turn may be incorporated into dihydropteroate (10). Sulfonamides may have a higher affinity for the microbial enzyme tetrahydropteroic acid synthetase than the natural substrate PABA. Richmond (11) has suggested that sulfonamides may act on bacterial repressor genes or by feedback inhibition to decrease formation of new enzyme. The ultimate result of decreased folic acid synthesis is a decrease in bacterial nucleotides with subsequent inhibition of bacterial growth.

Antimicrobial Activity In Vitro

Sulfonamides exhibit in vitro inhibitory activity against a broad spectrum of gram-positive and gram-negative bacteria as well as *Actinomyces, Chlamydia, Plasmodia,* and *Toxoplasma* (Table 1). The in vitro antimicrobial sensitivity of sulfonamides is strongly influenced by the size of the inoculum and the composition of the test media. High concentrations of PABA and thymidine inhibit sulfonamide activity.

Antimicrobial Resistance. Resistance to sulfonamides is widespread and is found in about 20–40 percent of community and nosocomial strains of bacteria, including staphylococci, Enterobacteriaceae, *Neisseria meningitidis,* and *Pseudomonas* sp. (12).

TABLE 1. In Vitro Activity of Sulfonamides Against Representative Organisms

	Range of MIC[a] (μg/ml)
Gram-positive	
Staphylococcus aureus	8–64
Streptococcus pneumoniae	4–128
Streptococcus pyogenes	0.5–16
Streptococcus faecalis	25–250
Corynebacterium diphtheriae	25–75
Listeria monocytogenes	3–75
Bacillus anthracis	12–100
Gram-negative	
Escherichia coli	4–64
Klebsiella spp.	8–128
Proteus mirabilis	8–128
Serratia marcescens	25–>1000
Salmonella sp.	16–128
Shigella sp.	2–32
Hemophilus influenzae	1–16
Neisseria gonorrhoeae	4–32
Neisseria meningitidis	0.25–>10
Pseudomonas aeruginosa	>100–200
Other	
Chlamydia trachomatis	0.1
Nocardia asteroides	2–16

SOURCE: Modified from Garrod et al. (21), Bushby (22), and Bach et al. (23).

[a] Minimum Inhibitory Concentration. Range is expressed for a variety of sulfonamide compounds.

Organisms may develop resistance or partial resistance by mutation, resulting in either microbial overproduction of PABA (13) or a structural change in a folic acid synthesizing enzyme that has lowered affinity for sulfonamide (14). The former mechanism has been implicated in resistant strains of *Neisseria gonorrhoeae* and *Staphylococcus aureus* (13,15), and the latter has been found in strains of *Escherichia coli* (16). Resistance also may be mediated by plasmids, episomal-resistance transfer factors (R factors) that may code for the production of drug-resistant enzymes, such as dihydropteroate synthetase (17) or may result in decreased bacterial cell permeability to sulfonamides (18). R-factor transfer can occur in the gastrointestinal tract as well as in vitro and has been seen especially with Enterobacteriaceae (19). More than one resistance mechanism may be operating simultaneously (20).

Pharmacology

Routes of Administration. Sulfonamides are usually administered orally, although sulfadiazine and sulfisoxazole are available for use as intravenous or subcutaneous preparations. These latter forms are used scarcely, if at all. Sulfacetamide is available as ophthalmic preparations, and silver sulfadiazine and mafenide acetate are applied topically in burn patients and are associated with significant absorption of sulfonamide percutaneously. Vaginal preparations are available for topical application.

Absorption. Most of the short- and medium-acting sulfonamides are absorbed rapidly and almost completely in the un-ionized state from the small intestine and stomach. Compounds with *N*-1 substitutions are absorbed poorly, as are more acidic compounds (e.g., phthalylsulfathiazole, Fig. 1f). Long-acting sulfonamides also are absorbed rapidly but have a much slower excretion rate. Topical sulfonamides are absorbed and may result in detectable blood levels.

Distribution. The sulfonamides generally are well distributed throughout the body, entering the cerebrospinal fluid and synovial, pleural, and peritoneal fluids with concentrations approaching 80 percent of serum levels. Blood and tissue levels are related to the degree of protein binding (Table 2) and lipid solubility. Sulfonamides administered in pregnancy readily cross the placenta and are present in the fetal blood and amniotic fluid (25).

Excretion. Acetylation and glucuronidation occur in the liver, and free and metabolized drug appear in the urine. Glomerular filtration is probably a route of excretion, although partial reabsorption and active tubular secretion also are involved, especially at low creatinine clearance rates. Urinary excretion is more rapid for those sulfonamides with low pKa values (e.g., sulfamethizole, sulfisoxazole), and alkalinization of the urine increases excretion by this route. Plasma half-lives vary widely and are related inversely to lipid solubility and directly to pKa but are not clearly related to the degree of protein binding (24). Small amounts of sulfonamides are found in bile, human milk, prostatic secretions, saliva, and tears.

Protein Binding and Blood or Tissue Levels. Sulfonamides are bound variably and not irreversibly to plasma albumin, and the bound drug is inactive (Table 2). Levels obtainable in cerebro spinal and other body fluids are inversely related

TABLE 2. Levels in Blood, Cerebrospinal Fluid, Plasma Half-life, and Protein Binding of Some Sulfonamides

Drug	*Peak Blood Level*[a] *(μg/ml)*	*% of Serum Level in CSF*	*Plasma Half-life (hours)*	*% Protein Binding*
Sulfadiazine	30–60	40–80	17	45
Sulfisoxazole	40–50	30–50	5–6	92
Sulfamethoxazole	80–100	25–30	11	70
Sulfadoxine	50–75	20–30	100–230	80–98

SOURCE: Modified from Anand (24) and Garrod et al. (21).

[a] Approximate free sulfonamide level after 2-g oral dose.

to the degree of protein binding. The amount of free drug in plasma is directly related to pKa (24).

Use in Renal Insufficiency. Sulfonamides can be used in renal failure; but therapeutic serum levels will persist longer because of reduced excretion, and the dosage must be reduced and the interval between doses extended proportional to the degree of renal impairment. Protein binding of sulfonamides is decreased in severe renal insufficiency (26). The *N*-4 acetylated metabolite of sulfonamides may accumulate in patients with renal failure especially during prolonged therapy. This derivative loses its antibacterial effect but still may have toxic properties. Plasma levels of sulfonamide should be measured every 3 days, and peak concentrations of sulfamethoxazole should be less than 120 μg/ml.

Toxicity and Adverse Reactions

Sulfonamides may cause nausea, vomiting, diarrhea, rash, fever, headache, depression, jaundice, hepatic necrosis, and a serum sicknesslike syndrome. Earlier, less soluble compounds (sulfadiazine, sulfathiazole) used in excessively high doses were associated with crystalluria and tubular deposits of sulfonamide crystals. These complications could be minimized by the maintenance of high urine flow and alkalinization of the urine. This complication usually is not seen with modern soluble sulfonamides. Tubular necrosis, interstitial nephritis, or necrotizing angiitis may be associated rarely with sulfonamide sensitivity (27).

More serious adverse reactions due to sulfonamides include acute hemolytic anemia (sometimes related to a deficiency in erythrocyte glucose-6-phosphate dehydrogenase—G6PD), aplastic anemia, agranulocytosis, thrombocytopenia, and leukopenia.

Sulfonamides should not be administered during the last month of pregnancy because they compete for bilirubin-binding sites on plasma albumin and may increase fetal blood levels of unconjugated bilirubin increasing the risk of kernicterus. Also, because of the immature fetal acetyl transferase system, blood levels of free sulfonamide may be increased, further adversely affecting the risk of kernicterus (24).

Finally, significant hypersensitivity reactions may occur to sulfonamides administered via any route. The most important of these include erythema nodosum, erythema multiforme (including Stevens-Johnson syndrome), drug eruption, vasculitis similar to periarteritis nodosa, and anaphylaxis. Long-acting sulfonamides have been associated with fatal hypersensitivity reactions, especially in children, and this severely limits their use. Locally applied sulfonamides (e.g., to skin) may be associated with any of these adverse reactions.

Drug Interactions

Sulfonamides may displace from albumin-binding sites drugs such as warfarin, thus increasing the effective activity of the displaced drug. Anticoagulant dosage therefore should be reduced during sulfonamide therapy. Sulfonamides also displace methotrexate from its bound protein, thereby increasing methotrexate toxicity. An increased hypoglycemic effect of chlorpropamide and tolbutamide may occur during sulfonamide therapy, possibly due to the same mechanism or to structural similarities. Sulfonamides may potentiate the action of some thiazide diuretics, phenytoin, and uricosuric agents. Conversely, sulfonamides themselves may be displaced from binding sites by indomethacin, phenylbutazone, salicylates, probenecid, and sulfinpyrazone, resulting in increased sulfonamide activity.

The activity of sulfonamides may be decreased by procaine and other local anesthetics derived from PABA. Methenamine compounds should not be used with sulfonamides because of the formation of insoluble urinary precipitates. Intravenous solutions of sulfonamides are physically incompatible with chloramphenicol, aminoglycosides, lincomycin, methicillin, tetracyclines, vancomycin, norepinephrine, insulin, procaine, Ringer's lactate solution, and others. Sulfonamides may decrease protein-bound iodine and ^{131}I uptake and may produce false-positive Benedict's tests for urine glucose and false-positive sulfosalicylic acid tests for urine proteins (28–30).

Major Clinical Use

Sulfonamides are primarily used in the treatment of acute urinary tract infections due to susceptible bacteria. Most first episodes of infection in the unobstructed urinary tract will be due to *E. coli* that are sensitive to sulfonamides. Sulfisoxazole is administered orally in a usual dosage of 1 g qid. For recurrent or chronic urinary tract infections, the infecting organism may or may not be sensitive to sulfonamides, and the choice of therapy should be based on appropriate sensitivity tests.

Sulfonamides are also quite effective in the therapy of infections due to *Nocardia asteroides.* Therapy must include 4–6 g or more daily after a loading dose of 4 g and should be continued for 4–6 months or longer if necessary.

Sulfonamides are effective in the prophylaxis of patients against recurrent attacks of rheumatic fever associated with group A β-hemolytic streptococcal infections, but they are not effective for therapy for established streptococcal pharyngitis. Sulfonamide prophylaxis of close contacts of patients with meningitis due to *N. meningitidis* is effective if the infecting organism is known to be sulfonamide sensitive (adult dose for sulfadiazine is 1 g q12h for 2 days). Sulfonamides have been used to treat toxoplasmosis and *P. falciparum* malaria (with pyrimethamine), meliodosis, dermatitis herpetiformis, lymphogranuloma venereum, and chancroid; and topical and systemic therapy is effective for trachoma and inclusion conjunctivitis (usually with topical tetracycline). Nongonococcal urethritis due to *Chlamydia,* but not *Ureaplasma urealyticum,* responds well to sulfonamide therapy. Currently, sulfonamides are used frequently in combination with trimethoprim (see below).

TRIMETHOPRIM

Structure and Derivation

Trimethoprim is a 2,4-diamino-5-(3′,4′,5′-trimethoxybenzyl) pyrimidine (Fig. 2). This drug was synthesized by Hitchings and coworkers as a dihydrofolate reductase inhibitor thought to potentiate the activity of sulfonamides by sequential inhibition of folic acid synthesis (2). In the United States, trimethoprim is now available as a single agent as well as in combination with sulfamethoxazole (see below). Trimethoprim does have antibacterial activity of its own, and its pharmacology will be reviewed.

Mechanism of Action

Trimethoprim owes its activity to powerful inhibition of bacterial dihydrofolate reductase, which is the enzyme step after the step in folic acid synthesis blocked by sulfonamides. Trimethoprim is 50,000–100,000 times more active against bacterial dihydrofolate reductase than against the human enzyme. Trimethoprim interferes with the conversion of dihydrofolate to tetrahydrofolate, the precursor of folinic acid and ultimately purine and DNA synthesis (Fig. 3). The sequential blockage of the same biosynthetic pathway by sulfonamides and trimethoprim results in a high degree of synergistic activity against a wide spectrum of microorganisms. Humans do not synthesize folic acid but require it in their diet and, therefore, human purine synthesis is not affected significantly by the enzyme inhibition by trimethoprim (31,32).

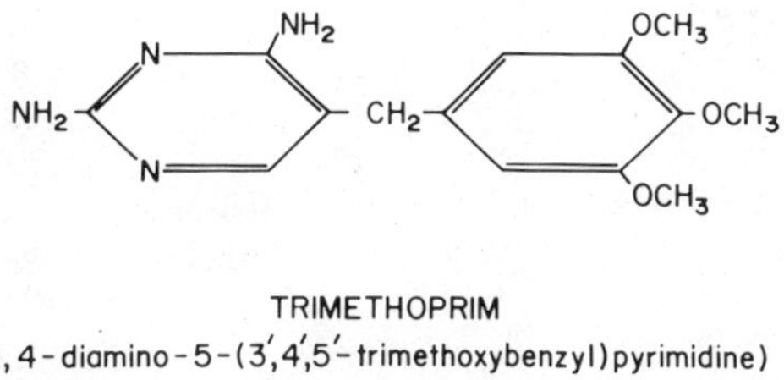

FIGURE 2. Chemical structure of trimethoprim.

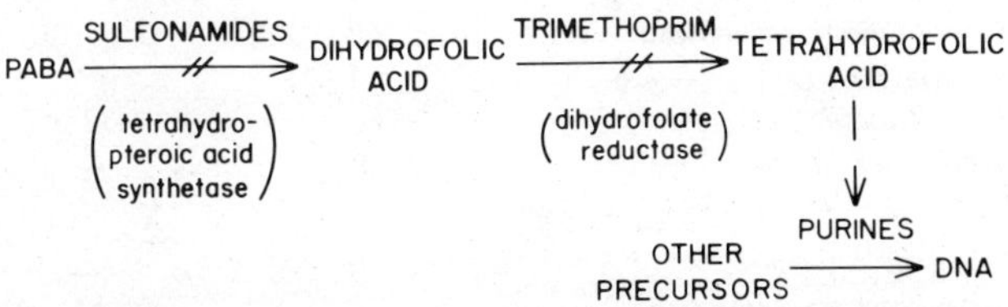

FIGURE 3. Action of sulfonamides and trimethoprim on the metabolic pathway of bacterial folic acid synthesis.

Antimicrobial Activity

Trimethoprim is quite active in vitro against most gram-positive cocci and most gram-negative rods except for *Pseudomonas aeruginosa* and *Bacteroides* sp. (Table 3). *Trepönema pallidum, Mycobacterium tuberculosis, Mycoplasma* sp., and most anaerobes are resistant. Thymidine will inhibit the in vitro activity of trimethoprim, but the addition of thymidine phosphorylase or 5 percent lysed horse blood to Mueller-Hinton or other sensitivity media removes this inhibition. The minimum inhibitory concentration (MIC) will vary considerably with the media used (33).

Potentiation of the action of trimethoprim is seen in combination with sulfamethoxazole (see below and Table 3). Antibacterial synergism has been demon-

TABLE 3. In Vitro Activity of Trimethoprim Against Representative Organisms

Organism	*MIC[a] Alone (μg/ml)*	*MIC with Sulfamethoxazole (μg/ml, 1:20)*
Gram-positive		
Staphylococcus aureus	0.15–2	0.04–1.6
S. epidermidis	0.02	—
Streptococcus pneumoniae	0.004–5	0.05–1.5
S. pyogenes	0.02–1	0.015–0.4
S. faecalis	0.15–0.5	0.015–0.4
Corynebacterium diphtheriae	0.15–0.5	0.05–0.15
Listeria monocytogenes	0.05–1.5	0.015–0.15
Clostridium perfringens	2–50	—
Propionibacterium acnes	0.07	—
Gram-negative		
Escherichia coli	0.01–>5	0.005–>5
Klebsiella sp.	0.15–5	0.05–3.1
Proteus mirabilis	0.15–1.5	0.05–0.15
Serratia marcescens	0.8–50	0.4–50
Salmonella sp.	0.01–0.4	0.05–0.15
Shigella sp.	0.04–0.8	0.02–0.5
Citrobacter freundii	0.2	—
Vibrio cholera	0.2	—
Hemophilus influenzae	0.1–12.5	0.04–50
Neisseria gonorrhoeae	0.2–128	0.15–3.1
N. meningitidis	3.1–50	0.01–1.6
Pseudomonas aeruginosa	50–1000	3.1–100
P. cepacia	1–2	—
P. maltophilia	>32	>32
Bacteroides fragilis	≥4.0	—
Other		
Nocardia asteroides	3–100	1.5
Chlamydia trachomatis	20	—

SOURCE: Modified from Garrod et al. (21), Bushby (22), Bach et al. (23), Phillips and Warren (38), Trehane et al. (39), and Moody and Young (40).

[a] MIC varies with the method, inoculum size, and media used.

strated in vitro for trimethoprim and polymyxins (34) and for trimethoprim and aminoglycosides against some gram-negative bacilli (35). The combination of trimethoprim-sulfamethoxazole is active in vitro against 90–95 percent of tested *S. aureus, Streptococcus pyogenes, Streptococcus pneumoniae, E. coli, Proteus mirabilis, Shigella* sp., *Salmonella* sp., *Pseudomonas cepacia, Pseudomonas pseudomallei, Yersinia enterocolitica,* and *N. gonorrhoeae* (36). Almost all strains of *P. aeruginosa* are resistant in vitro to trimethoprim-sulfamethoxazole. The optimal ratio for in vitro synergism of trimethoprim-sulfamethoxazole in combination is 1:20, but this ratio does not always obtain in vivo.

The synergism seen with trimethoprim-sulfamethoxazole depends somewhat on the sensitivity of the organism to each drug. In one study (37), over 95 percent of organisms sensitive to both drugs showed synergism, whereas 60 percent of sulfamethoxazole-resistant strains and 45 percent of trimethoprim-resistant strains showed synergism. Only 9 percent of strains resistant to both drugs showed in vitro potentiation. However, using an inoculum of a 10^{-3} dilution of an overnight broth culture, Bach et al. (23) reported that of the sulfamethoxazole-resistant strains tested, 90–100 percent of the following organisms were sensitive to less than 1 μg/ml of trimethoprim in combination with the sulfonamide: enterococci (25 strains), *H. influenzae* (35 strains), *Klebsiella pneumoniae* (33 strains), *Serratia marcescens* (27 strains), *Salmonella* sp. (34 strains), and *Shigella* sp. (31 strains).

Resistance to Trimethoprim. Bacteria may develop trimethoprim resistance by frequent passage in media containing the drug. Clinical resistance has increased. In one hospital in France (41) trimethoprim-resistant Enterobacteriaceae (MIC $\geq$ 4 μg/ml) increased from 18 to 25 percent of isolates. A decrease in the ratio of strains resistant to both sulfamethoxazole and trimethoprim compared to stains resistant only to trimethoprim may reflect an increase in independent trimethoprim resistance, and this might be a useful monitoring parameter in hospitals (42).

Trimethoprim resistance may be due to changes in cell permeability, loss of bacterial-drug binding capacity, and overproduction of or alterations in dihydrofolate reductase. However, the clinically most important mechanism is due to plasmid-mediated dihydrofolate reductases that are resistant to trimethoprim (43,44).

Resistance to both trimethoprim and sulfamethoxazole is less frequent, occurring in 4–8 percent of Enterobacteriaceae. Although permeability changes may occur in the bacterial cell, thymine requiring auxotrophs may also account for clinically significant resistance to both drugs. These mutants lack thymidylate synthetase and are probably less virulent than are sensitive strains (45,46).

Pharmacology

Routes of Administration. Trimethoprim is available as 100 mg tablets for oral use. Trimethoprim is absorbed readily and almost completely from the gastrointestinal tract. Peak serum levels after taking 100 mg appear 1–4 hours after ingestion and approach 1 μg/ml. The coadministration of sulfamethoxazole does not affect the rate of absorption or serum levels of trimethoprim.

Trimethoprim is also available in fixed combination with sulfamethoxazole in a ratio of 1:5 for oral use (trimethoprim, 80 mg; sulfamethoxazole, 400 mg; Bactrim, Septra); double-strength and quarter-strength pediatric tablets are available as is an oral suspension containing 40 mg trimethoprim and 200 mg sulfamethoxazole per 5 ml. Intravenous trimethoprim (16 mg/ml) plus sulfamethoxazole (80 mg/ml) is available. When administered intravenously, 10 ml or 160 mg trimethoprim (with 800 mg sulfamethoxazole) produces a peak serum trimethoprim concentration of 3.4 μg/ml in 1 hour. After repeated doses, the peak trimethoprim concentration may approach 9 μg/ml (47). Similar peak levels may be reached with oral therapy, but at 2–4 hours after taking the dose (48,49).

Distribution. Trimethoprim is widely distributed in tissues and may appear in kidney, lung, and sputum in higher concentrations than in plasma, as well as in bile, saliva, human breast milk, and seminal fluid (50). Trimethoprim is also found in prostatic fluid at two to three times the serum concentration, but lower levels may be present in patients with chronic prostatitis (51,52). Cerebrospinal fluid levels are about 40 percent of serum levels.

Metabolism and Excretion. Approximately 60–80 percent of an administered dose of trimethoprim is excreted in the urine via tubular secretion within 24 hours. The remainder of the drug is excreted by the kidney in one of four oxide- or hydroxyl-derivatives. The urinary metabolites are bacteriologically inactive (47). Trimethoprim is also excreted in the bile. The serum half-life ranges from 9 to 11 hours in healthy subjects and is prolonged in patients with renal insufficiency. Unlike sulfamethoxazole, the excretion rate of trimethoprim is increased with acidification of the urine, and serum protein binding (65–70 percent) does not decrease significantly with increasing degrees of uremia (26). Urine concentrations in healthy subjects (60–1000 μg/ml) are usually in excess of the MIC of most urinary pathogens (26). Trimethoprim-sulfamethoxazole can be given in the usual doses to patients with creatinine clearances of 30 ml/min or greater. One-half the usual daily dose can be given to patients with creatinine clearances of 15–30 ml/min, but trimethoprim-sulfamethoxazole is not recommended for use in patients with clearances less than 15 ml/min (26,53,54). Both trimethoprim and nonacetylated sulfamethoxazole are removed by hemodialysis (26). Patients needing chronic peritoneal dialysis can receive the equivalent of one double-strength trimethoprim-sulfamethoxazole tablet every 48 hours.

Toxicity and Side Effects

The toxic and undesired effects of trimethoprim-sulfamethoxazole include all those discussed above for sulfonamides. Nausea, vomiting, diarrhea, anorexia, and hypersensitivity reactions are the most frequent (55,56). Rash has been noted frequently in patients with acquired immunodeficiency syndrome. In addition, impaired folate utilization may be seen in humans with prolonged administration. This is usually manifest as a megaloblastic marrow, with hypersegmented polymorphonuclear leukocytes. Also leukopenia, thrombocytopenia, and granulocytopenia may be seen. The administration of folinic acid usually prevents or treats effectively the antifolate effects of trimethoprim, and the latter drug's antibacterial efficacy is not impaired except possibly against enterococci. Pseudomembranous colitis has been described with trimethoprim-sulfamethoxazole but is uncommon (57). Renal dysfunction may occur in patients with preexisting renal disease, but this is reversible with dose reduction (58). Trimethoprim-sulfamethoxazole may cause an increase in measured serum creatinine (59). Active levels of phenytoin may be increased markedly by trimethoprim-sulfamethoxazole (60).

Trimethoprim Plus Other Antimicrobial Agents

Other sulfonamides, such as sulfamoxole, sulfadiazine, sulfadimidine, and sulfametrol, have been combined with trimethoprim but more clinical studies are needed to recommend their use over the currently used combination (61). Combinations of trimethoprim with other agents such as rifampin (62–64) polymyxin (34), amikacin (65), and metronidazole (66) have been suggested or used. Extensive clinical experience with these combinations is lacking.

Clinical Use

Urinary Tract Infections. Trimethoprim-sulfamethoxazole is useful in the treatment of recurrent or chronic urinary tract infections due to sensitive organisms. Most Enterobacteriaceae are sensitive to the combined action of these drugs. Initially released for treatment of more complicated infections in the urinary tract, the combination is also effective in acute pyelonephritis and cystitis, although soluble sulfonamides alone would be appropriate for many cases.

Because trimethoprim accumulates in prostatic secretions, trimethoprim-sulfamethoxazole is often effective in bacterial prostatitis (52), as well as in orchitis and epididymitis due to susceptible bacteria.

The usual dosage in an adult for the treatment of acute prostate or urinary infection is two tablets every 12 hours or one double-strength tablet every 12 hours. The pediatric dose for urinary tract infection is 150–185 mg/m^2 for trimethoprim and 750–925 mg/m^2 for sulfamethoxazole daily in two divided doses. Single-dose therapy with one or two double-strength tablets may be effective in women with uncomplicated lower urinary tract infection (67,68). However, in patients with chronic tissue invasive urinary infections, longer-term therapy of up to 6 weeks might be required (69).

Trimethoprim-sulfamethoxazole has been shown to be useful in the long-term suppressive therapy of adults and children with chronic or recurrent urinary infections, and extremely low doses (one-half to one tablet at bedtime or every other night) are effective (70,71). Trimethoprim is thought to achieve effective concentrations in the vaginal secretions, and it is believed by some that it exerts its protective effect on reducing the number of recurrent infections in this manner despite the fact that trimethoprim-sulfamethoxazole-resistant organisms may be present in the vaginal and stool flora (72). Trimethoprim alone is effective therapy for uncomplicated and recurrent urinary infections in women. Usual doses are 100–200 mg bid (72–74), and nightly doses of 100 mg may be effective suppressive therapy (73,75). Reeves (76) has argued that trimethoprim alone is preferable to the combination of trimethoprim-sulfamethoxazole for acute urinary tract infections and possibly other infections as well; however, further studies are needed, and trimethoprim-resistant organisms might increase with extended use.

Respiratory Tract Infections. Trimethoprim-sulfamethoxazole is effective in the treatment of acute bronchitis and pneumonitis due to sensitive organisms, although it is not the treatment of choice for any single organism. Trimethoprim-sulfamethoxazole may be as effective as tetracyclines in the reduction of acute exacerbations in patients with chronic bronchitis (77,78), but full doses should be used. Although not usually considered for use in seriously ill patients with pneumonia, intravenously administered trimethoprim-sulfamethoxazole may be effective in patients with infections due to susceptible gram-negative bacteria (79).

Consistent with its antibacterial spectrum, trimethoprim-sulfamethoxazole may be as effective as ampicillin for the treatment of sinusitis and otitis media (80), and ampicillin-resistant strains of *H. influenzae* might be susceptible.

Gastrointestinal Infections. Although antibiotics per se prolong the carrier state in acute gastroenteritis due to *Salmonella* sp., trimethoprim-sulfamethoxazole is reasonably effective in eliminating chronic *Salmonella* carriage including carriers of *Salmonella typhi,* especially in patients over 2 years of age. Typhoid fever also may be treated successfully with this combination, although the development of resistant strains has been reported (81). Trimethoprim-sulfamethoxazole is effective in shigellosis, especially due to ampicillin-resistant strains (82). Intravenous administration may be necessary for patients with some of these infections. Trimethoprim-sulfamethoxazole also is effective in the treatment of diarrhea due to enteropathogenic *E. coli* and in the treatment and prophylaxis of traveler's diarrhea (83–85). The combination may be a useful adjunct to fluids in the treatment of cholera (86).

Sexually Transmitted Diseases. Trimethoprim–sulfamethoxazole is effective in the treatment of uncomplicated gonorrhea when used in several dosage regimens (e.g., 2 tabs po bid for 5 days, 4 tabs bid for 2 days, and a single dose of 8 tabs) (87–89). For pharyngeal gonorrhea, especially that due to penicillinase producing *N. gonorrhoeae,* nine tablets/day for 5 days has been recommended (90). Nongonococcal urethritis due to *Chlamydia trachomatis* may be treatable with the combination, but its activity is due to the sulfonamide (91). The combination is also effective therapy for chancroid and lymphogranuloma venereum. It is ineffective for syphilis.

Other Infections. Trimethoprim-sulfamethoxazole is useful against brucellosis (long-term therapy for 6 weeks) (92), biliary tract infections, acute and chronic osteomyelitis (93,94), periodontal infection (95), mycetoma due to paracoccidioidomycosis and other fungi (96), and nocardiosis (97). Individual cases of successful response to combination therapy have been described for melioidosis (98), *P. cepacia* bacteremia (99), and Whipple's disease (100).

Intravenous trimethoprim-sulfamethoxazole has been useful in treating gram-negative rod bacteremia and staphylococcal bacteremia and endocarditis, although other agents are clearly preferred for the latter (66,101,102). Meningitis due to susceptible organisms may be successfully treated, but other agents are usually preferred. The combination may be effective in meningitis due to *Listeria monocytogenes* (103).

Trimethoprim plus sulfalene and trimethoprim-sulfamethoxazole have been used in the treatment of susceptible *P. falciparum* infections, although these combinations are not very active against multiple-resistant strains. In vitro efficacy has been suggested for *Toxoplasma gondii* and *Mycobacterium kansasii, Mycobacterium marinum,* and *Mycobacterium scrofulaceum,* but clinical experience is limited (104,105).

PNEUMOCYSTIS CARINII INFECTIONS AND PROPHYLACTIC THERAPY FOR NEUTROPENIC PATIENTS. One of the most recent applications of combined trimethoprim-sulfamethoxazole has been in the treatment of infections due to *P. carinii.* High-dose oral or intravenous therapy (trimethoprim, 20 mg/kg/day; sulfamethoxazole, 100 mg/kg/day in two or three divided doses po or three or four doses IV) is quite effective in this infection with cures resulting in 70–80 percent of patients (106,107). Treatment should continue for 10–14 days. Hughes et al. (108) have shown that this drug combination is effective in the chemoprophylaxis of leukemic and other immunosuppressed cancer patients against *P. carinii* infections. (See Chapters 237, 263, 269, and 273 for further discussion of therapy for *P. carinii* infections.) Long-term therapy with 150 mg/m^2 of trimethoprim and 750 mg/m^2 of sulfamethoxazole daily in two divided doses almost eliminated this infection from their population, which consisted mostly of children with leukemia.

Gurwith et al. (109) presented evidence of a striking reduction in gram-negative rod bacteremia in neutropenic patients treated prophylactically with trimethoprim-sulfamethoxazole (2 tabs bid or more until stools were free of Enterobacteriaceae) compared with untreated control neutropenic patients. Similar data were reported recently by Kauffman et al. (110) and Gualtieri et al. (111), but other studies in progress do not universally show a benefit in preventing bacteremia in neutropenic patients with acute myelocytic leukemia (112). Trimethoprim-sulfamethoxazole may prolong recovery from induction-chemotherapy induced neutropenia as has been reported in some but not all studies (113,114).

Trimethoprim Use in Pregnancy. The teratogenicity of trimethoprim in humans is not clearly defined, but this drug is not recommended for use in pregnancy at this time.

REFERENCES

1. Carithers HA: The first use of an antibiotic in America. *Am J Dis Child* 128:207, 1974.
2. Bushby SRM, Hitchings GH: Trimethoprim, a sulphonamide potentiator. *Br J Pharmacol Chemother* 33:72, 1968.
3. Schwartz IK, Campbell CC: Indications for the use of Fansidar in malaria. *New Engl J Med* 307:194, 1982.
4. Ballin JC: Evaluation of a new topical agent for burn therapy: Silver sulfadiazine (Silvadene). *JAMA* 230:1184, 1974.
5. Mayer KH, Hopkins JD, Gillece ES, et al: Acquisition of an endemic antibiotic resistance plasmid by a new epidemic strain of *Enterobacter cloacae. Clin Res* 30:374, 1982.
6. McHugh G, Moellering RC Jr, Hopkins CC, et al: *Salmonella typhimurium* resistant to silver nitrate, chloramphenicol and ampicillin: A new threat in burn units? *Lancet* 1:231, 1975.
7. Woods DD: Relation of p-aminobenzoic acid to mechanism of action of sulphanilamide. *Brit J Exp Pathol* 21:74, 1940.
8. Fildes P: Rational approach to research in chemotherapy. *Lancet* 1:955, 1940.
9. Miller AK, Bruno P, Berglund RM: The effect of sulfathiazol on the in vitro synthesis of certain vitamins by *Escherichia coli. J Bacteriol* 54:9, 1947.
10. Brown GM: The biosynthesis of pteridines. *Adv Enzymol* 35:35, 1971.
11. Richmond MH: Structural analogy and chemical reactivity in the action of antibacterial compounds, in *Biochemical Studies of Antimicrobial Drugs.* Proc Sixteenth Symp Soc General Microbiology. London, Cambridge University Press, 1966, p 301.
12. Hamilton-Miller JMJ: Mechanisms and distribution of bacterial resistance to diaminopyrimidines and sulphonamides. *J Antimicrob Chemother* 5(suppl B):61, 1979.
13. Landy M, Larkun NW, Oswald EJ, et al: Increased synthesis of p-aminobenzoic acid associated with the development of resistance in *Staph aureus. Science* 97:265, 1943.
14. Wolf B, Hotchkiss RD: Genetically modified folic acid synthesising enzymes in *Pneumococcus. Biochemistry* 2:145, 1940.
15. Landy M, Gerstung RB: p-Aminobenzoic acid synthesis by *Neisseria gonorrhoeae* in relation to clinical and cultural sulfonamide resistance. *J Bacteriol* 47:448, 1944.
16. Swedberg G, Castensson S, Sköld O: Characterization of mutationally altered dihydropteroate synthase and its ability to form a sulfonamide-containing dihydrofolate analog. *J Bacteriol* 137:129, 1979.
17. Sköld O: R-factor mediated resistance to sulfonamides by a plasmid-borne, drug resistant dihydropteroate synthase. *Antimicrob Agents Chemother* 9:49, 1976.
18. Kabins SA, Panse MV, Cohen S: Role of R-factor and bacterial host in sulfonamide resistance mediated by R-factor in *Escherichia coli. J Infect Dis* 123:158, 1971.
19. Watanabe T: Infective heredity of multiple drug resistance in bacteria. *Bacteriol Rev* 27:87, 1963.
20. Then RL: Mechanisms of resistance to trimethoprim, the sulfonamides and trimethoprim-sulfamethoxazole. *Rev Infect Dis* 4:261, 1982.
21. Garrod LP, Lambert HP, O'Grady F: *Antibiotic and Chemotherapy,* ed 4. Edinburgh and London, Churchill Livingstone, 1973.
22. Bushby SRM: Trimethoprim-sulfamethoxazole: In vitro microbiologic aspects. *J Infect Dis* 128:S442, 1973.
23. Bach MC, Finland M, Gold W, et al: Susceptibility of recently isolated pathogenic bacteria to trimethoprim and sulfamethoxazole separately and combined. *J Infect Dis* 128:S508, 1973.

24. Anand N: Sulfonamides and sulfones, in Corcoran JW and Hahn FE (eds): *Antibiotics III: Mechanism of Action of Antimicrobial and Antitumor Agents.* Berlin, Springer-Verlag, 1975, p 668.
25. Sparr RA, Pritchard JA: Maternal and newborn distribution and excretion of sulfamethoxypyridazine (Kynex). *Obstet Gynecol* 12:131, 1958.
26. Craig WA, Kunin CM: Trimethoprim-sulfamethoxazole: Pharmacodynamic effects of urinary pH and impaired renal function. *Ann Intern Med* 78:491, 1973.
27. Weinstein L, Madoff MA, Samet CM: The sulfonamides IV. *New Engl J Med* 263:952, 1960.
28. Dunea G, Freedman P: Proteinuria. *JAMA* 203:973, 1968.
29. Hansten PD: *Drug Interactions,* ed 2. Philadelphia, Lea & Febiger, 1973.
30. Griffin JP, D'Arcy PF: *A Manual of Adverse Drug Interactions.* Bristol, John Wright and Sons, 1975, p 63.
31. Burchall JJ: Trimethoprim and pyrimethamine, in Corcoran JW and Hahn FE (eds): *Antibiotics III: Mechanism of Action of Antimicrobial and Antitumor Agents.* Berlin, Springer-Verlag, 1975, p 304.
32. Hitchings GT: The biochemical basis for the antimicrobial activity of septrin, in Bernstein LS, Salter AJ (eds): *Trimethoprim/Sulphamethoxazole in Bacterial Infections.* Edinburgh and London, Churchill Livingstone, 1973, p 7.
33. Dornbusch K, Moore WB: The effects of different media on the response of bacteria to sulphonamides and trimethoprim using the disc-diffusion method and regression line analysis, in Bernstein LS, Salter AJ (eds): *Trimethoprim/Sulphamethoxazole in Bacterial Infections.* Edinburgh and London, Churchill Livingstone, 1973, p 31.
34. Simmons NA: Colistin, sulphamethoxazole and trimethoprim in synergy against gram-negative bacilli. *J Clin Pathol* 23:757, 1970.
35. Parsley TL, Provonchee RB, Glicksman C, et al: Synergistic activity of trimethoprim and amikacin against gram-negative bacilli. *Antimicrob Agents Chemother* 12:349, 1977.
36. Bushby SRM: Sensitivity patterns and use of a combined disc of trimethoprim-sulphamethoxazole, in Bernstein LS, Salter AJ (eds): *Trimethoprim/Sulphamethoxazole in Bacterial Infections.* Edinburgh and London, Churchill Livingstone, 1973, p 31.
37. Bohni E: Vergleichende bakteriologishe untersuchungen mit der kombination trimethoprim sulfamethoxazole in vitro und in vivo. *Chemotherapy* 14(suppl):1, 1969.
38. Phillips I, Warren C: Activity of sulfamethoxazole and trimethoprim against *Bacteroides fragilis. Antimicrob Agents Chemother* 9:736, 1976.
39. Trehane JD, Day J, Yeo CK, et al: Susceptibility of chlamydiae to chemotherapeutic agents, in Hobsen D and Holmes KK (eds): *Nongonococcal Urethritis and Related Infections.* Am Soc Microbiology. Washington, DC, 1077, pp 214–222.
40. Moody MR, Young VM: In vitro susceptibility of *Pseudomonas cepacia* and *Pseudomonas maltophilia* to trimethoprim and trimethoprim-sulfamethoxazole. *Antimicrob Agents Chemother* 7:836, 1975.
41. Acar JF, Goldstein FW: Genetic aspects and epidemiologic implications of resistance to trimethoprim. *Rev Infect Dis* 4:270, 1982.
42. O'Brien TF, Acar JF, Altmann G, et al: Laboratory surveillance of synergy between and resistance to trimethoprim and sulfonamides. *Rev Infect Dis* 4:351, 1982.
43. Richards HN, Datta N, Sojka NJ, et al: Trimethoprim resistance plasmids and transposons in Salmonella. *Lancet* 2:1194, 1978.
44. Burchall JJ, Pelwell L, Fling ME: Molecular mechanisms of resistance to trimethoprim. *Rev Infect Dis* 4:246, 1982.
45. Smith HW, Tucker JF: The virulence of trimethoprim resistant thymine-requiring strains of Salmonella. *J Hyg* (*Lond*) 76:97, 1976.
46. Maskell R, Okubadejo OA, Payne RH, et al: Human infections with thymine-requiring bacteria. *J Med Microbiol* 11:33, 1978.
47. Grose WE, Bodey GP, Loo TL: Clinical pharmacology of intravenously administered trimethoprim-sulfamethoxazole. *Antimicrob Agents Chemother* 15:447, 1979.
48. Bach MC, Gold O, Finland M: Absorption and urinary excretion of trimethoprim, sulfamethox-

azole, and trimethoprim-sulfamethoxazole: Results with single doses in normal young adults and preliminary observations during therapy with trimethoprim-sulfamethoxazole. *J Infect Dis* 128:S584, 1973.

49. Kaplan SA, Weinfeld RE, Abruzzo CW, et al: Pharmacokinetic profile of trimethoprim-sulfamethoxazole in man. *J Infect Dis* 128:S547, 1973.
50. Pater RB, Welling PG: Clinical pharmacokinetics of co-trimoxazole (trimethoprim/sulfamethoxazole). *Clin Pharmacokinet* 5:405, 1980.
51. Winningham DG, Nemoy NJ, Stamey TA: Diffusion of antibiotics from plasma into prostatic fluid. *Nature* 219:139, 1968.
52. Meares EM Jr: Prostatitis: Review of pharmacokinetics and therapy. *Rev Infect Dis* 4:475, 1982.
53. Welling PG, Craig WA, Amidon GL, et al: Pharmacokinetics of trimethoprim and sulfamethoxazole in normal subjects and in patients with renal failure. *J Infect Dis* 128(suppl):556, 1973.
54. Salter AJ: Trimethoprim sulfamethoxazole: An assessment of more than 12 years of use. *Rev Infect Dis* 4:190, 1982.
55. Jick H: Adverse reactions to trimethoprim-sulfamethoxazole in hospitalized patients. *Rev Infect Dis* 4:426, 1982.
56. Lawson DH, Paice BJ: Adverse reactions to trimethoprim-sulfamethoxazole. *Rev Infect Dis* 4:429, 1982.
57. Cameron A, Thomas M: Pseudomembranous colitis and co-trimoxazole. *Br Med J* 1:1321, 1977.
58. Bailey RR, Little PJ: Deterioration in renal function in association with co-trimoxazole therapy. *Med J Aust* 1:914, 1976.
59. Trollfors B, Wahl, Alestig K: Co-trimoxazole, creatinine and renal function. *J Infect* 2:221, 1980.
60. Hansen JM, Kampmann JP, Siersbaek-Nielsenk, et al: The effect of different sulfonamides on phenytoin metabolism in man. *Acta Med Scand* [*Suppl*] 624:106, 1979.
61. Bernstein LS: Combination of trimethoprim with sulfonamides other than sulfamethoxazole. *Rev Infect Dis* 4:411, 1982.
62. Brumfitt W, Hamilton-Miller JMT: Rifamprim (rifampicin plus trimethoprim): Pharmacokinetics and effects on the normal flora of man. *Biopharmocol Drug Dispos* 2:157, 1981.
63. Kerry DW, Hamilton-Miller JMT, Brumfitt W: Trimethoprim and rifampicin: In vitro activities separately and in combination. *J Antimicrob Chemother* 1:417, 1975.
64. Alvarez S, DeMaria A Jr., Kulkarni R, et al: Interactions of rifampin and trimethoprim in vitro. *Rev Infect Dis* 4:390, 1982.
65. Zinner SH, Lagast H, Kasry A, Klastersky J: Synergism of trimethoprim combined with aminoglycosides in vitro and in serum of volunteers. *Eur J Clin Microbiol* 1:144, 1982.
66. Salter AJ: Trimethoprim-sulfamethoxazole in treatment of severe infections. *Rev Infect Dis* 4:338, 1982.
67. Tolkoff-Rubin NE, Weber D, Fang LST, et al: Single dose therapy with trimethoprim-sulfamethoxazole for urinary tract infection in women. *Rev Infect Dis* 4:444, 1982.
68. Counts GW, Stamm WE, McKevitt M, et al: Treatment of cystitis in women with a single dose of trimethoprim-sulfamethoxazole. *Rev Infect Dis* 4:484, 1982.
69. Gleckman R, Crowley M, Natsios GA: Treatment of recurrent invasive urinary-tract infections of men. *New Engl J Med* 301:878, 1979.
70. Harding GK, Ronald AR: A controlled study of antimicrobial prophylaxis of recurrent urinary infection in women. *New Engl J Med* 291:597, 1974.
71. Harding GKM, Ronald AR, Nicolle LE, et al: Long-term antimicrobial prophylaxis for recurrent urinary tract infection in women. *Rev Infect Dis* 4:438, 1982.
72. Brumfitt W, Pursell R: Double-blind trial to compare ampicillin, cephalexin, co-trimoxazole and trimethoprim in treatment of urinary infection. *Br Med J* 2:673, 1972.
73. Kasanen A, Toivanen P, Sourander L, et al: Trimethoprim in the treatment and long-term control of urinary tract infection. *Scand J Infect Dis* 6:91, 1974.
74. Iravani A, Richard GA, Baer H: Treatment of uncomplicated urinary tract infection with

trimethoprim versus sulfisoxazole with special reference to antibody-coated bacteria and faecal flora. *Antimicrob Agents Chemother* 19:824, 1981.

75. Stamm WE, Counts GW, Wagner KR, et al: Antimicrobial prophylaxis of recurrent urinary tract infections. *Ann Intern Med* 92:770, 1980.
76. Reeves D: Sulphonamides and trimethoprim. *Lancet* 2:370, 1982.
77. Pandy GJ: Trimethoprim/sulphamethoxazole and doxycycline in acute exacerbations of chronic bronchitis in general practice: A comparative study. *Med J Aust* 1:264, 1979.
78. Pines A: Trimethoprim-sulfamethoxazole in the treatment and prevention of purulent exacerbations of chronic bronchitis. *J Infect Dis* 128:S706, 1973.
79. Schmidt U, Sen P, Kapila R, et al: Clinical evaluation of intravenous trimethoprim sulfamethoxazole for serious infections. *Rev Infect Dis* 4:333, 1982.
80. Shurin PA, Pelton SI, Donner A, et al: Trimethoprim-sulfamethoxazole compared with ampicillin in the treatment of acute otitis media. *J Pediatr* 96:1081, 1980.
81. Datta N, Richards H, Datta C: *Salmonella typhi* in vivo acquires resistance to both chloramphenicol and cotrimoxazole. *Lancet* 1:1181, 1981.
82. Nelson JD, Kusmiesz H, Shelton S: Oral or intravenous trimethoprim-sulfamethoxazole therapy for shigellosis. *Rev Infect Dis* 4:546, 1982.
83. Thoren A, Wolde-Mariam I, Stintzing G, et al: Antibiotics in the treatment of gastroenteritis caused by enteropathogenic *Escherichia coli. J Infect Dis* 141:27, 1980.
84. DuPont HL, Evans DG, Rios N, et al: Prevention of travelers' diarrhea with trimethoprim-sulfamethoxazole. *Rev Infect Dis* 4:533, 1982.
85. DuPont. HL, Reves RR, Galindo E, et al: Treatment of travelers' diarrhea with trimethoprim/sulfamethoxazole and with trimethoprim alone. *N Engl J Med* 307:841, 1982.
86. Francis TI, Lewis EA, Oyediran ABOO, et al: Effect of chemotherapy on the duration of diarrhoea, and on vibrio excretion by cholera patients. *J Trop Med Hyg* 74:172, 1971.
87. Svindland HB: Treatment of gonorrhoea with sulphamethoxazole-trimethoprim. Lack of effect on concomitant syphilis. *Br J Vener Dis* 49:50, 1973.
88. Lawrence A, Phillips E, Nicol C: Various regiments of trimethoprim-sulfamethoxazole in the treatment of gonorrhea. *J Infect Dis* 128(suppl):S673, 1973.
89. Rahim G: Single dose treatment of gonorrhoea with cotrimoxazole. A report on 1,223 cases. *Br J Vener Dis* 51:179, 1975.
90. Centers for Disease Control: Sexually Transmitted Diseases Treatment Guidelines, 1982. *Morbidity and Mortality Weekly Report* 31:35S–62S, 1982.
91. Hammerschlag MR: Activity of trimethoprim-sulfamethoxazole against *Chlamydia trachomatis* in vitro. *Rev Infect Dis* 4:500, 1982.
92. Daikos GK, Papapolyzos N, Marketos N, et al: Trimethoprim-sulfamethoxazole in brucellosis. *J Infect Dis* 128(suppl):S731, 1973.
93. Bajpai J, Chaturvedi SN, Khanuja SPS: Chemotherapy of acute bone and joint infections. *Int Surg* 62:172, 1977.
94. Millard FJC: Trimethoprim/sulphamethoxazole in the treatment of chronic osteomyelitis, in Bernstein LS, Salter AJ (eds): *Trimethoprim-Sulphamethoxazole in Bacterial Infections.* Churchill Livingstone, Edinburgh, 1973, pp 195–199.
95. Lakshmanan CDS: Comparative evaluation of cotrimoxazole and demeclocycline in periodontal bacterial infection, abstract no. 128. *J Dent Res* 55(special issue D):D137, 1976.
96. Mahgoub ES: Medical management of mycetoma. *Bull WHO* 54:303, 1976.
97. Wallace RJ: Septimus EJ, Williams JH, et al: Use of trimethoprim-sulfamethoxazole for the treatment of infections due to Noccardia. *Rev Infect Dis* 4:315, 1982.
98. Morrison IM: Chronic melioidosis. *Proc R Soc Med* 63:239, 1970.
99. Neu HC, Garvey GJ, Bleach MP: Successful treatment of Pseudomonas cepacia endocarditis in a heroin addict with trimethoprim sulfamethoxazole. *J Infect Dis* 128(suppl):768, 1973.
100. Viteri AL, Greene JF Jr, Chandler JB Jr: Whipple's diseases, successful response to sulfamethoxazole-trimethoprim. *Am J Gastroenterol* 75:309, 1981.
101. Geddes AM, Ball AP, Farrell ID: Co-trimoxazole for the treatment of serious infections. *J Antimicrob Chemother* 5(suppl B):221, 1979.

102. Bengtsson E, Svanbom M, Tunevall G: Trimethoprim-sulphamethoxazole treatment in staphylococcal endocarditis and gram-negative septicemia. *Scand J Infect Dis* 6:177, 1974.

103. Scheer M, Hirschman SZ: Oral and ambulatory treatment of Listeria bacteremia and meningitis with trimethoprim-sulfamethoxazole. *Mt Sinai J Med* (*NY*) 49:411, 1982.

104. Grossman PL, Krahenbuhl JL, Remington JS: In vivo and in vitro effects of trimethoprim and sulfamethoxazole on Toxoplasma infection, in Siegenthaler W, Lüthy R (eds): *Current Chemotherapy 1.* American Society for Microbiology, Washington, DC, 1978, pp 135–137.

105. Wallace RJ, Wissk, Bushby MB, et al: In vitro activity of trimethoprim and sulfamethoxazole against nontuberculosis mycobacteria. *Rev Infect Dis* 4:326, 1982.

106. Sattler RF, Remington JS: Intravenous trimethoprim-sulfamethoxazole therapy for *Pneumocystis carinii* pneumonia. *Am J Med* 70:1215, 1981.

107. Young LS: Trimethoprim-sulfamethoxazole in the treatment of adults with pneumonia due to *Pneumocystis carinii. Rev Infect Dis* 4:608, 1982.

108. Hughes WT, Kuhn S, Chaudhary S, et al: Successful chemoprophylaxis for *Pneumocystis carinii* pneumonitis. *New Engl J Med* 267:1419, 1977.

109. Gurwith M, Brunton J, Lank B, et al: A prospective controlled investigation of prophylactic trimethoprim/sulfamethoxazole in hospitalized granulocytopenic patients. *Am J Med* 66:248, 1979.

110. Kauffman CA, Liepman MA, Bergman AG, et al: Trimethoprim/sulfamethoxazole prophylaxis in neutropenic patients: Reduction of infections and effect on bacterial and fungal flora. *Am J Med* 74:599, 1983.

111. Gualtieri RJ, Donowitz GR, Kaiser DC, et al: Double-blind randomized study of prophylactic trimethoprim/sulfamethoxazole in granulocytopenic patients with hematologic malignancies. *Am J Med* 74:934, 1983.

112. EORTC International Antimicrobial Therapy Project Group. Trimethoprim-sulfamethoxazole in the prevention of infection in neutropenic patients (in press).

113. Wade JC, Schimpff SC, Hargadon MT, et al: A comparison of trimethoprim-sulfamethoxazole plus nystatin with gentamicin plus nystatin in the prevention of infections in acute leukemia. *N Engl J Med* 304:1057, 1981.

114. Wade JC, de Jongh CA, Newman KA, et al: Selective antimicrobial modulation as prophylaxis against infection during granulocytopenia: Trimethoprim-sulfamethoxazole vs. nalidixic acid. *J Infect Dis* 147:624, 1983.

14

URINARY TRACT AGENTS: QUINOLONES, NITROFURANTOIN, AND METHENAMINE

VINCENT T. ANDRIOLE

Several antibacterial drugs are concentrated primarily in the urinary tract, that is, in the renal tubules with back diffusion into the renal parenchyma, and/or in the urine of the renal pelves and bladder. Since effective plasma concentrations are not obtained with safe doses of these agents (with the possible exceptions of norfloxacin and ciprofloxacin) they cannot be used to treat patients with systemic infections but only to treat patients with infections of the urinary tract. For this reason these drugs (nalidixic acid, oxolinic acid, cinoxacin, norfloxacin, nitrofurantoin, and methenamine) are known as urinary tract antiseptics. Ciprofloxacin, a newer quinolone, will also be available in an injectable preparation and may be used to treat systemic infections.

QUINOLONES: NALIDIXIC ACID, OXOLINIC ACID, CINOXACIN, NORFLOXACIN, AND CIPROFLOXACIN

Nalidixic acid (1-ethyl-7-methyl-1, 8-napthyridine-4-one-3-carboxylic acid) is one of a series of 1, 8 napthyridine derivatives first described by Lesher and colleagues in 1962 (1). This compound is only slightly soluble in water but is readily soluble in dilute alkali and is stable in urine. Nalidixic acid is marketed as Negram (Winthrop, 1964). Oxolinic acid (5-ethyl-5, 8-dihydro-8-oxo-1, 3-dioxolo-[4,5-g]-quinoline-7-carboxylic acid), a quinolone derivative, is a crystalline substance that is a weak organic acid (2–4). Oxolinic acid is marketed as Utibid (Warner/Chilcott, 1975). Cinoxacin [1-ethyl-1, 4-dihydro-4-oxo (1,3) dioxolo (4,5-g) cinnoline-3-carboxylic acid] is a new synthetic antibacterial agent similar to nalidixic acid (5). It is a yellow-white crystalline solid with a pKa of 4.7, which is insoluble in water and poorly lipid soluble but is soluble in alkaline solution. Cinoxacin is marketed as Cinobac (Dista/Lilly, 1981). Norfloxacin [1-ethyl-6-fluoro-1,4 dihydro-4-oxo-7-(1-piperazinyl)-3-quinoline carboxylic acid (AM 715 or MK-0366)] is another new synthetic antibacterial agent similar to nalidixic acid (5a,5b). It is a yellow white crystalline solid only slightly soluble in water. Norfloxacin is under development and it is planned for it to be marketed as Noroxin (Merck). Ciprofloxacin [1-cyclopropyl-6-fluoro-1, 4-dihydro-4-oxo-7-(1-piperazinyl)-3-quinoline carboxylic acid hydrochloride (Bay 09867)] is also a new quinolone derivative similar to nalidixic acid (5c). It is a light yellow crystalline substance slightly soluble in water. Ciprofloxacin is under development and will be marketed (Miles/Bayer). Nalidixic acid, oxolinic acid, cinoxacin, norfloxacin, and ciprofloxacin are synthetic chemotherapeutic agents and are structurally similar (Fig. 1).

Mechanism of Action

The exact mechanism of action of nalidixic acid is unknown. Early studies have shown that nalidixic acid rapidly inhibits DNA synthesis in susceptible bacterial cells, although not in mammalian cells, whereas protein and RNA synthesis continue (6). However, the exact mechanism by which nalidixic acid inhibits DNA synthesis has not been definitively determined. Inhibition of DNA synthesis by nalidixic acid has been shown to be reversible, since bacterial cells exposed to the drug will resume growth when placed in a drug-free medium (7). Nalidixic acid does not bind to purified DNA (8), nor does it inhibit those enzymes known to be involved in the synthesis of DNA precursors or in the modification of DNA (9,10). The drug has been shown to affect replication at

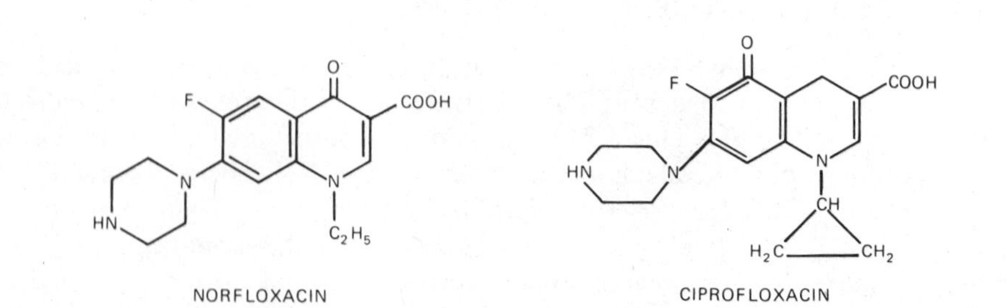

FIGURE 1. Structure of nalidixic acid, oxolinic acid, cinoxacin, norfloxacin, and ciprofloxacin.

a stage beyond the production of deoxynucleoside triphosphates and to inhibit synthesis taking place on the double stranded DNA template but not through any known enzyme involved in DNA metabolism (11). Recent studies indicate that the mode of action of nalidixic acid affects bacterial DNA topoisomerases (gyrases), of which four subunits (2α, 2β) have been defined (11a), and DNA nicking-closing enzyme (11b). The topoisomerases are required to supercoil strands of bacterial DNA into the bacterial cell.

The mechanism of action of oxolinic acid is probably similar to that of nalidixic acid. Studies emphasizing uptake of precursors labeled with ^{14}C have shown that oxolinic acid does not significantly inhibit protein, lipid, or ribonucleic acid synthesis, nor does it affect the bacterial cell membrane, but it appears to inhibit bacterial deoxyribonucleic acid synthesis (3).

The mechanism of action of cinoxacin is comparable to that of nalidixic acid. Cinoxacin inhibits DNA synthesis during bacterial replication (12,13). The mechanism of action of norfloxacin and ciprofloxacin appears to be comparable to that of nalidixic acid (5c).

Antimicrobial Activity

Nalidixic acid has greater antimicrobial activity against gram-negative rods than it does against gram-positive bacteria. It is active against most of the Enterobacteriaceae, to the extent that approximately 99 percent of the strains of *Escherichia coli,* 98 percent of *Proteus mirabilis,* 75–97 percent of other *Proteus* sp., 92 percent of *Klebsiella* and *Enterobacter* sp., and 80 percent of other coliform bacteria are sensitive to the drug at concentrations that are easily achieved in the urine, that is, 16 μg/ml or lower (1,14). Some strains of *Salmonella* and *Shigella* are also sensitive, and *Brucella* sp. may be sensitive. *Pseudomonas* sp. are resistant. Acquired resistance of sensitive gram-negative bacteria to the drug can be induced in vitro by serial passage of these bacteria in increasing concentrations of nalidixic acid (15), but it does not seem to be transferable. Resistance may also be acquired during treatment of bacteriuria, so repeat urine culture and sensitivity testing are of practical clinical importance (16). Gram-positive bacteria including *Staphylococcus aureus, Streptococcus pneumoniae,* and *Streptococcus faecalis* are resistant to nalidixic acid (1,14).

The antibacterial spectrum of activity of oxolinic acid is similar to that of nalidixic acid in that it is primarily active against gram-negative bacteria with the exception of *Pseudomonas* sp. Oxolinic acid is significantly more active than nalidixic acid in vitro and is two to four times more active in vivo (2). Oxolinic acid inhibits 95 percent of the strains of *E. coli,* 92 percent of *P. mirabilis,* 89 percent of other *Proteus* sp., 91 percent of other coliform bacteria, and 64 percent of *Klebsiella-Enterobacter* isolates, at concentrations of 1.56 μg/ml or less (17). Although *Klebsiella-Enterobacter* isolates are less susceptible, 93 percent are inhibited by 6.25 μg/ml, an amount of oxolinic acid easily achieved in urine (17). *Neisseria gonorrhoeae* and *Neisseria meningitidis* are also inhibited at concentrations of 0.01–0.19 μg/ml of the drug (2). Except for *S. aureus* strains that are inhibited at concentrations of 6.25 μg/ml, oxolinic acid has no significant activity against other gram-positive bacteria or fungi (2). Sensitive gram-negative bacteria can acquire resistance to oxolinic acid in a stepwise manner in vitro similar to that observed with nalidixic acid. Cross resistance between these two agents has been demonstrated, that is, oxolinic acid-resistant strains are also resistant to nalidixic acid and vice versa. Also resistance is not reversed in vitro even after 10–12 consecutive passages in drug-free media (3). As with nalidixic acid, resistance to oxolinic acid may also be acquired during treatment of patients with bacteriuria so follow-up urine culture and sensitivity testing are clinically important (18).

The antibacterial spectrum of activity of cinoxacin, although similar to that of nalidixic acid, is somewhat greater against some bacterial species (5,19). However, the activity of cinoxacin appears to be somewhat less than that of oxolinic acid (20). Cinoxacin is active against most strains of gram-negative bacteria that cause urinary tract infections at concentrations that are readily attained in the urine. Cinoxacin is most active against *E. coli* and inhibits more than 90 percent of strains at a concentration of 16 μg/ml. It is active against all *Proteus* sp. and most strains of *Klebsiella, Enterobacter, Citrobacter, Providencia,* and *Serratia* sp. Cinoxacin also demonstrates in vitro activity against *Salmonella, Shigella, Alcaligenes, Acinetobacter, Moraxella,* and *Hemophilus* sp., as well as against *Clostridium perfringens, Clostridium tetani, N. meningitidis,* and *Pseudomonas pseudomallei.* Cinoxacin has negligible activity against *Pseudomonas aeruginosa* and gram-positive cocci such as *S. aureus, Staphylococcus saphrophyticus, Streptococci* sp., and enterococci (5,19,20,21). Cross resistance among bacterial isolates develops among cinoxacin, naladixic acid, and oxolinic acid (12,20). Resistance to cinoxacin of organisms that are usually susceptible can be induced in vitro and is mediated presumably via chromosomes, since there is no evidence that resistance is transferred as an extrachromosomal plasmid (13).

Norfloxacin is 100 times more active than nalidixic acid, with a spectrum that includes enterococci and staphylococci as well as *Pseudomonas* (5a). Norfloxacin is active against most strains of gram-negative and gram-positive bacteria that cause urinary tract infections at concentrations that are readily attained in the urine. Norfloxacin inhibits more than 90 percent of strains of *E. coli* at a concentration of 0.2 μg/ml, *Klebsiella* species at 0.4 μg/ml, *Salmonella* and *Shigella* species at 0.1 μg/ml, *Citrobacter* species at 0.4 μg/ml, *Enterobacter cloacae* at 0.2 μg/ml, *Enterobacter aerogenes* at 0.4 μg/ml, *Enterobacter agglomerans* at 0.2 μg/ml, *Proteus mirabilis* at 0.1 μg/ml, *Morganella* species at 0.2 μg/ml, *Proteus vulgaris* at 0.8 μg/ml, *Proteus rettgeri* at 0.3 μg/ml, *Providencia* species at 1.6 μg/ml, *Pseudomonas aeruginosa,* including gentamicin-resistant strains, at 0.8 μg/ml, *Pseudomonas maltophilia* at 3.1 μg/ml, *Serratia marcescens* at 3.1 μg/ml, *Acinetobacter calcoaceticus* at 6.3 μg/ml, and *Yersinia, Arizona, Aeromonas,* and *Campylobacter* at concentrations below 1 μg/ml. Norfloxacin is also active against *Hemophilus influenzae* at concentrations of 0.12 μg/ml and *Neisseria gonorrhoeae,* regardless of β-lactamase activity, at 0.016 μg/ml. Norfloxacin is somewhat less active against gram-positive species, with 90 percent of strains of *Staphylococcus aureus* inhibited at concentrations of 1.6 μg/ml, methicillin-resistant strains of *S. aureus* at 4.0 μg/ml, *S. saprophyticus* at 4 μg/ml, *S. epidermidis* at 1 μg/ml, *Streptococcus pyogenes* at 6.3 μg/ml, *Streptococcus agalactiae* at 3.1 μg/ml, *Streptococcus faecalis* at 12.5 μg/ml, *Streptococcus pneumoniae* at 4 μg/ml, and *Listeria* species at 3.1 μg/ml. Members of the *Bacteroides fragilis* group of anaerobes are relatively resistant to norfloxacin, since they are inhibited at concentrations of 8 to 128 μg/ml, as are most other anaerobes. Norfloxacin has some activity against *Gardnerella vaginalis,* inhibiting 90 percent of isolates at 32 μg/ml, and *Ureaplasma urealyticum* at concentrations of 8 mg/ml (5b,21a–e).

Ciprofloxacin, though similar in antibacterial activity, is even more potent than norfloxacin. Ciprofloxacin is active against most strains of gram-negative and gram-positive bacteria that cause urinary tract infections at concentrations that are easily attained in the urine. Ciprofloxacin inhibits more than 90 percent of strains of *E. coli* at a concentration of 0.06 μg/ml, *Klebsiella* species at 0.25 μg/ml, *Salmonella* and *Shigella* species at 0.015 and 0.008 μg/ml, respectively, *Citrobacter diversus* at 0.03 μg/ml, *Citrobacter freundii* at 0.125 μg/ml, *Enterobacter cloacae* at 0.03 μg/ml, *Enterobacter aerogenes* at 0.06 μg/ml, *Proteus mirabilis* at 0.06 μg/ml, *Proteus vulgaris* at 0.06 μg/ml, *Morganella morganii* at 0.016 μg/ml, *Providencia stuartii* at 0.5 μg/ml, *Pseudomonas aeruginosa* at 0.25 μg/ml, *Pseudomonas maltophilia* at 4 μg/ml, *Pseudomonas cepacia* at 8 μg/ml, *Serratia marcescens* at 0.13 μg/ml, *Acinetobacter calcoaceticus* at 0.5 μg/ml, *Yersinia enterocolitica* at 0.06 μg/ml, *Aeromonas hydrophilia* at 0.008 μg/ml, and *Pasteurella multocida* at 0.016 μg/ml. Ciprofloxacin is also active against *H. influenzae* at concentrations of 0.015 μg/ml and *Neisseria gonorrhoeae,* regardless of β-lactamase activity, at 0.004 μg/ml. In contrast to norfloxacin, ciprofloxacin is more active against *Bacteroides fragilis,* with 90 percent of strains inhibited at concentrations of 4 μg/ml. Similarly, ciprofloxacin is more active than norfloxacin against gram-positive bacteria, with 90 percent of strains of *Staphylococcus aureus,* including methicillin-resistant strains, inhibited at concentrations of 0.5 μg/ml, *Staphylococcus epidermidis* at 0.25 μg/ml, *Streptococcus pyogenes* at 0.2 μg/ml, *Streptococcus agalactiae* at 1 μg/ml, *Streptococcus faecalis* at 2 μg/ml, *Streptococcus pneumoniae* at 2 μg/ml, viridans streptococci at 4 μg/ml, and *Listeria monocytogenes* at 1 μg/ml. Compared to norfloxacin, ciprofloxacin has increased activity against all bacterial species studied. Ciprofloxacin has excellent activity against *Chlamydia trachomatis,* inhibiting 90 percent of isolates at 1 μg/ml (5c, 21f–i).

Pharmacology

Nalidixic acid is administered by the oral route and is almost completely (96 percent) absorbed from the gastrointestinal tract (22). It is rapidly metabolized in the liver to hydroxynalidixic acid that is biologically active and to antibacterially inactive monoglucoronide conjugates both of which, along with the parent compound, are rapidly excreted by the kidney into the urine. The biologically active drug in the plasma consists of the hydroxylated metabolite (one-third) and the parent compound (two-thirds), which are 63 percent and 93 percent, respectively, bound to plasma proteins (23). Plasma levels of 20–50 μg/ml may be attained 2 hours after a single oral dose of 1 g of the drug (24). The drug does not accumulate in tissues even after prolonged administration, and the kidney is the only organ in which tissue concentrations may exceed plasma levels (22). Nalidixic acid does not distribute into prostatic fluid (25). It will appear in human milk of lactating mothers and therefore may be harmful to the newborn (26). Excretion is almost completely via the kidney into the urine. About 85 percent of the drug in the urine is in the conjugated inactive form. Most of the remainder is present as biologically active hydroxynalidixic acid, which is 16 times more active than the parent compound, nalidixic acid, and is primarily responsible for the therapeutic effect of this drug in the treatment of urinary tract infection (23). Urine concentrations of the active drug, following a 0.5–1.0-g single oral dose in adults, range from 25 to 250 μg/ml and remain between 100 and 500 μg/ml with a 1-g oral dose administered every 6 hours (15,24). Bactericidal levels of the drug are also attained in the urine of patients with moderate or advanced renal failure (24). The antibacterially active component of the drug does not accumulate in the serum of azotemic patients during continuous therapy (24) as do the inactive monoglucuronides that may also contribute to toxicity (27). Although increased toxicity has not been observed in patients with advanced renal failure given usual doses of nalidixic acid, the drug should be used cautiously in these patients as well as in patients with liver disease, since conjugation of the drug may be impaired in this latter group.

Oxolinic acid is also administered orally after which active and inactive metabolites are excreted in the urine and eliminated in the feces. Plasma levels of oxolinic acid after oral administration are low or borderline with respect to antimicrobic activity against susceptible bacteria. An effective bactericidal concentration for most susceptible microorganisms is achieved in the urine within 4 hours and is sustained for 12 hours after the recommended oral dose. The concentration of oxolinic acid attained in 24-hour urine collections after an oral dose of 2 g/day averaged 38 μg/ml with a range of 16–64 μg/ml (28). Although oxolinic acid given to patients with moderate or advanced renal failure did not further impair or damage the kidney nor interfere with the drug's renal excretion, it should be used cautiously in patients with severely impaired renal function. Since oxolinic acid is excreted in human milk, it is contraindicated in nursing mothers.

Cinoxacin is also administered orally and is rapidly and almost completely absorbed from the gastrointestinal tract. Peak plasma levels usually occur in 2–3 hours and are in the range of <4–14.8 and 2.8–28 μg/ml after an oral dose of 250 and 500 mg, respectively. Approximately 70 percent of cinoxacin is bound to plasma proteins. It has a serum half-life of approximately 1 hour, which may increase threefold in patients with creatinine clearances of less than 30 m/min/1.73 m^2. Although the concomitant ingestion of food delays the absorption of cinoxacin and causes a 30 percent reduction in mean peak plasma levels, the overall recovery of the drug in urine is not affected significantly. Peak urine concentrations in the range of 88–925 μg/ml occur within 4–6 hours and are decreased in patients with impaired renal function. Cinoxacin concentrations in human prostatic tissue range from 0.6 to 6.3 μg/g, whereas concentrations in renal tissue exceed those in serum (29). Approximately 60 percent of an orally administered dose is excreted into the urine unchanged in patients with normal renal function, whereas about 40 percent is metabolized by the liver. Urine metabolism studies have shown that in addition to the parent compound, cinoxacin is metabolized to at least four microbiologically inactive metabolites that represent approximately 30–40 percent of the ingested dose (30). The renal clearance of cinoxacin exceeds the glomerular filtration rate, and probenecid inhibits cinoxacin excretion by the kidney. These observations suggest that this drug is excreted by both glomerular filtration and tubular secretion (31). Also, changes in urinary pH do not appear to influence cinoxacin excretion significantly. It is not known whether cinoxacin is excreted into human milk. Because other drugs in this class are excreted into human milk and because of the potential for serious adverse reactions from cinoxacin in nursing infants, the drug should not be used in nursing women.

Norfloxacin is also administered orally and is readily absorbed from the gastrointestinal tract. Peak plasma levels usually occur 1 to 2 hours after each dose and are in the range of 0.75, 1.58, 2.41, 3.15, and 3.87 μg/ml for doses of 200, 400, 800, 1200, and 1600 mg, respectively. The elimination half-life of norfloxacin is about 7 hours and is similar for all doses studied. Concentrations of norfloxacin in urine also peak at 1 to 2 hours after dosage. Mean peak values for increasing doses of norfloxacin (200, 400, 800, 1200, and 1600 mg) are 200, 478, 697, 992, and 1045 μg/ml, respectively. Renal clearances approximate 285 ml/min. Approximately 30 percent of each dose is excreted into urine as unmetabolized norfloxacin, with lesser quantities of glucuronide conjugate and six active metabolites with modifications in the piperazine ring being excreted. Crystals of norfloxacin are occasionally observed during microscopic examination of freshly voided urine collected after the 1200 and 1600 mg doses. However, crystalluria is not encountered at lower doses (31a). It is not known whether norfloxacin is excreted into human milk.

Ciprofloxacin is also administered orally and is rapidly absorbed from the gastrointestinal tract. Peak plasma levels usually occur in 1 to 1.5 hours and are approximately 2 μg/ml after an oral dose of 500 mg. Approximately 36 percent of ciprofloxacin is bound to plasma proteins. It has a serum half-life of approximately 3.9 hours. Peak urine concentrations occur within 4 hours. Approximately 20 percent of the administered dose can be recovered as active drug in the urine during the first 4 hours, an additional 5 percent between 4 to 8 hours, 3 percent more between 8 to 12 hours, and an additional 2 percent between 12 to 24 hours. Thus, 30 percent of active drug is recovered in the urine during a period of 24 hours. Ciprofloxacin also penetrates blister fluid well, with 57 percent of the serum concentration recoverable. Also, the concentration of ciprofloxacin in blister fluid exceeds that in serum about 3 hours after administration (31b). It is not known whether ciprofloxacin is excreted into human milk. A parenteral preparation of ciprofloxacin is also available and is currently under investigation.

Toxicity and Adverse Reactions

Oral nalidixic acid is usually well tolerated although a number of adverse reactions have been reported.

Gastrointestinal side effects include nausea, vomiting, diarrhea, and abdominal pain.

Dermatologic reactions include pruritis, nonspecific rashes, and urticaria associated with eosinophilia, as well as photosensitivity reactions involving skin surfaces exposed to sunlight that are most commonly manifested as a sunburn and rarely as a bullous eruption (32–34). Patients receiving the drug should be cautioned to avoid excessive exposure to direct sunlight.

Ophthalmologic side effects include blurred vision, diplopia, photophobia, abnormal accommodation, and changes in color perception, all of which disappear with cessation of therapy.

Central nervous system reactions include headaches, drowsiness, asthenia, giddiness, vertigo, syncope, sensory changes, grand mal seizures, and acute reversible toxic psychosis (35–37), as well as pseudotumor cerebri with intracranial hypertension, papilledema, and bulging fontanelles in infants and young children (38–41), which reverses after cessation of therapy. Also, convulsions, hyperglycemia, and glycosuria without abnormal serum ketones has been reported in one patient who took an overdose of nalidixic acid (42). Therefore, the drug should not be given to patients with convulsive disorders, preexisting mental instability, parkinsonism, or cerebral vascular insufficiency, nor to infants or pregnant women in the first trimester, and it probably should not be used in children.

Nalidixic acid has rarely been associated with blood dyscrasias and hemolytic anemia that sometimes is associated with glucose-6-phosphate dehydrogenase (G6PD) deficient red blood cells (26,43). The drug has also rarely been associated with cholestatic jaundice and possibly may precipitate acute respiratory failure in patients with impaired respiratory function (44).

Oxolinic acid has been associated frequently with excitative central nervous system responses, which include restlessness, insomnia, nervousness, dizziness, headache, and nausea (22). This potential is increased in elderly patients and is more common with oxolinic acid than with nalidixic acid. Less frequent reactions include abdominal pain, vomiting, anorexia, diarrhea, constipation, pruritis, and weakness. Abnormal liver function tests and reduced leucocyte counts have also been observed. Rare reactions include photophobia, palpitations, swelling of extremities, reduction in hematocrit or hemoglobin values, eosinophilia, urticaria, rash, soreness of mouth and gums, and metallic taste. A seizure occurred in one patient with known epilepsy, and hallucinations and hysteria occurred in one patient who received a larger dose than recommended. All reactions are reversible with cessation of treatment.

Oral cinoxacin is well tolerated, and adverse reactions occur infrequently (4.4 percent) and are reversible (31). Gastrointestinal reactions are the most common side effects, and nausea is the most frequent (3 percent of patients), followed by vomiting, anorexia, abdominal cramps, and diarrhea. The frequency of adverse central nervous system reactions is less than 1 percent. These consist of headache, dizziness, insomnia, paresthesias, perineal burning, photophobia, and tinnitus. Hypersensitivity reactions (less than 3 percent) include urticaria, morbilliform rash, pruritis, and edema. Abnormal liver [serum glutamic-oxaloacetic transaminase (SGOT), serum glutamic-pyruvic transaminase (SGPT), and alkaline phosphatase] and renal [blood urea nitrogen (BUN) and serum creatinine] function values have been observed in less than 1 percent of patients who have received cinoxacin. This drug should be used with caution in patients with a history of liver disease. Also, the use of cinoxacin in prepubertal children and during pregnancy is not recommended.

Drug Interactions

Nalidixic acid glucuronide conjugates may produce a false-positive reaction for urine glucose when tested with Benedict's solution such as Clinites, but not with glucose oxidase test strips such as Clinistix. Diabetic patients treated with this drug should be so alerted. Nitrofurantoin interferes with the therapeutic action of nalidixic acid.

The safety of the concomitant use of oxolinic acid and other central nervous system stimulants has not been established. Also, oxolinic acid may enhance the effects of the oral anticoagulants, bishydroxycoumarin and warfarin, by displacing these drugs from serum albumin-binding sites. Nitrofurantoin also interferes with the therapeutic action of oxolinic acid (45).

NITROFURANTOIN

Nitrofurantoin, *O*-(5-nitrofurfurylideneamino)-hydantoin, is one of a series of synthetic nitrofuran compounds that belong to a class of organic substances characterized by a heterocyclic ring consisting of four carbon atoms and one oxygen atom (Fig. 2). This compound has been available for clinical use in a microcrystalline form since 1953 and is marketed as Furadantin (Eaton). Since nitrofurantoin is of limited solubility in water, a macrocrystalline form of the drug was prepared in 1967 and is marketed as Macrodantin (Eaton).

Mechanism of Action

The precise mechanism of action of nitrofurantoin is not known, although there is evidence that the drug inhibits a variety of enzyme systems in bacteria (46). Nitrofurans can also enter mammalian cells and have been shown to affect several enzymes in these cells, the most notable of which is to arrest spermatogen-

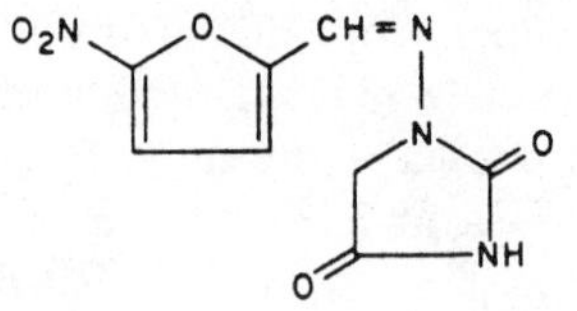

FIGURE 2. Structure of nitrofurantoin.

esis in animals (47). Also, at high local concentrations nitrofurantoin immobilizes human sperm (48).

Antimicrobial Activity

Nitrofurantoin is active against a wide spectrum of gram-positive and gram-negative bacteria and particularly against many strains of the common urinary tract pathogens (Table 1).

Bacterial species with a minimum inhibitory concentration (MIC) of 32 μg/ml or less of nitrofurantoin are considered sensitive since this concentration of the drug can easily be achieved in the urine with usual therapeutic doses. *Escherichia coli* are very sensitive (96 percent) to nitrofurantoin at this concentration, as are other coliform bacteria (68 percent), whereas *Enterobacter* and *Klebsiella* sp. are less susceptible (36 percent) (49). The majority of *Proteus* sp. (92 percent) are moderately resistant, and *P. aeruginosa* is almost always resistant (49). The usual minimum inhibitory concentration of nitrofurantoin for *E. coli* is 16 μg/ml, whereas *Enterobacter* and *Klebsiella* sp. may require 100 μg/ml, and *P. mirabilis,* 200 μg/ml (49). The drug is also active against staphylococci and enterococci, and the minimum inhibitory concentrations are lower, 4.0 μg/ml for *S. aureus* and 25.0 μg/ml for *S. faecalis* (46). Salmonellae, shigellae, and *Neisseria* sp. are also susceptible to nitrofurantoin, as are *S. pyogenes, S. pneumoniae,* and *Corynebacterium* sp., including *C. diphtheriae,* but their susceptibility to the drug is of little practical importance (46). In contrast to nalidixic and oxolonic acid, microorganisms sensitive to nitrofurantoin do not readily become resistant to this drug.

Pharmacology

Nitrofurantoin is usually administered orally and is rapidly and completely absorbed from the gastrointestinal tract. The drug crosses the blood-brain and the placental barrier. Only very low levels of antibacterial activity are attained in serum after usual oral doses of the drug, and nitrofurantoin does not accumulate in the serum of patients with normal renal function when given continuously in recommended doses. Also therapeutically active concentrations of the drug are not attained in most body tissues. The serum half-life is about 20 minutes in patients with normal renal function because about two-thirds of the drug is rapidly metabolized in tissues with inactivation apparently occurring in all body

TABLE 1. Nitrofurantoin Antibacterial Spectrum In Vitro

Gram-positive organisms
Bacillus subtilis
Corynebacterium sp. (diphtheroids)
Staphylococcus aureus
Streptococcus faecalis
Gram-negative organisms
Enterobacter aerogenes
Alcaligenes faecalis
Escherichia coli
Klebsiella pneumoniae
Proteus mirabilis
Proteus morganii
Proteus rettgeri
Proteus vulgaris
Pseudomonas aeruginosa

tissues although the liver may play a major role (50). One-third of the drug is rapidly excreted into the urine by both glomerular filtration and tubular secretion with significant reabsorption when the urine is acid (50). Nitrofurantoin acts as a weak acid, so in an acid urine more of the drug is in the undissociated form and more of the drug is reabsorbed, with less appearing in the urine. In an alkaline urine, more of the drug is in the dissociated or ionized form, little of the drug is reabsorbed, and more appears in the urine (51), but the antibacterial efficacy is decreased (11). Therefore, the urine should not be alkalinized. Nitrofurantoin has been shown to diffuse into the interstitial tissue of the renal medulla (52) and to be present in higher concentrations in the lymphatics draining the medulla than in serum (53). Since one-third of an orally administered dose of the drug is excreted unchanged (i.e., in a therapeutically active form) into the urine (50), an average dose of nitrofurantoin yields a urine concentration of approximately 200 (range 50–250) $\mu g/ml$ in patients with normal renal function. (Nitrofurantoin may color the urine brown.) However, recovery of the drug from the urine is linearly related to creatinine clearance so the concentration of the drug in the urine of uremic patients may be insufficient to inhibit common urinary tract pathogens when the glomerular filtration rate is less than 30 ml/min (54). Furthermore, nitrofurantoin accumulates in the serum of patients with creatinine clearances of less than 60 ml/min (54), and blood levels may range between 5 and 6.5 $\mu g/ml$ in severe uremia (55), which increases the danger of developing systemic toxicity particularly peripheral neuropathy (56). Although nitrofurantoin is removed by hemodialysis, it is contraindicated in patients with significant renal impairment, as well as in newborn and premature infants who may also develop toxic blood levels.

The macrocrystalline form of nitrofurantoin (Macrodantin) was introduced to delay absorption from the gastrointestinal tract. Since nitrofurantoin is of limited solubility in water, an increase in size of the drug particles might significantly retard its solution rate in, and consequently its absorption from, the alimentary tract. Delaying the drug's entrance into body fluids was hoped to lower its peak serum concentration and to decrease the incidence and severity of nausea and vomiting without significantly affecting its concentration in the urinary tract (57). Studies on humans have shown that although the urinary excretion of the macrocrystals is prolonged, there is no difference between macrocrystals and fine particles in the percentage of dose recovered from the urine. The macrocrystalline form results in maximum urinary concentrations of about 150 μg/ml after a dose of 100 mg and is probably associated with a lower incidence of side effects and better patient tolerance than the microcrystalline form (58). The mechanism of action, antimicrobic activity, and pharmacology of the macrocrystalline form is otherwise similar to conventional microcrystalline nitrofurantoin.

Toxicity and Adverse Reactions

Gastrointestinal irritation is the most common side effect of nitrofurantoin therapy, particularly anorexia, nausea, and vomiting, which may be controlled by reduction in dosage or by concomitant administration of food or milk, although sometimes it is severe enough to require discontinuation of the drug. Diarrhea and abdominal pain occur less frequently. Gastrointestinal intolerance appears to occur less frequently in patients receiving nitrofurantoin macrocrystals than in those receiving microcrystalline tablets (58). The crystalline and macrocrystalline forms are therapeutically equivalent.

Hypersensitivity reactions occur occasionally and may involve the skin, lungs, blood, and liver. Also chills, drug fever, arthralgia, a lupus erythematosis syndrome, and anaphylaxis have been observed.

Dermatologic allergic manifestations include maculopapular, erythematous, or eczematous rashes, urticaria, angioneurotic edema, and pruritis and usually subside when the drug is stopped (46). Pulmonary reactions include asthmatic attacks in patients with a history of asthma, as well as acute, subacute, or chronic reactions. Acute pneumonitis is commonly manifested by the sudden onset of fever, chills, cough, dyspnea, chest pain, pulmonary infiltration with consolidation or pleural effusion on x-ray films, and eosinophilia (59). This syndrome is more common in elderly patients, and the symptoms usually occur within the first week of treatment but may become evident within hours or days or in some cases after a prolonged period after starting nitrofurantoin therapy. This pneumonitis is probably immunologically mediated and is rapidly reversible with cessation of therapy. Corticosteroid treatment may be beneficial and necessary in severe cases (60). The syndrome rapidly recurs after rechallenge with the drug (61), and there is some evidence that cell-mediated immunity is implicated in this type of nitrofurantoin sensitivity (62). In *subacute* pneumonitis the symptoms are more insidious, fever and eosinophilia are observed less often, and recovery may be slower. *Chronic* pulmonary reactions are rare and usually occur in patients on continuous therapy for 6 months or more. Insidious onset of malaise, dyspnea on exertion, cough, altered pulmonary function, and roentgenographic and histologic findings of interstitial fibrosis with or without interstitial pneumonitis are common (63,64). Fever is rarely prominent. This syndrome may also have an immunologic basis. In some cases improvement occurs with cessation of nitrofurantoin and institution of steroid therapy. However, the severity of this reaction and the degree of resolution appear to be related to the amount of time therapy is continued after the onset of clinical signs and symptoms. Permanently impaired pulmonary function may occur even after the drug is discontinued, especially when the syndrome is not recognized early.

Hematologic reactions include leukopenia, granulocytopenia, eosinophilia, megaloblastic anemia, and hemolytic anemia. Megaloblastic anemia is rare and appears to be due to folic acid deficiency, particularly when repeated courses of the drug are used (65). Nitrofurantoin can precipitate an acute hemolytic anemia in patients with glucose-6-phosphate dehydrogenase deficient red blood cells, which is found in 10 percent of blacks and a small percentage of Mediterranean and Near-Eastern ethnic groups. Also the drug should not be given to infants with immature red cell enzyme systems.

Hepatotoxic reactions are very rare and include cholestatic jaundice with prodromal fever, rash and eosinophilia (66), and hepatocellular damage (67).

Neurologic reactions include headache, drowsiness, dizziness, nystagmus, which is readily reversible, and peripheral polyneuropathy. This peripheral neuritis is an ascending sensorimotor neuropathy, which may be progressive if the drug is continued and is one of the most serious side effects of nitrofurantoin therapy (68). Although it occurs more commonly in patients with renal failure (56), it also occurs in patients with normal blood urea nitrogen levels and low creatinine clearances (69), as well as in patients, especially the elderly, with normal renal function who receive prolonged courses of nitrofurantoin. The mechanism is unknown (70), but demyelination and degeneration of both sensory and motor nerves occur. The drug should be stopped at the earliest signs of neuritis such as paresthesiae.

Transient alopecia may occur. Also, a 17-month-old infant who received nitrofurantoin for 68 days developed permanent yellow discoloration of those teeth that erupted during therapy (71).

Drug Interactions

Nitrofurantoin antagonizes the action of nalidixic acid.

METHENAMINE

Methenamine (hexamethylenetetramine, hexamethyleneamine, hexamine) is a tertiary amine and has the properties of a monoacidic base in its salt formation and can be combined with an unlimited number of organic and inorganic compounds. It is a colorless, odorless compound that is readily soluble in water, forming weakly basic solutions of pH 8.0–8.5. Its chemical structure is shown in Figure 3.

Methenamine was introduced by Nicolaier in 1895 for the treatment of urinary infections (72) and is available, as the pure base, in 0.5-g tablets as methenamine, *National Formulary* (NF) (Lilly). Methenamine has also been combined with mandelic acid, apparently because of Rosenheim's observations in 1935 (73) that mandelic acid is excreted in the urine unchanged and, when given in large doses, renders the urine bactericidal. The combination of methenamine and mandelic acid is marketed as methenamine mandelate under the trade name Mandelamine (Warner-Chilcott). Methenamine has also been combined with hippuric acid to form the salt methenamine hippurate, and this combination is marketed as Hiprex (Merrell-National) and Urex (Riker).

Mechanism of Action

Methenamine itself is not bactericidal nor, regardless of concentration, is it antibacterial in alkaline solutions. Its mechanism of action is due to its hydrolysis, at acid pH, to ammonia and formaldehyde according to the following reaction:

$$N_4(CH_2)_6 + 6H_2O + 4H^+ \rightleftarrows 4NH_4^+ + 6HCHO$$

Formaldehyde is the active degradation product of methenamine (72) and can only be liberated from methenamine at a pH below 7.0 (74), for example, 6 percent is yielded at pH 6 and 20 percent at pH 5. Only two body fluids, gastric juice and urine, are capable of releasing formaldehyde from methenamine (74–77). Although methenamine has no antimicrobial activity in the presence of alkaline fluids, formaldehyde is equally bactericidal at acid and alkaline pHs (76). Nevertheless, the degradation of methenamine to formaldehyde is entirely dependent on two factors: proper acidification of the urine and time for hydrolysis of methenamine to occur. Furthermore, the ultimate antibacterial effect of methe-

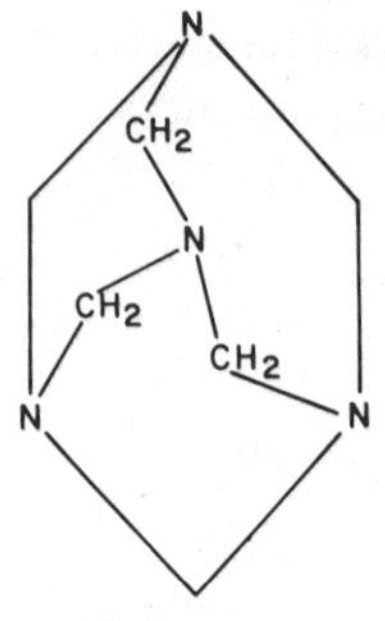

FIGURE 3. Structure of methenamine.

namine, that is, through the generation of formaldehyde, is also dependent on the concentration of methenamine in the urine, as well as on the urine pH and the time the drug remains in the urine (78,79). Specifically, at an average urinary methenamine concentration of 0.75 mg/ml and in a quite acid urine (pH 5.0–5.5), at least 1 hour is needed to generate approximately 25 μg/ml of free formaldehyde, 2 hours more reliably produces bactericidal levels of free formaldehyde, and 3 hours is required to reach 90 percent of the final equilibrium (79). Low concentrations of methenamine in the urine are inadequate to generate bactericial levels of free formaldehyde regardless of urine pH and time (79).

Since the proper function of methenamine is dependent on an acid urine, various poorly metabolized acids have been used to acidify the urine putatively during therapy with methenamine. The acids most commonly used are mandelic acid, hippuric acid, ascorbic acid, and acid-producing foods such as cranberry juice. Also, low pH alone is bacteriostatic so acidification could possibly serve a double function. Furthermore, mandelic acid and hippuric acid are bacteriostatic in vitro aside from their effect on pH. These organic acids inhibit the metabolism of bacteria by means of their un-ionized molecules (80). For these reasons, these acids are widely thought to contribute to the lowering of urinary pH, as well as to producing an antibacterial effect in urine, which, if true, would be an advantage. However, it is important to emphasize that to achieve this effect, that is, bacteriostasis, in urine it is necessary to administer these acids (mandelic, hippuric, ascorbic, and cranberry juice) in prohibitively large doses, otherwise the urine is not rendered inhibitory. Equally important is that the prepared combinations of the methenamine salts of organic acids, methenamine mandelate and hippurate, when given as currently recommended, contain only a fraction of the dosage of the organic acid (mandelic or hippuric) that is required to either exert an antibacterial effect in the urine or to influence the pH of the urine. Unfortunately, there is little evidence that the acid forms (mandelic or hippuric) of the methenamine salt contribute in any way to the antibacterial activity of methenamine (81). Fortunately, in most circumstances normal urine, in the absence of diuresis, is sufficiently acid to liberate free formaldehyde from methenamine (82).

Antimicrobial Activity

Methenamine, through the liberation of free formaldehyde into the urine, is active against all gram-positive and gram-negative bacteria and also against fungi. Almost all bacteria are susceptible to free formaldehyde at about the same concentration, that is, 20 μg/ml (81). However, urinary tract infections due to urea-splitting organisms such as *Proteus* sp. may not respond to methenamine because it is difficult to acidify the urine in the presence of these infections, and free formaldehyde is not liberated. Significant resistance cannot be induced in vitro (83) and is not a problem with methenamine because bacteria and fungi do not become resistant to formaldehyde.

Pharmacology

Methenamine, methenamine mandelate, and hippurate are rapidly absorbed from the gastrointestinal tract, but 10–30 percent is hydrolyzed by the gastric juice in the stomach unless the drug is protected by enteric coating. Because of the ammonia produced, methenamine is contraindicated in patients with hepatic insufficiency. Antimicrobial activity is not achieved in the blood since methenamine does not liberate formaldehyde in serum, and mandelic or hippuric acid serum levels are too low to produce any antibacterial effect. Methenamine distributes widely into body fluids, since it is distributed through total body water including that of red blood cells; cerebrospinal, synovial, and pericardial fluids; and both aqueous and vitreous humors of the eye (74). Only methenamine, not formaldehyde, is present in these body fluids since almost no formaldehyde is generated at physiologic pH, so there is no antibacterial activity in tissues, body fluids, or blood. Methenamine is rapidly excreted into urine. Its clearance from the blood is considerably less than glomerular filtration rate (84), and its half-life in blood is quite long. Also, in the presence of an optimally acid urine, only 2–20 percent of the methenamine present is converted to free formaldehyde. Over 90 percent of an administered dose will be excreted into the urine within 24 hours. Although some antibacterial activity may be demonstrated within half an hour, adequate antibacterial activity through the generation of sufficient formaldehyde does not occur, even in a properly acid urine (pH 5.0–5.5), until at least 1 hour, and more likely 2 hours, after the administration of methenamine. This antibacterial activity is not found in urine from the renal pelvis or ureter but only in bladder urine because the transit time down the renal tubules, calyces, and pelvis into the bladder is too short to allow generation of significant amounts of formaldehyde (75,81,85). Exceptions may occur in extremely dehydrated patients with highly acid urine or in those with some degree of obstructive renal residual urine. The antibacterial activity in bladder urine may be maintained for at least 6 hours or until the patient voids, after which hydrolysis of new methenamine will have to occur to render newly formed urine bactericidal (81). It is probably best not to force fluids in a patient receiving methenamine because a diuretic urine may be more alkaline, and diuresis may reduce the concentration of free formaldehyde to a noninhibitory (<20 μg/ml) level. Except for urine, so little methenamine decomposes in body fluids and tissues that it is virtually nontoxic systemically, and renal insufficiency is no contraindication to methenamine alone. Also, since the acidifying ability of the renal tubules functions in azotemia, these patients can convert methenamine to formaldehyde. However, the acid salts are contraindicated, and methenamine mandelate may precipitate crystalluria.

Toxicity

Methenamine is usually well tolerated, as are both the methenamine salts, mandelate and hippurate, but some patients develop gastrointestinal side effects such as gastric distress, nausea, vomiting, and diarrhea. Some patients complain of bladder irritation, with dysuria, frequency, albuminuria, and hematuria, particularly with high doses or prolonged administration. Various rashes may also occur. The methenamine salts should be avoided in patients with gout because these drugs may precipitate urate crystals in the urine.

Drug Interactions

Methenamine combines with sulfamethizole and possibly other sulfonamides in the urine, which results in mutual antagonism.

MAJOR USES AND DOSAGE

In addition to the general uses and doses described in Table 2, these urinary tract agents have also been used as prophylactic and suppressive agents in patients with recurrent urinary tract infections, as well as in catheterized patients with bacteriuria and in chronically infected patients with neurogenic bladders on long-term indwelling catheter drainage. Nalidixic acid has been used as long-term therapy for frequently recurrent bacteriuria in adults, as well as in children with bacteriuria associated with urinary tract abnormalities (16,86). The follow-up cure rate was disappointingly similar to that observed with other antimicrobial agents, and resistance to nalidixic acid commonly emerged during treatment (16). Nitrofurantoin has also been used for long-term suppressive therapy, particularly during pregnancy and in children with persistent or frequently recurrent bacteriuria, with reasonably good results (87,88). In contrast to nalidixic acid, bacterial resistance was not a problem with nitrofurantoin. Methenamine has also been used successfully as prophylactic therapy in men with recurrent bacteriuria (89), as well as in patients with recurrent bacteriuria caused by multiply antibiotic-resistant gram-negative bacilli or by yeasts, because these pathogens are susceptible to formaldehyde (11,84,90). In addition, it has been successfully used as a prophylactic agent in otherwise healthy girls and women who have recurring urinary tract infection in the absence of structural abnormalities of the urinary tract (90,91), although it does not appear to be as effective as trimethoprim-sulfamethoxazole administered once daily in these patients (91). In short, nitrofurantoin, methenamine, or trimethoprim-sulfamethoxazole appear to be the better agents as compared with nalidixic or oxolinic acid for prophylaxis of frequently recurrent urinary tract infections.

Cinoxacin has been shown to be as effective as nalidixic acid, nitrofurantoin, and trimethoprim-sulfamethoxazole in the treatment of uncomplicated acute symptomatic urinary tract infections, asymptomatic bacteriuria, and recurrent urinary tract infections (31). In contrast to nalidixic acid, rapid emergence of resistant organisms during acute and long-term treatment with cinoxacin has not been observed. The efficacy of cinoxacin prophylaxis for frequently recurrent urinary tract infections is less clear. A comparison of placebo versus cinoxacin

TABLE 2. Urinary Tract Agents

Agent	*Dosage*	*Use*
Nalidixic acid	Adults: 1 g qid for 1–2 weeks; thereafter, if needed, 0.5 g qid for periods longer than 2 weeks Children: 55 mg/kg/day in 4 divided doses for 1–2 weeks; thereafter, if needed, 33 mg/kg/day for periods longer than 2 weeks	Acute and recurrent uncomplicated urinary tract infections due to susceptible organisms; or long-term suppressive therapy for frequently recurrent bacteriuria (single daily dose of 1 g). Do not use in infants <3 months of age or in patients with renal carbuncle or perinephric abscess.
Oxolinc acid	Adults: 750 mg bid for 2 weeks Children: Not recommended	Acute and recurrent uncomplicated urinary tract infections due to susceptible organisms. Do not use in patients with renal insufficiency, renal carbuncle, or perinephric abscess or in infants or nursing mothers.
Cinoxacin	Adults: 250 mg qid or 500 mg bid for 1–2 weeks Children: Not recommended	Acute and recurrent uncomplicated urinary tract infections and asymptomatic bacteriuria due to susceptible organisms. Dose must be reduced in patients with renal insufficiency. Do not use in patients with renal carbuncle or perinephric abscess, in nursing mothers, or in prepubertal children.

Nitrofurantoin	Adults: 50 or 100 mg qid for 1–2 weeks Children: 1.25–1.75 mg/kg qid for 1–2 weeks	Acute and recurrent uncomplicated urinary tract infections due to susceptible organisms; or long-term suppressive therapy for frequently recurrent bacteriuria (single dose of 50–100 mg in adults, or 1 mg/kg bid in children). Do not use in patients with renal insufficiency, renal carbuncle, perinephric abscess, or in infants.
Methenamine	Adults: 0.5–2 g (usually 1 g) qid or bid Children: 15 mg/kg qid	Chronic suppressive treatment of urinary tract infections when urine pH is 5.5 or less. Not a primary drug for acute urinary tract infections.
Methenamine mandelate	Adults: 1 g qid Children: 15 mg/kg qid	Chronic suppressive treatment of urinary tract infections when urine pH is 5.5 or less. Not a primary drug for acute urinary tract infections.[a]
Methenamine hippurate	Adults: 1 g bid Children age 6–12 years: 0.5–1 g bid	Chronic suppressive treatment of urinary tract infections when urine pH is 5.5 or less. Not a primary drug for acute urinary tract infections.[a]

[a] One gram of methenamine mandelate or hippuric acid contains only 480 mg of methenamine and 520 mg of mandelic or hippuric acid. These combinations contain an amount of acid that is unlikely to contribute significant antibacterial activity to the urine. Also, there is little evidence that these acid forms contribute to the antibacterial activity of methenamine.

prophylaxis in the prevention of frequently recurrent urinary infection indicated that cinoxacin (single tablet nightly prophylaxis) reduced the frequency of recurrent urinary tract infections in women (92). However, another study failed to confirm this observation (93).

Norfloxacin has been shown to be as effective as trimethoprim-sulfamethoxazole in the treatment of uncomplicated acute symptomatic urinary tract infections and has significantly fewer side effects. Norfloxacin was effective in infections due to *Pseudomonas aeruginosa* and other multiresistant pathogens (93a). Ciprofloxacin is currently being studied in patients with acute uncomplicated symptomatic urinary tract infections as well as in patients with infections caused by *Pseudomonas* and other multiresistant pathogens. Preliminary data suggest that ciprofloxacin will be as effective as norfloxacin and trimethoprim-sulfamethoxazole in the treatment of certain urinary tract infections.

Methenamine has also been used regularly to treat patients with chronic bacteriuria in the presence of indwelling bladder catheters or who are receiving intermittent bladder catheterization, as well as to treat patients with neurogenic bladders with indwelling catheters. There is little evidence that methenamine, when given as methenamine mandelate or hippurate, prevents the acquisition of or eradicates bacteriuria in patients with suprapubic or indwelling Foley catheters (94,95). This is understandable since the mechanism of action of methenamine requires the generation of formaldehyde, which takes a minimum of 1 hour to be made in sufficient antibacterial concentrations. It is unlikely that urine remains in the bladder long enough for this reaction to occur in patients with constant bladder drainage. On the other hand, methenamine could potentially be effective in patients with neurogenic bladders receiving intermittent catheterization since urine would remain in the bladder for sufficient periods of time. However, recent observations indicate that methenamine, when given as the mandelic acid salt, methenamine mandelate, was ineffective as either a suppressive or prophylactic agent in patients on intermittent catheterization (95). It is important to emphasize that the methenamine used in all these studies was combined with mandelic or hippuric acid as mandelamine mandelate or hippurate. The actual amount of methenamine in these combinations is less than half of the total dose administered, which may have provided inadequate urine concentrations of methenamine for the generation of sufficient formaldehyde.

In summary, the urinary tract agents discussed in this chapter seem to be effective in treating acute, uncomplicated symptomatic bacteriuria of the lower urinary tract. Nitrofurantoin is effective in treating upper tract infection and frequently recurrent bacteriuria as well as a long-term suppressive agent in children and pregnant women. Methenamine, used properly, is also effective in women with uncomplicated recurrent bacteriuria, including those that are multiply antibiotic resistant, and as a prophylactic agent in men with recurrent infection. There is little convincing evidence that methenamine combined with mandelic or hippuric acid has any advantage over the use of methenamine alone. In fact, there is a strong possibility that when these salts are used in the doses currently recommended, insufficient methenamine is delivered to the urine to generate adequate concentrations of formaldehyde. Nalidixic acid may be effective in some patients with recurrent infections, but the problem of the development of antibacterial resistance to this agent is significant. Since cinoxacin, norfloxacin, and ciprofloxacin avoid most of the disadvantages of nalidixic acid (i.e., low urinary concentrations that require large dosage schedules and rapid emergence of resistant organisms during therapy) while maintaining all of its benefits, cinoxacin, norfloxacin, and ciprofloxacin may well replace nalidixic acid in the treatment of urinary tract infections. Although much more remains to be learned about these drugs, the quinolones have established themselves as an interesting group of agents, particularly since their activity is unrelated to that of other common antibiotics and bacterial resistance is not plasmid-borne. Current clinical investigation will surely determine their efficacy, toxicity, and value in the treatment of all types of urinary tract infections.

REFERENCES

1. Lesher GY, Froelich EJ, Gruett MD, et al: 1,8-naphthyridine derivatives. A new class of chemotherapeutic agents. *J Med Pharm Chem* 5:1063, 1962.
2. Turner FJ, Ringel SM, Martin JF, et al: Oxolinic acid, a new synthetic antimicrobial agent. I. In vitro and in vivo activity. *Antimicrob Agents Chemother* 1967: 475.
3. Ringel SM, Turner FJ, Lindo FL, et al: Oxolinic acid, a new synthetic antimicrobial agent. II. Bactericidal rate and resistance development. *Antimicrob Agents Chemother* p 480, 1967.
4. Ringel SM, Turner FJ, Roemer S, et al: Oxolinic acid, a new synthetic antimicrobial agent. III. Concentrations in serum, urine, and renal tissue. *Antimicrob Agents Chemother* p 486, 1967.
5. Wick WE, Preston DS, White WA, et al: Compound 64716, a new synthetic antibacterial agent. *Antimicrob Agents Chemother* 4:415, 1973.

5a. Ito A, Hirai K, Inoue M, et al: In vitro antibacterial activity of AM-175, a new nalidixic acid analog. *Antimicrob Agents Chemother* 17:103, 1980.

5b. Downs JT, Andriole VT, Ryan JL: In vitro activity of MK-0366 against clinical urinary pathogens including gentamicin-resistant *Pseudomonas aeruginosa. Antimicrob Agents Chemother* 21:670, 1982.

5c. Wise R, Andrew JM, Edwards LJ: In vitro activity of Bay 09867, a new quinoline derivative, compared with those of other antimicrobial agents. *Antimicrob Agents Chemother* 23:559, 1983.

6. Goss WA, Deitz WH, Cook TM: Mechanism of action of nalidixic acid on *Escherichia coli.* II. Inhibition of deoxyribonucleic acid synthesis. *J Bacteriol* 89:1068, 1965.
7. Deitz WH, Cook TM, Goss WA: Mechanism of action of nalidixic acid on Escherichia coli. III. Conditions required for lethality. *J Bacteriol* 91:768, 1966.
8. Bourguignon GJ, Levitt M, Sternglanz R: Studies on the mechanism of action of nalidixic acid. *Antimicrob Agents Chemother* 4:479, 1973.
9. Boyle JV, Cook TM, Goss WA: Mechanism of action of nalidixic acid on *Escherichia coli.* VI. Cell-free studies. *J Bacteriol* 97:230, 1969.
10. Pedrini AM, Geroldi D, Siccardi A, et al: Studies on the mode of action of nalidixic acid. *Eur J Biochem* 25:359, 1972.
11. Pratt WB: The urinary tract antiseptics, in Pratt WB (ed): *Chemotherapy of Infection.* New York, Oxford University Press, 1977, p 215.

11a. Pedrini A: Nalidixic acid, Hahn FE (ed), *Antibiotics.* Berlin, Springer-Verlag, Vol 5, 1979, p 154.

11b. Sugino A, Peebles CL, Krenzer KN, Cozzarelli NR: Mechanism of action of nalidixic acid: Purification of *E. coli* Nal A gene production and its relationship to DNA gyrase and a novel nicking-closing enzyme. *Proc Natl Acad Sci USA* 74:4767, 1977.

12. Goss WA, Dietz WH, Book TM: Mechanism of action of nalidixic acid on Escherichia coli. II. Inhibition of deoxyribonucleic acid synthesis. *J Bacteriol* 10:918, 1965.

13. Ott JL, Gordee RS: Inhibition of R-factor transfer by cinoxacin. Current chemotherapy. *Proc 10th Int Cong Chemother* 1:688, 1978.

14. Barlow AM: Nalidixic acid in infections of urinary tract. *Br Med J* 2:1308, 1963.

15. Buchbinder M, Webb JC, Anderson LV, et al: Laboratory studies and clinical pharmacology of nalidixic acid (WIN 18,320). *Antimicrob Agents Chemother* p 308, 1962.

16. Ronald AR, Turck M, Petersdorf RG: A critical evaluation of nalidixic acid in urinary tract infections. *New Engl J Med* 275:1081, 1966.

17. Cox CE: Oxolinic acid therapy of recurrent urinary tract infections. *Del Med J* 42:327, 1970.

18. D'Alessio DJ, Olexy VM, Jackson GG: Oxolinic acid treatment of urinary tract infections. *Antimicrob Agents Chemother* p 490, 1967.

19. Mardh PA, Colleen S, Andersson KE: Studies in cinoxacin. I. In vitro activity of cinoxacin as compared to nalidixic acid, against urinary tract pathogens. *J Antimicrob Chemother* 3:411, 1977.

20. Gordon RG, Stevens LI, Edmiston CE, et al: Comparative in vitro studies of cinoxacin, nalidixic acid, and oxolinic acid. *Antimicrob Agents Chemother* 10:918, 1976.

21. Jones RN, Fuchs PC: In vitro antimicrobial activity of cinoxacin against 2,968 clinical bacterial isolates. *Antimicrob Agents Chemother* 10:146, 1976.

21a. King A, Warren C, Shannon K, Phillips I: In vitro antibacterial activity of Norfloxacin (MK-0366). *Antimicrob Agents Chemother* 21:604, 1982.

21b. Neu HC, Labthavikul P: In vitro activity of norfloxacin, a quinoline-carboxylic acid, compared with that of β-lactams, aminoglycosides, and trimethoprim. *Antimicrob Agents Chemother* 22:23, 1982.

21c. Norrby SR, Jonsson M: Antibacterial activity of Norfloxacin. *Antimicrob Agents Chemother* 23:15, 1983.

21d. Corrado ML, Cherubin CE, Shulman M: The comparative activity of norfloxacin with other antimicrobial agents against gram-positive and gram-negative bacteria. *J Antimicrob Chemother* 11:369, 1983.

21e. Gadebusch HH, Shungu DL, Weinberg E, Chung SK: Comparison of the antibacterial activity of norfloxacin (MK 0366, AM 715), a new organic acid, with that of other orally absorbed chemotherapeutic agents. *Infection* 10:41, 1982.

21f. Bauernfeind A, Petermuller C: In vitro activity of ciprofloxacin, norfloxacin and nalidixic acid. *Eur J Clin Microbiol* 2:111, 1983.

21g. Muytjens HL, van der Ros-van de Repe J, van Veldhuizen G: Comparative activities of ciprofloxacin (Bay 09867), norfloxacin, pipemidic acid, and nalidixic acid. *Antimicrob Agents Chemother* 24:302, 1983.

21h. Fass RJ: In virtro activity of ciprofloxacin (Bay 09867). *Antimicrob Agents Chemother* 24:568, 1983.

21i. Heessen FWA, Muytjens HL: In vitro activities of ciprofloxacin, norfloxacin, pipemidic acid, cinoxacin, and nalidixic acid against *Chlamydia trachomatis. Antimicrob Agents Chemother* 25:123, 1984.

22. McChesney EW, Froelich EJ, Lesher GY, et al: Absorption, excretion and metabolism of a new antibacterial agent, nalidixic acid. *Toxicol Appl Pharmacol* 6:292, 1964.

23. Portmann GA, McChesney EW, Stander H., et al: Pharmacokinetic model for nalidixic acid in man. II. Parameters for absorption, metabolism and elimination. *J Pharm Sci* 55:72, 1966.

24. Stamey TA, Nemoy NJ, Higgins M: The clinical use of nalidixic acid. A review of some observations. *Invest Urol* 6:582, 1969.

25. Stamey TA, Meares EM, Winningham DG: Chronic bacterial prostatitis and the diffusion of drugs into prostatic fluid. *J Urol* 103:187, 1970.

26. Belton EM, Jones RV: Haemolytic anaemia due to nalidixic acid. *Lancet* 2:691, 1965.

27. Adam WR, Dawborn JK: Plasma levels and urinary excretion of nalidixic acid in patients with renal failure. *Aust NZ J Med* 1:126, 1971.
28. Atlas E, Clark H, Silverblatt F, et al: Nalidixic acid and oxolinic acid in the treatment of chronic bacteriuria. *Ann Intern Med* 70:713, 1969.
29. Burt RAP, Morgan T, Payne JP, et al: Cinoxacin concentrations in plasma, urine, and prostatic tissue after oral administration to man. *Br J Urol* 49:147, 1977.
30. Black HR, Israel KS, Wolen RL, et al: Pharmacology of cinoxacin in humans. *Antimicrob Agents Chemother* 15:165, 1979.
31. Scavone JM, Gleckman RA, Fraser DG: Cinoxacin: mechanism of action, spectrum of activity, pharmacokinetics, adverse reactions, and therapeutic indications. *Pharmacotherapy* 2:266, 1982.
31a. Swanson BN, Boppana VK, Vlasses PH, et al: Norfloxacin disposition after sequentially increasing oral doses. *Antimicrob Agents Chemother* 23:284, 1983.
31b. Crump B, Wise R, Dent J: Pharmacokinetics and tissue penetration of ciprofloxacin. *Antimicrob Agents Chemother* 24:784, 1983.
32. Zelickson AS: Phototoxic reaction with nalidixic acid. *JAMA* 190:556, 1964.
33. Burry JN, Crosby RWL: A case of phototoxicity to nalidixic acid. *Med J Aust* 2:698, 1966.
34. Mathew TH: Nalidixic acid. *Med J Aust* 2:243, 1966.
35. Cahal DA: Reactions to nalidixic acid. *Br Med J* 2:590, 1965.
36. Finegold SM, Miller LG, Posnick D, et al: Nalidixic acid: Clinical and laboratory studies. *Antimicrob Agents Chemother* p 189, 1966.
37. Kremer L, Walton M, Wardle EN: Nalidixic acid and intracranial hypertension. *Br Med J* 4:488, 1967.
38. Boreus LO, Sundstrom B: Intracranial hypertension in a child during treatment with nalidixic acid. *Br Med J* 2:744, 1967.
39. Fisher OD: Nalidixic acid and intracranial hypertension. *Br Med J* 3:370, 1967.
40. Cohen DN: Intracranial hypertension and papilledema associated with nalidixic acid therapy. *Am J Ophthalmol* 76:680, 1973.
41. Rao KG: Pseudotumor cerebri associated with nalidixic acid. *Urology* 4:204, 1974.
42. Islam MA, Sreedharan T: Convulsions, hyperglycaemia, and glycosuria from overdose of nalidixic acid. *JAMA* 192:1100, 1965.
43. Mandal BK, Stevenson J: Haemolytic crisis produced by nalidixic acid. *Lancet* 1:614, 1970.
44. Today's Drugs: Nalidixic acid. *Br Med J* 1:741, 1967.
45. Westwood GPC, Hooper WL: Antagonism of oxolinic acid by nitrofurantoin. *Lancet* 1:460, 1975.
46. Kucers A, Bennett NM: Nitrofurans, in Kucers A, Bennett NM (eds): *The Use of Antibiotics.* Philadelphia, JB Lippincott Co., 1979, p 749.
47. Paul HE, Paul, MF: The nitrofurans—chemotherapeutic properties, in Schnitzer RJ, Hawking F (eds): *Experimental Chemotherapy.* New York, Academic Press, 1966, p 521.
48. Albert PS, Mininberg DJ, Davis JE: Nitrofurans: sperm-immobilizing agents. Their tissue toxicity and clinical application. *Urology* 4:307, 1974.
49. Turck M, Ronald AR, Petersdorf RG: Susceptibility of Enterobacteriaceae to nitrofurantoin correlated with eradication of bacteriuria. *Antimicrob Agents Chemother* p 446, 1966.
50. Reckendorf HK, Castringius RG, Spingler HK: Comparative pharmacodynamics, urinary excretion, and half-life determinations of nitrofurantoin sodium. *Antimicrob Agents Chemother* 1962:531, 1963.
51. Andriole VT: Factors affecting antibiotic concentrations in urine and kidney tissue. *Proc 4th Int Congr Nephrol,* Stockholm 3:338, 1969.
52. Currie GA, Little PJ, McDonald SJ: The localization of cephaloridine and nitrofurantoin in the kidney. *Nephron* 3:282, 1966.
53. Katz YJ, Cockett ATK, Moore RS: Renal lymph and antibacterial levels in the treatment of pyelonephritis. *Life Sci* 3:1249, 1964.
54. Sachs J, Geer T, Noell P, et al: Effect of renal function on urinary recovery of orally administered nitrofurantoin. *New Engl J Med* 278:1032, 1968.
55. Loughridge L: Peripheral neuropathy due to nitrofurantoin. *Lancet* 2:1133, 1962.

56. Felts JH, Hayes DM, Gergen JA, et al: Neural, hematologic and bacteriologic effects of nitrofurantoin in renal insufficiency. *Am J Med* 51:331, 1971.
57. Hailey FJ, Glascock HW: Gastrointestinal tolerance to a new macrocrystalline form of nitrofurantoin: A collaborative study. *Curr Therap Res* 9:600, 1967.
58. Kalowski S, Radford N, Kincaid-Smith, P: Crystalline and macrocrystalline nitrofurantoin in the treatment of urinary tract infection. *New Engl J Med* 290:385, 1974.
59. Dawson RB: Pulmonary reactions to nitrofurantoin. *New Engl J Med* 274:522, 1966.
60. Morgan LK: Nitrofurantoin pulmonary hypersensitivity. *Med J Aust* 2:136, 1970.
61. Murray MJ, Kronenberg R: Pulmonary reactions simulating cardiac pulmonary edema caused by nitrofurantoin. *New Engl J Med* 273:1185, 1965.
62. Pearsall HR, Ewalt J, Tsoi MS, et al: Nitrofurantoin lung sensitivity: Report of a case with prolonged nitrofurantoin lymphocyte sensitivity and interaction of nitrofurantoin-stimulated lymphocytes with alveolar cells. *J Lab Clin Med* 83:728, 1974.
63. Rosenow EC, DeRemee RA, Dines DE: Chronic nitrofurantoin pulmonary reaction: Report of five cases. *New Engl J Med* 279:1258, 1968.
64. Holmberg L, Boman G, Bottiger LE, et al: Adverse reactions to nitrofurantoin. Analysis of 921 reports. *Am J Med* 69:733, 1980.
65. Bass BH: Megaloblastic anaemia due to nitrofurantoin. *Lancet* 1:530, 1963.
66. Ernaelsteen D, Williams R: Jaundice due to nitrofurantoin. *Gastroenterology* 41:590, 1961.
67. Bhagwat AG, Warren RE: Hepatic reaction to nitrofurantoin. *Lancet* 2:1369, 1969.
68. Ellis FG: Acute polyneuritis after nitrofurantoin therapy. *Lancet* 2:1136, 1962.
69. Craven RS: Furadantin neuropathy. *Aust NZ J Med* 1:246, 1971.
70. Toole JF, Parrish ML: Nitrofurantoin polyneuropathy. *Neurology* 23:554, 1973.
71. Ball JS, Ferguson AW: Permanent discoloration of primary dentition by nitrofurantoin. *Br Med J* 2:1103, 1962.
72. Nicolaier A: Ueber die therapeutische verwendung des urotropin (Hexamethylente tramin). *Deut Med Wochenschr* 21:541, 1895.
73. Rosenheim ML: Mandelic acid in the treatment of urinary infections. *Lancet* 1:1032, 1935.
74. Hanzlik PJ, Collins AB: Hexamethylenamine: The liberation of formaldehyde and the antiseptic efficiency under different chemical and biological conditions. *Arch Intern Med* 12:578, 1913.
75. Levy LH, Strauss A: A clinical and bacteriological study of hexamethylenamin as a urinary antiseptic. *Arch Intern Med* 14:730, 1914.
76. Shohl AT, Deming CL: Hexamethylenamin: Its quantitative factors in therapy. *J Urol* 4:419, 1920.
77. De Eds F: Fate of hexamethylenamin in the body and its bearing on systemic antisepsis. *Arch Intern Med* 34:511, 1924.
78. Heathcote RSA: Hexamine as an urinary antiseptic. I. Its rate of hydrolysis at different hydrogen ion concentrations. II. Its antiseptic power against various bacteria in urine. *Br J Urol* 7:9, 1935.
79. Jackson J, Stamey TA: The Riker method for determining formaldehyde in the presence of methenamine. *Invest Urol* 9:124, 1971.
80. Draskoczy P, Weiner N: Effect of organic acids on oxidative metabolism of Escherichia coli. *Fed Proc* 19:140, 1960.
81. Stamey TA: General and specific principles of therapy, in Stamey TA (ed): *Urinary Infections.* Baltimore, Williams & Wilkins, 1972, p 253.
82. Elliot JS, Sharpe RF, Lewis L: Urinary pH. *J Urol* 81:339, 1959.
83. Duca CJ, Scudi JV: Some antibacterial properties of Mandelamine (methenamine mandelate). *Proc Soc Exp Biol Med* 66:123, 1947.
84. Scudi JV, Reinhard JF: Absorption, distribution and renal excretion of Mandelamine (methenamine mandelate). *J Lab Clin Med* 33:1304, 1948.
85. Hinman F: An experimental study of the antiseptic value in the urine of the internal use of hexamethylenamin. *JAMA* 61:1601, 1913.
86. Kneebone GM: A clinical appraisal of nalidixic acid in urinary tract infection in childhood. *Med J Aust* 2:947, 1965.

87. Marshall M, Johnson SH: Use of nitrofurantoin in chronic and recurrent urinary tract infections in children. *JAMA* 169:919, 1959.

88. Normand ICS, Smellie JM: Prolonged maintenance chemotherapy in the management of urinary infection in childhood. *Br Med J* 1:1023, 1965.

89. Freeman RB, Smith WM, Richardson JA, et al: Long-term therapy for chronic bacteriuria in men: U.S. Public Health Service cooperative study. *Ann Intern Med* 83:133, 1975.

90. Holland NH, West CD: Prevention of recurrent urinary tract infections in girls. *Am J Dis Child* 105:560, 1963.

91. Harding GK, Roland AR: A controlled study of antimicrobial prophylaxis of recurrent urinary infection in women. *New Engl J Med* 291:597, 1974.

92. Landes RR: Long term low dose cinoxacin therapy for the prevention of recurrent urinary tract infections. *J Urol* 123:47, 1980.

93. Schaeffer AJ, Jones JM, Flynn SS: Prophylactic efficacy of cinoxacin in recurrent urinary tract infection: biologic effects on the vaginal and fecal flora. *J Urol* 127:1118, 1982.

93a. Panichi G, Pantosti A, Testore GP: Norfloxacin (MK-0366) treatment of urinary tract infections in hospitalized patients. *J Antimicrob Chemother* 11:589, 1983.

94. Gerstein AR, Okun R, Gonick HC, et al: The prolonged use of methenamine hippurate in the treatment of chronic urinary tract infections. *J Urol* 100:767, 1968.

95. Vainrub B, Musher DM: Lack of effect of methenamine in suppression of, or prophylaxis against, chronic urinary infection. *Antimicrob Agents Chemother* 12:625, 1977.

15

ANTIMYCOBACTERIAL AGENTS

ROBERT H. ALFORD

Drugs for mycobacterial infections will be categorized under three headings: those primarily for *Mycobacterium tuberculosis,* drugs for "atypical" mycobacterial infections, and agents primarily for treatment of leprosy. Traditionally, antimicrobics for tuberculosis have been classified further as "first line drugs" by virtue of superior efficacy with acceptable toxicity, and "second line" drugs either having less efficacy, greater toxicity, or both (1–4).

Antituberculous drugs vary according to bactericidal function and site of action in tuberculous lesions (4). All of the first-line agents are bactericidal except ethambutol. The bactericidal action of pyrazinamide (PZA) against actively metabolizing tubercle bacilli was overlooked initially because infections in PZA-treated animals relapsed due to metabolically inactive organisms ("persisters") that subsequently regrew. In site of action, drugs may exert their effects against mycobacteria either within cavities, intracellularly, or intermittantly replicating in closed caseous lesions: (*1*) Four agents have activity against the large, actively dividing extracellular populations in cavities—isoniazid (INH), rifampin, streptomycin, and ethambutol. Pyrazinamide is rendered inactive at the neutral or slightly alkaline pH encountered in such areas. (*2*) Against intracellular mycobacteria at acid pH, isoniazid, rifampin, and pyrazinamide are active whereas streptomycin, other aminoglycosides, and capreomycin lose their activity at low pH. (*3*) Slowly replicating organisms in caseous lesions are killed only by rifampin and, somewhat less readily, by isoniazid. Thus, the combination of INH and rifampin is bactericidal for all three populations in tuberculous lesions (*4*). These principles are especially important in designing "short course" chemotherapy and for resistant or relapsing infections (4).

FIRST-LINE ANTITUBERCULOSIS DRUGS

Isoniazid

Derivation and Structure. Isoniazid, isonicotinic acid hydrazide (INH), a synthetic agent, was demonstrated in 1952 to be effective in treatment of human tuberculosis (5). Its structure is indicated in Figure 1.

Mechanism of Action. Isoniazid, cidal against growing *Mycobacterium tuberculosis* in vitro, is static against "resting" organisms. It acts primarily by inhibition of synthesis of mycolic acid (3), an important component of mycobacterial cell walls. Against certain "atypical" mycobacteria, isoniazid in higher concentration appears to have a second mechanism of action affecting energy-requiring metabolic pathways (6).

Antimicrobial Activity. Against *M. tuberculosis,* 0.025–0.05 μg/ml of isoniazid is inhibitory. It is active against intracellular organisms. Tubercle bacilli become resistant to isoniazid administered alone. Initially susceptible isolates will become isoniazid-resistant in 71 percent of cases treated for 3 months with INH alone (5). Resistance results from selection under antimicrobic pressure of less susceptible variants of *M. tuberculosis* that initially comprise 1 in 10^6 bacilli among untreated mycobacterial populations. Surviving bacilli exhibit decreased INH uptake. Large populations like the 10^9–10^{10} bacilli in open pulmonary cavities are especially likely to have included among them significant numbers of resistant mycobacteria that subsequently overgrow leading to secondary resistance. Emergence of resistance depends on the type and duration of prior therapy (7). Significant primary resistance to INH in untreated cases occurs in approximately 6 percent of isolates in the United States of America, and should be anticipated particularly in immigrants from regions having high levels of endemic drug resistance. Primary resistance has been documented in 43 percent of Korean isolates of *M. tuberculosis* (8).

Pharmacology. Isoniazid, well absorbed orally or intramuscularly, is subsequently distributed throughout the body including the cerebrospinal fluid. CSF levels are usually about 20 percent of plasma levels but may equal plasma concentrations in the presence of meningeal inflammation.

Metabolism of isoniazid is initially by liver *N*-acetyl transferase. Its rate of

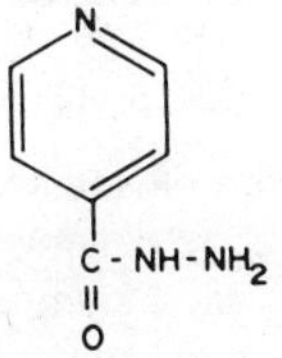

FIGURE 1. Structure of isonizid.

acetylation is determined genetically with slow acetylation inherited as an autosomal recessive trait (3). Five percent of Canadian eskimos are slow acetylators compared with 83 percent of Egyptians. Ten to 15 percent of orientals are slow acetylators as are 58 percent of American caucasians (3). Six hours after a 4 mg/kg oral dose, slow acetylators have isoniazid serum levels of > 0.8 μg/ml and rapid acetylators < 0.2 μg/ml (1). The striking bimodal distribution of serum half-lives caused by acetylation status is depicted in Figure 2. Acetylator status does not affect outcome with daily therapy because plasma levels are well above inhibitory concentrations. However, weekly intermittent therapy may be adversely affected with rapid acetylators faring less well. Primarily excreted as metabolically altered drug in the urine, some unaltered INH appears there as well. Dosage modification in hepatic or renal failure is not usually necessary, but in the presence of severe hepatic insufficiency, reduction in dosage by one-half is recommended, and with significant renal failure, dosage reduction to 150–200 mg/day is recommended for slow acetylators (9).

Adverse Reactions. Isoniazid has infrequent major toxicities that include hepatitis. Approximately 15 percent of isoniazid recipients will have some elevation in SGOT that resolves with continued therapy. Although fatal INH hepatitis had been clearly documented by 1970 (10), early reports did not elucidate its frequency. Documentation of the incidence of major isoniazid hepatotoxicity awaited a large prophylactic trial reported in 1972 in which 19 of 2321 recipients developed serious hepatitis associated with two deaths (11). Hepatotoxicity occurs at any time but is most likely to occur 4 to 8 weeks after the onset of treatment. Isoniazid hepatotoxicity is clearly correlated with age, as is indicated

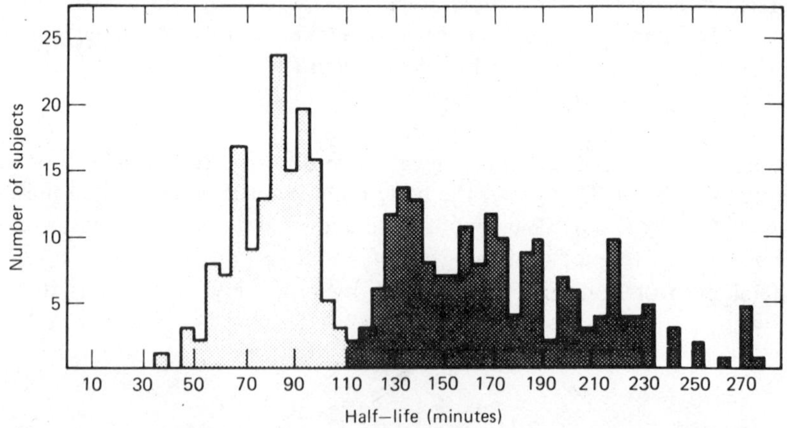

FIGURE 2. Bimodal distribution of isoniazid half-lives as related to acetylation status. 5 mg/kg administered to patients intravenously. Light bars indicate rapid acetylators and dark bars slow acetylators [From Pratt (3). From Tiiten H: Isoniazid and ethionamide serum levels and inactivation in Finnish subjects. *Scand J Resp Dis* 50:110, 1969.]

TABLE 1. Age-Related Incidence of Isoniazid Hepatotoxicity

Age (Years)	*Serious Hepatotoxicity (% Patients)*
<20	"Rare"
20–34	0.3
35–49	1.2
50>	2.3

SOURCE: Data from Center for Disease Control (14)

in Table 1, presumably due to diminished capacity for repair of INH hepatocellular damage in the elderly. Hepatotoxicity is also more likely to occur in alcoholics with preexisting liver damage (11–12), causing varying degrees of hepatocellular damage histologically that may become extensive, resembling viral hepatitis with acute yellow atrophy (13). Cholestasis as the predominant feature is infrequent.

Isoniazid hepatotoxicity was initially thought to reflect acetylation status with increased prevalence of toxicity in rapid acetylators due to an acetylhydrazine metabolite. Subsequent studies have failed to verify this association. The need for monitoring serum hepatic enzyme concentrations is controversial, but patients should be advised to discontinue isoniazid at the onset of symptoms consistent with hepatitis.

Appreciation of the frequency of isoniazid hepatotoxicity has not significantly limited therapeutic indications but has had a major impact on "chemoprophylactic" usage. No longer is "routine" INH chemoprophylaxis of adult PPD skin test converters recommended, with special caution indicated in people over age 35 (14).

Neurotoxicity. Peripheral neuropathy occurs in 17 percent of people receiving 6 mg/kg/day of isoniazid, but less frequently with conventional dosage. Neuropathy is especially likely in people with poor nutrition or underlying neuropathy resulting from alcoholism, diabetes, or uremia, and is more frequent in slow acetylators who have higher serum levels of unaltered drug. Increased pyridoxine excretion occurs with isoniazid administration. Pyridoxine replacement does not affect the INH antimicrobial action (3), but does ameliorate the neuropathy.

Central nervous system isoniazid toxicity may cause aberrations ranging from memory loss to psychosis, or seizures. Particular caution should be exercised when administering isoniazid to people with convulsive disorders. Optic neuropathy has been reported. Toxic CNS reactions are not related directly to pyridoxine deficiency for certain but have responded to its administration (1).

Hypersensitivity Reactions. Fever that may be sustained or "spiking," skin eruptions, or hematologic abnormalities may occur. A substantial number of

INH recipients will develop positive antinuclear antibody (ANA) tests, and some will manifest an isoniazid-induced lupuslike syndrome that is usually reversible upon discontinuation of the drug.

Other Reactions. Arthritic disorders associated with isoniazid administration have included Dupuytren's contracture and the "shoulder-hand" syndrome. Pellagra may occur in malnourished recipients of INH (1,3). Pyridoxine deficiency-related anemia can occur.

Significant Drug Interactions. Phenytoin (Dilantin) toxicity is potentiated by isoniazid. Mental changes, nystagmus, and ataxic gait can occur especially in slow acetylators in whom high isoniazid levels inhibit phenytoin metabolism. Combined INH and rifampin therapy predisposes to elevation of serum hepatic enzymes in up to 29 percent of recipients of that combination. Isoniazid plasma levels are increased by concurrent para-aminosalicylic acid (PAS) because of interference with acetylation.

Use. Isoniazid is indicated for all forms of tuberculosis. In 1952, pulmonary disease was found to respond favorably to isoniazid (5). Tuberculous meningitis was almost always fatal before the advent of chemotherapy. Isoniazid-containing regimens produced 83 percent survival compared with 45 percent with streptomycin plus PAS (15). Survival in miliary disease reached 77 percent with INH compared with 22 percent with streptomycin plus PAS (16). Indications for isoniazid include preventive therapy or "chemoprophylaxis" of selected PPD skin test converters.

Availability and Dosage. Isoniazid is available as INH, Nydrazid, Hyzyd, and Niconyl. Dosage forms include 100- and 300-mg tablets, syrup containing 10 mg/ml, and a 100 mg/ml solution for parenteral injection. The usual dosage is 5–10 mg/kg/day (often 300 mg/day), with the lower dosage range used routinely in adults for most therapy or "prophylaxis." The higher dosage schedules may be used for serious infections and for infants and children. Therapeutic regimens should include one or more companion drugs to discourage emergence of isoniazid-resistant bacilli.

Intermittent therapy, twice weekly high-dose isoniazid (15 mg/kg orally) combined with streptomycin (25–30 mg/kg IM), ethambutol (50 mg/kg PO), low-dose rifampin (600 mg PO), or pyrazinamide is being used more frequently after an initial period of daily drug administration (17). Such intermittant regimens are less expensive and encourage compliance.

Although not recommended for intravenous infusion, isoniazid for injection has been administered intravenously (9) and can be so given cautiously if other routes of administration are contraindicated.

Ethambutol

Derivation and Structure. Ethambutol was discovered in 1961 among synthetic compounds being screened for antituberculous activity. Its structure is indicated in Figure 3.

Mechanism of Action. Ethambutol is tuberculostatic. Its precise mechanism of action is not known, although it is probably an antimetabolite affecting RNA synthesis. Seventy-five percent of human strains of tubercle bacilli are susceptible to 1 μg/ml.

Pharmacology. Orally administered ethambutol is 75 to 80 percent absorbed, yielding peak plasma levels of 5 μg/ml after a dose of 25 mg/kg. It is distributed throughout the body, including the cerebrospinal fluid. Although little ethambutol crosses normal meninges, 10 to 50 percent of serum levels appear in CSF with meningeal inflammation. After conversion of approximately 15 percent of absorbed ethambutol to inactive metabolites, approximately 80 percent of the parent and metabolized drug is excreted in the urine. Thus, it is necessary to modify dosage in the presence of significant renal failure.

Antimicrobial Activity. Ethambutol is bacteriostatic at concentrations of less than 8 μg/ml against most strains of *M. tuberculosis,* even those that are isoniazid-resistant. Resistance of a stepwise nature occurs when ethambutol is administered without companion drugs. Only occasional primary resistance has been reported, and cross-resistance with other antimycobacterial drugs is unusual. Thus, ethambutol's principal role is as a "companion" drug to retard emergence of resistance.

Adverse Reactions. The major toxicity of ethambutol is neuropathic. Peripheral neuropathy may occur but more common is retrobulbar neuritis which is reported regularly with a dosage of 50 mg/kg/day. Characteristically, impairment of visual acuity or color vision develops, and there may be constriction of visual fields. More likely in association with high dose or prolonged ethambutol administration, retrobulbar neuritis is usually reversible. Blindness has occurred in the elderly with as little as 15 mg/kg/day. Consequently, patients receiving ethambutol should be instructed to report optic symptoms, and visual acuity and color perception should be tested every 4 to 6 weeks. Gastrointestinal intolerance is infrequent. Hyperuricemia occurs secondary to decreased urinary uric

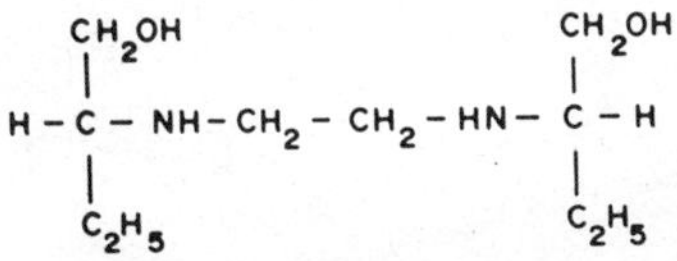

FIGURE 3. Structure of ethambutol.

acid excretion. Infrequent hypersensitivity reactions include dermatitis, arthralgias, and fever.

Usage. Ethambutol is indicated as therapy for infections due to *M. tuberculosis.* With combined therapy, resistance develops slowly. Because of its greater activity, lower incidence of side effects, and better record of compliance, ethambutol has largely replaced para-amino salicylic acid (PAS) in the United States as a bacteriostatic companion drug for isoniazid.

Availability and Dosage. Ethambutol is available as ethambutol hydrochloride (Myambutol). It is supplied in 100- and 400-mg tablets. Usual dosage is 15–25 mg/kg/day initially, followed after 60 days by 15 mg/kg/day as a single daily dose.

Rifampin

Derivation and Structure. Rifampin (termed rifampicin in the United Kingdom) is a semisynthetic derivative of a complex macrocyclic antibiotic, rifamycin B, produced by *Streptomyces mediterranei.* In 1967, it was introduced for clinical trials against mycobacterial infections. The complex structure is indicated in Figure 4.

Mechanism of Action. Rifampin affects mycobacterial growth by inhibiting bacillary DNA-dependent RNA-polymerase. Human RNA-polymerase is insensitive to rifampin's action. It is bactericidal against *M. tuberculosis* at 0.005–0.2 μg/ml. Rifampin's lipid solubility enhances intracellular penetration.

Unlike any other combination, rifampin and isoniazid have consistently sterilized tissue in experimental murine tuberculosis.

Pharmacology. Rifampin is well absorbed orally, yielding peak levels of 7–8 μg/ml after 600 mg PO. It is widely distributed throughout the body including the cerebrospinal fluid. CSF levels have been undetectable to 0.5 μg/ml in normal people and as high as 50 percent of the plasma concentration with

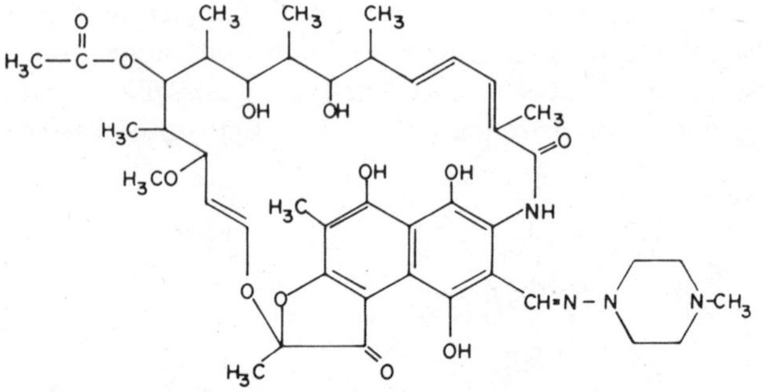

FIGURE 4. Structure of rifampin.

meningeal irritation. Rifampin is metabolized to a deacetylated active form that undergoes biliary excretion and enterohepatic recirculation. Due to induction of rifampin's own metabolizing enzymes (cytochrome P-450-coupled), biliary excretion increases with continued therapy. Excretion is primarily into the gastrointestinal tract, with the drug also excreted in the urine. Both serum concentrations and urinary excretion increase in the presence of hepatic failure (18). Probenecid causes decreased excretion by blocking hepatic uptake. In liver failure, some dosage reduction is indicated, but full dosage can be administered in renal failure.

Antimicrobial Activity. Rifampin is active against *M. tuberculosis* to a degree comparable with isoniazid. It affects intracellular, slowly replicating bacilli in caseous foci or intracavitary organisms, as noted previously. In vitro, rapid, one-step resistance emerges with a low frequency precluding rifampin's use alone. Resistance has been reported among clinical isolates of *Mycobacterium tuberculosis* (19).

Hepatotoxicity. Adverse reactions are rather frequent with rifampin, but only 6 of 372 patients taking the drug for 20 weeks had to discontinue it because of adverse effects (20). The major adverse effect is hepatotoxicity, which resulted in 16 deaths in 500,000 rifampin recipients (1).

Minimal abnormalities of liver function tests are common in people receiving rifampin and usually resolve even with continuation of the drug. Characteristically, elevations of bilirubin and alkaline phosphatase are noted (21), whereas elevations of hepatocellular enzymes such as SGOT may be a consequence of rifampin, isoniazid, or both. Rifampin-induced toxic liver changes occur earlier and produce a patchier cellular abnormality with less marked periportal inflammation than hepatitis caused by isoniazid (22). Alcoholics with preexisting liver damage appear to be especially prone to serious rifampin-induced liver toxicity. Concomitant INH may increase chances of rifampin-related hepatotoxicity. It has been suggested that rifampin not be given to alcoholics with underlying liver damage "unless other drug combinations are contraindicated (22)." Such advice is hard to follow since alcoholism also predisposes to isoniazid hepatitis, and because other alternatives such as PZA, PAS, and ethionamide also may be hepatotoxic. Children appear to be at increased risk of serious rifampin-associated hepatotoxicity perhaps in part because of their relatively higher doses. Jaundice has been frequent (27 percent) in children with tuberculous meningitis treated with rifampin in combination regimens but could have been potentiated by phenytoin or other seizure medications (23).

Effects on Immune Parameters. The effects of rifampin on humoral and cell-mediated immunity appear to be extensive, but are of uncertain significance. Light chain proteinuria occurs in 85 percent of people receiving rifampin (24). It inhibits blastic transformation of phytohemagglutinin-stimulated lymphocytes and interferes with cutaneous reactivity to intradermal tuberculin (25).

Hypersensitivity Reactions. Flushing, fever, pruritis without rash, urticaria, eosinophilia, hemolysis, and renal failure due to interstitial nephritis (26) may occur after rifampin administration. A systemic flulike syndrome, at times associated with thrombocytopenia, may have an immunologic basis and has been described most often with intermittent high-dose rifampin (21). However, regimens employing 600 mg of rifampin twice weekly have recently produced the flulike syndrome very infrequently (27).

Other Side Effects. Widespread systemic distribution of rifampin is reflected in the orange color appearing in urine, feces, saliva, sputum, pleural fluid, tears, sweat, semen, and CSF of people receiving the drug. Patients should be appropriately forewarned. With overdosage, a "red man" syndrome caused from drug discoloration has occurred. Infrequent gastrointestinal intolerance to the point of nausea with vomiting may result.

Significant Drug Interactions. By potentiating cytochrome P-450-related enzymatic reactions, rifampin induces increased hepatic excretion of a number of drugs metabolized by the liver. In this manner, it causes decreased activity of the coumarin-type anticoagulants that persists 5 to 7 days after rifampin is discontinued. Menstrual irregularities and decreased efficacy of oral contraceptives have been reported due to potentiation of steroid hormone metabolism. On the other hand, competition for excretion with contrast materials used in cholecystography may result in failure of gallbladder visualization. Rifampin crosses the placenta readily and consequently is not approved for use in pregnancy. There is interference with gastrointestinal absorption of rifampin by PAS. Probenecid administration causes increased plasma rifampin concentrations.

Usage. In pulmonary tuberculosis, rifampin's efficacy is indicated by sputum conversion 2 weeks earlier with rifampin than with non-rifampin-containing regimens (20). Because of rifampin's potent antimycobacterial action, combination regimens containing it have yielded gratifying results in short-duration therapy and in retreatment of drug-resistant tuberculosis. Rifampin in combination with isoniazid has been recommended for extrapulmonary tuberculous infections including tuberculous meningitis.

Availability and Dosage. Rifampin is available in the United States under the brand names Rifadin and Rimactane, supplied as 300-mg capsules. The usual dose is 600 mg once daily for adults and 10–20 mg/kg/day for children (not to exceed 600 mg/day). Twice weekly 1200- and 900-mg dosage regimens have largely been abandoned due to unacceptably high numbers of toxic reactions. A 600-mg twice weekly regimen has been generally well tolerated. Rifampin capsules can be opened, and the drug suspended in simple sugar syrup for pediatric administration. The suspension can be refrigerated for up to 2 weeks.

Ansamycin

In addition to rifampin, several other rifamycin antibiotics possess a high degree of activity against mycobacteria including *M. tuberculosis, M. avium-intracellulare* complex, and *M. fortuitum* (28,29). Ansamycin (LM-427), a derivative of rifamycin-S, is among a group of spiropiperidyl rifamycins that are quite active in vitro and effective in experimental murine tuberculosis (28). Investigations are underway to define ansamycin's role in treating tuberculosis and atypical mycobacterial infections.

Streptomycin

Derivation and Structure. Streptomycin, an aminoglycoside antimicrobic introduced in the 1940s, was the first drug to reduce tuberculosis mortality. Its structure, mechanism of action, and pharmacology are given in Chapter 6. Briefly, the drug is administered intramuscularly yielding serum levels of 25–30 μg/ml after a 1-g injection. It is practically excluded from the central nervous system. Streptomycin's toxicities are similar to other aminoglycoside antibiotics with less nephrotoxicity and greater vestibular toxicity than most aminoglycosides used clinically at present.

Antimicrobial Activity. In vitro, streptomycin is bactericidal for *M. tuberculosis,* but in animals it can be only suppressive and is inactive against intracellular tubercle bacilli. Concentrations of 0.4–10 μg/ml are inhibitory. Rapid emergence of resistance has long been recognized as a hazard of single drug therapy with streptomycin. Approximately 1 bacterium in 10^6 is primarily resistant to streptomycin. Such high concentrations of tubercle bacilli most often reside in cavitary pulmonary lesions. Primarily occurring cross-resistance to streptomycin is found most often among patient populations having a high incidence of INH resistance. Among other aminoglycosides, amikacin appears to possess superior activity to streptomycin against *M. tuberculosis* (30). However, familiarity, low toxicity, and reasonable price will enable streptomycin to remain the aminoglycoside of choice for tuberculosis.

Usage. Streptomycin is indicated in multiple drug therapy for tuberculosis. Caution must be exercised with prolonged dosage of greater than 1 g/day and with administration to the elderly or to people with impaired renal function. Care must also be taken if streptomycin is used in combination with other nephrotoxic or ototoxic antibiotics.

Availability and Dosage. Streptomycin sulfate for injection is provided in 0.5 g/ml single injection vials and multidose vials. The customary dose in adults ranges from 2 g daily to 1 g twice weekly (most often 500 mg–1 g daily). The higher dosage schedules are indicated for initial short-term (2 to 4 weeks) therapy with subsequent reduction to 1 g/day or less. Children should receive 20–40 mg/kg/day in two divided doses q 12 hours.

Pyrazinamide

Derivation. Pyrazinamide (PZA) is a synthetic analog of nicotinamide that has been elevated to first line usage for "short course" therapy regimens because of its bactericidal action (4) plus acceptable toxicity at relatively low doses. Its structure is indicated in Figure 5.

Mechanism of Action. PZA is bactericidal for the tubercle bacillus at 12.5 μg/ml. Its maximal activity is at acid pH like that often present in tuberculous lesions, especially intracellularly. Its precise action is unknown. Resistance will evolve rapidly when the drug is used alone. Metabolically inactive tubercle bacilli are resistant to pyrazinamide rendering it inappropriate for long-term therapy (4).

Pharmacology. Well absorbed orally, pyrazinamide is widely distributed throughout the body in levels that exceed the inhibitory concentration for the tubercle bacillus. It also enters CSF across inflamed meninges. PZA is metabolized by the liver. Its metabolic products are excreted largely in the urine so it is best avoided in renal failure.

Toxicity. Hepatotoxicity occurring in up to 15 percent of people receiving pyrazinamide in initial trials long ago discouraged its use. Early trials of PZA employed dosage of 40–50 mg/kg/day for prolonged periods. Currently recommended regimens of 20–35 mg/kg/day appear to be much safer (31,32). Patients with preexisting liver disease probably should not receive the drug; symptoms and hepatic function tests should be monitored in those receiving pyrazinamide. Other side effects include urate retention in 56 percent of PZA recipients in one series (32). Photosensitivity and rash have been reported.

Usage. Because of fear of hepatotoxicity, pyrazinamide has been reserved in the United States for treatment of patients with drug-resistant infections. In other nations, it has played a role in initial therapy, particularly in areas of high primary resistance. Low in price, it can be administered once weekly, favoring its usage in developing nations. Now pyrazinamide is receiving attention worldwide as a component of multidrug short course chemotherapy (4,27,32).

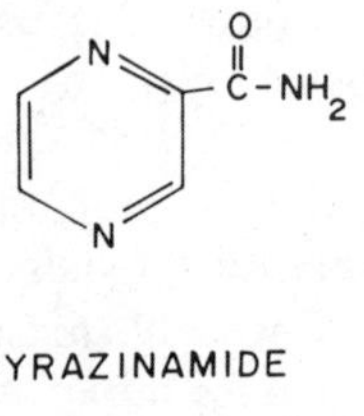

PYRAZINAMIDE

FIGURE 5. Structure of pyrazinamide.

Availability and Dosage. Pyrazinamide is available in 500 mg tablets. The usual dose is 20–35 mg/kg/day orally in two to four spaced doses equivalent to 1.5–2.0 g daily. Apparently it has been well tolerated in a twice weekly dosage of 50 mg/kg, not to exceed 3 g/day, for short course regimens. It has even been administered in a 90 mg/kg dose once weekly with little overt hepatotoxicity.

SECOND-LINE ANTITUBERCULOUS DRUGS

Para-Aminosalicylic Acid (PAS)

This synthetic compound, supplied as a sodium or calcium salt or resin, inhibits growth of mycobacteria by impairment of folate synthesis. Para-aminosalicylic acid is incompletely absorbed orally. A 4-g oral dose yields plasma concentrations of 7–8 μg/ml. Eighty-five percent of absorbed PAS is excreted in urine in the form of various degradation products.

Toxicity. Chief among side effects of para-aminosalicylic acid is gastrointestinal intolerance which may be severe and thus often causes poor patient compliance with treatment regimens. PAS can cause a reversible drug-induced lupuslike syndrome or can produce lymphoreticular hyperplasia. Recipients can develop a mononucleosislike syndrome with fever, rash, lymphadenopathy, hepatosplenomegaly, and occasionally toxic hepatitis. Hypersensitivity to para-aminosalicylic acid is frequent, occurring in 5 to 10 percent of its recipients. Further, it seems to cross-sensitize to streptomycin and isoniazid in patients who are receiving multidrug regimens. Readministration of any of the components in a combination regimen after PAS hypersensitivity may subsequently result in reaction to the companion drug. Increased toxicity of isoniazid in association with para-aminosalicylate may result from PAS inhibition of INH acetylation.

Usage. Para-aminosalicylic acid was once included in standard combination therapy for *M. tuberculosis.* In the United States, it has, to a large extent, been supplanted by ethambutol. Due to its low cost, PAS retains a place in multidrug therapy in developing countries but is becoming less favored because of the need for close supervision to prevent poor compliance.

Availability and Dosage. Para-aminosalicylic acid is provided as acid salts (Pamisyl), as a sodium-potassium-free ascorbate (Pascorbic), and as a resin (Resipas). Dosage forms include 500-mg tablets and 4-g resin packets. The customary dose is 10–12 g/day in three to four divided doses for adults (6–8 g/day of the sodium-potassium-free ascorbate) and in children 200–300 mg/kg/day in divided doses.

Cycloserine

Derivation. Initially produced by fermentation, cycloserine is now synthesized. By virtue of inhibition of cell wall synthesis, cycloserine possesses antimicrobial activity against a broad range of prokaryotic microorganisms, including mycobacteria. Five to 20 μg/ml is inhibitory for *M. tuberculosis.*

Pharmacology. Cycloserine is readily absorbed orally with peak serum levels of 20–50 μg/ml. Widely distributed among tissues, no blood-brain barrier exists to cycloserine (1). Approximately two-thirds of the drug is excreted unchanged in urine, and the remainder is metabolized to inactive forms.

Side Effects. Peripheral neuropathy or central nervous system dysfunction can be caused by cycloserine. Behavioral alterations or seizures can result. In patients with latent seizures, the drug is contraindicated.

Usage. Cycloserine is one of several agents to choose from for retreatment regimens or for primarily resistant *M. tuberculosis.*

Availability and Dosage. Cycloserine is provided as Seromycin in 250-mg capsules. The usual dose is 500—1000 mg/day in two divided doses, with 500 mg daily used most frequently.

Ethionamide

Derivation. Ethionamide, a derivative of isonicotinic acid, was synthesized in 1956. It is tuberculostatic at 0.6–2.5 μg/ml against susceptible strains.

Pharmacology. Ethionamide is absorbed well orally, yielding peak plasma concentrations of 20 μg/ml. It is widely distributed and penetrates both normal and inflamed meninges, yielding CSF concentrations approximately the same as in serum. The drug is metabolized by the liver with metabolites excreted mainly in the urine. Ethionamide interferes with isoniazid acetylation.

Side Effects. Most people taking ethionamide will experience gastrointestinal irritation with nausea and, frequently, vomiting. Various neurologic disorders can be caused by ethionamide, including peripheral neuropathy or psychiatric disturbances that may require discontinuation of the drug and reportedly are alleviated by pyridoxine and nicotinamide. Reversible hepatotoxicity, heralded by increasing SGOT values, may occur in approximately 5 percent of ethionamide recipients. Hypersensitivity-type rash or poor diabetic control are infrequent complications.

Usage. Ethionamide is among the choices of agents for retreatment or treatment of primarily resistant tuberculosis.

Availability and Dosage. Ethionamide is available as Trecator-SC in 250-mg tablets. The usual initial dosage is 250 mg twice daily (or as a single dose on retiring) and is increased by 125 mg/day until 1 g/day is reached. Commonly, 500–750 mg becomes the maximum dose because of gastrointestinal intolerance.

Kanamycin, Viomycin, Capreomycin, Amikacin

These agents are considered as a group because they all must be administered by intramuscular injection, have similar pharmacokinetics, similar toxicities, and are excreted by the kidneys. The first three have been employed principally as alternative agents in retreatment regimens for resistant tuberculosis. These agents have additive oto- and nephrotoxicity and should not be given, as a rule, in combination with each other, streptomycin, or another aminoglycoside.

Kanamycin. Kanamycin is an aminoglycoside antibiotic described in Chapter 20 to which some resistant tubercle bacilli are susceptible. Except for lower price, kanamycin probably should be superceded by amikacin as an alternative in retreatment schedules. (See amikacin.)

AVAILABILITY AND DOSAGE. Kanamycin sulfate is supplied as Kantrex, 0.5 g/2ml; 1 g/3ml; or 75 mg/2 ml (pediatric dose form) for intramuscular injection. The usual dose is 15 mg/kg/day which, for practical purposes, is 1 g/day in most adults.

Viomycin. Viomycin is a complex basic polypeptide antibiotic for injection (2). Certain resistant *M. tuberculosis* strains are susceptible. Cross-resistance to viomycin and capreomycin occurs regularly and less consistently between viomycin and kanamycin (33). Susceptible strains of *M. tuberculosis* are inhibited by 1–10 μg/ml.

AVAILABILITY AND DOSAGE. Viomycin sulfate for injection is available as Viocin in 1- and 5-g vials. The usual dosage is 2 g twice weekly, administered as 1 g every 12 hours on the days of injection. One to 2 g daily has been used for periods of not longer than 1 to 2 weeks.

Capreomycin. Capreomycin is a polypeptide antibiotic produced by *Streptomyces capreolus.* Susceptible *M. tuberculosis* strains are susceptible to 1–50 μg/ml (usually 10 μg/ml), depending on the culture medium. Average peak serum concentrations of 30 μg/ml are achieved. Cross-resistance occurs chiefly between capreomycin and viomycin, but also between capreomycin and kanamycin. According to some authorities, capreomycin is less toxic than viomycin, and especially less toxic than kanamycin (33). Capreomycin may be employed in retreatment of resistant tuberculosis as one component of a multiple drug regimen.

AVAILABILITY AND DOSAGE. Capreomycin sulfate is supplied as Capastat. Dosage is 1 g intramuscularly daily for 2 to 4 months, reduced to 1 g two to three times weekly thereafter.

Amikacin. In vitro and animal trials have indicated that amikacin is among the most active, if not the most active aminoglycoside against *M. tuberculosis* (30). It has not been used extensively clinically in tuberculosis. Due to expense and toxicity, it should not supplant streptomycin as the first line aminoglycoside for initial treatment of susceptible tuberculosis. It probably should replace its congener, kanamycin, except for cost since both have similar pharmacokinetics and toxicities. In renal failure, amikacin might be chosen because assays for it are more generally available.

USAGE. Amikacin appears to have merit as an alternative drug for retreatment of resistant *M. tuberculosis* infections.

Amithiozone

Amithiozone (thiacetazone), a thiosemicarbazole, is quite active against most strains of *M. tuberculosis.* Susceptible strains are inhibited by 1 μg/ml (1,2). Peak serum concentrations are 1–2 μg/ml. Resistance to amithiozone readily develops with single drug therapy necessitating combination regimens. Toxicity (gastrointestinal irritation and marrow suppression) has precluded use of this agent in Europe and the United States. (The drug is unavailable in the U.S.A.) Gastrointestinal toxicity is comparable to that of PAS. Additionally, hepatic damage has occurred usually in patients receiving isoniazid concomitantly. Apparently there is a lower incidence of untoward effects in people from Africa. Consequently, because of its low price, amithiozone has been used as a "first line" drug particularly in East African developing nations (2). Amithiozone (Panthrone, Tibione) is administered orally in a dose of 150 mg/day or 450 mg twice weekly.

Amoxicillin-Clavulanic Acid

The combination of amoxicillin and a broadly active inhibitor of bacterial betalactamases, clavulanic acid, is reportedly bactericidal for most strains of *M. tuberculosis* in concentrations of both drugs that could be clinically achieved in plasma (34). Although in very early stages of investigation, this raises the exciting prospect of someday using relatively nontoxic and inexpensive betalactam antibiotics for tuberculosis by pharmacologically rendering beta-lactamases of tubercle bacilli inactive.

DRUGS FOR TREATMENT OF ATYPICAL MYCOBACTERIAL INFECTIONS

"Atypical" mycobacteria vary greatly in susceptibility to antimicrobics. Some are susceptible to agents used principally for treatment of tuberculosis; other atypicals respond to various antibiotics used more commonly for treating pyogenic bacterial infections; and still others, especially among the *M. avium-intra-*

cellulare group, are frequently resistant to virtually all available drugs. Mycobacteria of the avium-intracellulare complex often contain plasmids that contribute to their broad antimicrobial resistance (35). Choosing appropriate therapy for atypicals is further confounded because methodology for susceptibility testing has not been standardized. For example, two laboratories have reported that *M. avium-intracellulare* bacilli are susceptible to a combination of rifampin and ethambutol (36,37), but resistance to that combination was detected in another laboratory (38). Standardization of atypical mycobacterial identification and susceptibility testing methods has just begun (39). Rational chemotherapy for atypical mycobacterial infections based on susceptibility results is now becoming feasible (40).

ANTITUBERCULOUS DRUGS USED FOR TREATMENT OF ATYPICAL MYCOBACTERIA

Several agents used principally for treatment of *M. tuberculosis* were evaluated years ago for activity against "atypical" mycobacteria (41). Isoniazid inhibits nearly 40 percent of strains of *M. kansasii* at a concentration of 1–5 μg/ml contrasted to only 10 to 30 percent of *M. avium-intracellulare* strains that are inhibited by that concentration. Some authorities include isoniazid in multidrug regimens for treatment of many atypical mycobacterial infections even in the face of in vitro INH resistance. Because of border-line susceptibilities of most atypical mycobacteria, doses of isoniazid up to 10–15 mg/kg/day have often been used with accompanying increased toxicity.

Rifampin is used for treatment of many atypical mycobacterial infections. Its in vitro activity is such that 93 to 100 percent of *M. kansasii* strains are inhibited by 0.25–1 μg/ml, and virtually all *M. marinum* are susceptible (42,43). About one-half of *M. scrofulaceum* strains are inhibited in vitro by 4–16 μg/ml of rifampin, as are a similar percentage of *M. avium-intracellulare* strains (36,37). *M. fortuitum* complex is universally resistant to rifampin, although *M. ulcerans* bacilli are generally susceptible. The response of *M. marinum* infections to rifampin has been particularly encouraging. Synergy of rifampin and other agents is often demonstrable in vitro. Its role as a single agent is discouraged to prevent emergence of resistant mycobacteria (36,37). Treatment with rifampin alone has resulted in acquired resistance by *M. kansasii* (44).

Aminoglycosides have been extensively used for treatment of atypical mycobacterial infections. Eighty-six percent of *M. kansasii* strains are streptomycin-susceptible, as are 93 percent of *M. scrofulaceum.* Forty-four percent of strains of *M. avium-intracellulare* have been streptomycin-sensitive. *M. fortuitum* complex is generally resistant whereas *M. ulcerans* strains demonstrate universal susceptibility to streptomycin in vitro (45). Despite in vitro susceptibility, streptomycin has not been efficacious for *M. ulcerans* infections probably because of inactivity against bacilli located intracellularly, and, indeed, surgical excision of Buruli ulcers remains the only effective treatment. Kanamycin is not active in vitro against most *M. kansasii* strains, whereas most *M. scrofulaceum* isolates are kanamycin-susceptible, and *M. avium-intracellulare* and *M. fortuitum* are not predictably kanamycin-sensitive.

Amikacin, a congener of kanamycin, appears to have greater activity against atypical mycobacteria than the parent compound. Many atypicals are susceptible to 12.5 μg/ml of amikacin (30). However, marked variability exists between mycobacteria in susceptibility to amikacin. Virtually all *M. marinum* strains are susceptible to 3 μg/ml of amikacin (43), but only 50 percent of the *M. fortuitum* group are susceptible to 12.5 μg/ml (46). Susceptibility of *M. avium-intracellulare* varies between laboratories from virtually complete susceptibility in vitro and in murine infections (47) to in vitro resistance at 10 μg/ml (29).

Ethambutol, ethionamide, and cycloserine possess variable activity against *M. avium-intracellulare* and have been employed in combination for infections caused by that group. Capreomycin frequently is the only antituberculous drug showing activity against *M. fortuitum.*

MISCELLANEOUS ANTIMICROBIALS FOR TREATMENT OF ATYPICAL MYCOBACTERIA

Erythromycin

Nearly all strains of *M. kansasii* and *M. scrofulaceum* and a minority of those of *M. avium-intracellulare* are susceptible to concentrations of erythromycin that can be achieved in plasma by conventional therapy (48). Additional therapeutic trials with erythromycin against organisms with documented in vitro susceptibility are needed (40).

Tetracyclines

Some strains included in the *M. fortuitum-chelonei* complex are tetracycline-susceptible. Although extensive in vitro testing has not been performed, encouraging clinical results have occurred with tetracyclines, especially minocycline (Minocin) in *M. marinum* infections (49).

Other Antimicrobics

Although *M. marinum* infections have responded to therapy with trimethoprim-sulfa, most strains are resistant to achievable plasma concentrations (43).

Clofazimine, discussed more fully under antileprosy drugs, has shown promising in vitro activity against *M. avium-intracellulare.* Most strains tested are inhibited by 1.6–2.0 μg/ml of clofazimine (29,50). However, a clinical trial of clofazimine in combination therapy against *M. avium-intracellulare* yielded disappointing results.

Active chemotherapeutic agents for serious *M. fortuitum* and *M. avium-intra-*

cellulare infections are greatly needed. Cefoxitin (Mefoxin), cefmetazole, and *N*-forminidoyl thienamycin, apparently because of resistance to *M. fortuitum* beta-lactamase, are active in vitro against approximately 80 percent of *M. fortuitum* strains at achievable plasma concentrations (51). Ansamycin (LM-427), a congener of rifamycin-S, was inhibitory against all strains of *M. avium-intracellulare* tested, in a concentration of < 2 μg/ml (29).

A summary of in vitro susceptibility data of atypical mycobacteria is supplied in Table 2. The table is to serve as a guide only. It is a compilation of data from a number of laboratories using nonstandard methodology. In many studies, a small number of strains were tested. Furthermore, in vitro susceptibility of atypical mycobacteria to an antimicrobial agent fails to guarantee therapeutic efficacy. Above-cited failures of clofazimine in *M. avium-intracellulare* infections and of streptomycin in *M. ulcerans* infections indicate limitations of extrapolating in vitro data to clinical experience. As a rule, however, good therapeutic outcomes are more likely when agents are used to which atypical mycobacteria are susceptible in vitro. Especially in treatment of more resistant atypical mycobacterial infections like those caused by *M. avium-intracellulare* or *M. fortuitum* complex, well-designed clinical trials with antimicrobials known to be active in vitro have not been done. Readily available analyses of plasma levels of the antimycobacterial agents are also greatly needed to assess efficacy and toxicity of drug regimens. Polypharmacy of atypical mycobacterial infections without confirmatory susceptibility testing and plasma concentrations fosters unnecessary toxicity and expense.

DRUGS FOR TREATMENT OF LEPROSY

Background

Chemotherapy for leprosy has, over the past 40 years, consisted, for all practical purposes, of dapsone alone. This has produced gratifying clinical results and has been economically affordable. Because of monotherapy, however, resistance of leprosy bacilli, both secondary and now primary, has emerged as a worldwide concern (53) leading to long overdue use of multidrug therapeutic regimens for leprosy (54).

Dapsone and Other Sulfones

Derivation and Structure. Diaminodiphenyl sulfone (dapsone, DDS) is a synthetic compound demonstrated to be effective against rat leprosy in 1941 and soon thereafter used successfully in human trials. Its structure is indicated in Figure 6.

Mechanism of Action. Sulfones are bacteriostatic presumably by the same mechanism by which sulfonamides interfere with folate synthesis.

TABLE 2. Antimicrobials for "Atypical" Mycobacteria: Likelihood of In Vitro Susceptibilities Being Within Range of Achievable Serum Concentrations

Category	*Runyon Group*	*Mycobacterial Species*	*Likelihood of Susceptibility to Antimicrobial*[a]
Photochromogens	I	*M. kansasii*	Erythromycin (4+), rifampin (4+), streptomycin (4+), ethionamide (4+), amikacin (3+), cycloserine (3+), ethambutol (3+), viomycin (3+), INH (2+)
		M. marinum	Rifampin (4+), amikacin (4+), kanamycin (4+), minocycline (3+)
Scotochromogens	II	*M. scrofulaceum*	Amikacin (4+), erythromycin (4+), kanamycin (4+), streptomycin (4+), rifampin (3+), ethionamide (2+), INH (1+)
Nonchromogens	III	*M. avium-intracellulare*	Amikacin (4+), ansamycin (4+), clofazimine (3+), ethionamide (2+), rifampin (2+), streptomycin (2+), cycloserine (2+), kanamycin (1+), INH (1+), ethambutol (1+), viomycin (1+), erythromycin (1+)
Rapid growers	IV	*M. fortuitum*	Cefoxitin (3+), cefmetazole (3+), N-formimidoyl thienamycin (3+), amikacin (3+), minocycline (2+), capreomycin (2+), kanamycin (2+), ethionamide (1+), gentamicin (1+), viomycin (1+)
		M. chelonei	Amikacin (2+), kanamycin (2+), erythromycin (2+)
Other		*M. ulcerans*	Rifampin (4+), streptomycin (4+), clofazimine (2+)

[a] Compilation of data from published sources (29,30, 36–38, 40–43, 45–52) ranked according to percentage of tested strains that were found susceptible to achievable serum concentrations of the antimicrobials: 81–100% = (4+), 61–80% = (3+), 41–60% = (2+), 21–40% = (1+).

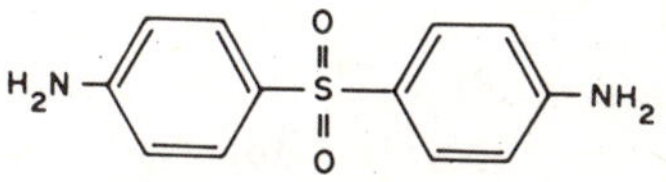

FIGURE 6. Structure of dapsone.

Antimicrobial Activity. By mouse foot-pad inoculation, as little as 0.003 μg/ml of dapsone inhibits *Mycobacterium leprae* (55). Dapsone appears "weakly bactericidal" for the majority of leprosy bacilli. It has been estimated that 99.9 percent of bacillary populations are killed after 3 to 4 months of therapy with dapsone (54). However, despite initial susceptibility, "persister" bacilli apparently exist for years. Secondary dapsone resistance is evident principally in lepromatous (multibacillary) patients in whom resistance has emerged as long as 5 to 24 years after commencing therapy (56). The incidence of secondary resistance varies widely between geographic regions, now occurring in 2 to 7 percent of cases. Fully resistant *M. leprae* should be suspected when patients supervised on 100 mg dapsone daily relapse during treatment (53). Apparently because of infection from secondarily resistant cases, primary dapsone resistance is now encountered at least as frequently as secondary resistance. Of newly diagnosed multibacillary cases, partial (the usual situation) to fully developed (infrequent) primary dapsone resistance is reported in from 4 percent (Phillipines) to 55 percent (Ethiopia) of cases, depending on geographic origin (53). It has been assumed that primary resistance exists as frequently in tuberculoid (paucibacillary) cases as lepromatous ones (53).

Pharmacology. Oral dapsone is well absorbed. Distributed throughout body fluids, tissue levels are approximately 2 μg/ml. Serum half-life of dapsone is 21 to 44 hours, with drug retention for up to 3 weeks. Dapsone is acetylated, with 70 to 80 percent being excreted as metabolites in the urine. Dosage thus should be reduced in significant renal failure.

Side Effects and Adverse Reactions. Dapsone, an oxidant drug, can produce minor hemolysis in patients receiving 200–300 mg/day. Insignificant hemolysis occurs at doses under 100 mg/day in normal people or at doses of 50 mg/day or less in people with glucose-6-phosphate dehydrogenase (G6PD) deficiency. Methemaglobinemia is common. Gastrointestinal intolerance occurs, manifested by anorexia with occasional nausea and vomiting. Hematuria, fever, pruritus, and skin rashes can occur.

Reactions encountered with dapsone or other sulfones may be difficult to extricate from the reactions that occur because of the disease itself. A *sulfone syndrome* has been reported 5 to 6 weeks after initiation of therapy and is characterized by fever, jaundice, dermatitis, and lymphadenopathy producing a picture somewhat like infectious mononucleosis (57). Its likelihood is diminished by gradual increase in dapsone doses until full therapeutic dosage is attained. Also, during dapsone administration, erythema nodosum leprosum

(ENL) reactions commonly become manifest in people with multibacillary disease. In borderline or intermediate cases, lepra reactions may be accentuated by dapsone therapy. Finally, although apparently infrequent, hypersensitivity reactions to dapsone may be difficult to recognize due to the complexity of the illness.

Usage. Dapsone continues to be the basic therapeutic agent for *M. leprae* infections, often as a component of multidrug programs.

Availability and Dosage. Dapsone (DDS) is available as Alvosulfon tablets of 25 or 100 mg. To avoid untoward reactions, it is begun in a dose of 1 25-mg tablet per week with a gradual increase by 1 tablet per week or so until a full therapeutic dose is reached—usually 100 mg/day. Appropriately reduced dosage is given to children.

Acedapsone

Derivation. Acedapsone (4,4'-diacetyldiaminodiphenylsulfone) is a long-acting repository derivative of dapsone.

Pharmacology. Slow absorption of acedapsone occurs from injection sites, with peak concentrations occurring between 22 and 35 days later. The parent compound has little activity against *M. leprae* but is converted into active dapsone. Its half-life is 46 days and 43 days for the derived dapsone (58). Because of its long half-life, injections only five times yearly have been used. A 300 mg IM dose maintained dapsone levels in volunteers above the inhibitory concentration for *M. leprae,* measured in mice for approximately 100 days.

Usage. This repository drug has been employed in *M. leprae* infections with promising results. Microbiologic and clinical responses are somewhat slower than with daily dapsone, raising the concern that resistance may become a problem. Long-term studies with acedapsone by injection five times yearly have yielded encouraging results, indicated by the fact that 91 percent of patients improved or "healed" after 6 years (59). Acedapsone shows promise especially in areas where other routes of therapy are not feasible. Trials incorporating widely spaced doses of rifampin plus acedapsone are in progress with the hope of reducing the burden of *M. leprae* more rapidly, thus lessening the likelihood of acedapsone-dapsone resistance.

Rifampin

Mechanism of Action and Resistance. The mechanism of action of rifampin against *M. leprae* is presumed to be by inhibition of DNA-dependent RNA-polymerase producing a relatively rapid bactericidal effect. The inhibitory concentration of rifampin for human strains of *M. leprae* tested in mice is 0.3

TABLE 3. Efficacy of Antileprosy Agents in Rendering Tissue Free of Bacilli[a]

Antimicrobial	Adult Human Dosage	Time Until Tissue Negative by Mouse Foot Pad Assay (Days)	
		Range	*Median*
Rifampin	1500 mg once	<3–<5	<3
Rifampin	600 mg/day	3–<14	<7
Dapsone	50 mg/day[b]	21–>134	61
Clofazimine	200 mg/day[c]	94–138	113
Acedapsone	225 mg/q 75 days	44–>306	214

[a] Modified from tabulation of Shepard, Levy, and Fasal (60).
[b] Dosage raised to 50 mg/day over period of 4 weeks.
[c] Dosage decreased to 100 mg/day in some patients having excessive skin pigmentation.

μg/ml. A tabulation of relative activity of antileprosy drugs in clearing tissue of viable bacilli is shown in Table 3.

Usage. Clinical trials of rifampin have indicated that rifampin differs by several orders of magnitude in its initial effectiveness compared with other antileprosy drugs (60). Demonstration by skin biopsy that a single dose of 1500 mg of rifampin can reduce viability of leprosy bacilli to undetectable levels by 3 to 5 days is truly remarkable. However, limitations of biopsy evaluations are inherent, since the method can only account for a decrease to about 10^8 total leprosy bacilli (60). Prolonged therapy of multibacillary lepromatous disease with 600 mg of rifampin daily has failed to eradicate large bacterial populations. Evidently, in leprosy as in other infections, rifampin as a solitary therapeutic agent promotes bacterial resistance. Despite generally satisfactory clinical results with rifampin alone, relapse has occurred in a minority of cases after 4 years of treatment with 300–600 mg daily (54). Although it causes a rapid decrease in *M. leprae* populations, rifampin should be employed with another, preferably two, companion drugs including dapsone for multibacillary disease. The high cost of rifampin has discouraged its use in economically deprived areas. However, once monthly therapy with 600–1200 mg of rifampin in combination drug regimens has produced satisfactory preliminary clinical responses without adverse reactions (54,61). Lepra and ENL reactions have been comparable or less severe with rifampin-containing regimens.

Clofazimine (B-663)

Derivation and Structure. The structure of clofazimine, a phenazine dye, is indicated in Figure 7.

Mechanism of Action and Antimicrobial Activity. Clofazimine's precise mechanism of action is not known. It is weakly bactericidal against *M. leprae.* The

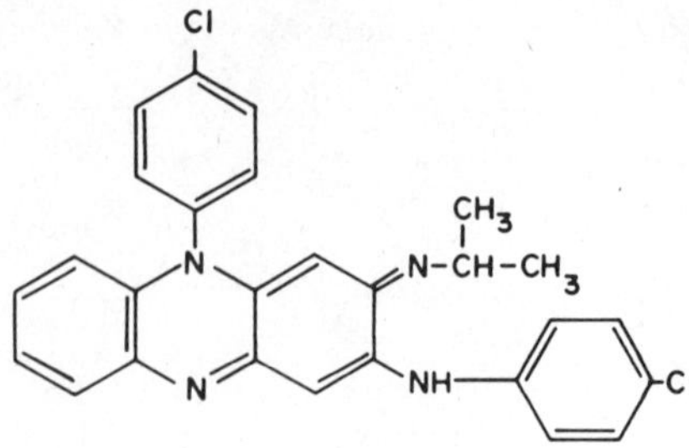

FIGURE 7. Structure of clofazimine.

inhibitory concentration of clofazimine in mouse tissue is between 0.1 and 1 mg/kg (62). A delay of some 50 days ensues before tissue antimicrobic activity can be demonstrated in man.

Pharmacology. Clofazimine's pharmacokinetics are complex. Absorption is quite variable with 9 to 74 percent of an administered dose appearing in feces. The route of administration is oral, resulting in plasma concentrations of 0.4–3 μg/ml with a half-life of approximately 70 days. Clofazimine is widely distributed throughout reticuloendothelial tissues, especially in liver, spleen, lung, adrenals, adipose tissue, and in skin lesions. Red-orange crystals of clofazimine can be observed microscopically in phagocytic reticuloendothelial cells. Precise concentrations in tissues can only be estimated because of very uneven distribution of the drug. It is largely unmetabolized and subsequently excreted slowly, with less than 1 percent of a dose appearing in urine. Biliary excretion appears to be the major route of disposition of clofazimine. A dose of 100 mg/day has been calculated to eventually result in total accumulation of at least 10 g of drug in human tissue (62).

Adverse Reactions. Gastrointestinal intolerance that is usually not severe may occur. Skin pigmentation is the major side effect from drug accumulation, resulting in red-brown to almost black skin discoloration in susceptible people. Other side effects are negligible.

Usage. Clofazimine is expensive. Its principal role has been as therapy for sulfone-resistant infections and for people who are sulfone-intolerant usually because of severe sulfone-associated ENL or lepra reactions. These reactions occur much less frequently with clofazimine than with dapsone (63).

Availability and Dosage. Clofazimine is available as Lamprene in 100-mg capsules. For monotherapy, its dose has ranged from 300 mg monthly to 600 mg daily and has usually been 100–300 mg/day. Administration of clofazimine alone once weekly or less frequently has resulted in diminished efficacy (63). In combination therapeutic regimens for multibacillary disease, recommended dosage has been either 300 mg monthly or 50–100 mg daily.

ADDITIONAL DRUGS FOR TREATMENT OF MULTIBACILLARY LEPROSY

Amithiozone (Thiacetazone)

Derivation, structure, pharmacokinetics, untoward reactions, and dosage of this thiosemicarbazone are described under second-line drugs for tuberculosis.

Usage. Amithiozone's efficacy is greater in tuberculoid than lepromatous (multibacillary) disease. The drug can be administered when sulfones cannot be tolerated. Considerable cross-resistance with sulfones occurs. Amithiozone is not available in the United States.

Long-Acting Sulfonamides

Hypersensitivity reactions, including erythema multiforme (Stevens-Johnson syndrome) may result from long-acting sulfonamides. Used with varying degrees of success for treatment of leprosy, they have no particular advantage over sulfones, share cross-resistance with them, and consequently have been supplanted by the sulfones (64).

Ethionamide and Prothionamide

Ethionamide has been described under second-line agents for tuberculosis. It and its congener, prothionamide, possess similar pharmacokinetics and dosing and provide alternatives to clofazimine in multidrug regimens for multibacillary disease principally in people who are unable to tolerate or who will not accept clofazimine due to skin pigmentation (54). Ethionamide and prothionamide are apparently weakly cidal for *M. leprae.* Both drugs are available as 125- or 250-mg tablets. Dosage with either is 375–500 mg daily (54). Both agents are expensive, cause a considerable degree of gastrointestinal intolerance, and rarely cause drug-induced hepatitis.

CHEMOTHERAPY: ASSOCIATED REACTIONS IN LEPROSY

Febrile reactions in people with leprosy can be treated with acetylsalicylic acid (aspirin) in conventional dosages. Chloroquine phosphate (Aralen, Avloclor, Resochin) in a dose of 250–500 mg of diphosphate daily has been used in some centers for treatment-associated reactions. Methylprednisolone, 60 mg daily initially, followed by tapering of dosage, has been reasonably efficacious (65). Thalidomide in an initial dosage of 400 mg daily has been used to lessen therapy-associated reactions. Thalidomide should not be abruptly discontinued due to exacerbations of reactions. Consequently, gradually tapering dosage and even maintenance with 50 mg/day has been recommended (64). Because of teratogenic potential, thalidomide should never be administered to pregnant women or those of childbearing age. Patients who manifest severe reactions are best managed by a specialist.

REFERENCES

1. Mandell GL, Sande MA: Drugs used in the chemotherapy of tuberculosis and leprosy, in Gilman AS, Goodman LS, Gilman A (eds) *The Pharmacological Basis of Therapeutics,* ed. 6. New York, MacMillan Publishing Co, 1980, pp 1200–1221.
2. Kucers A, Bennett NM: Drugs mainly for tuberculosis, in *The Use of Antibiotics,* ed. 3. London, Heinemann Medical Books, 1979, pp 798–862.
3. Pratt WB: Chemotherapy of tuberculosis, in *Chemotherapy of Infection.* New York, Oxford University Press, 1977, pp 231–262.
4. Stead WW, Dutt AK: Chemotherapy for tuberculosis today. *Am Rev Resp Dis* 125(3) suppl.:94, 1982.
5. Tuberculosis Chemotherapy Trials Committee: Interim report to the Medical Research Council; the treatment of pulmonary tuberculosis with isoniazid. *Br Med J* 2:735, 1952.
6. Herman RP, Weber MM: Site of action of isoniazid on the electron transport chain and its relationship to nicotinamide adenine dinucleotide regulation in *Mycobacterium phlei. Anitmicrob Agents Chemother* 17:450, 1980.
7. Costello HD, Caras GJ, Snider DE: Drug resistance among previously treated tuberculosis patients: A brief report. *Am Rev Resp Dis* 121:313, 1980.
8. Carpenter JL, Covelli HD, Avant ME, et al: Drug-resistant *Mycobacterium tuberculosis* in Korean isolates. *Am Rev Resp Dis* 126:1092, 1982.
9. Bowerson DW, Winterbauer RH, Steward GL, et al: Isoniazid dosage in patients with renal failure, *N Engl J Med* 289:84, 1973.
10. Grossman LA, Kaplan HJ, Brittingham TE: Jaundice and death from isoniazid. *J Tenn Med Assoc* 63:23, 1970.
11. Kopanoff DE, Snider DE, Caras GJ: Isoniazid-related hepatitis. *Am Rev Respir Dis* 117:991, 1978.
12. Gronhagen-Riska C, Hellstrom PE, Froseth B: Predisposing factors in hepatitis induced by isoniazid-rifampin treatment of tuberculosis. *Am Rev Respir Dis* 118:461, 1978.
13. Mitchell JR, Zimmerman HJ, Ishak KG, et al: Isoniazid liver injury: clinical spectrum, pathology, and probable pathogenesis. *Ann Intern Med* 84:181, 1976.
14. Center for Disease Control: Isoniazid-associated hepatitis: summary of the report of the Tuberculosis Advisory Committee and special consultants to the directory. *Morbidity and Mortality Weekly Report* 23:97, 1974.
15. Falk A: US Veterans Administration-Armed Forces cooperative study on the chemotherapy of tuberculosis. XIII. Tuberculous meningitis in adults with special reference to survival, neurologic residuals, and work status. *Am Rev Respir Dis* 91:823, 1965.
16. Falk A: US Veterans Administration-Armed Forces cooperative study on the chemotherapy of tuberculosis. XII. Results of treatment in miliary tuberculosis: a followup study of 570 adult patients. *Am Rev Respir Dis* 91:6, 1965.
17. American Thoracic Society: Intermittent therapy for adults with tuberculosis. *Am Rev Respir Dis* 110:374, 1974.
18. Acocella G, Bonollo M, Garimoldi M, et al: Kinetics of rifampicin and isoniazid administered alone and in combination to normal subjects and patients with liver disease. *Gut* 13:47, 1972.
19. Stottmeier KD: Emergence of rifampin-resistant *Mycobacterium tuberculosis* in Massachusetts. *J Infect Dis* 133:88, 1976.
20. Newman R, et al: Rifampin in initial treatment of pulmonary tuberculosis. A US Public Health Service tuberculosis therapy trial. *Am Rev Respir Dis* 109:216, 1974.
21. Sanders WE Jr: Rifampin. *Ann Intern Med* 85:82, 1976.

22. Thompson JE: The effect of rifampicin on liver morphology in tuberculous alcoholics. *Aust NZ J Med* 6:111, 1976.
23. Rahajoe NN, Rahajoe N, Boediman I, et al: The treatment of tuberculous meningitis in children with a combination of isoniazid, rifampicin, and streptomycin—preliminary report. *Tubercle* 60:245, 1979.
24. Graber CD, Jebaily J, Galphin RL, et al: Light chain proteinuria and humoral immunocompetence in tuberculosis patients treated with rifampin. *Am Rev Respir Dis* 107:713, 1973.
25. Grassi GG, Pozzi E: Effect of rifampin on delayed hypersensitivity reactions. *J Infect Dis* 126:542, 1972.
26. Flynn CT, Rainford DJ, Hope E: Acute renal failure and rifampin: Danger of unsuspected intermittent dosage. *Br Med J* 2:482, 1974.
27. Dutt AK, Stead WW: Present chemotherapy for tuberculosis. *J Infect Dis* 146:698, 1982.
28. Sanfilippo A, Della Bruna C, Marsili L, et al: Biological activity of a new class of rifamycins, spiro-piperidyl-rifamycins. *J Antibiot* (Tokyo) 33:1193, 1980.
29. Greene JB, Sidhu GS, Lewin S, et al: *Mycobacterium avium-intracellulare:* A cause of disseminated life-threatening infection in homosexuals and drug abusers. *Ann Intern Med* 97:539, 1982.
30. Sanders WE Jr, et al: Activity of amikacin against mycobacteria in vitro and in experimental infections with *M tuberculosis. Am Rev Respir Dis* 113:(4)suppl.59, 1976.
31. Girling DJ: The hepatic toxicity of antituberculous regimens containing isoniazid, rifampicin, and pyrazinamide. *Tubercle* 59:13, 1978.
32. Zierski M, Bek E: Side effects of drug regimens used in short-course chemotherapy for pulmonary tuberculosis. A controlled clinical study. *Tubercle* 61:41, 1980.
33. McClatchy JK, et al: Cross-resistance in *M. tuberculosis* to kanamycin, capreomycin, and viomycin. *Tubercle* 58:29, 1977.
34. Cynamon MH, Palmer GS: In vitro activity of amoxicillin in combination with clavulanic acid against *Mycobacterium tuberculosis. Antimicrob Agents Chemother* 24:429, 1983.
35. Crawford JT, Bates JH: Isolation of plasmids from mycobacteria. *Infect Immun* 24:979, 1979.
36. Heifets LB: Synergistic effect of rifampin, streptomycin, ethionamide, and ethambutol on *Mycobacterium intracellulare. Am Rev Respir Dis* 125:43, 1982.
37. Zimmer BL, DeYoung DR, Roberts GD: In vitro synergistic activity of ethambutol, isoniazid, kanamycin, rifampin, and streptomycin against *Mycobacterium avium-intracellulare* complex. *Antimicrob Agents Chemother* 22:148, 1982.
38. Dutt AK, Stead EW: Long-term results in medical treatment in *Mycobacterium intracellulare* infection. *Am J Med* 67:449, 1979.
39. Sommers HM, McClatchy JK: Laboratory diagnoses of the Mycobacterioses. *Cumitech 16, Cumulative Techniques and Procedures in Microbiology,* Morello JA, (ed) *Am Soc Microbiol,* Washington DC, March 1983.
40. Irwin RS, Pratter MR, Corwin W, et al: Pulmonary infection with *Mycobacterium chelonei:* successful treatment with one drug based on disk diffusion susceptibility data. *J Infect Dis* 145:772, 1982.
41. Hobby GL, Redmond WB, Runyon EH, et al: A study on pulmonary disease associated with mycobacteria other than *Mycobacterium tuberculosis:* identification and characterization of the mycobacteria. XVIII. A report of the Veterans Administration-Armed Forces cooperative study. *Am Rev Respir Dis* 95:954, 1967.
42. Rynearson TK, Shronts JS, Wolinsky E: Rifampin: in vitro effect on atypical mycobacteria. *Am Rev Respir Dis* 104:272, 1971.
43. Sanders WJ, Wolinsky E: In vitro susceptibility of *Mycobacterium marinum* to eight antimicrobial agents. *Antimicrob Agents Chemother* 18:529, 1980.
44. Davidson PT, Waggoner R: Acquired resistance to rifampicin by *Mycobacterium kansasii. Tubercle* 57:271, 1976.
45. Leach RH, Fenner F: Studies on *Mycobacterium ulcerans* and *Mycobacterium balnei.* III. Growth in semisynthetic culture media of Dubos and drug sensitivity in vitro and in vivo. *Aust J Exp Biol Med Sci* 32:835, 1954.

46. Sanders WE Jr, Hartwig EC, Schneider NJ, et al: Susceptibility of organisms in the *Mycobacterium fortuitum* complex to antituberculous and other antimicrobial agents. *Antimicrob Agents Chemother* 12:295, 1977.
47. Sanders WE Jr: Personal communication.
48. Molavi A, Weinstein L: In vitro activity of erythromycin against atypical mycobacteria. *J Infect Dis* 123:216, 1971.
49. Loria PR: Minocycline hydrochloride treatment for atypical acid-fast infection. *Arch Dermatol* 112:517, 1976.
50. Gangadharam PRJ, Candler ER: Activity of some antileprosy compounds against *Mycobacterium intracellulare* in vitro. *Am Rev Respir Dis* 115:705, 1977.
51. Cynamon MH, Palmer GS: In vitro susceptibility of *Mycobacterium fortuitum* to N-formimidoyl thienamycin and several cephamycins. *Antimicrob Ag Chemother* 22:1079, 1982.
52. Swenson JM, Thornsberry C, Silcox VA: Rapidly growing mycobacteria: testing of susceptibility to 34 antimicrobial agents by broth microdilution. *Antimicrob Agents Chemother* 22:186, 1982.
53. USPHS Centers for Disease Control: Increase in prevalence of leprosy caused by dapsone-resistant *Mycobacterium leprae. MMWR* 30:637, 1982.
54. WHO Study Group: Chemotherapy of leprosy for control programmes. World Health Organization, Geneva, 1982.
55. Levy L, Peters JH: Susceptibility of *Mycobacterium leprae* to dapsone as a determinant of patient response to acedapsone. *Antimicrob Agents Chemother* 9:102, 1976.
56. Pearson JMH, Rees RJW, Waters MFR: Sulphone resistance in leprosy. A review of one hundred proven clinical cases. *Lancet* 2:69, 1975.
57. Editorial: Adverse reactions to dapsone. *Lancet* 2:184, 1981.
58. Peters JH, Murray JF, Gordon GR, et al: Acedapsone treatment of leprosy patients: response versus drug disposition. *Am J Trop Med Hyg* 26:127, 1977.
59. Russell DA, Shepard CC, McRae DH, et al: Acedapsone (DADDS) treatment of leprosy patients in the Karimui of Papua New Guinea: status at six years. *Am J Trop Med Hyg* 24:485, 1975.
60. Shepard CC, Levy L, Fasal P: Further experience with the rapid bactericidal effect of rifampin on *Mycobacterium leprae. Am J Trop Med Hyg* 23:1120, 1974.
61. Yawalkar SJ, Languillon J, Hajra SK, et al: Once-monthly rifampicin plus dapsone in initial treatment of lepromatous leprosy. *Lancet* 1:1199, 1982.
62. Levy L: Pharmacologic studies of clofazimine. *Am J Trop Med Hyg* 23:1097, 1974.
63. US Leprosy Panel: Spaced clofazimine therapy of lepromatous leprosy. *Am J Trop Med Hyg* 25:437, 1976.
64. Convit J, Browne SG, Languillon J, et al: Therapy of leprosy. *Bull WHO* 42:667, 1970.
65. Grove DI, Warren, KS, Mahmoud AAF: Algorithms in the diagnosis and management of exotic diseases. XV. Leprosy. *J Infect Dis* 134:205, 1976.

16

ANTIFUNGAL AGENTS

JOHN E. BENNETT

This chapter concerns agents used primarily for treatment of systemic mycoses. Topical imidazole drugs will be included here because of features common to systemic imidazoles. Topical ciclopirox olamine, marketed as a 1 percent cream, appears interchangeable with topical imidazoles (clotrimazole, econazole, miconazole) but is a unique synthetic drug, not included in the following discussion. Oral iodide therapy is used almost exclusively for cutaneous sporotrichosis and will not be considered here. Hydroxystilbamidine is not discussed because its usage has been eclipsed completely by better drugs.

POLYENE MACROLIDE ANTIBIOTICS

Currently three drugs of the class polyene macrolide antibiotics are commercially available in the United States: nystatin, amphotericin B, and natamycin. Overseas, natamycin is marketed as a topical preparation, interchangeable with nystatin. In the United States, only a 5 percent ophthalmic suspension is available. It is used for mycotic conjunctivitis and keratitis.

These three drugs are members of a large group of antibiotics, all sharing certain features of structure, mechanism of action, and toxicity (1). Polyene refers to the conjugated double bonds and macrolide to the internal ester in the ring structure (Fig. 1). The lipophilic polyene structure is probably the major site responsible for the mechanism of action. Combination of the polyene with certain cytoplasmic membrane sterols, principally ergosterol, in fungi causes the membrane to become porous (2). Mechanisms for drug-induced resistance to polyenes include decrease in membrane ergosterol and modification of membrane sterols to those that combine less well with polyenes (2–5). In patients, secondary drug resistance has been very uncommon and usually of small magnitude. Most polyene-resistant mutants in clinical specimens have been isolated from sites in which pathogenicity of the isolate was unclear, such as isolates from urine, sputum, or stool. A few exceptions are notable (5,6). Polyene-resistant

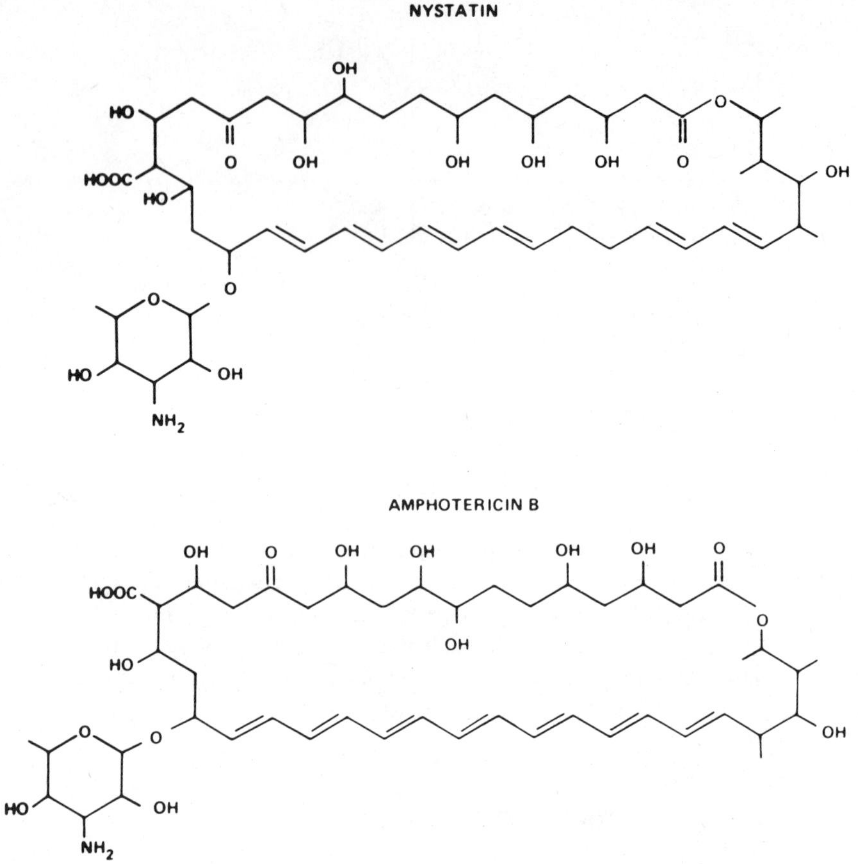

FIGURE 1. Proposed structures for amphotericin B and one of the major components of nystatin (see ref. 1).

mutants created in vitro often have altered appearance, slower growth, and decreased virulence (5,7).

Polyene antibiotics are, in general, poorly soluble in water at neutral pH, very soluble in dimethylsulfoxide or dimethylformamide, poorly absorbed from the gastrointestinal tract, and toxic on parenteral administration. Many polyenes have been tested for possible clinical value, but none offers clear advantages over amphotericin B or nystatin. Cross resistance between polyenes is essentially complete (7,8).

Nystatin

Nystatin, named for New York State, is produced by *Streptomyces noursei.* Toxicity after parenteral administration to animals has led to its use only topically and orally. No systemic absorption occurs from these sites. Superficial penetration is adequate to treat mucocutaneous candidiasis unless the epidermis is markedly hypertrophic. Ringworm and subcutaneous mycoses fail to respond. Each nystatin preparation is tailored for a particular form of candidiasis. Vaginal tablets are designed for vaginal candidiasis but have also been used as troches for oral and esophageal infection. For vaginitis due to *Candida,* one 100,000 unit tablet is inserted high in the vagina, using an applicator, once or twice daily for 14 days. The failure rate of approximately 20 percent appears to be somewhat higher than a 7-day regimen of miconazole or clotrimazole cream, as discussed later. Esophageal candidiasis sometimes responds to four times daily use of either the suppository, sucked on like a troche, or nystatin suspension (100,000 units/ml). The suspension is used in the same way for either oral or esophageal candidiasis. The patient is instructed to take 5 ml four times a day, swishing the suspension around the mouth and then swallowing it. This regimen is highly effective for oral candidiasis, making the older, messy gentian violet therapy obsolete. Nystatin is also marketed as cream, lotion, ointment, and powder formulations for cutaneous candidiasis. These preparations are not indicated for ringworm. Oral tablets (500,000 units) have been used in conjunction with vaginal tablets to treat vaginal candidiasis, the hope being to decrease the likelihood of recolonization of the vagina with fecal *Candida.* Although this appears logical, the contribution of the oral tablet is not well established, and the nystatin-induced decrease in fecal colony count of *Candida* is seldom more than 10-fold. Incorporation of nystatin into tetracycline tablets is done with a closely related goal, that is, to decrease the incidence of tetracycline-induced vaginal candidiasis. Although an occasional study with a tetracycline and either nystatin or amphotericin B has been interpreted to show a decrease in the incidence of tetracycline-induced vaginal candidiasis (9), the majority have failed to confirm this beneficial effect. Other tetracycline side effects, such as diarrhea, are not mitigated (10). The expense of these combinations must be balanced against their questionable efficacy.

Other than the bitter taste of nystatin suspension, adverse reactions to conventional treatment courses of oral or topical nystatin are inconsequential. Oral administration of 20–30 million units per day in divided doses has been used in bowel sterilization regimens for patients in protected environments. No systemic absorption is detectable.

Amphotericin B

Amphotericin B is produced by *Streptomyces nodosus.* The complete structure, as discovered by Ganis and coworkers (11), includes seven conjugated double bonds, a free carboxyl, and a glycosidic side chain with a primary amino group. The drug is amphoteric, hence the name, and is soluble but chemically unstable at extremes of pH. Intravenous administration of microparticulate suspensions at neutral pH gave low blood levels. A marked increase in therapeutic effect, toxicity, and blood level occurred when the drug was complexed with bile salt (desoxycholate) and injected as a colloidal suspension (12). The commercially available preparation of amphotericin B for parenteral use (Fungizone for Infusion) is marketed in 50-mg vials that also contain 41 mg of desoxycholate and 25.2 mg of sodium phosphate buffer. A small percentage of the preparation is amphotericin A and other impurities, but these seem to have a negligible effect on toxicity. The vial is reconstituted with distilled water or aqueous dextrose and administered intravenously in 5 percent dextrose in water. The drug decomposes slowly in solution, but the effect is negligible under the usual conditions of intravenous administration. The infusion bottle need not be light shielded (13). Addition of an electrolyte, such as potassium or sodium salts, to the solution causes the colloid to aggregate. The aggregated colloidal solution slowly becomes cloudy and probably gives a suboptimal therapeutic effect on infusion. Even without aggregation the colloidal solution is partially retained by a 0.22-μm pore membrane filter (14). Hyperalimentation lines should use 0.45-μm pore filters.

Concentrations of amphotericin B in biologic fluids have usually been measured by bioassay (15), but high-pressure liquid chromatography (16), rubidium 86 release (17), and radiometric respirometry (18) have been described. Despite the proliferation of methods, routine determination of amphotericin B serum, urine, or cerebrospinal fluid concentrations has no definite clinical value. Nonetheless, amphotericin B assays have revealed some remarkable pharmacologic properties of this drug. When colloidal amphotericin B is admixed in serum, desoxycholate separates from amphotericin B (19), and more than 95 percent of the latter binds to serum proteins (20), principally to β-lipoprotein (21). Presumably the drug is bound to the cholesterol carried on this protein. The majority of the drug leaves the circulation promptly, perhaps bound to cholesterol-containing cytoplasmic membranes. Amphotericin B is stored in the liver and other organs; the drug appears to reenter the circulation slowly (22). Most of the drug is degraded in situ with only a small percentage being excreted in urine (15,22) or bile (23). Blood levels are uninfluenced by hepatic or renal failure (20,23). Hemodialysis does not alter blood levels except for an occasional patient with lipemic plasma who may be losing drug by adherence to the dialysis membrane (20). Concentrations of amphotericin B in fluids from inflamed areas, such as pleura, peritoneum, joint, vitreous humor (24), and aqueous humor, are roughly two-thirds of the trough serum level. Cord blood from one infant contained amphotericin B concentration of 0.37 μg/ml, half the simultaneous maternal trough blood level. Amphotericin B penetrates poorly into either normal or inflamed meninges, vitreous humor, or normal amniotic fluid. Urine concentrations are similar to serum concentrations. Peak serum concentrations with conventional intravenous doses are roughly 0.5–2.0 μg/ml but fall rapidly initially to slowly approach a plateau of roughly 0.2–0.5 μg/ml (15).

Toxicity of intravenous amphotericin B is formidable, but nearly all patients can complete a conventional course of therapy. Therapy is best begun with a small test dose, such as 1 mg in adults, to assess the patient's febrile response. This dose can be given in 20 ml of 5 percent dextrose over 10–20 minutes. The patient's temperature, pulse and respiration rates, and blood pressure are recorded every 30 minutes for 4 hours. The amount of the next dose and the addition of hydrocortisone to the infusion is determined by the extent of fever, chills, hypotension, and dyspnea, as well as by the rate of progression of the mycosis, by the cardiopulmonary status of the patient, and by concomitant adrenal corticosteroid therapy. A patient with a rapidly progressing infection, with good cardiopulmonary status, and with a mild reaction to the test dose can for the next dose be given amphotericin B, 0.3 mg/kg, with hydrocortisone hemisuccinate, approximately 0.7 mg/kg. Patients already receiving supraphysiologic doses of adrenal corticosteroids receive little or no benefit from additional steroid in the infusion. A smaller second dose is appropriate for fragile patients with marked reactions to the test dose. Therapy for indolent mycoses may also be initiated slowly and without the addition of hydrocortisone. Tolerance to the febrile reactions develops with time, allowing diminution and eventual discontinuance of the hydrocortisone. The amphotericin B dose is advanced progressively to about 0.5 mg/kg/day by the third to fifth day in patients with prior normal renal function. This dose is maintained or advanced slowly to 0.6 mg/kg/day or, at most, 0.7 mg/kg/day while biweekly determinations of blood creatinine, hematocrit, potassium, and bicarbonate levels are observed. Each infusion is given over 2–4 hours in 500 ml of 5 percent dextrose in water. We prefer to add heparin, 1000 units, to this infusion, although there is no proof this decreases phlebitis.

Azotemia is a normal concomitant of amphotericin B therapy (25). The azotemia reaches a plateau during therapy at a level commensurate with the daily dose. Other nephrotoxic drugs, including cyclosporine (26), increase azotemia. Salt repletion can improve renal function in the sodium depleted patient (27). A therapeutic course of amphotericin B is usually followed by a permanent reduction in glomerular filtration rate. This reduction is unrelated to the azotemia during therapy but is correlated with the total dose (25). Dosage reduction during therapy to keep the serum creatinine level below 3.5 mg/dl is recommended only to help keep nausea and vomiting from causing dehydration and cachexia. Adequate oral intake of high potassium foods, such as certain fruits and meat, can help prevent hypokalemia.

During an average course of therapy, the patient's serum creatinine level will rise to 2.0–3.0 mg/dl, cyllindruria occurs, the hematocrit falls to 20–30 percent and, in one-fourth of the patients, hypokalemia necessitates oral potassium supplements. Weight loss of 15 lb is common. Renal tubular acidosis may occur but rarely requires treatment (28). Headache and phlebitis are common. Rare side effects include thrombocytopenia, mild leukopenia, anaphylaxis, and burning sensations on the soles of the feet. Neither rash nor hepatotoxicity has been clearly documented. Side effects disappear in the first 3 months after therapy. The slow disappearance of side effects perhaps reflects the slow catabolism of the drug, which can be found in serum and urine up to 6 weeks after a course of therapy. Several pregnant patients have received intravenous amphotericin B during the second or third trimester without fetal damage. However, safety in pregnancy is not clearly established.

Mechanisms for the toxic reactions are not fully understood. Amphotericin-B-induced cell permeability probably accounts for the loss of intracellular potassium into the blood and out the urine. Ventricular tachycardia in experimental animals given rapid injections of 5 mg/kg may also result from membrane damage. Renal damage morphologically is primarily injury to both proximal and distal tubular cells (29). Glomerular damage is subtle or absent. Conceivably, nephrotoxicity in humans results from renal vascular constriction, such as occurs in dogs (30). Anemia is normocytic, normochromic, and accompanied by a normal appearing bone marrow. Erythrocyte survival is normal (31). The serum erythropoietin level is abnormally low for the degree of anemia (32). Acute respiratory deterioration was thought to have occurred in one institution when amphotericin B was given during or right after leukocyte transfusion (33). Aggregation of leukocytes by amphotericin B (34) with trapping in the lung has been proposed. Rarity of this phenomenon has raised consideration of a third factor, perhaps bacterial endotoxin, necessary to create the syndrome.

Administration of amphotericin B on alternate days rather than daily does not reduce nephrotoxicity if the alternate day dose is doubled. The number of venipunctures is decreased, and ambulation is facilitated by an alternate-day double-dose schedule, but more febrile reactions may be encountered. Therapeutic effects of both regimens are indistinguishable. Adequate hydration and salt replacement remain the best measures to minimize azotemia.

Mycoses with a useful response to amphotericin B include blastomycosis, candidiasis, histoplasmosis, cryptococcosis, paracoccidioidomycosis, coccidioidomycosis, aspergillosis, mucormycosis, and extracutaneous sporotrichosis. Daily doses range from 0.4 to 0.6 mg/kg/day, depending on mycosis. Lower doses (0.2–0.3 mg/kg) have been used largely in situations in which spontaneous recovery is a good possibility, such as esophagitis due to *Candida*. The duration of therapy in systemic mycoses is 6–12 weeks in most patients. Esophagitis due to *Candida* is often treated for only 5–7 days.

Localized injections of amphotericin B may be useful. Sporotrichosis or coccidioidomycosis of joints may benefit by intra-articular injections of 5–15 mg, depending on joint size. Intrathecal amphotericin B is essential in coccidioidal meningitis. After test doses of 0.05 and 0.1 mg, doses of 0.2–0.5 mg are given from one to three times per week into the lumbar, cisternal, or ventricular cerebrospinal fluid. Hydrocortisone, 5–15 mg, in the injection helps decrease the resulting fever, headache, and nausea. Lumbar injections may cause temporary radicular pain and loss of motor function in the legs, rectum, and bladder (35). Use of 10 percent glucose as a diluent and positioning the patient during injection to permit hyperbaric flow toward the brain may decrease local myelopathy (36). Injections into the lateral cerebral ventricle through a subcutaneous siliconized rubber reservoir are useful, but the complication rate is high (37). Bladder irrigations with amphotericin B, 50 μg/ml, in distilled water have been used in *Candida*-induced cystitis (38). Corneal baths with 1 mg/ml are irritating but beneficial in keratomycosis.

Attempts to improve the therapeutic ratio of amphotericin B led to synthesis of several derivatives (39), the most promising of which seemed to be the methyl ester. Occurrence of leukoencephalopathy in humans essentially halted further studies on this compound (40). Interest has now turned to liposome-packaged colloidal amphotericin B.

Amphotericin B in Combination with Other Drugs

Under certain conditions, the antifungal activity of amphotericin B can be enhanced with flucytosine, rifampin, or tetracycline. Use of the amphotericin B–flucytosine combination will be discussed in the section dealing with the latter drug. Rifampin, which is not antifungal when used alone, decreases the in vitro concentration of amphotericin B necessary to inhibit growth of *Candida* (41), *Histoplasma* (42), *Cryptococcus* (43), and *Aspergillus* species (44). The amount of reduction is roughly from twofold to fourfold. In experimental mouse infections with *Histoplasma* (45), *Blastomyces* (45), and *Aspergillus* (46) but not *Coccidioides* (47) or *Candida* (48), rifampin therapy resulted in a significant decrease in the dose of amphotericin B necessary to prolong life. Perhaps significant is the fact that the combination did not result in a therapeutic effect superior to that obtainable with optimum doses of amphotericin B alone. This would suggest an amphotericin-B-sparing rather than amphotericin-B-enhancing effect. Anecdotal clinical experiences with this combination have surfaced neither a noticeable improvement in therapeutic efficacy nor a definite synergistic toxicity.

Tetracycline provided an amphotericin-B-sparing effect in experimental murine coccidioidomycosis (49). In vitro, minocycline decreased the concentration of amphotericin B necessary to inhibit many strains of *Candida* and *Cryptococcus* (50). This combination has attracted little clinical attention thus far because of all the potential toxic interactions between tetracyclines and amphotericin B.

Combinations of amphotericin B with antitumor agents have received clinical trial based on favorable experience in experimental animals (51).

Amphotericin B combined with ketoconazole has not appeared particularly promising in vitro or in vivo. The effect in vitro is very method dependent (52). Under some conditions, antagonism can be demonstrated (53). In experimentally infected mice, the effect of the combination in candidiasis (54), histoplasmosis (55), and cryptococcosis (54,55) was not superior to the better single drug.

FLUCYTOSINE

Flucytosine [5-fluorocytosine (5-FC), Ancobon] is the fluorine analogue of a normal body constituent, cytosine (Fig. 2). The drug was synthesized as a potential antitumor agent, but that property was lacking. Routine screening discovered the antifungal effect, which became the sole use of this drug (56). Flucytosine is a white powder, moderately soluble in water, very stable on dry storage,

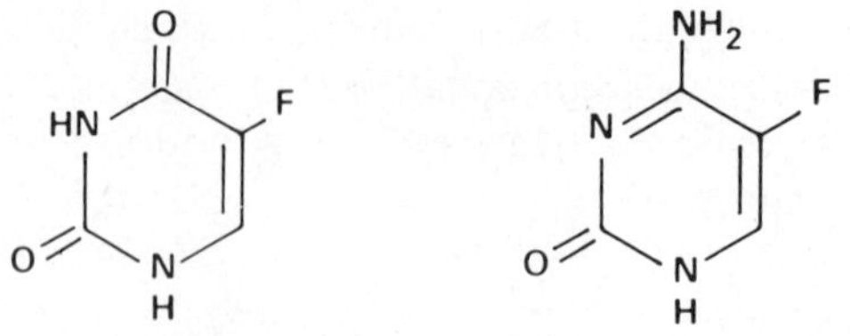

5-Fluorouracil
(5-FU)

5-Fluorocytosine
(5-FC)

FIGURE 2. Structural formulas of 5-fluorocytosine (5-FC) and 5-fluorouracil (5-FU), a closely related antitumor agent.

and marketed as 250- and 500-mg capsules. Absorption from the gastrointestinal tract is rapid and complete. Approximately 90 percent is excreted unchanged in the urine. Protein binding is barely measurable (20). Cerebrospinal fluid concentrations approximate 74 percent of simultaneous serum concentrations. The drug is readily cleared by hemodialysis (20). Peritoneal dialysis also removes flucytosine from the body.

Half-life of the drug in the serum of patients with normal renal function is 3–5 hours (57). Abnormal hepatic function has no influence, but decreased renal function can prolong the half-life to beyond 24 hours.

Mechanism of flucytosine's antifungal action appears to be by deamination to 5-fluorouracil (5-FU) (Fig. 2) and then conversion through several steps to 5-fluorodeoxyuridylic acid monophosphate, a noncompetitive inhibitor of thymidylate synthetase (58). This interferes with DNA synthesis. Additional mechanisms of action may also be operative (59).

Flucytosine is usually given as 150 mg/kg/day in four divided doses. Patients with a serum creatinine level of 1.7 mg/dl or greater usually require dose reduction. As a rough rule, the dose can be estimated by dividing 150 mg/kg/day by the serum creatinine in milligrams per deciliter. Ideally, the blood level should be measured in azotemic patients 2 hours after the last dose and immediately before the next dose. These values should range between 50 and 100 μg/ml. Patients receiving hemodialysis may be given a single postdialysis dose of 37.5 mg/kg. Further doses are adjusted by blood level. Reliable biologic (60) and physical (61) methods are available to assay flucytosine, even in the presence of amphotericin B.

Flucytosine given alone to patients with normal renal, hematologic, and gastrointestinal function is associated with very infrequent adverse effects. These include rash, diarrhea, and, in about 5 percent, hepatic dysfunction. In the presence of azotemia or concomitant amphotericin B, leukopenia, thrombocytopenia, and enterocolitis may appear and can be fatal. These complications seem to be far more frequent among patients whose flucytosine blood levels exceed 100–125 μg/ml (62). Patients receiving flucytosine should have their leukocyte count and platelet count determined twice a week. Serum alkaline phosphatase and transaminase levels should be followed weekly. Appearance of loose stools or dull abdominal pain should prompt withholding the drug to evaluate progression of symptoms. Patients with bone marrow and gastrointestinal toxicity from flucytosine often tolerate the drug at reduced dosages. Patients with rash or hepatotoxicity have not been rechallenged. Flucytosine is teratogenic for rats and is contraindicated in pregnancy.

Conversion of flucytosine to 5-fluorouracil within the human body occurs in sufficient degree to be a possible explanation for toxicity to bone marrow and gastrointestinal tract (63). It is possible that secretion of the drug into the colon occurs, where flucytosine becomes deaminated by intestinal bacteria and is reabsorbed as 5-fluorouracil.

Flucytosine has a beneficial effect in cryptococcosis, candidiasis, and chromomycosis. It is not the drug of choice for any infection except chromomycosis because the clinical efficacy in the first three mycoses is inferior to amphotericin B and because secondary drug resistance is common in all four infections. Although the frequency and clinical significance of primary drug resistance is debatable, drug resistance arising during therapy is usually profound and accompanied by clinical deterioration. Mechanisms for the drug resistance may include loss of deaminase and decreased permeability to the drug. This problem has been significant enough to cause flucytosine to be used largely in combination with amphotericin B.

Flucytosine in Combination with Amphotericin B

Flucytosine and amphotericin B are additive or synergistic in their effects in vitro against doubly sensitive isolates of *Candida* and *Cryptococcus* (64,65). Results with *Aspergillus* are contradictory (44,66). In experimental mouse infections with these three fungi, the effects were at least additive (46,67–69) except for one report with *Aspergillus* (55). Like other combinations with amphotericin B, the combination was not superior in animals to the effect obtainable by amphotericin B alone. Still, the ability of flucytosine to permit lower doses of amphotericin B and the ability of the latter to prevent drug resistance against the former seemed reason enough to warrant clinical trials. Initial favorable experience with this combination in cryptococcal meningitis (70) led to a prospective multicenter trial in which 10 weeks of amphotericin B therapy was compared with 6 weeks of the combination (71). Amphotericin B was used as 0.4 mg/kg/day when used alone or as 0.3 mg/kg/day in the combination. Flucytosine was used as 150 mg/kg/day, divided into four daily doses, with appropriate dose reductions for azotemia. Among the 51 patients with cryptococcal meningitis who were randomized, who met the diagnostic criteria, and who received their drugs according to protocol, the 6-week combination regimen was as effective or more so by all measurements than the 10-week amphotericin B regimen. Nephrotoxicity was significantly less with the combination, although side effects of flucytosine, none fatal, did occur frequently.

Clinical experience with flucytosine–amphotericin B therapy for systemic candidiasis has generated cautious enthusiasm. Enough experience with the combination has occurred to warrant a few generalities.

Physicians not familiar with the combination are likely to encounter more serious toxicity with the combination than with amphotericin B. Prevention of serious or fatal flucytosine toxicity is most difficult in patients with either moderate or rapidly changing azotemia or bone marrow damage from tumor or antitumor therapy. The combination probably should be used with caution in patients having inflammatory bowel disease or altered intestinal motility. Flucytosine blood levels should be determined twice weekly and analyzed promptly when patients are receiving hemodialysis or when the serum creatinine level exceeds roughly 2.5 mg/dl. Use of a nomogram (see above) to adjust flucytosine dosage and frequent assessment of bone marrow and bowel toxicity are adequate for lesser and slowly changing azotemia.

Combination regimens with amphotericin B doses in excess of 0.3 mg/kg/day or 0.6 mg/kg every other day encounter sufficient azotemia to make the safe administration of flucytosine difficult. The amphotericin-B-sparing function of flucytosine in this setting is lost. At present, there are no clear indications for adding flucytosine to amphotericin B regimens containing these higher doses.

Flucytosine resistance has occurred, albeit uncommonly, during combination therapy. Use of the combination in such patients incurs the risk of toxicity without evidence that flucytosine adds to the therapeutic effect. Whenever flucytosine is used to treat a patient who has received that drug before, the isolate should be tested for susceptibility. In most laboratories, a minimum inhibitory concentration (MIC) of 15 μg/ml or less is considered sensitive.

IMIDAZOLES

The *N*-substituted imidazole ring (Fig. 3) confers antifungal activity upon a variety of synthetic organic compounds. Unlike the 5-nitroimidazoles such as metronidazole, activity against bacteria and protozoa, although measurable, has not been clinically significant. Most of the imidazoles reaching clinical trials have had similar in vitro activity, encompassing a broad range of superficial and deep pathogens (72,73). Determination of activity in vitro has shown a marked dependence of the result upon inoculum size, pH, culture medium, and incubation time (72–75). There are no widely accepted methods for measuring in vitro activity, and no firm indications for performing such tests can be offered. Secondary drug resistance has been encountered but is extremely rare (76).

Knowledge about the imidazoles is most extensive for ketoconazole. This drug will be discussed first, with the implicit understanding that information gleaned about this compound may apply to many other systemic imidazoles now coming to clinical trial in the United States, such as the triazole, itraconazole, and the topical imidazoles such as terconazole, bifonazole, and econazole, the last being identical to miconazole except for the absence of the chlorine atom on the 2 position of the benzyloxy group.

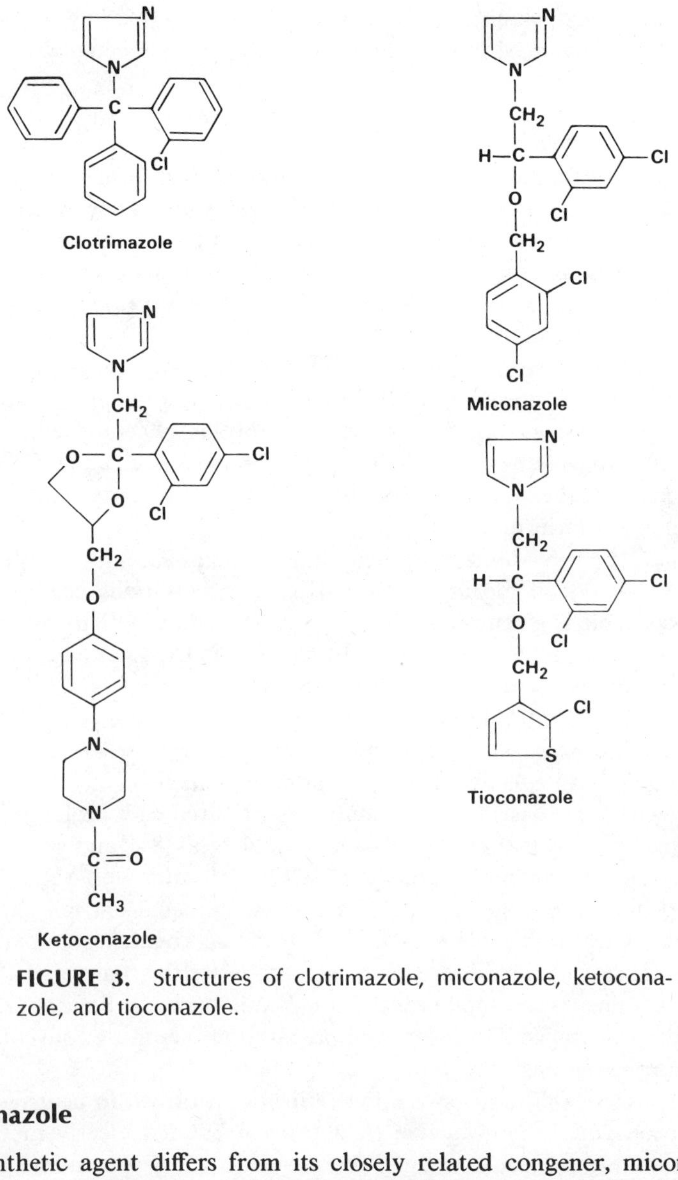

FIGURE 3. Structures of clotrimazole, miconazole, ketoconazole, and tioconazole.

Ketoconazole

This synthetic agent differs from its closely related congener, miconazole, in its solubility at pH less than 3. Solubility in acidic aqueous solutions is conferred in large part by the basic piperazine ring. The mechanism of action appears to be both interference with formation of membrane sterol and other membrane lipids (77). The membrane sterol defect is at the level of ^{14}C demethylation. This sterol and lipid effect can be seen only in cells growing aerobically. Cytotoxicity at high drug concentrations with anaerobic, resting cells involves another mechanism (78). Interference with germ tube formation of *Candida albicans* (79) is much more marked at low concentrations than decreased budding of yeast cells, accounting for two striking effects of the drug in vitro: adherence of *C. albicans* to squamous mucosal cells is decreased and killing of this fungus by leukocytes is enhanced (80) in the presence of low ketoconazole concentrations.

Ketoconazole pharmacology has been reviewed (73). The drug is metabolized in the liver and excreted as inactive drug in the bile and, to a small extent, in the urine. Very little biologically active drug appears in urine. Serum protein binding exceeds 90 percent. The drug is not removed significantly by hemodialysis or peritoneal dialysis. Decreased renal or hepatic function does not alter plasma drug levels. Based on studies of oral ingestion by volunteers, initial half-life is approximately 2 hours, with a β-phase half-life of about 9 hours commencing 8–12 hours after ingestion.

Oral absorption is variable among people but markedly impaired in patients receiving cimetidine, presumably due to increased gastric pH. Simultaneous ingestion of antacid but not food impairs absorption. Therapy with rifampin decreases ketoconazole blood levels by roughly a third. Ketoconazole does not appear to increase hepatic microsomal enzymes as do some imidazoles and does not alter warfarin metabolism.

Penetration of cerebrospinal fluid is minimal, perhaps accounting for the negligible activity in fungal meningitis (81). High concentrations occur in sebum when ketoconazole is given orally, in accord with clinical activity against fungi proliferating in keratin (73). The drug also appears in exudates and breast milk. Low concentrations occur in vaginal secretions (82) and saliva.

Ketoconazole is available at present only in a 200-mg tablet, scored for pediatric use. Topical preparations and suspensions for oral use are experimental.

Ketoconazole is an effective drug in a variety of cutaneous mycoses. Chronic mucocutaneous candidiasis has been controlled or cured with prolonged courses of approximately 3–5 mg/kg/day (83). Oral, esophageal (84), and vaginal thrush respond in the nonimmunosuppressed host (73). Results with vaginal thrush treated by ketoconazole 400 mg/day for 5 days are equal but not superior to results with topical imidazole creams (73). Concern about hepatotoxicity and possible teratogenicity in the pregnant woman as well as failure of the Food and Drug Administration to approve this indication prevent ketoconazole from being the drug of choice. However, oral preparations are more convenient than are vaginal preparations.

In the treatment (85) and prevention (86) of oral thrush in neutropenic patients, ketoconazole is more active than placebo but not clearly more active than nystatin (87), a level of activity often considered disappointing. Doses of ketoconazole ranging from 200 to 600 mg/day have not been clearly effective in preventing disseminated candidiasis in neutropenic patients.

Ketoconazole 200–400 mg/day has improved griseofulvin-resistant ringworm, although relapse is common when the drug is discontinued. There is some effect on onychomycosis, but the potential toxicity and expense makes this drug inappropriate for that indication. Similarly, the drug is probably not indicated for tinea versicolor, although response is usual and relapse is uncommon.

Ketoconazole is effective at doses of 400–800 mg/day in the treatment of nonmeningeal blastomycosis and histoplasmosis. Both chronic pulmonary and disseminated histoplasmosis respond. The usual course of therapy has been 6–12 months. Paracoccidioidomycosis has responded to 200–400 mg/day (88). Coccidioidomycosis responds less well to ketoconazole, with the response in the skin being best and response in cavitary pulmonary or meningeal disease being negligible (89). Useful improvement can be seen when doses of 400–800 mg have been used to treat coccidioidal skin abscess, arthritis, and pneumonia. Bone lesions rarely have improved radiologically, but sinuses that are draining from bone lesions may close. In all these mycoses, the clinical response tends to be manifest over a period of weeks. Treatment of critically ill patients with an oral slowly acting drug is generally inadvisable, making intravenous amphotericin B the drug of choice.

Pulmonary cryptococcosis has been said to respond to ketoconazole, but this response may not exceed the natural rate of pulmonary resolution (90). Relapse in the cerebrospinal fluid is not prevented by ketoconazole (91).

The major toxicity of ketoconazole is dose-dependent nausea and vomiting. In patients without other causes of gastrointestinal upset, doses below 10 mg/kg/day only occasionally cause sufficient distress to necessitate discontinuing therapy. When lower doses of the drug are given with food, nausea is less and usually transient or nonexistent. Gynecomastia (92) and a temporary dose-dependent depression of both serum testosterone (93,94) and adrenocorticotropic hormone (ACTH)-stimulated cortisol response (95,96) can be seen. Asymptomatic elevation of serum transaminase occurs in 2–5 percent of patients (97) often returning to normal spontaneously. In perhaps 1 in 10,000 cases, progressive symptomatic hepatotoxicity ensues and can be fatal if the drug is not discontinued (97–99). Eighty percent of cases occur within 3 months of starting the drug. Rechallenge has reproduced the disease (98). Patients should be instructed to discontinue the drug and report to the physician for hepatic function tests should anorexia, abdominal pain, jaundice, or increased nausea occur. The manufacturer recommends periodic liver function tests. The illness can be mistaken for viral hepatitis.

Clotrimazole

Clotrimazole is available as a 1 percent solution for cutaneous candidiasis, ringworm, or pityriasis versicolor. Vaginal cream (1 percent) and a 100-mg tablet are marketed and effective for vaginal candidiasis (100,101). The 10-mg oral lozenge is well tolerated and comparable in efficacy to nystatin suspension for the treatment (102) or prevention (103) of oral thrush in immunosuppressed patients.

Miconazole

The intravenous preparation of miconazole has been eclipsed by ketoconazole and is useful only in rare and marginal circumstances, such as the critically ill patient with *Pseudallescheria boydii* infection (104). The vaginal cream (2 percent) or suppository is equal in efficacy to clotrimazole, either of these two drugs being treatment of choice for vulvovaginal candidiasis (105). The topical cream or lotion (2 percent) is comparable to clotrimazole or econazole topical preparations for ringworm, cutaneous candidiasis, or pityriasis versicolor (106).

REFERENCES

1. Hamilton-Miller JMT: Chemistry and biology of the polyene macrolide antibiotics. *Bacteriol Rev* 37:166, 1973.
2. Hamilton-Miller JMT: Fungal sterols and the mode of action of the polyene antibiotics. *Adv App Microbiol* 17:109, 1974.
3. Pesti M, Ferenczy L: Protoplast fusion hybrids of *Candida albicans* sterol mutants differing in nystatin resistance. *J Gen Microbiol* 128:123, 1982.
4. Merz WG, Sandford GR: Isolation and characterization of a polyene-resistant variant of *Candida tropicalis. J Clin Microbiol* 9:677, 1979.
5. Drutz DJ, Lehrer RI: Development of amphotericin B-resistant *Candida tropicalis* in a patient with defective leukocyte function. *Am J Med Sci* 276:77, 1978.
6. Pappagianis D, Collins MS, Hector R, et al: Development of resistance to amphotericin B to *Candida lusitaniae* infecting a human. *Antimicrob Agents Chemother* 16:123, 1979.
7. Hebeka EK, Solotorovsky M: Development of resistance to polyene antibiotics in *Candida albicans. J Bacteriol* 89:1533, 1965.
8. Kim SJ, Kwon Chung KJ: Polyene-resistant mutants of *Aspergillus fennelliae:* Sterol content and genetics. *Antimicrob Agents Chemother* 6:102, 1974.
9. Silverman M, Okun R: Oxytetracycline-nystatin in the prevention of candida vaginitis. *Am J Obstet Gynecol* 111:398, 1971.
10. Clinical Trials Subcommittee of the British Tuberculosis Association: Comparison of side-effects of tetracycline and tetracycline plus nystatin. *Br Med J* 2:411, 1968.
11. Ganis P, Avitabile G, Mechlinski W, et al: Polyene macrolide antibiotic amphotericin B. Crystal structure of the *N*-iodoacetyl derivative. *J Am Chem Soc* 93:4560, 1971.
12. Bennett JE, Hill GJ, Butler WT, et al: Correlation of particle size of intravenous amphotericin B with toxic and chemotherapeutic effects. *Antimicrobial Agents and Chemotherapy—1963.* Ann Arbor, Mich, American Society for Microbiology, 1964, p 745.
13. Block ER, Bennett JE: Stability of amphotericin B in the infusion bottle. *Antimicrob Agents Chemother* 4:648, 1973.
14. Tipple M, Shadomy S, Espinel-Ingroff A: Availability of active amphotericin B after filtration through membrane filters. *Am Rev Respr Dis* 115:879, 1977.
15. Bindschadler DD, Bennett JE: A pharmacologic guide to the clinical use of amphotericin B. *J Infect Dis* 120:427, 1969.
16. Mayhew JW, Fiore C, Murray T, et al: An internally standardized assay for amphotericin B in tissues and plasma. *J Chromatog* 274:271, 1983.
17. Cosgrove RF, Fairbrother JE: Bioassay method for polyene antibiotics based on the measurement of rubidium efflux from rubidium-loaded yeast cells. *Antimicrob Agents Chemother* 11:31, 1977.
18. Merz WG, Fay D, Thumar B, et al: Susceptibility testing of filamentous fungi to amphotericin B by a rapid radiometric method. *J Clin Microbiol* 19:54, 1984.
19. Jagdis FA, Monji N, Lawrence RM, et al: Distribution of radiolabeled amphotericin B methyl ester and amphotericin B in nonhuman primates. Sixteenth Interscience Conference of Antimicrobial Agents and Chemotherapy. Washington, DC, American Society of Microbiology, 1976, abstract 305.
20. Block ER, Bennett JE, Livoti LG, et al: Flucytosine and amphotericin B: Hemodialysis effects on the plasma concentration and clearance. *Ann Intern Med* 80:613, 1974.

21. Bennett JE: Amphotericin B binding to serum betalipoprotein, in Iwata (ed): *Recent Advances in Medical and Veterinary Mycology.* Tokyo, University of Tokyo Press, 1977, p 107.
22. Atkinson AJ, Bennett JE: Amphotericin B pharmacokinetics in humans. *Antimicrob Agents Chemother* 13:271, 1978.
23. Craven PC, Ludden TM, Drutz DJ, et al: Excretion pathways of amphotericin B. *J Infect Dis* 140:329, 1979.
24. Fisher JF, Taylor AT, Clark J, et al: Penetration of amphotericin B into the human eye. *J Infect Dis* 147:164, 1983.
25. Butler WT, Bennett JE, Alling DW, et al: Nephrotoxicity of amphotericin B. Early and late effects in 81 patients. *Ann Intern Med* 61:175, 1964.
26. Kennedy MS, Deeg HJ, Siegel M, et al: Acute renal toxicity with combined use of amphotericin B and cyclosporine after marrow transplantation. *Transplantation* 35:211, 1982.
27. Heidemann HT, Gerkens JF, Spickard WA, et al: Amphotericin B nephrotoxicity in humans decreased by salt repletion. *Am J Med* 75:475, 1983.
28. McCurdy DK, Frederic M, Elkinton JR: Renal acidosis due to amphotericin B. *N Engl J Med* 278:124, 1968.
29. Utz JP, Bennett JE, Brandriss MW, et al: Amphotericin B toxicity. *Ann Intern Med* 61:334, 1964.
30. Gerkens JF, Heidemann HT, Jackson EK, et al: Effect of aminophylline on amphotericin B nephrotoxicity in the dog. *J Pharmacol Exp Ther* 224:609, 1983.
31. Brandriss M, Wolff S, Moores R, et al: Anemia induced by amphotericin B. *JAMA* 189:663, 1964.
32. MacGregor RR, Bennett JE, Erslev AJ: Erythropoietin concentration in amphotericin B-induced anemia. *Antimicrob Agents Chemother* 14:270, 1978.
33. Wright DG, Robichaud KJ, Pizzo PA, et al: Lethal pulmonary reactions associated with the combined use of amphotericin B and leukocyte transfusions. *N Engl J Med* 304:1185, 1981.
34. Boxer LA, Ingraham LM, Allen J, et al: Amphotericin-B promotes leukocyte aggregation of nylon-wool-fiber-treated polymorphonuclear leukocytes. *Blood* 58:518, 1981.
35. Carnevale NT, Galgiani JN, Stevens DA, et al: Amphotericin B-induced myelopathy. *Arch Intern Med* 140:1189, 1980.
36. Alazraki NP, Fierer J, Halpern SE, et al: Use of a hyperbaric solution for administration of intrathecal amphotericin B. *N Engl J Med* 290:641, 1974.
37. Diamond RD, Bennett JE: A subcutaneous reservoir for intrathecal therapy of fungal meningitis. *N Engl J Med* 288:186, 1973.
38. Wise GJ, Wainstein S, Goldberg P, et al: *Candida* cystitis. Management by continuous bladder irrigation with amphotericin B. *JAMA* 224:1636, 1973.
39. Mechlinski W, Schaffner CP: Polyene macrolide derivatives. I. *N*-Acylation and esterification reactions with amphotericin B. *J Antibiot (Tokyo)* 25:256, 1972.
40. Ellis WG, Sobel RA, Nielsen SL: Leukoencephalopathy in patients treated with amphotericin B methyl ester. *J Infect Dis* 146:125, 1982.
41. Edwards JE, Morrison J, Henderson DK, et al: Combined effect of amphotericin B and rifampin on *Candida* species. *Antimicrob Agents Chemother* 17:484, 1980.
42. Kobayashi GS, Medoff G, Schlessinger D, et al: Amphotericin B potentiation of rifampicin as an antifungal agent against the yeast phase of *Histoplasma capsulatum. Science* 177:709, 1972.
43. Fujita NK, Edwards JE: Combined in vitro effect of amphotericin B and rifampin on *Cryptoccus neoformans. Antimicrob Agents Chemother* 19:196, 1981.
44. Kitahara M, Seth UK, Medoff G, et al: Activity of amphotericin B, 5-fluorocytosine and rifampin against six clinical isolates of *Aspergillus. Antimicrob Agents Chemother* 9:915, 1976.
45. Kitahara M, Kobayashi GS, Medoff G: Enhanced efficacy of amphotericin B and rifampicin in treatment of murine histoplasmosis and blastomycosis. *J Infect Dis* 133:663, 1976.
46. Arroyo J, Medoff G, Kobayashi GS: Therapy of murine aspergillosis with amphotericin B in combination with rifampin or 5-fluorocytosine. *Antimicrob Agents Chemother* 11:21, 1977.

47. Huppert M, Pappagianis D, Sun SH, et al: Effect of amphotericin B and rifampin against *Coccidioides immitis* in vitro and in vivo. *Antimicrob Agents Chemother* 9:406, 1976.
48. Graybill JR, Ahrens J: Interaction of rifampin with other antifungal agents in experimental murine candidiasis. *Rev Infect Dis* 5:S620, 1983.
49. Huppert M, Sun SH, Vukovich KR: Combined amphotericin B-tetracycline therapy for experimental coccidioidomycosis. *Antimicrob Agents Chemother* 5:473, 1974.
50. Lew M, Beckett KM, Levin MJ: Combined activity of minocycline and amphotericin B in vitro against medically important yeasts. *Antimicrob Agents Chemother* 14:465, 1978.
51. Presant CA, Klahr C, Santala R: Amphotericin B induction of sensitivity to adriamycin, 1,3-bis (2-chloroethyl)-1-nitrosourea (BCNU) plus cyclophosphamide in human neoplasia. *Ann Intern Med* 86:47, 1977.
52. Brajtburg J, Kobayashi D, Medoff G, et al: Antifungal action of amphotericin B in combination with other polyene or imidazole antibiotics. *J Infect Dis* 146:138, 1982.
53. Sud IJ, Feingold DS: Effect of ketoconazole on the fungicidal action of amphotericin B in *Candida albicans. Antimicrob Agents Chemother* 23:185, 1983.
54. Graybill JR, Williams DM, Cutsem EV, et al: Combination therapy of experimental histoplasmosis and cryptococcosis with amphotericin B and ketoconazole. *Rev Infect Dis* 2:551, 1980.
55. Polak A, Scholer HJ, Wall M: Combination therapy of experimental candidiasis and aspergillosis in mice. *Chemotherapy* 28:461, 1982.
56. Bennett JE: Flucytosine. *Ann Intern Med* 86:319, 1977.
57. Cutler RE, Balir, AD, Kelly MR: Flucytosine kinetics in subjects with normal renal function. *Clin Pharmacol Ther* 24:333, 1978.
58. Diasio RB, Bennett JE, Myers CE: Mode of action of 5-fluorocytosine. *Biochem Pharmacol* 27:703, 1978.
59. Oliver SO, Williamson DH: The molecular events involved in the induction of petite yeast mutants by fluorinated pyrimidines. *Mol Gen Genet* 146:253, 1976.
60. Kaspar RL, Drutz DJ: Rapid, simple bioassay for 5-fluorocytosine in the presence of amphotericin B. *Antimicrob Agents Chemother* 7:462, 1975.
61. Harding SA, Johnson GF, Solomon HM: Gas chromatographic determination of 5-fluorocytosine in human serum. *Clin Chem* 22:772, 1976.
62. Kauffman C, Frame PT: Bone marrow toxicity associated with 5-fluorocytosine therapy. *Antimicrob Agents Chemother* 11:244, 1977.
63. Diasio RB, Lakings DE, Bennett JE: Evidence for conversion of 5-fluorocytosine to 5-fluorouracil in humans. Possible factor in 5-fluorocytosine clinical toxicity. *Antimicrob Agents Chemother* 14:903, 1978.
64. Medoff G, Comfort M, Kobayashi GS: Synergistic action of amphotericin B and 5-fluorocytosine against yeast-like organisms. *Proc Soc Exp Biol Med* 138:571, 1971.
65. Polak A: Synergism of polyene antibiotics with 5-fluorocytosine. *Chemotherapy* 24:2, 1978.
66. Lauer BA, Reller LB, Schröter GPJ: Susceptibility of *Aspergillus* to 5-fluorocytosine and amphotericin B alone and in combination. *J Antimicrob Chemother* 4:375, 1978.
67. Block ER, Bennett JE: The combined effect of 5-fluorocytosine and amphotericin B in the therapy of murine cryptococcosis. *Proc Soc Exp Biol Med* 142:476, 1973.
68. Rabinovich S, Shaw BD, Bryant T, et al: Effect of 5-fluorocytosine and amphotericin B on *Candida albicans* in mice. *J Infect Dis* 130:28, 1974.
69. Titsworth E, Grunberg E: Chemotherapeutic activity of 5-fluorocytosine and amphotericin B against *Candida albicans* in mice. *Antimicrob Agents Chemother* 4:306, 1973.
70. Utz JP, Garriques IL, Sande MA, et al: Therapy of cryptococcosis with a combination of flucytosine and amphotericin B. *J Infect Dis* 132:368, 1975.
71. Bennett JE, Dismukes WE, Duma RJ, et al: A collaborative study comparing amphotericin B-5-fluorocytosine versus amphotericin B alone in the treatment of cryptococcal meningitis. *N Engl J Med* 301:126, 1979.
72. Custem JV: The antifungal activity of ketoconazole. *Am J Med* 74(suppl):9, 1983.
73. Heel RC, Brogden RN, Carmine A, et al: Ketoconazole: A review of its therapeutic efficacy in superficial and systemic fungal infections. *Drugs* 23:1, 1982.

74. Minagawa H, Kitaura K, Nakamizo N: Effects of pH on the activity of ketoconazole against *Candida albicans. Antimicrob Agents Chemother* 23:105, 1983.
75. Brass C, Shainhouse JZ, Stevens DA: Variability of agar dilution-replicator method of yeast susceptibility testing. *Antimicrob Agents Chemother* 15:763, 1979.
76. Ryley JF, Wilson RG, Barrett-Bee KJ: Azole resistance in *Candida albicans. Sabouraudia* 22:53, 1984.
77. Borgers M, Bossche HV, Brabender MD: The mechanism of action of the new antimycotic ketoconazole. *Am J Med* 74:2, 1983.
78. Sud IJ, Feingold DS: Mechanisms of action of the antimycotic imidazoles. *J Invest Dermatol* 76:438, 1981.
79. Borgers M, Bossche HVD, Brabander MD, et al: Promotion of pseudomycelium formation of *Candida albicans* in culture: A morphological study of the effects of miconazole and ketoconazole. *Postgrad Med J* 55:687, 1979.
80. Brabander MD, Aerts F, Cutsem JV, et al: The activity of ketoconazole in mixed cultures of leukocytes and candida albicans. *Sabouraudia* 18:197, 1980.
81. Craven PC, Graybill JR, Jorgensen JH, et al: High-dose ketoconazole for treatment of fungal infections of the central nervous system. *Ann Intern Med* 98:160, 1983.
82. Nusch W, Plempel M: Microbiological determination of bay N 7133 and ketoconazole after oral application in cervical and vaginal smears of patients. *Mykosen* 26:12, 1983.
83. Horsburgh CR, Kirkpatrick CH: Long-term therapy of chronic mucocutaneous candidiasis with ketoconazole: Experience with twenty-one patients. *Am J Med* 74:23, 1983.
84. Fazio RA, Wickremesinghe PC, Arsure EL: Ketoconazole treatment of Candida esophagitis: A prospective study of 12 cases. *Am J Gastroenterol* 78:261, 1983.
85. Hughes WT, Bartley DL, Patterson GG, et al: Ketoconazole and candidiasis: A controlled study. *J Infect Dis* 147:1060, 1983.
86. Brincker H: Prevention of mycosis in granulocytopenic patients with prophylactic ketoconazole treatment. *Mykosen* 26:242, 1983.
87. Jones PG, Kauffman CA, McAuliffe LS, et al: Efficacy of ketoconazole vs. nystatin in prevention of fungal infections in neutropenic patients. *Arch Intern Med* 144:549, 1984.
88. Restrepo A, Gomez I, Cano LE, et al: Post-therapy status of paracoccidioidomycosis treated with ketoconazole. *Am J Med* 74:53, 1983.
89. Galgiani JN: Ketoconazole in the treatment of coccidioidomycosis. *Drugs* 26:355, 1983.
90. Dismukes WE, Stamm AM, Graybill JR, et al: Treatment of systemic mycoses with ketoconazole: Emphasis on toxicity and clinical response in 52 patients. *Ann Intern Med* 98:13, 1983.
91. Perfect JR, Durack DT, Hamilton JD, et al: Failure of ketoconazole in cryptococcal meningitis. *JAMA* 247:3349, 1982.
92. DeFelice R, Johnson DG, Galgiani JN: Gynecomastia with ketoconazole. *Antimicrob Agents Chemother* 19:1073, 1981.
93. Schurmeyer TH, Nieschlag E, Ketoconazole-induced drop in serum and saliva testosterone. *Lancet* 2:1098, 1982.
94. Grosso DS, Boyden TW, Pamenter RW, et al: Ketoconazole inhibition of testicular secretion of testosterone and displacement of steroid hormones from serum transport proteins. *Antimicrob Agents Chemother* 23:207, 1983.
95. Pont A, Williams PL, Loose DS, et al: Ketoconazole blocks adrenal steroid synthesis. *Ann Intern Med* 97:370, 1982.
96. Loose DS, Kan PB, Hirst MA, et al: Ketoconazole blocks adrenal steroidogenesis by inhibiting cytochrome P450-dependent enzymes. *J Clin Invest* 71:1495, 1983.
97. Lewis JH, Zimmerman HJ, Benson GD, et al: Hepatic injury associated with ketoconazole therapy. *Gastroenterology* 86:503, 1984.
98. Heiberg JK, Svejgaard E: Toxic hepatitis during ketoconazole treatment. *Br Med J* 2:283, 1981.
99. Tkach JR, Rinaldi MG: Severe hepatitis associated with ketoconazole therapy for chronic mucocutaneous candidiasis. *Cutis* 29:482, 1982.

100. Svendsen E, Lie S, Gunderson TH, et al: Comparative evaluation of miconazole, clotrimazole and nystatin in the treatment of Candida vulvo-vaginitis. *Curr Therapy Res* 23:666, 1978.
101. Franklin R: Seven day clotrimazole therapy for vulvovaginal candidiasis. *South Med J* 71:141, 1978.
102. Shechtman LB, Funaro L, Robin T, et al: Clotrimazole treatment of oral candidiasis in patients with neoplastic disease. *Am J Med* 76:91, 1984.
103. Owens NJ, Nightingale CH, Schweizer RT, et al: Prophylaxis of oral candidiasis with clotrimazole troches. *Arch Intern Med* 144:290, 1984.
104. Lutwick LI, Rytel MW, Yañez JP, et al: Deep infections from *Petriellidium boydii* treated with miconazole. *JAMA* 241:272, 1979.
105. Culbertson C: Monistat: A new fungicide for treatment of vulvovaginal candidiasis. *Am J Obstet Gynecol* 120:973, 1974.
106. Van Cutsem J, Reyntjens A: Miconazole therapy of pityriasis versicolor. A Review. *Mykosen* 21:87, 1978.

17

ANTIVIRAL AGENTS

FREDERICK G. HAYDEN
R. GORDON DOUGLAS, JR.

GENERAL PRINCIPLES

Antiviral drugs with proven effectiveness are currently available for a number of common and, in some instances, clinically severe viral infections (Table 1). The recent availability of alternative agents has already led to comparative testing of drug efficacy in infections due to influenza A, herpes simplex (HSV), and varicella zoster viruses (VZV).

Mechanisms of Action

Chemotherapeutic agents for viral infections can be categorized into three broad groups: agents that directly inactivate intact viruses (virucidal), those that inhibit viral replication at the cellular level (antiviral), and those that augment or modify the host response to infection (immunomodulating). Virucidal agents may cause direct inactivation in a single step, such as detergents, organic solvents like ether or chloroform, and ultraviolet light, or in multiple steps, as with photodynamic inactivation. However, despite extensive study of mucocutaneous HSV infections (1–4), such agents have not proven clinically useful in the treatment of established infections. Treatments that destroy both the host tissues and the virus simultaneously, such as cryotherapy, cautery, or podophyllin treatment of warts, are useful only in discrete mucocutaneous infections. One potential use of virucidal agents may be in preventing transmission of certain viral infections. This approach is currently under study in rhinovirus colds where hand contamination and self-inoculation of infectious secretions may occur.

Antivirals. Since viral replication depends primarily on host cell metabolic functions, the challenge has been to identify agents that inhibit virus-specific events such as attachment to the cell, uncoating of the viral genome, or assembly of progeny virions, or that preferentially inhibit virus-directed, as contrasted to host cell-directed, macromolecular synthesis. While many compounds exist

TABLE 1. Viral Infections in Which Antiviral Agents Have Proven Therapeutic Efficacy

Type of Infection	*Antiviral Drug*	*Route of Administration*	*Usual Dosage*
HSV encephalitis	Vidarabine	IV	15 mg/kg/day for 10 days. Constant infusion over 12–24 hours.
Neonatal HSV	Vidarabine[a]	IV	15 mg/kg/day for 10 days. Constant infusion over 12–24 hours. Higher dosages (30 mg/kg/day) under study.
Herpes zoster (immunocompromised hosts)[b]	Vidarabine	IV	10 mg/kg/day for 5–7 days. Constant infusion over 12–24 hours.
	Acyclovir[a]	IV	500 mg/M^2/8 hours for 7 days[d]. Constant infusion over 1 hour. Alternative dosage and oral route of administration under study.
Herpes zoster (normal hosts)	Acyclovir[a]	IV	5–10 mg/kg/8 hours for 5 days. See above.
Varicella (immunocompromised hosts)	Vidarabine[a]	IV	10 mg/kg/day for 5 days. Constant infusion over 12–24 hours.
	Acyclovir[a]	IV	500 mg/kg/8 hours for 7 days[d].
Genital HSV (primary)	Acyclovir	IV	5 mg/kg/8 hours for 5–7 days. Constant infusion over 1 hour. Indicated in severe initial infections.
	Acyclovir[a]	Oral	1,000 mg/day in 5 divided doses for 10 days.
	Acyclovir	Topical	4–6 applications/day for 7–14 days. Longer treatment may prevent delayed new lesion formation. One-half inch ribbon of ointment per 4 square inches applied with gloved finger.

Genital HSV (recurrent)	Acyclovir[a]	Oral	1,000 mg/kg/day in 5 divided doses for 5 days.
HSV keratoconjunctivitis[c]	Idoxuridine	Topical	One drop of 0.1% solution every 1 hour while awake and every 2 hours at night. Instillation of 0.5% ointment 5 times/day.
	Vidarabine	Topical	One-half inch ribbon of 3% ointment 5 times/day.
	Trifluridine	Topical	One drop of 1% solution every 2 hours (up to 9 drops/day).
	Acyclovir[a]	Topical	One-half inch ribbon of 3% ointment 5 times/day.
Mucocutaneous HSV (immunocompromised hosts)	Acyclovir	IV	250 mg/M²/8 hours for 7 days.
	Acyclovir	Topical	6 applications/day for 7 days. One-half inch ribbon of ointment per 4 square inches applied with gloved finger. Useful only in limited, non-life-threatening infections.
Influenza A virus[e]	Amantadine	Oral	200 mg/day for 5–7 days. 2–4 mg/lb/day in children $\leq$9 years.
	Rimantadine[a]	Oral	200–300 mg/day for 5–7 days. Optimal dosage under study.

[a] Not currently approved by the Food and Drug Administration for this indication.

[b] Antiviral therapy is most effective in localized herpes zoster $\leq$3 days duration.

[c] Treatment of HSV ocular infections should be supervised by an ophthamologist. Duration of therapy and dosage depends on response.

[d] Dosage recommendations are those used in studies that show efficacy in this condition. Acyclovir dosage of 250 mg/M^2 is approximately 6.2 mg/kg, and 500 mg/M^2 is approximately 12.4 mg/kg in a 70 kg adult.

[e] Efficacy documented only in uncomplicated influenza $\leq$48 hours duration.

that exhibit antiviral activity in vitro, most affect some host cell function and are associated with low therapeutic ratios or unacceptable toxicity in humans.

Currently useful antivirals selectively inhibit specific events in viral replication, and consequently, most have a restricted spectrum of antiviral activity. Similarly, since these agents inhibit ongoing replication at the host cell level, they are not effective in the elimination of nonreplicating or latent viruses.

Drug Resistance. A related problem that may limit the effectiveness of an antiviral drug is the development of viral resistance to the inhibitory action of the drug. Indeed, the selection of a drug-resistant strain of virus implies that the drug has a specific antiviral mechanism (5). Although a well-documented laboratory phenomenon for a variety of antiviral agents, in vivo development of drug resistance has been found during use of idoxuridine in HSV keratitis (6,7) and during acyclovir therapy of mucocutaneous HSV infection (8–11).

Combination Chemotherapy. The combined use of antiviral agents with different mechanisms of action has been investigated as a means of increasing antiviral activity without increasing toxicity. Combination therapy has been used successfully in experimental infections due to enteroviruses (12), influenza (13,14), and various herpesviruses (15–17). Combined treatment with vidarabine and human leukocyte interferon has been found to be clinically useful in chronic hepatitis B virus infections (18,19). However, this combination has also been associated with an increased risk of vidarabine toxicity in hepatitis patients (20,21).

Host Immune Response. Since antivirals are virustatic or inhibitory in their activity, viral infection may resume when the compound is removed. Intact host immunologic responses remain essential for recovery from virus infections. Antivirals that impair host responses to infection, such as cytosine arabinoside in herpes zoster (22), may actually prolong the course of infection. Factors other than inhibition of viral replication alone are important in healing certain viral diseases, particularly mucocutaneous HSV infections, where it has been possible to demonstrate antiviral effects without clinical benefit (23).

Immunomodulation. Immunomodulating agents used for treating viral infections include those that supplement deficient host immune responses, such as exogenous antibody in chronic echovirus infection (24) or interferon in herpes zoster of immunocompromised hosts (25). Administration of transfer factor from persons recovering from chickenpox has been shown to transfer CMI responses and to protect susceptible leukemic children from varicella (26). Chemical agents that appear to augment cell-mediated immune (CMI) responses, such as levamisole or inosiplex, have been used with variable success (27).

Drug Administration

Prophylaxis Versus Therapy. Prophylactic administration, as in amantadine hydrochloride for influenza A virus infection or methisazone in smallpox, is generally more effective than therapeutic. Since most antivirals probably serve to protect uninvolved cells and limit the spread of infection, rapid etiologic diagnosis and early administration of antiviral drugs are necessary for therapeutic efficacy.

Clinical and Laboratory Evaluation. Clinical efficacy depends on achieving effective antiviral concentrations at the site of infection, and specifically, adequate intracellular concentrations of the antiviral agent or its active metabolites. Pharmacokinetic studies that define absorption, stability in body fluids, tissue distribution, and metabolic fate of antiviral drugs are important in selecting the proper dosage. Unfortunately, no standardized or generally accepted correlations exist between in vitro inhibitory concentrations, achievable blood or body fluid concentrations of antiviral agents, and clinical response (reviewed in 27a). For example, although cytosine arabinoside appears more active against HSV than vidarabine in vitro, the reverse has been found in clinical trials (22,28–30). Similarly, intravenous administration of vidarabine does not consistently result in plasma concentrations that inhibit viral replication in vitro, yet vidarabine has proven efficacious in severe HSV infections. Animal models are useful in the testing of antiviral agents, but may differ from the corresponding human infection in regard to pathogenesis, drug sensitivity of the virus, drug pharmacology, or toxicity (31).

Topical Administration. Topical application of antivirals to the cornea, skin, mucus membranes, or respiratory tract attempts to provide high concentrations at the site of infection and to avoid the possible toxicity of systemic administration. Topically applied drugs must be able to penetrate such barriers as stratified epithelium or local secretions to reach the site of active viral replication. For example, although beneficial in the treatment of HSV keratitis, topically applied vidarabine and its monophosphate derivative are ineffective in recurrent genital or labial HSV infections (32–35).

Delivery of antiviral drugs to the respiratory tract in the form of small particle aerosols has been used with some benefit in influenza A, influenza B, and respiratory syncytial virus infections (36–39), and the use of intranasally administered interferon has been shown to be protective in both experimentally-induced and naturally-occurring rhinovirus colds.

SPECIFIC ANTIVIRAL AGENTS

Acyclovir (9-[2-hydroxyethoxymethyl]guanine, acycloguanosine, ACV, Zovirax)

Spectrum. Acyclovir is a purine nucleoside analogue that has an acyclic side chain instead of the cyclic sugar moiety of natural nucleosides (Fig. 1). Its antiviral activity is limited to herpesviruses, including HSV types 1 and 2, VZV, and Epstein-Barr virus (40–43). Depending on the type of cell culture, acyclovir concentrations causing 50 percent reduction in plaque formation average 0.02–

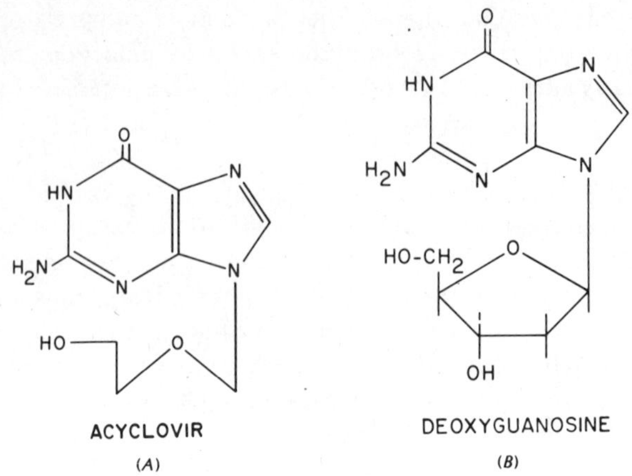

FIGURE 1. Chemical structure of (*A*) acyclovir and the natural nucleoside (*B*) deoxyguanosine.

0.2 μg/ml for type 1 HSV, 0.2–0.4 μg/ml for type 2 HSV, and 0.8–1.2 μg/ml for VZV. Concentrations of approximately 1.6 μg/ml inhibit the replication of Epstein-Barr virus DNA in productively infected cells (43), but higher concentrations do not affect latent or persistent infection (44). Much higher concentrations, 22.7 μg/ml and greater, are required for inhibition of CMV plaque formation (42,45). Acyclovir has shown antiviral activity in various animal models of HSV infection when administered topically, parenterally, or orally (46–48). In HSV-induced skin infections of mice, early topical application prevents both lesions and the development of latent infection in sensory ganglia (49,50).

Mechanism of Action. The antiviral mechanism of action of acyclovir involves inhibition of viral DNA synthesis. Acyclovir uptake and intracellular phosphorylation to the monophosphate derivative are facilitated by HSV-induced thymidine kinase (51). Cellular enzymes convert the monophosphate to acyclovir triphosphate, which is present in 40- to 100-fold higher concentrations in HSV-infected cells than in uninfected cells (51). The triphosphate form selectively inhibits viral DNA polymerase, and to a much smaller extent cellular α-DNA polymerase, and competes with guanosine triphosphate as a substrate for this enzyme (52). Acyclovir triphosphate is also incorporated into viral DNA where it acts as a chain terminator (53). The DNA polymerases of various herpesviruses differ in their degree of inhibition by acyclovir triphosphate; the polymerase of the Epstein-Barr virus appears to be especially sensitive to its inhibitory action (54).

Experimental studies have shown that alterations in either the viral thymidine kinase (TK) or DNA polymerase can cause acyclovir resistance in vitro (55,56). In animal models, acyclovir-resistant mutants with deficient TK activity appear to be less virulent and less likely to cause latent CNS infection than wild type strains (50,57,58), but the virulence of these strains in immunocompromised patients is uncertain. Strains that are acyclovir-resistant because of an altered TK substrate specificity but that retain neurovirulence have also been described (59). One study found that 40 percent of HSV strains that had not been exposed to acyclovir contained acyclovir-resistant virus, accounting for at least one percent of the total virus population (11,11a). Acyclovir-resistant strains of HSV with diminished TK activity have been isolated from immunocompromised patients given intravenous acyclovir for mucocutaneous HSV infections (8–10) and from patients with genital HSV infections before and after topical therapy (60). One study of bone marrow transplant patients treated with intravenous acyclovir for recurrent mucocutaneous HSV infections recovered acyclovir-resistant virus in 1 of 52 first treatment courses and 2 of 22 second courses (10a). Currently, the clinical significance of these observations is not resolved, but the use of acyclovir should be limited to circumstances where clinical efficacy has been established.

Pharmacology. The plasma $T_{1/2}$ of systemic acyclovir averages 2.9 hours (range 1.5–6.3 hours) in adults with normal renal function, but is slightly longer (mean 3.8 hours) in neonates and increases to 19.5 hours in anuric patients (61–63). Peak and trough plasma concentrations at the end of a 1-hour infusion average 9.8 μg/ml and 0.7 μg/ml after 5 mg/kg/8 hr and 20.7 and 2.3 after 10 mg/kg/8 hr, respectively (61). The bioavailability of oral acyclovir is low (15–30%) and decreases with increasing doses (64). Peak concentrations of 0.3–0.9 μg/ml occur between 1.5 and 4 hours after 200 mg oral doses taken every 4 hours (65), and steady-state peak concentrations averaged 1.4 (range 0.9–1.8) μg/ml in adults ingesting 200 mg five times per day for therapy of genital herpes (80). Cerebrospinal fluid concentrations are approximately one-half of plasma values (61). After oral administration, salivary concentrations average 13 percent of simultaneous plasma concentrations, but vaginal secretion concentrations range from 15 to 170 percent of plasma values (65). Percutaneous absorption of acyclovir after topical administration appears to be low; plasma concentrations ranging from <0.01 to 0.3 μg/ml have been detected in herpes zoster patients treated topically. In patients with genital HSV infections treated with topical acyclovir, concentrations in genital lesions at 4 to 12 hours after application range widely (0.002–38 μg/ml), and no detectable acyclovir is present in cervicovaginal secretions (60).

Renal excretion of unmetabolized acyclovir by glomerular filtrations and tubular secretion accounts for 60 to 91 percent of an administered dose, while less than 15 percent is excreted as 9-carboxymethoxymethylguanine or minor metabolites (61, 66, 67). By competing for the organic acid secretory pathway, acyclovir may decrease the renal clearance of other drugs eliminated by active renal secretion, such as methothexate (64). Dosage reductions are indicated in patients with creatinine clearances less than 50 ml/minute/1.73 M^2 (see Table 2). Acyclovir is readily hemodialyzable, and 60 percent of the drug in the body is removed during a 6-hour hemodialysis (63,68).

TABLE 2. Acyclovir Dosage Adjustments Suggested for Patients With Impaired Renal Function

Creatinine Clearance	*Standard Dose (%)*	*Dosing Interval (Hours)*
ml/minute/1.73 M^2		
>50	100	8
25–50	100	12
10–25	100	24
0–10[a,b]	50	24

SOURCE: Recommendations taken from Blum et al (62) and Laskin et al (63).

[a] An alternative in patients with end-stage renal disease is administration of 14 percent of standard dose every 8 hours after loading with 37 percent of the standard dose (63).

[b] Postdialysis administration of 60–100 percent of standard dose (64,68).

Toxicity. Topical acyclovir may cause transient burning when applied to genital lesions, more commonly in first episodes and in female patients (60). The polyethylene glycol base of topical acyclovir may cause vaginal erythema and is not approved for intravaginal use.

Intravenous acyclovir is generally well tolerated, although phlebitis may occur at the injection site, especially following extravasation of the alkaline solution (pH 9–11). Uncommonly reported side effects include rash, diaphoresis, hematuria, hypotention, headache, and nausea (69). Approximately 1 percent of patients receiving intravenous acyclovir have manifested encephalopathic changes characterized by lethargy, obtundation, tremors, confusion, hallucinations, delerium, seizures, or coma (69,70). Concurrent interferon administration or intrathecal methotrexate may be risk factors. A recent study found that 4 percent of bone marrow transplant recipients developed one or more of these symptoms after 2 to 18 days of intravenous acyclovir therapy (750–3,000 mg/M^2/day) for herpesvirus infection (71). Most had diffuse EEG abnormalities and increased cerebrospinal fluid concentrations of myelin basic protein (71). Improvement or resolution of symptoms occurred within 1 to 2 weeks after stopping treatment with acyclovir, but two patients developed neurologic symptoms again after reinstitution of therapy.

Reversible renal dysfunction has been observed in approximately 5 percent of patients treated with intravenous acyclovir at a dosage of 5 mg/kg/8 hr. In animals acyclovir can cause a crystalline nephropathy, and in humans solubility decreases to 2.5 mg/ml at 37°C. Bolus infusion, dehydration, preexisting renal insufficiency, and high doses appear to be associated risk factors. One study found that one-half of adults receiving 500 mg/M^2/dose for treatment of herpes zoster had reversible increases in serum creatinine of at least 25 percent (72), although a subsequent study at the same dosage found renal dysfunction in only 6 percent of acyclovir recipients (73). Oral acyclovir has been associated infrequently with nausea, and headache.

Acyclovir has shown mutagenic activity in some in vitro assays at high concentrations. Acyclovir (20 μg/ml) did not alter cell-mediated immune responses of human peripheral blood leukocytes (PBL) (74) or affect human granulocyte progenitor cell growth (75) in vitro. Other studies found that concentrations of 6.4–22.7 μg/ml inhibited the proliferative responses of human PBL to mitogens or herpesvirus antigens (76,77). No significant immunosuppressive activity or teratogenicity has been noted in animal studies (78), but safety in the pregnant human has not been established.

Clinical Studies. A number of placebo-controlled, double-blind clinical trials have demonstrated the therapeutic efficacy of acyclovir in primary genital HSV infections (79–83). Topical acyclovir is associated with therapeutic and antiviral effects of a smaller magnitude than oral or intravenous administration (see Table 3) and does not influence the frequency of new lesion formation after initiation of treatment. Because some patients treated with topical acyclovir develop new lesions and/or increased symptoms after stopping therapy, longer durations of application (10–14 days) have been advocated (60,81). Topical acyclovir has minimal clinical efficacy in patients with preexisting HSV antibodies (nonprimary initial infection), such as people with a history of orofacial HSV infection, and although associated with an antiviral affect, topical acyclovir offers no significant clinical benefit in recurrent genital HSV infections (81,84).

Intravenous acyclovir has been shown to reduce markedly the duration of viral shedding, time to healing, and duration of symptoms in patients hospitalized with severe primary genital HSV infections (79). Similarly, in outpatients with initial genital HSV infections, oral acyclovir has been associated with significant reductions in virus shedding, symptoms, time to healing, as well as prevention of new vesicle formation compared to placebo (80,83). Neither of these regimens has been associated with reductions in the frequency of recurrent genital lesions. Oral acyclovir appears to offer the best outpatient regimen for initial genital HSV infections at the present time. Controlled clinical trials have also shown that oral acyclovir is associated with antiviral activity and statistically significant but modest clinical affects in recurrent genital HSV infections (83). One study found that when therapy was initiated by patients during the prodrome or at the first sign of lesions, oral acyclovir was associated with significant reductions in the durations of shedding (mean 2.1 vs. 3.9 days), time to healing (5.7 vs. 7.2 days), time to crusting (2.4 vs. 3.9 days), frequency of new lesion formation (7 vs. 22 percent), but no difference in the duration of pain (85). Another study found that chronic oral acyclovir (600 mg/day for 4 months) significantly reduced the frequency of recurrences (27 vs. 94 percent in patients with frequently recurring genital HSV infection, although following completion of acyclovir administration, all patients experienced recurrent infection (85a). In a placebo-controlled trial of recurrent labial HSV infection, topical acyclovir was found to reduce duration of virus shedding in patients treated with 8 hours of the onset of lesions but was not associated with clinical benefit compared to placebo (23). Topical application of 5 percent acyclovir in a cream formulation, not

TABLE 3. Acyclovir Therapy of Primary Genital HSV Infection

	Intravenous (*Inpatient*[b])		*Oral* (*Outpatient*[c])		Topical (*Outpatient*[d])	
	ACV ($n = 14$)	*P* ($n = 13$)	*ACV* ($n = 13$)	*P* ($n = 10$)	*ACV* ($n = 26$)	*P* ($n = 23$)
Duration of virus shedding from						
Genital lesions (days)	2[a]	13	F 5[a]	15	4[a]	7
			M 6[a]	15		
Cervix (days)	1[a]	9	5	17	NS	NS
Time to crusting (days)	6[a]	13	F 9[a]	15	9	12
			M 5[a]	15		
Time to healing (days)	9[a]	21	F 10[a]	16	11	14
			M 12[a]	21		
Duration of pain (days)	3[a]	7	F 3	3	6	9
			M 2[a]	4		
Duration of systemic symptoms (days)	4	7	2	3	NS	NS
Percent with complications (extragenital lesions, urine retention)	0[a]	31	NS	NS	NS	NS
Percent with new vesicle formation after day 2 of treatment	20[a]	69	4[a]	44	No difference	
Percent with recurrences	60	88	68	72	No difference	
Median time to recurrence (days)	126	55	94	101	116	116

[a] $P < 0.05$, acyclovir versus placebo; F: female; M: male; NS: not stated. Time intervals are reported as medians for intravenous and as means for topical and oral acyclovir.
[b] Data taken from L Corey et al (79). Acyclovir dose: 5 mg/kg/8 hours for 5 days.
[c] Data taken from YJ Bryson et al (80). Acyclovir dose: 200 mg 5 times/day for 10 days.
[d] Data taken from L Corey et al (81). Acyclovir dose: applications every 4 hours while awake for 7 days.

currently available in the United States, has been reported to be therapeutically effective in both recurrent labial and genital HSV infections (86a,86b), which suggests that penetration of intact skin is the crucial factor in effectiveness.

Systemic acyclovir has been used successfully for both the prevention and treatment of mucocutaneous HSV infections in immunosuppressed patients. Prophylactic intravenous acyclovir (250 mg/M^2/8 hr), begun before transplantation and continued for 18 days, was effective in reducing the incidence of HSV disease in seropositive bone marrow transplant recipients (87). However, the majority of patients developed mild or asymptomatic HSV infections after acyclovir therapy was discontinued, and no effect on CMV infections was found. Similar results have been observed in seropositive leukemia patients receiving intensive chemotherapy (87a). Chronic oral acyclovir has been found to reduce the frequency of recurrent mucocutaneous HSV infections in immunosuppressed hosts (86), and controlled studies indicate that oral acyclovir is useful for prophylaxis during intense periods of immunosuppression (87a). In a therapeutic trial in patients with established mucocutaneous HSV infection, intravenous acyclovir (250 mg/M^2/8 hr for 7 days) shortened the median healing time (9.3 vs. 13.5 days), duration of pain (8.9 vs. 13.1 days), and the period of virus shedding (2.8 vs. 16.8 days) when compared to placebo (87b), but recurrences are common after cessation of therapy. Topical acyclovir therapy of labial or facial HSV infections in immunocompromised patients diminishes the duration of virus shedding (88) and in one recent study was found to shorten significantly the time to loss of pain and healing of lesions (88a). However, topical acyclovir should be used only in limited, extraoral mucocutaneous HSV infections in such patients.

In immunocompetent hosts several studies have found that intravenous acyclovir is associated with significant reductions in the time to healing of skin lesions and the duration of pain during the acute phase of herpes zoster, if administered within 72 to 96 hours of the onset of symptoms (72,89,90). In one study, acyclovir therapy (500 mg/M^2/8 hr for 5 days) significantly shortened the duration of virus shedding (2 vs. 5 days), duration of pain (2 vs. 5 days), duration of new lesion formation (2 vs. 4 days), and time to 50 percent healing (7 vs. 14 days) compared to placebo (72). No effect on the incidence or severity of postherpetic neuralgia has been documented in these studies. Uncontrolled trials suggest that topically applied acyclovir is therapeutically effective in ocular herpes zoster (91), and a randomized study to compare topical acyclovir and corticosteroids is in progress. In immunocompromised patients intravenous acyclovir (500 mg/M^2/8 hr for 7 days) in patients with localized zoster reduced the frequency of cutaneous dissemination (4 vs. 21 percent) and visceral complications (0 vs. 8 percent) compared to placebo (73). Similar trends were seen in patients who had disseminated zoster at the time of initiating therapy, but no significant differences were observed in resolution of lesions or pain (73). In immunosuppressed children with varicella, intravenous acyclovir (500 mg/M^2/8 hours for 7 days) was associated with a lower frequency of visceral complications (0 vs. 45 percent) compared to placebo, although the number of patients studied was small (92). The relative effectiveness of vidarabine and acyclovir in VZV infections of immunocompromised hosts remains to be determined.

Trials of intravenous acyclovir in CMV infections have shown no consistent clinical benefit, although reductions in viremia and viral titers in the urine have been observed in some patients (70, 93,94). In an uncontrolled study of bone marrow transplant recipients with pneumonia, high-dose acyclovir was associated with possible bone marrow and neurologic toxicity but no clinical benefit (70). In one case of Epstein-Barr virus-related posttransplant lymphoma, acyclovir therapy appeared to suppress orofacial shedding of virus and to induce transient remissions, although the patient ultimately died from a polyclonal B cell lymphoma (95). Several other cases of severe Epstein-Barr virus infections have not responded to acyclovir (96). Controlled trials in infectious mononucleosis of normal hosts are in progress.

Amantadine (1-adamantanamine hydrochloride, Symmetrel)

Spectrum. Amantadine hydrochloride is a symmetric tricyclic amine (Fig. 2) that specifically inhibits the replication of influenza A viruses. By plaque assay, the 50 percent inhibitory concentrations of amantadine range from 0.2–0.4 μg/ml for contemporary strains of influenza A viruses including H1N1, H2N2, and H3N2 subtypes (97,98). Higher concentrations (25–50 μg/ml) have variable in vitro inhibitory activity against some influenza B, rubella, paramyxo-, and arenaviruses (99), but these concentrations are too high to be clinically relevant. Both prophylactic and therapeutic activity has been demonstrated in experimental influenza A virus infection of animals. Studies in experimental animals have found that delivery of amantadine directly to the respiratory tract in aerosol form has greater efficacy than systemic administration (13,100,101).

Mechanism of Action. The exact mechanism of action of amantadine is undefined, but it appears to inhibit an early stage in viral replication, possibly uncoat-

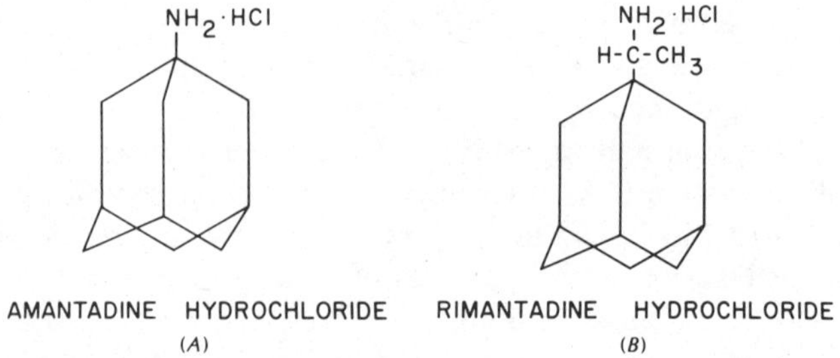

FIGURE 2. Chemical structures of (*A*) amantadine hydorchloride and (*B*) rimantadine hydrochloride.

ing of the viral genome (102–105). Electron microscopy studies have found that attachment and penetration of influenza virus appear to proceed normally in the presence of amantadine (102), and no direct effect on virus-associated RNA dependent RNA polymerase activity has been found (103). Studies of neutral-red-labeled virus have found that amantadine prolongs the period of photosensitivity, an effect that indicates inhibition of uncoating (104). Other in vitro studies have found that, although amantadine is readily concentrated in the lysosomes and cytosol of mammalian cells, its antiviral effect is quickly lost on its removal from surrounding medium (106). These findings indicate that the fraction of amantadine accounting for its antiviral activity is readily exchanged with the extracellular medium and that most of the cell-associated amantadine does not contribute to its antiviral action (106).

Resistance to amantadine is readily achieved in the laboratory by serial passage of influenza A virus strains in the presence of amantadine in vitro or in animals (107). One study concluded that susceptibility to amantadine is influenced by the gene coding for the matrix protein (108), but other studies have found that the genetics of amantadine resistance are more complex (109). Amantadine-resistant influenza A viruses have not yet been isolated from treated patients. However, one study reported recovering several relatively amantadine and rimantadine resistant H3N2 strains from untreated patients (109a), and more studies are needed.

Pharmacokinetics. Amantadine is well absorbed after oral administration of capsule, tablet, or syrup forms. The time to peak plasma level averages 3–4 hours, but ranges vary widely in healthy adults (110). Peak plasma concentrations average 0.3–0.4 μg/ml after administration of 100 mg doses and are approximately twofold higher after 200 mg doses in healthy adults (111–113). After administration of 200 mg/day for 5–7 days, plasma concentrations average 0.7–0.8 μg/ml (111,112,114). In children with cystic fibrosis mean plasma concentrations were 0.6 μg/ml during longterm ingestion of 6 mg/kg/day (114a). One study has concluded that nasal secretion levels of amantadine approximate those found in the serum (115), although some evidence suggests that amantadine is concentrated in pulmonary tissues (110,115a). After intermittent, small particle aerosol administration, nasal wash concentrations range from 2–19 μg/ml (36), and the drug readily appears in the urine indicating rapid absorption (116).

Amantadine is excreted unmetabolized in the urine by glomerular filtration and probably tubular secretion (117). The mean plasma half-life is 12–17 hours but has ranged from 7–31 hours in apparently healthy adults (113,117). Plasma half-life increases in elderly people (118) and in patients with impaired renal function in whom plasma concentrations from 1.0–5.0 μg/ml have been associated with confusion, delirium, hallucinations, seizures, and other signs of neurotoxicity (117,119). Dosage guidelines for patients with renal insufficiency are summarized in Table 4. Amantadine is poorly excreted in hemodialysis patients, and the amount removed by a single dialysis is only a small portion of the total body stores (117,120).

TABLE 4. Amantadine Dosage Adjustments Suggested in Patients With Impaired Renal Function

Creatinine Clearance	*Suggested Maintenance Regimen*
ml/minute/1.73 m^2	
≥100	100 mg twice daily or 200 mg once daily
80	100 mg twice daily
60	200 mg/100 mg alternate days
40	100 mg daily
30	200 mg twice weekly
20	100 mg thrice weekly
10[a]	200 mg/100 mg alternating every 7 days

SOURCE: Recommendations taken from Horadam et al (117).

[a] or thrice weekly hemodialysis.

Toxicity. Orally administered amantadine is generally well tolerated, and no serious renal, hepatic, or hematopoetic toxicity has been documented. Long-term amantadine ingestion has been associated with livido reticularis, peripheral edema, orthostatic hypotension, and possibly congestive heart failure, vision loss, and urinary retention (121–124). The most common side effects related to amantadine ingestion are minor gastrointestinal and central nervous system complaints that often resolve despite continued administration. These include nervousness, lightheadedness, difficulty concentrating, insomnia, and loss of appetite or nausea (125). Amantadine-associated side effects are related to dosage and duration of administration. Although higher doses have been used in the treatment of parkinsonian symptoms (121,122), dosages of 300 mg/day are poorly tolerated by healthy working adults and are also associated with significantly decreased performance on psychomotor tests designed to measure sustained attention and problem-solving ability (125). In contrast, dosages of 200 mg/day have not been associated with changes in psychomotor or academic performance in healthy adults (125–127). The potential for neurotoxicity appears to be increased by concommitent ingestion of antihistamines or anticholinergic drugs (126,128). In recent studies of long-term prophylaxis of influenza A virus infections (200 mg/day), the excess dropout rate because of side effects has ranged from 6 to 11 percent of amantadine recipients as compared to placebo (129–131). Serious neurotoxic reactions may be transiently reversed by physostigmine administration (132).

In vitro studies have found that high concentrations (25–50 μg/ml) of amantadine can inhibit lymphocyte transformation responses to mitogen and specific antigens (133,134). High dosages are teratogenic in certain laboratory animals.

Clinical Studies. The clinical usefulness of amantadine as an antiviral agent is limited to the prevention and treatment of influenza A virus infections. Early studies showed that amantadine was ineffective in the prophylaxis of influenza B or experimentally induced measles virus infections (135). A number of placebo-controlled, blinded studies have documented the prophylactic efficacy of amantadine at a dosage of 200 mg/day against the development of clinical illness in experimentally induced and naturally occurring influenza A virus infections (129,130,136,137). The efficacy of amantadine in preventing illness documented to be secondary to influenza infection has ranged from 50 to over 90 percent, rates comparable to those obtained with inactivated influenza A virus vaccines. Prophylactic efficacy has been demonstrated in both nosocomial influenza (138) and in the household setting (139). Dosages of 100 mg/day have been shown to be highly protective against influenza A infection in a semiclosed population of teenaged students (139a).

Prophylactic administration is recommended in elderly (≥65 years) or chronically ill patients who have not received vaccine due to contraindication, unavailability, or other reasons; unvaccinated persons who provide essential community services; and in those at increased risk of exposure, such as household contacts of persons with influenza or hospital staff with patient contact. Prophylaxis should be begun as soon as influenza is identified in a community or region and should be continued throughout the period of risk (usually 4–8 weeks) since any beneficial effects diminish rapidly after discontinuation of the drug (139a,140). Alternatively, since amantadine does not interfere with the response to inactivated vaccine, the drug can be started in conjunction with immunization and continued for 2 weeks until protective antibody develops.

A series of placebo, blinded trials have demonstrated that amantadine is also an effective therapeutic agent in naturally occurring influenza A virus infection of previously healthy, young adults (141–145). When begun within 1–2 days of onset of symptoms, a dosage of 200 mg/day has been shown to reduce the duration of fever and systemic complaints by approximately 50 percent and in some studies to decrease the duration of virus shedding compared to placebo (141,145). One study found that amantadine-treated students were able to return to class more rapidly compared to placebo recipients (145). Other studies of adults with infection due to H3N2 subtype influenza viruses have found that certain abnormalities of peripheral airways function resolve more quickly in amantadine-treated patients (146,147), but to date, no controlled trials have documented that amantadine prevents the pulmonary complications of influenza or that it is therapeutically useful in patients with established pulmonary complications. A recent study comparing the efficacy of aspirin and amantadine treatment of naturally occurring H1N1 subtype influenza found that aspirin-treated patients defervesced more rapidly but experienced significantly higher rates of drug-related side effects and slower symptomatic improvement than amantadine recipients (148). In addition, in this study (148), 100 mg per day was found to be as effective as 200 mg per day. Intermittent aerosol administration of amantadine has also proven to be therapeutically useful in uncomplicated, naturally occurring influenza (36). An injectable formulation is not available.

Bromovinyl Deoxyuridine (E-5-(2-bromovinyl)-deoxyuridine, BVDU)

BVDU is a halogenated thymidine analogue that selectively inhibits HSV and VZV replication in vitro (149–151). One in vitro study found that BVDU was approximately 55-fold more active than acyclovir against HSV type 1 strains but 25-fold less active against type 2 strains (150). For VZV, the average 50 percent plaque inhibitory concentrations are 0.001–0.004 μg/ml (151). BVDU inhibits HSV type 2 replication only at 100- to 200-fold higher concentrations than for HSV type 1, and this differential activity has been used presumptively to identify HSV types in the clinical laboratory (152). BVDU inhibits EBV genome replication in productively infected cells and, unlike acyclovir, causes prolonged inhibition of viral replication in persistently infected cells after drug removal (44). BVDU has shown therapeutic activity in various animal models of HSV infection following topical, oral, or parenteral administration (153–156) and, depending on the time of initiating treatment, can prevent latent infections (155). In experimental simian varicella virus infection of monkeys, oral or parenteral BVDU demonstrated both prophylactic and therapeutic activity, even when begun as late as day 4–6 following virus inoculation (156).

BVDU is selectively phosphorylated by HSV- or VZV-specific thymidine kinases (TK), so that virus strains resistant to acyclovir because of TK deficiency are also BVDU-resistant (157–159). The triphosphate inhibits the activity of viral DNA polymerase and appears to be incorporated in the place of deoxythymidine-5′-triphosphate in viral DNA (158,159). Single oral doses of 60 or 125 mg are associated with peak plasma concentrations of 0.4 μg/ml that are cleared within 4 hours of dosing; the principal metabolite appears to be bromovinyl uracil, which remains detectable for at least 24 hours (159a). Because of its potent, selective anti-VZV activity, BVDU is an especially promising agent for treatment of varicella and herpes zoster. An uncontrolled study suggested that orally administered BVDU was effective in herpes zoster of immunocompromised hosts (160), and other studies are in progress.

Idoxuridine (5-iodo-2′-deoxyuridine, IDU, IUDR, Stoxil, Herplex, Dendrid)

Idoxuridine is an iodinated thymidine analogue (Fig. 3) that inhibits the in vitro replication of various DNA viruses, particularly herpesviruses and poxviruses (162). Plaque production by most clinical isolates of HSV type 1 is inhibited by concentrations of 2–10 μg/ml (6,7,163). The antiviral mechanism of action of idoxuridine is not completely defined, but the phosphorylated derivatives interfere with various enzyme systems, and the triphosphate inhibits viral DNA synthesis and is incorporated into both viral and cellular DNA (162). Resistance to the antiviral effect of idoxuridine readily develops under laboratory conditions and has occurred in viral isolates recovered from idoxuridine-treated patients

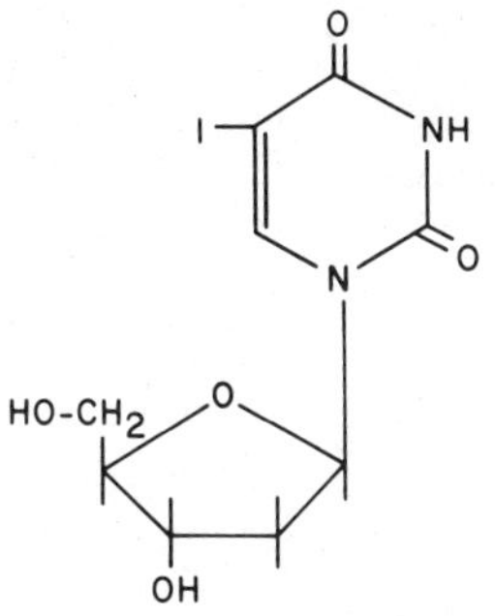

IDOXURIDINE

FIGURE 3. Chemical structure of idoxuridine.

with HSV keratitis (6,7). Idoxuridine is teratogenic, mutagenic, and immunosuppressive in certain experimental systems (162).

Clinical Studies. A double-blind, randomized study of systemically administered idoxuridine (100 mg/kg/day for 5 days) found not only lack of efficacy in HSV encephalitis but also side effects of liver function abnormalities and serious bone marrow toxicity (165).

The therapeutic usefulness of topically applied idoxuridine depends on the site of infection and the vehicle of administration. Idoxuridine in ointment or solution form was ineffective in recurrent herpes labialis, varicella, or localized herpes zoster (166,167). In contrast, several studies concluded that frequent application of idoxuridine dissolved in dimethyl sulfoxide (5–40 percent idoxuridine in 100 percent DMSO) hastened the healing of skin lesions and shortened the duration of pain in localized herpes zoster (168,169) but minimal beneficial effects were found in a more recent study (164). A double-blind, placebo controlled trial found that topical application of 30% idoxuridine in DMSO appeared to shorten the duration of viral shedding in recurrent or primary genital HSV infections, but did not reduce the duration of symptoms or lesions compared to DMSO alone or to saline (170). Mild, local burning after topical application of DMSO is common, and headache, dizziness, sedation, nausea, localized and generalized dermatitis have also been reported (170,171). DMSO is teratogenic and can cause adverse ocular effects in laboratory animals.

In the United States, idoxuridine is approved by the FDA only for topical treatment of HSV keratitis. Controlled trials (172) and extensive clinical experience (173) have indicated greater efficacy in epithelial infections, especially initial episodes, than in stromal infections. Adverse reactions include pain, pruritis, inflammation, or edema involving the eye or lids, and, rarely, allergic reactions.

Methisazone (N-methylisatin-B-thiosemicarbazone, Marboran)

Methisazone and its parent compound isatin-B-thiosemicarbazone inhibit poxvirus replication in vitro through interference with translation of late viral messenger RNA, protein synthesis, and subsequent virus assembly (174).

The oral formulation of methisazone, a suspension in sucrose, is associated with a high incidence of gastrointestinal side effects (175). Several studies have shown prophylactic effectiveness against alastrim in Brazil and smallpox in India, but these studies were neither randomized nor blinded (175–177). A randomized, placebo-controlled study found a trend toward prophylactic efficacy against smallpox (178), but therapeutic administration in smallpox is ineffective (175). Uncontrolled studies suggest that methisazone may ameliorate complications of vaccination, including vaccinia ganrenosa and eczema vaccinatum (179,180). When given at the time of vaccination, methisazone may depress the local reaction and possibly impair the antibody response (181). Methisazone is not approved for use in the United States, and the eradication of smallpox has made this drug less important.

Phosphonoformate Trisodium (PFA, Foscarnet)

PFA and phosphonoacetate (PAA) are pyrophosphate analogues that selectively inhibit replication of herpes viruses. They preferentially inhibit viral, as compared to cellular, DNA polymerase activity and DNA polymerization, probably by affecting the pyrophosphate-binding site of DNA polymerases (182–185). HSV mutants that are cross-resistant to PAA and PFA because of an altered DNA polymerase are readily isolated under laboratory conditions (186,187). Topical application of either agent is associated with therapeutic and antiviral activity in HSV-induced skin and genital tract infections of experimental animals, but PAA causes dermal toxicity after topical application (188). Systemically administered PAA and PFA are retained in the bone matrix of experimental animals (189,190). Unlike acyclovir or PAA, topically applied PFA does not prevent development of latent infection in sensory ganglia following HSV skin infection of mice (191). One placebo-controlled, multicentered trial reported that application of a 3 percent PFA ointment six times per day for 4 days provided therapeutic benefit in patients with recurrent labial herpes (192).

Ribavirin (1-b-D-ribofuranosyl-1,2,4-triazole-3-carboxamide, Virazole)

The synthetic nucleoside ribavirin is a guanosine analogue in which both the triazole-caboximide moiety and the D-ribose sugar are necessary for antiviral activity. Ribavirin inhibits the in vitro replication of a wide range of RNA and DNA viruses, including myxo-, paramyxo-, arena-, bunya-, RNA tumor, herpes, adeno-, and poxviruses (193,194). By plaque assay the ED_{50} concentrations range from 3–10 μg/ml for influenza A and B (97) and respiratory syncytial (RS) (195) viruses. Inhibitory concentrations for a particular virus differ markedly in different cell types (193), and the ability of cells to take up ribavirin and form active metabolites may be important determinants of antiviral activity (196). Ribavirin is generally not active against viruses with single-stranded RNA genomes that act directly as messenger RNA, such as entero- and rhinoviruses. A structurally related selenazole carboxamide nucleoside (2-b-D-ribofuranosylselenazole-4-carboxamide) has been recently reported to have significantly greater in vitro inhibitory activity than ribavirin against a wide range of pathogenic viruses (196a).

Mechanism of Action. The antiviral mechanism of action of ribavirian is not defined but relates to alteration of nucleotide pools and messenger RNA formation. Intracellular phosphorylation to the mono-, di-, and triphosphate derivatives is mediated by host cell enzymes (197,198). Ribavirin monophosphate competitively inhibits inosine-5′-phosphate dehydrogenase and interferes with the synthesis of guanine nucleotides and thus nucleic acid synthesis (198,199). However, inhibition of this normal cellular enzyme would not fully account for a selective antiviral action. Low concentrations of ribavirin (2–10 μg/ml) reversibly inhibit macromolecular synthesis and the proliferation of certain rapidly dividing, uninfected mammalian cells (200,200a–202).

Synthesis of influenza virus RNA and protein has been reported to be inhibited by ribavirin concentrations that do not affect cellular RNA or protein synthesis (203,204), although some studies of influenza- or togavirus-infected cells have not found a distinction between concentrations that inhibit viral replication and those inhibiting cellular RNA synthesis (200,200a,205). Ribavirin triphosphate has been reported to selectively inhibit influenza virus RNA polymerase activity in a cell-free assay system (206). Studies of vaccinia virus replication found that ribavirin triphosphate is a competitive inhibitor of the capping guanylation of viral messenger RNA (207). In contrast to other synthetic antiviral agents, resistance to ribavirin has not been produced under experimental conditions (208).

Ribavirin has biologic activities beyond its antiviral and cytotoxic effects. In rodents, parenteral ribavirin inhibited the serum antibody but not cellular immune responses to inactivated influenza vaccine (209) and diminished in vivo primary antibody responses and memory cell generation to T-dependent and T-independent antigens (210). Ribavirin suppresses nucleic acid synthesis in quiescent and mitogen-stimulated human peripheral blood lymphocytes in vitro (211), and ribavirin treatment is associated with fewer CF, but not HI, antibody conversions in patients with naturally acquired influenza A virus infection (212). In experimental animals, ribavirin has therapeutic activity against transplantable virus-induced tumors (209,213,214) and autoimmune diseases (215). Ribavirin is teratogenic and embryotoxic in small mammals during the first trimester of pregnancy (216).

Pharmacology and Toxicity. The human pharmacology of ribavirin is incompletely defined. Oral administration of ^{14}C-labeled ribavirin (approximately 3 mg/kg) demonstrated that radioactive urinary excretion averaged 33 percent of dose at 24 hours and 53 percent at 72 hours (217). Peak plasma levels equivalent to 1–2 μg/ml ribavirin occurred at 1–1.5 hours and decayed in a complex manner. Radioactivity concentrated in RBC in the form of ribavirin or its metabolites (3 percent of total dose) and decayed gradually with an apparent $T_{1/2}$ of about 40 days (217). In children with bronchiolitis treated with aerosolized ribavirin, peak plasma levels of about 0.3 μg/ml and respiratory secretions levels of 50–200 μg/ml have been observed (218). Plasma concentrations depend on the duration of aerosol exposure and average 0.2 and 2.0 μg/ml for exposures of 2.5 and 20 hours, respectively (218a). By radioimmunoassay plasma $T_{1/2}$ averages approximately 9 hours (range 5–13.5 hours) (218).

Reversible increases of serum bilirubin (up to 25–29 percent of recipients), serum iron, and uric acid concentrations occur during short-term administration of oral ribavirin 800–1,000 mg/day (212,219,220). Prolonged administration causes a dose-dependent macrocytic anemia in animals (216); increased reticulocyte counts occur in ribavirin-treated patients after cessation of oral therapy (212). Aerosolized ribavirin has been well tolerated except for mild conjunctival injection in some recipients (37–39) and specifically has not caused deterioration in pulmonary function (39).

Clinical Studies. Prophylactic oral administration of ribavirin of 600 mg/day showed marginal effectiveness in experimental influenza B (221) but no effectiveness in experimental influenza A virus infection (222). Higher oral doses (1,000 mg/day) were reported to reduce symptoms and fever in experimental influenza A virus infection (220), but this dose had no clinical or antiviral activity in naturally occurring influenza A virus infection of adults (212). Oral ribavirin (600 mg/day for 14 days) was reportedly associated with more rapid resolution of bilirubin and transaminase elevations and with more rapid weight gain in patients with acute hepatitis of undetermined type (223). Another study (800 mg/day for 10 days) reported reductions in pain and new lesion formation in recurrent genital herpes (224), but confirmation of these observations is needed.

Aerosol administration has greater therapeutic activity than the parenteral route in animal models of influenza (13,100) and RSV infection (225). In humans, ribavirin administered in small-particle aerosol form for an average of 23 (37) or 39 (38) hours over 3 days was associated with reductions in viral titers, fever, and systemic illness compared to aerosolized saline in young adults with naturally acquired influenza A (37) or B (38) virus infection of less than 24 hours duration. The relative therapeutic activity of aerosolized ribavirin and oral amantaine or rimantadine in influenza A virus infections and the value of aerosolized ribavirin in high-risk groups, such as infants or adults hospitalized with influenza, need study.

A placebo-controlled, double-blind study found that aerosolized ribavirin reduced fever and systemic symptoms in experimental RSV infection of young adults (39). A recent controlled trial found that aerosolized ribavirin (exposure periods averaging 20 hours/day for 3–6 days) shortened the duration of virus shedding and improved clinical measures, including arterial oxygen saturation, in infants hospitalized with RSV pneumonia (226). A similar study of infants with RSV bronchiolitis found that aerosolized ribavirin (12 hours/day for 5 days) was associated with reductions in illness severity but not in duration of hospitalization or virus shedding (226a).

Parenterally administered ribavirin has antiviral and therapeutic activity in animal models of Lassavirus, other arenaviruses, and bunyavirus infections (196,227) and is undergoing clinical trials. Ribavirin is commercially available in several Latin American countries but not currently in the United States.

Rimantadine Hydrochloride (α-methyl-1-adamantanemethylamine hydrochloride)

Rimantadine hydrochloride is a structural analog of amantadine (Fig. 2) and shares its antiviral spectrum and mechanism of action. In vitro and animal model studies have found that rimantadine has somewhat greater antiviral activity than amantadine against influenza A viruses (97,228–231). Rimantadine concentrations that cause 50 percent inhibition of influenza A virus plaque formation range from 0.1–0.4 μg/ml (97). Rimantadine also appears to block the intracellular uncoating of influenza viruses, possibly inhibiting the release of M protein from virus ribonucleoproteins and preventing penetration into the cell nucleus (232,232a).

Pharmacology and Toxicity. The pharmacokinetics of orally administered rimantadine are incompletely defined. Maximum plasma concentrations averaging 0.3 μg/ml occur at 4.5 hours after administration of single 200 mg doses in adults (233). Plasma rimantadine concentrations average 48 percent of amantadine values at 4 hours after single 100 or 200 mg doses and 61–65 percent after multiple doses (111). Steady-state peak serum rimantadine concentrations range from 0.6–2.6 μg/ml (mean 1.2 μg/ml) in elderly adults ingesting 200 mg per day for several months (233a). In healthy adults the plasma half-life of rimantadine averages approximately 28 hours, nearly twofold longer than that of amantadine. Less than 10 percent of the administered rimantadine dose is recovered in the urine, as contrasted to over 90 percent with amantadine (233). Approximately 30 percent of orally administered rimantadine is recovered as hydroxylated metabolites in the urine.

Rimantadine administration is associated with side effects similar to those observed with amantadine, but except for gastrointestinal complaints, side effects are less frequent with rimantadine when the drugs are given in equal doses (125,145). Rimantadine (300 mg/day) is associated with higher rates of gastrointestinal complaints, but not central nervous system or sleep disturbances as compared to placebo, nor is it associated with alterations of psychomotor test performance (125). Studies to date indicate that amantadine and rimantadine differ in their pharmacokinetics but not in their potential for side effects at comparable plasma concentrations.

Clinical Studies. Placebo-controlled, double-blinded trials have shown that rimantadine is effective in preventing both experimentally induced and naturally occurring influenza virus infection (130,234–236,236a). One field trial comparing equivalent 200 mg/day dosages of rimantadine and amantadine found that the drugs were 65 and 78 percent effective, respectively, in preventing influenza-like illness and 85 and 91 percent effective, respectively, in preventing laboratory-documented influenza (130). A study of previously vaccinated nursing home patients found that rimantadine (200 mg/day) had 80 percent efficacy in preventing influenza-like illness compared to placebo (236a).

Both oral and aerosolized rimantadine have been shown to be therapeutically useful in experimentally induced influenza (237). Oral rimantadine (300 mg/day) has therapeutic effects in uncomplicated, naturally occurring influenza A virus infection comparable to those of amantadine (200 mg/day) (142). One study employing equivalent 200 mg/day dosages found that amantadine-treated patients tended to improved more rapidly than rimantadine-treated patients, but that by 48 hours after initiating therapy, both groups had significantly less fever, greater symptomatic improvement, and lower frequencies of virus shedding than placebo-treated patients (145). Most clinical trials employing equal dosages of amantadine and rimantadine (200 mg/day) have found that amantadine is somewhat, although not significantly, more effective than rimantadine, but is also associated with higher frequencies of central nervous system side effects (130,145,235).

Trifluridine (5-trifluoromethyl-2′-deoxyuridine, trifluorothymidine, Viroptic)

Trifluridine is a fluorinated pyrimidine nucleoside (Fig. 4) that has in vitro inhibitory activity against HSV types 1 and 2, cytomegalovirus, vaccinia, and some strains of adenovirus (238–240). Its antiviral mechanism of action is undefined but involves inhibition of viral DNA synthesis. It also inhibits cellular DNA synthesis at relatively low concentrations (238,239). The triphosphate derivative is incorporated into viral, and to a lesser extent cellular, DNA in competition with deoxythymidine triphosphate. Trifluridine is active against thymidine-kinase-negative strains of HSV, which indicates that this enzyme is not essential to its action. It also exhibits mutagenic, teratogenic, and antineoplastic activities in experimental systems (238).

The use of trifluridine as an antiviral agent is currently limited to topical therapy of ocular HSV infections, in which it is approved by the Food and Drug Administration for treatment of primary keratoconjuctivitis and recurrent epithelial keratitis due to HSV types 1 and 2. Topical trifluridine has been found to be more active than idoxuridine, but trials comparing its efficacy with that of topical vidarabine have generally found no significant differences (241,

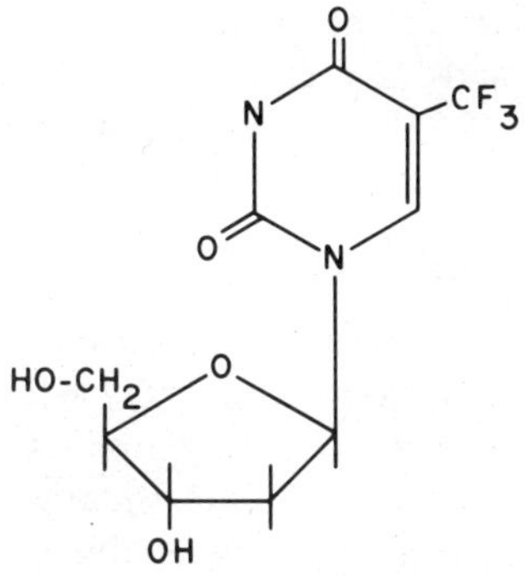

TRIFLUOROTHYMIDINE

FIGURE 4. Chemical structure of trifluorothymidine.

242). Topical trifluridine has been effective in some patients that have not responded clinically to idoxuridine or vidarabine (243,244). Adverse reactions include discomfort on instillation, palpebral edema, and uncommonly hypersensitivity reactions, irritation, superficial punctate or epithelial keratopathy.

Vidarabine (9-b-D-ribofuranosyladenine, ara-A, adenine arabinoside, Vira-A)

Spectrum. Vidarabine is an analogue of adenine deoxyriboside (Fig. 5), which has in vitro antiviral activity against HSV types 1 and 2, VZV, Epstein-Barr virus, animal herpesviruses, vaccinia and variola viruses, rhabdo, and some RNA tumor viruses (245–250). Vidarabine also inhibits the in vitro replication of idoxuridine or acyclovir-resistant HSV strains and acyclovir-resistant VZV

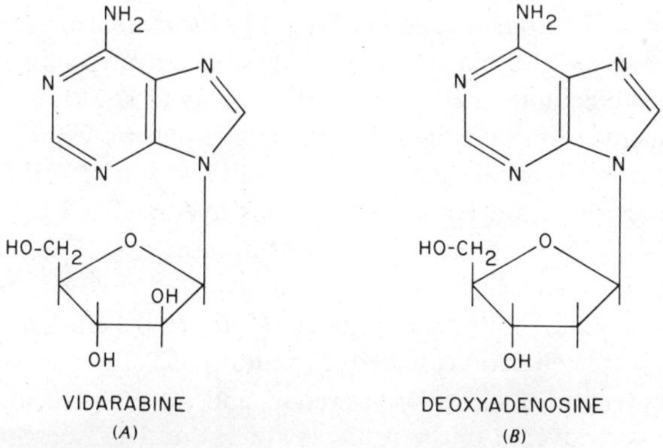

FIGURE 5. Chemical structures of (*A*) vidarabine and the natural nucleoside (*B*) deoxyadenosine.

strains (248,250), but has variable activity against cytomegalovirus (249). Plaque formation by most HSV and VZV strains is completely inhibited by 3.0 μg/ml or less of vidarabine (245,246). The 50 percent plaque inhibitory concentrations are approximately 0.2 μg/ml for HSV-2 and 0.04 μg/ml for vaccinia virus (245).

Mechanism of Action. The antiviral mechanisms of vidarabine are not completely understood. Vidarabine is phosphorylated by cellular enzymes to the triphosphate derivative, which competitively inhibits HSV, and to a lesser extent cellular, DNA polymerase activity (245,251). Vidarabine triphosphate is incorporated into both cellular and viral DNA, where it may act as a chain terminator for newly synthesized HSV nucleic acid (251–253). The principal metabolite in vivo and in cell culture is hypoxanthine arabinoside (ara-Hx), a compound with 30- to 50-fold less antiviral activity than vidarabine (246,249). However, ara-Hx appears to enhance the antiviral activity of vidarabine both in vitro and in specimens from patients receiving vidarabine (254). The carbocyclic analog of vidarabine (Cyclaradine) is resistant to the action of adenosine deaminase and retains comparable antiviral activity in vitro and in animal models (254a,254b).

Vidarabine, but not ara-Hx, also inhibits S-adenosylhomocysteine hydrolase, an enzyme involved in transmethylation reactions, both in vitro and in RBC collected from treated patients (255,256). This effect continues for over 1 week following cessation of therapy and has been postulated to contribute to the antiviral and toxic effects of vidarabine.

Pharmacology. Following intravenous infusion, vidarabine is rapidly deaminated to ara-Hx by adenosine deaminase (258,259). This enzyme is widely distributed through body tissues but in animals is present in relatively low concentrations in blood and brain (260). Samples for measurement of vidarabine levels need to be collected in the presence of an inhibitor of adenosine deaminase, such as 2-deoxycorformicin, and quickly frozen to prevent in vitro deamination. During a constant 12-hour infusion (10 mg/kg/12hr), plasma ara-Hx concentrations peak at 3–6 μg/ml, but no or minimal concentrations of vidarabine (0.2–0.4 μg/ml) are detectable in adults by HPLC assay (259,261). Ara-Hx is present in CSF at concentrations averaging 35 percent of plasma values, although CSF/plasma ratios over 90 percent have been found in infants (259,262,263). Another study found that peak ara-Hx concentrations averaged 3.7 μg/ml in full-term infants and 8.5 μg/ml in preterm infants at a dosage of 15 mg/kg/12 hr (263). These findings indicate that higher weight-adjusted dosages may be required in full-term infants. In four infants given 35 mg/kg/12 hr, mean plasma and CSF vidarabine concentrations were 0.275 and 0.353 μg/ml, respectively (262).

The primary route of clearance is renal, and 40–53 percent of the total of the daily dose is recovered in the urine as ara-Hx and 1–3 percent as the parent drug (259). The serum half-life of ara-Hx is approximately 3.5 hours in adults. Studies with labeled vidarabine have found accumulation of radioactivity in

RBC over 5–7 days and lasting up to 3 weeks (259). In patients with impaired renal function, plasma ara-Hx concentrations rise and may be associated with neurologic or other side effects (264). A dosage reduction of 25 percent has been recommended for patients with severe renal insufficiency (264), but guidelines of proven value have not been established. Ara-Hx is readily cleared during hemodialysis (50 percent over 6 hours), so that dosages should be given after dialysis (264).

Toxicity. Dose-related gastrointestinal toxicity is common with vidarabine and may be manifested by anorexia, nausea, vomiting, diarrhea and/or weight loss (259,265). The principal difficulty encountered during systemic administration of vidarabine relates to its poor solubility ($\leq$0.45 mg/ml) and the consequent infusion of large fluid volumes, often 1.5–2.5 liters at a dosage of 15 mg/kg/day.

At dosages higher than normally used (20 mg/kg/day), vidarabine is associated with megaloblastic bone marrow changes and sometimes with anemia, leukopenia, or thrombocytopenia (265). Infusion-related thrombophlebitis, weakness, hypokalemia, rash, and the syndrome of inappropriate secretion of antidiuretic hormone (SIADH) have been described (265–267), but controlled trials in serious herpes virus infections at dosages of 10–15 mg/kg/day have not documented serious bone marrow, liver, or renal toxicity.

A variety of neurologic side effects have been reported during vidarabine therapy. High dosages, concurrent interferon (20) or possibly allopurinol (268) therapy, and the presence of preexisting hepatic or renal insufficiency have been predisposing risk factors (20,267–270). The reported neurotoxicities include pain syndromes, usually in the extremities and sometimes lasting up to 6 months after cessation of therapy; tremor, often accentuated by intention and at times associated with facial grimacing, myoclonus, ataxia, or dysgraphia; and alterations in behavior or mentation, including disorientation, depression, aphasia, akinetic mutism, agitation, hallucinations, and rarely, coma or siezures (20, 267,270). Electroencephalograms have shown diffuse changes consistent with metabolic encephalopathy in some cases, but were reported to correlate poorly with clinical manifestations in one study (20). This study also found that serum ara-Hx concentrations were significantly higher in toxic patients than in asymtomatic ones (22). In several patients, an unusual brain pathology consisting of chromatolysis and neuronal degeneration has been described (270). Monitoring of ara-Hx concentrations in patients with hepatic or renal insufficency is advisable, but is not routinely available in most laboratories.

In contrast to cytosine arabinoside, vidarabine (3 μg/ml) did not inhibit mytogen- or antigen-induced lymphocyte blastogenesis or lymphocyte cytotoxicity to herpesvirus-infected target cells in vitro (271). Simularly, cell-mediated immune responses are not reduced in peripheral blood leukocytes collected from patients receiving vidarabine (271). In mice, vidarabine administration augments humoral immune responses and delayed hypersensitivity reactions and prolongs survival in cryptococcal infection (257). This enhancement of host responses may be mediated by interference with normal suppressor cell functions (257). Vidarabine has been shown to be mutagenic, teratogenic, and oncogenic in experimental systems, and its use should be restricted to serious infections.

Clinical Studies. The most notable successes with vidarabine have been observed in patients with HSV and VZV infections. The efficacy of vidarabine administered topically in HSV keratoconjunctivitis is well established and is superior to idoxuridine, in that topical vidarabine is effective in patients who cannot receive idoxuridine because of allergy, toxicity, or clinical drug resistance (272). However, when applied locally as a 3 percent ointment, vidarabine provided no benefit in genital or orofacial HSV infections (32–35).

Several multicenter, controlled trials have documented the therapeutic efficacy of intravenous vidarabine in severe HSV infections (see Table 1). Vidarabine (15 mg/kg/day for 10 days) increased survival in biopsy-proven HSV encephalitis from 30 percent in the placebo group to 72 percent at one month and 56 percent at 6 months (273). A follow up, open trial involving 75 patients with biopsy-proven disease confirmed long-term survival rates of 61 percent in vidarabine-treated patients (274). The most favorable prognosis was for younger patients who were treated early in the course of disease, as reflected by the level of consciousness at the time of initiating therapy (Fig. 6). At the same dosage vidarabine treatment reduced the mortality of neonatal HSV infection complicated by visceral dissemination or CNS involvement to 38 percent, compared to 74 percent in placebo recipients (275). Collaborative randomized trials comparing the efficacy of acyclovir and vidarabine (30 mg/kg/day for neonatal infection) in HSV encephalitis and neonatal infection are currently in progress. A recent double-blind, cross-over study found that vidarabine (10 mg/kg/day for 7 days) was of limited usefulness in mucocutaneous HSV infections of immunocompromised hosts (276). Significant but clinically modest reductions in the durations of pain, fever, and shedding of HSV type 1 were observed in vidarabine recipients (276).

In a cross-over, double-blind study of immunosuppressed patients with herpes zoster, accelerated clearance of virus from vesicles, more rapid cessation of new vesicle formation, and more frequent relief of acute pain were demonstrated in vidarabine recipients (10 mg/kg/day) compared to placebo recipients during the first 5 days of study (29). A subsequent placebo-controlled study of immunocompromised patients with localized herpes zoster of less than 72 hours duration found that vidarabine (10 mg/kg/day for 7 days) decreased the frequency of cutaneous dissemination (8 vs. 24 percent), visceral complications (5 vs. 19 percent), the time to healing, and the total duration of postherpetic neuralgia (Table 5) (30). A similar study in immunocompromised patients with varicella found that vidarabine accelerated the resolution of new vesicle formation and fever and reduced the risk of varicella-related complications (277) (Table 5).

Vidarabine therapy in selected patients with chronic hepatitis B virus infection is associated with reductions in plasma HBV-specific DNA polymerase activity and titers of HBsAg and HBeAg in some patients (278). However, greater

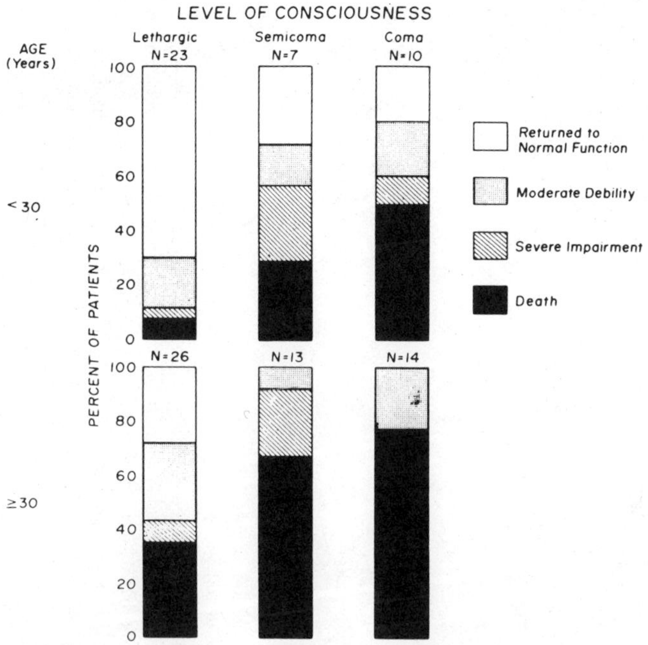

FIGURE 6. Influence of level of consciousness and age on morbidity and mortality in vidarabine-treated, biopsy-proven herpes simplex encephalitis. [Reprinted by permission from Whitley et al (274).]

TABLE 5. Effect of Vidarabine Therapy on Visceral Complications of Herpes Zoster or Varicella of Immunocompromised Patients

	Varicella		*Herpes zoster*	
Complication	*Vidarabine* (*n* = *19*)	*Placebo* (*n* = *15*)	*Vidarabine* (*n* = *63*)	*Placebo* (*n* = *58*)
Uveitis (blindness)			1	3
Neuropathy			0	2
Hepatitis	0	4	0	3
Pneumonitis (hepatitis)	1	4	0	0
Encephalitis	0	0	2	3
Total complications posttreatment (%)	1(5)[a]	8(53)[a]	3(5)[b]	11(19)[b]
Deaths	0	2	0	0

SOURCE: Data are taken from Whitley et al (30,277).

[a] $P < 0.01$, vidarabine vs. placebo.

[b] $P = 0.015$, vidarabine vs. placebo.

TABLE 6. Other Antiviral Agents of Investigational Interest

Antiviral Agent	*Antiviral Spectrum*	*Mechanism of Action*	*Comment/Clinical Studies*
Acyclic nucleosides DHPG(9-[1,3 dihydroxy-2-propoxymethyl]guanine; BIOLF-62; 2'NDG)[a]	HSV types 1 and 2, CMV, VZV, EBV, adenovirus	Inhibition of DNA synthesis—phosphorylation by HSV thymidine kinsase. Reduced activity against thymidine kinase deficient HSV.	More active than acyclovir in certain animal models of HSV infection. Highly active against CMV in vitro but mechanism of anti-CMV action undefined.
Arildone (4-[6-(2-chloro-4-methoxy)phenoxy]hexyl-3,5 heptanedione)[b]	Picornaviruses, paramyxoviruses, HSV types 1 and 2	Prevention of poliovirus uncoating—direct interaction with capsid protein. Mechanism of action against DNA viruses uncertain.	Clinical studies in progress.
Enviroxime (2-amino-1-[isopropylsulphonyl]-6-benzimidazole phenyl ketone oxime)[c]	Picornaviruses	Inhibition of viral macromolecular synthesis—prevents formation of functional viral RNA polymerase complex.	Intranasal enviroxime—modest prophylactic and/or therapeutic activity in experimentally induced rhinovirus infection. Oral formulation—high rate of gastrointestinal side effects.
2-fluoroarabinosyl nucleosides FIAC (2'-fluoro-5-iodo-1-b-D arabinofuranosyl-cytosine) FIAU (2'-fluoro-5-iodo-1-b-*D* arabinofuranosyl-uracil)	HSV types 1 and 2, VZV, EBV, CMV	Inhibition of DNA synthesis—specificity of action relates to phosphorylation by viral nucleoside kinases. Deamination of FIAC to	In vitro activity similar to acyclovir. More active than acyclovir and vidarabine in certain animal models of HSV infection. Clinical

FMAU (2′-fluoro-5-methyl-1-b-D arabinofuranosyl-uracil)[d]		FIAU, which has lower therapeutic index.	studies in progress. One randomized trial found that intravenous FIAC (400 mg/M^2/day for 5 days) provided greater clinical benefit than vidarabine in localized herpes zoster of immunocompromised hosts. Gastrointestinal side effects; reversible SGOT elevations; hematopoietic toxicity at higher doses.
Rifampicin[e]	Poxviruses, adenoviruses, CMV	Inhibition of late viral protein synthesis and assembly.	Topical application inhibited the vaccination reaction in volunteers. Oral administration—not effective in subacute sclerosing panencephalitis.
Zinc[f]	Picornaviruses, vaccinia, HSV	Inhibition of HSV DNA polymerase and inhibition of late viral protein cleavage in other viruses.	Topical applications of zinc solutions active in animal models of genital HSV infection. Reported activity in human mucocutaneous HSV infections and common colds.

[a] See references 288–291.
[b] See references 292–295.
[c] See references 296–300.
[d] See references 301–306a.
[e] See references 307–311.
[f] See references 312–316.

antiviral and clinical benefits appear to be derived from combined or sequential administration of vidarabine and interferon (18–21).

No therapeutic benefit has been observed in smallpox (279), despite use of high vidarabine doses (20 mg/kg/day for 7 days), or in patients with advanced progressive multifocal leukoencephalopathy (280). Uncontrolled studies in patients with congenital cytomegalovirus (CMV) infection or the CMV mononucleosis syndrome found transient suppression of virus excretion in the urine during vidarabine therapy (281). A randomized study of bone marrow transplant recipients found that intermittent administration of low vidarabine doses (5 mg/kg/day) did not reduce the frequency of interstitial pneumonia or CMV isolations (282). Administration of higher doses (10 mg/kg/day) to renal transplant patients with CMV-associated illness was associated not only with lack of therapeutic effect compared to placebo, but also with neurologic toxicity in 29 percent of recipients (270). Uncontrolled trials of high-dose vidarabine (20 mg/kg/day) suggested possible efficacy in CMV retinitis of immunocompromised hosts (283).

Vidarabine Monophosphate (adenine arabinoside 5′-monophosphate, ara-AMP, Vira-MP)

The phosphorylated ester of vidarabine, ara-AMP, is much more water soluble than the parent drug and can be administered intravenously or intramuscularly. The antiviral activity and the pharmacokinetics, metabolism, and toxicities of ara-AMP in humans are similar to those of vidarabine (245,284,285). Ara-AMP is quickly converted to vidarabine and further metabolized to ara-Hx, the major metabolite of ara-AMP in plasma and urine (285,286). Peak plasma levels of ara-Hx occur at 0.5 hours after intravenous and at 3 hours after intramuscular injection, and plasma $T_{1/2}$ averages 3.5–4 hours (range 1.8–6.2 hours) in adults. After intravenous or intramuscular injection of 25 mg/kg/day in four divided doses, peak plasma concentrations of ara-Hx average 6.7–8.9 μg/ml and those of vidarabine 1.3 μg/ml (285). CSF concentrations of ara-Hx are comparable to those obtained with vidarabine. Nearly 45 percent of the administered drug is recovered as ara-Hx and approximately 4–5 percent as vidarabine in the urine. Higher plasma ara-Hx concentrations are observed in patients with renal insufficiency (creatinine clearance $\leq$50 ml/minute/1.73 M^2) and may be associated with CNS side effects. Intramuscular injections may be associated with mild to moderate local pain and elevations in transaminases and creatine phosphokinase levels (286). Increased bone marrow toxicity and severe pain syndromes, typically involving lower extremity muscles and sometimes lasting more than 3 months after therapy, have been described in hepatitis B virus infected patients treated with doses of 7.5 mg/kg/day or higher (286).

Double-blind, placebo-controlled trials of topical ara-AMP (10 percent gel applied 5 times/day) found that it was ineffective in recurrent HSV genital (34) or labial (35) infections. Because it offers a possibility of ambulatory therapy, intramuscular ara-AMP is currently being studied for treatment of herpes zoster in older adults or immunocompromised hosts, hepatitis B virus, and genital HSV infections. Preliminary studies in chronic hepatitis B virus infection have found that ara-AMP treatment, alternating with courses of interferon, is associated with decreases in DNA polymerase activity (287).

Other Antiviral Agents

Other agents of investigational interest are presented in Table 6.

REFERENCES

1. Myers MG, Oxman MN, Clark JE, et al: Failure of neutral-red photodynamic inactivation in recurrent herpes simplex virus infections. *N Engl J Med* 293:945, 1975.
2. Corey L, Reeves WC, Chiang WT, et al: Ineffectiveness of topical ether for the treatment of genital herpes simplex virus infection. *N Engl J Med* 299:237, 1978.
3. Vontver LA, Reeves WC, Rattray M, et al: Clinical course and diagnosis of genital herpes simplex virus infection and evaluation of topical surfactant therapy. *Am J Obstet Gynecol* 133:548, 1979.
4. Guinan ME, MacCalman J, Kern ER, et al: Topical ether and herpes simplex labialis. *JAMA* 243:1059, 1980.
5. Herrmann EC Jr, Herrmann JA: A working hypothesis virus resistance development as an indicator of specific antiviral activity. *Ann NY Acad Sci* 284:632, 1977.
6. Coleman VR, Tsu E, Jawetz E: "Treatment-resistance" to idoxuridine in herpetic keratitis. *Proc Soc Exp Biol Med* 129:761, 1968.
7. Hirano A, Yumura K, Kurimura T, et al: Analysis of herpes simplex virus isolated from patients with recurrent herpes keratitis exhibiting "treatment-resistance" to 5-iodo-2′-deoxyuridine. *Acta Virol* 23:226, 1979.
8. Crumpacker CS, Schnipper LE, Marlowe SI, et al: Resistance to antiviral drugs of herpes simplex virus isolated from patients treated with acyclovir. *N Engl J Med* 306:343, 1982.
9. Burns WH, Saral R, Santos GW, et al: Isolation and characterization of resistant herpes simplex virus after acyclovir therapy. *Lancet* 1:421, 1982.
10. Sibrack CD, Gutman LT, Wilfert CM, et al: Pathogenicity of acyclovir-resistant herpes simplex virus type 1 from an immunodeficient child. *J Infect Dis* 146:673, 1982.

10a. Wade JC, McLaren C, Myers JD: Frequency and significance of acyclovir-resistant herpes simplex virus isolated from marrow transplant patients receiving multiple courses of treatment with acyclovir. *J Infect Dis* 148:1077, 1983.

11. Parris DS, Harrington JE: Herpes simplex virus variants resistant to high concentrations of acyclovir exist in clinical isolates. *Antimicrob Agents Chemother* 22:71, 1982.

11a. Smith KO, Kennell WL, Poirier RH, et al: In vitro and in vivo resistance of herpes simplex virus to 9-(2-hydroxy-ethoxymethyl) guanine (Acycloguanosine). *Antimicrob Agents Chemother* 17:144, 1980.

12. Eggers HJ: Successful treatment of enterovirus-infected mice by 2-(a-hydroxybenzyl)-benzimidazole and guanidine. *J Exp Med* 143:1367, 1976.
13. Wilson SZ, Knight V, Wyde PR, et al: Amantadine and ribavirin aerosol treatment of influenza A and B infection in mice. *Antimicrob Agents Chemother* 17:642, 1980.
14. Hayden FG, Douglas RG Jr, Simons R: Enhancement of activity against influenza viruses by combinations of antiviral agents. *Antimicrob Agents Chemother* 18:536, 1980.
15. Lerner AM, Bailey EJ: Synergy of 9-b-D-arabinofuranosyladenine and human interferon against herpes simplex virus, type 1. *J Infect Dis* 130:549, 1974.
16. Stanwick TL, Schinazi RF, Campbell DE, et al: Combined antiviral effect of interferon

and acyclovir on herpes simplex virus types 1 and 2. *Antimicrob Agents Chemother* 19:672, 1981.

17. Schinazi RF, Peters J, Williams CC, et al: Effect of combinations of acyclovir with vidarabine or its 5′-monophosphate on herpes simplex viruses in cell culture and in mice. *Antimicrob Agents Chemother* 22:499, 1982.
18. Scullard GH, Pollard RB, Smith JL, et al: Antiviral treatment of chronic hepatitis B virus infection. I. Changes in viral markers with interferon combined with adenine arabinoside. *J Infect Dis* 143:772, 1981.
19. Scullard GH, Andres LL, Greenberg HB, et al: Antiviral treatment of chronic hepatitis B virus infection: Improvement in liver disease with interferon and adenine arabinoside. *Hepatology* 1:228, 1981.
20. Sacks SL, Scullard GH, Pollard RB, et al: Antiviral treatment of chronic hepatitis B virus infection: pharmacokinetics and side effects of interferon and adenine arabinoside alone and in combination. *Antimicrob Agents Chemother* 21:93, 1982.
21. Smith CI, Kitchen LW, Scullard GH, et al: Vidarabine monophosphate and human leukocyte interferon in chronic hepatitis B infection. *JAMA* 247:2261, 1982.
22. Stevens DA, Jordan GW, Waddell TF, et al: Adverse effect of cytosine arabinoside on disseminated zoster in a controlled trial. *N Engl J Med* 289:873, 1973.
23. Spruance SL, Schnipper LE, Overall JC, Jr., et al: Treatment of herpes simplex labialis with topical acyclovir in polyethylene glycol. *J Infect Dis* 146:85, 1982.
24. Mease PJ, Ochs HD, Wedgwood RJ: Successful treatment of echovirus meningoencephalitis and myositisfasciitis with intravenous immune globulin therapy in a patient with X-linked agammaglobulinemia. *N Engl J Med* 304:1278, 1981.
25. Merigan TC, Rand KH, Pollard RB, et al: Human leukocyte interferon for the treatment of herpes zoster in patients with cancer. *N Engl J Med* 298:981, 1978.
26. Steele RW, Myers MG, Vincent MM, et al: Transfer factor for the prevention of varicella-zoster infection in childhood leukemia. *N Engl J Med* 303:355, 1980.
27. Werner GH: Immunopotentiating substances with antiviral activity. *Pharmacol Ther* 6:235–273, 1979.

27a. Hayden FG, Laskin OL, Douglas RG, Jr.: Antiviral agents in Lourian V (ed) *Antibiotics in Laboratory Medicine* 2nd Ed. Williams and Wilkins, Baltimore, Md. (in press).

28. De Clercq E, Descamps J, Verhelst G, et al: Comparative efficacy of antiherpes drugs against different strains of herpes simplex virus. *J Infect Dis* 141:563, 1980.
29. Whitley RJ, Ch'ien LT, Dolin R, et al: Adenine arabinoside therapy of herpes zoster in the immunosuppressed. *N Engl J Med* 294:1193, 1976.
30. Whitley RJ, Soong S-J, Dolin R, et al: Early vidarabine therapy to control the complications of herpes zoster in immunosuppressed patients. *N Engl J Med* 307:971, 1982.
31. Glasgow LA: Advantages and limitations of animal models in the evaluation of antiviral substances. *J Infect Dis* 133:A73, 1976.
32. Adams HG, Benson EA, Alexander ER, et al: Genital herpetic infection in men and women: Clinical course and effect of topical application of adenine arabinoside. *J Infect Dis* 133:A151, 1976.
33. Hilton AL, Bushell TEC, Waller D, et al: A trial of adenine arabinoside in genital herpes. *Br J Vener Dis* 54:50, 1978.
34. Spruance SL, Crumpacker CS, Haines H, et al: Ineffectiveness of topical adenine arabinoside 5′-monophosphate in the treatment of recurrent herpes simplex labialis. *N Engl J Med* 300:1180, 1979.
35. Hatcher VA, Friedman-Kien AE, Marcus EL, et al: Arabinosyladenine monophosphate in genital herpes: A double-blind, placebo-controlled study. *Antiviral Res* 2:283, 1982.
36. Hayden FG, Hall WJ, Douglas RG, Jr.: Therapeutic effects of aerosolized amantadine in naturally acquired infection due to influenza A virus. *J Infect Dis* 141:535, 1980.
37. Knight V, Wilson SZ, Quarles JM, et al: Ribavirin small-particle aerosol treatment of influenza. *Lancet* 2:945, 1981.

38. McClung HW, Knight V, Gilbert BE, et al: Ribavirin aerosol treatment of influenza B virus infection. *JAMA* 249:2671, 1983.
39. Hall CB, Walsh EE, Hruska JF, et al: Ribavirin treatment of experimental respiratory syncytial viral infection. *JAMA* 249:2666, 1983.
40. Schaeffer HJ, Beauchamp L, de Miranda P, et al: 9-(2-Hydroxyethoxymethyl) guanine activity against viruses of the herpes group. *Nature* 272:583, 1978.
41. Biron KK, Elion GB: In vitro susceptibility of varicellazoster virus to acyclovir. *Antimicrob Agents Chemother* 18:443, 1980.
42. Crumpacker CS, Schnipper LE, Zaia JA, et al: Growth inhibition by acycloguanosine of herpesviruses isolated from human infections. *Antimicrob Agents Chemother* 15:642, 1979.
43. Colby BM, Shaw JE, Elion GB, et al: Effect of acyclovir [9-(2-hydroxyethoxymethyl)guanine] on Epstein-barr virus DNA replication. *J Virol* 34:560, 1980.
44. Lin J-C, Smith MC, Cheng YC, Pagano JS: Epstein-Barr virus: Inhibition of replication by three new drugs. *Science* 221:578, 1983.
45. Lang DJ, Cheung K-S: Effectiveness of acycloguanosine and trifluorothymidine as inhibitors of cytomegalovirus infection in vitro. *Am J Med* 73(suppl):49, 1982.
46. Kern ER: Acyclovir treatment of experimental genital herpes simplex virus infections. *Am J Med* 73(suppl):100, 1982.
47. Collins P, Oliver NM: Acyclovir treatment of cutaneous herpes in guinea pigs and herpes encephalitis in mice. *Am J Med* 73(suppl):96, 1982.
48. Kern ER, Richards JT, Glasgow LA, et al: Optimal treatment of herpes simplex virus encephalitis in mice with oral acyclovir.
49. Field HJ, Bell SE, Elion GB, et al: Effect of acycloguanosine treatment on acute and latent herpes simplex infections in mice. *Antimicrob Agents Chemother* 15:554, 1979.
50. Klein RJ, Friedman-Kein AE, DeStefano E: Latent herpes simplex virus infections in sensory ganglia of hairless mice prevented by acycloguanosine. *Science* 221:723, 1979.
51. Elion GB: Mechanism of action and selectivity of acyclovir. *Am J Med* 73(suppl):7, 1982.
52. Derse D, Cheng Y-C, Furman PA, et al: Inhibition of purified human and herpes simplex virus-induced DNA polymerases by 9-(2-hydroxyethoxymethyl)granine triphosphate. *J Biol Chem* 256:11,447, 1981.
53. McGuirt PV, Furman PA: Acyclovir inhibition of viral DNA chain elongation in herpes simples virus-infected cells. *Am J Med* 73(suppl):67, 1982.
54. Pagano JS, Datta AK: Perspectives on interactions of acyclovir with Epstein-Barr and other herpes viruses. *Am J Med* 73(suppl):18, 1982.
55. Schnipper LE, Crumpacker CS: Resistance of herpes simplex virus to acycloguanosine: Role of viral thymidine kinase and DNA polymerase loci. *Proc Natl Acad Sci* 77:2270, 1980.
56. Coen D, Schaffer PA: Two distinct loci confer resistance to acycloguanosine in herpes simplex virus type 1. *Proc Natl Acad Sci* 77:2265, 1980.
57. Field HJ, Darby G: Pathogenicity in mice of strains of herpes simplex virus which are resistant to acyclovir in vitro and in vivo. *Antimicrob Agents Chemother* 17:209, 1980.
58. Field HJ: Development of clinical resistance to acyclovir in herpes simplex virus-infected mice receiving oral therapy. *Animicrob Agents Chemother* 21:744, 1982.
59. Darby G, Field HJ: Altered substrate specificity of herpes simplex virus thymidine kinase confers acyclovir-resistance. *Nature* 289:81, 1981.
60. Corey L, Holmes KK: Genital herpes simplex virus infections: Current concepts in diagnosis, therapy, and prevention. *Ann Intern Med* 98:973, 1983.
61. Blum RM, Liao SHT, de Miranda P: Overview of acyclovir pharmacokinetic disposition in adults and children. *Am J Med* 73(suppl):186, 1982.
62. Hintz M, Connor JD, Spector SA, et al: Neonatal acyclovir pharmacokinentics in patients with herpes virus infections. *Am J Med* 73(suppl):210, 1982.
63. Laskin OL, Longstreth, Whelton A, et al: Effect of renal failure on the pharmacokinetics of acyclovir. *Am J Med* 73(suppl):197, 1982.
64. Laskin OL: Clinical pharmacokinetics of acyclovir. *Clin Pharmacokinetics* 8:187, 1983.

65. Van Dyke RB, Connor JD, Wyborny C, et al: Pharmacokinetics of orally administered acyclovir in patients with herpes progenitalis. *Am J Med* 73(suppl):172, 1982.

66. De Miranda P, Good SS, Laskin OL, et al: Disposition of intravenous radioactive acyclovir. *Clin Pharmacol Ther* 30:662, 1981.

67. De Miranda P, Good SS, Krasny HC, et al: Metabolic fate of radioactive acyclovir in humans. *Am J Med* 73(suppl):215, 1982.

68. Krasny HC, Liao SHT, de Miranda P, et al: Influence of hemodialysis on acyclovir pharmacokinetics in patients with chronic renal failure. *Am J Med* 73(suppl):202, 1982.

69. Keeney RE, Kirk LE, Bridgen D: Acyclovir tolerance in humans. *Am J Med* 73(suppl):176, 1982.

70. Wade JC, Hintz M, McGuffin RW, et al: Treatment of cytomegalovirus pneumonia with high-dose acyclovir. *Am J Med* 73(suppl):249, 1982.

71. Wade JC, Meyers JD: Neurologic symptoms associated with parenteral acyclovir treatment after marrow transplantation. *Ann Intern Med* 98:921, 1983.

72. Bean B, Braun C, Balfour HH Jr: Acyclovir therapy for acute herpes zoster. *Lancet* 2:118, 1982.

73. Balfour HH, Jr, Bean B, Laskin OL, et al: Acyclovir halts progression of herpes zoster in immunocompromised patients. *N Engl J Med* 308:1448, 1983.

74. Steele RW, Marmer DJ, Keeney RE: Comparative in vitro immunotoxicology of acyclovir and other antiviral agents. *Infect Immun* 28:957, 1980.

75. McGuffin RW, Shiota FM, Meyers JD: Lack of toxicity of acyclovir to granulocyte progenitor cells in vitro. *Antimicrob Agents Chemother* 10:471, 1980.

76. Levin MJ, Leary PL, Arbeit RD: Effect of acyclovir on the proliferation of human fibroblasts and peripheral blood mononuclear cells. *Antimicrob Agents Chemother* 17:947, 1980.

77. Wingard JR, Hess AD, Stuart RK, et al: Effect of several antiviral agents on human lymphocyte functions and marrow progenitor cell proliferation. *Antimicrob Agents Chemother* 23:593, 1983.

78. Quinn RP, Wolberg G, Medzihradsky J, et al: Effect of acyclovir on various murine in vivo and in vitro immunologic assay systems. *Am J Med* 73(suppl):62, 1982.

79. Corey L, Fife KH, Benedetti JK, et al: Intravenous acyclovir for the treatment of primary genital herpes. *Ann Intern Med* 98:914, 1983.

80. Bryson YJ, Dillon M, Lovett M, et al: Treatment of first episodes of genital herpes simplex virus infection with oral acyclovir. *N Engl J Med* 308:916, 1983.

81. Corey L, Nahmias AJ, Guinan ME, et al: A trial of topical acyclovir in genital herpes simplex virus infections. *N Engl J Med* 306:1313, 1982.

82. Mindel A, Adler MW: Intravenous acyclovir treatment for primary genital herpes. *Lancet* 1:697, 1982.

83. Nilsen AE, Aasen T: Efficacy of oral acyclovir in the treatment of initial and recurrent genital herpes. *Lancet* 2:571, 1982.

84. Reichman RC, Badger GJ, Guinan ME, et al: Topically administered acyclovir in the treatment of recurrent herpes simplex genitalis: A controlled trial. *J Infect Dis* 147:336, 1983.

85. Reichman RC, Badger GJ, Mertz GJ, et al: Treatment of recurrent genital herpes simplex infections with oral acyclovir. *J Am Med Asso* 251:2103, 1984.

85a. Straus S, Seidlin M, Takiff H, et al: Suppression of recurrent genital herpes with oral acyclovir. *Clin Res* 31:543A, 1983.

86. Straus S, Seidlin M, Takiff H, et al: Oral acyclovir to suppress recurrent herpes simplex virus infections in immunodeficient patients. *Ann Intern Med* 100:522, 1984.

86a. Fiddian AP, Yeo JM, Kinghorn GR, et al: Successful treatment of recurrent herpes simplex infections with topical acyclovir. Proceedings of the Thirteenth International Congress of Chemotherapy, 1983. No. 4.7, p 2.

86b. Kinghorn GR, Turner EB, Barton IG, et al: Efficacy of topical acyclovir cream in first and recurrent episodes of genital herpes. *Antiviral Res* 3:291, 1983.

87. Saral R, Burns WH, Laskin OL, et al: Acyclovir prophylaxis of herpes-simplex-virus infections. *N Engl J Med* 305:63, 1981.

87aa. Saral R, Ambinder RF, Burns WH, et al: Acyclovir prophylaxis against herpes simplex virus infection in patients with leukemia. *Ann Intern Med* 99:773, 1983.

87a. Gluckman E, Devergie A, Melo R, et al: Prophylaxis of herpes infections after bone marrow transplantation by oral acyclovir. *Lancet* 2:706, 1983.

87b. Wade JC, Newton B, McLaren C, et al: Intravenous acyclovir to treat mucocutaneous herpes simplex infection after marrow transplantation. *Ann Intern Med* 96:265, 1982.

88. Whitley R, Barton N, Collins E, et al: Mucocutaneous herpes simplex virus infections in immunocompromised patients. *Am J Med* 73(suppl):236, 1982.

88a. Whitley RJ, Barton NH, Levin M, et al: Topical acyclovir, ACV, therapy of mucocutaneous herpes simplex virus, HSV, infections in the immunocompromised host. Program and abstracts of the Twenty-third Interscience Conference on Antimicrobial Agents and Chemotherapy, 1983. No. 563.

89. Peterslund NA, Ipsen J, Schonheyder H, et al: Acyclovir in herpes zoster. *Lancet* 2:827, 1981.

90. McGill J, MacDonald DR, Fall C, et al: Intravenous acyclovir in acute herpes zoster infection. *J Infect* 6:157, 1983.

91. McGill JI: The use of acycloguanosine in herpes zoster ocular infection. *Br J Ophthalmol* 65:524, 1981.

92. Prober CG, Kirk LE, Keeney RE: Acyclovir therapy of chickenpox in immunosuppressed children: A collaborative study. *J Pediatr* 101:622, 1982.

93. Balfour HH Jr, Bean B, Mitchell CD, et al: Acyclovir in immunocompromised patients with cytomegalovirus disease. Proceedings of a Symposium of Acyclovir sponsored by Burroughs Wellcome Co and The NIAID. July 20, 1983. *Am J Med* p 241.

94. Plotkin SA, Starr SE, Bryan CK: In vitro and in vivo responses of cytomegalovirus to acyclovir. *Am J Med* 73(suppl):257, 1982.

95. Hanto DW, Frizzera G, Gajl-Peczalska KJ, et al: Epstein-Barr virus-induced B-cell lymphoma after renal transplantation. *N Engl J Med* 306:913, 1982.

96. Sullivan JL, Bryon KS, Brewster FE, et al: Treatment of life-threatening Epstein-Barr virus infections with acyclovir. *Am J Med* 73(suppl):262, 1982.

97. Hayden FG, Cote KM, Douglas RG Jr: Plaque inhibition assay for drug susceptibility testing of influenza viruses. *Antimicrob Agents Chemother* 17:865, 1980.

98. Browne MJ, Moss MY, Boyd MR: Comparative activity of amantadine and ribavirin against influenza virus in vitro: Possible clinical relevance. *Antimicrob Agents Chemother* 23:503, 1983.

99. Koff WC, Elm JL Jr, Halstead SB: Inhibition of dengue virus replication by amantadine hydrochloride. *Antimicrob Agents Chemother* 18:125, 1980.

100. Walker JS, Stephen EL, Spertzel RO: Small-particle aerosols of antiviral compounds in treatment of type A influenza pneumonia in mice. *J Infect Dis* 133:A140, 1976.

101. Fenton RJ, Bessell C, Spilling CR, et al: The effects of peroral or local aerosol administration of 1-aminoadamantane hydrochloride (amantadine hydrochloride) on influenza infections of the ferret. *J Antimicrob Chemother* 3:463, 1977.

102. Dourmashkin RR, Tyrrell DA: Electron microscopic observations on the entry of influenza virus into susceptible cells. *J Gen Virol* 24:129, 1974.

103. Oxford JS, Galbraith A: Antiviral activity of amantadine: A review of laboratory and clinical data. *Pharmacol Ther* 11:181, 1980.

104. Kato N, Eggers HJ: Inhibition of uncoating of fowl plague virus by 1-adamantanamine hydrochloride. *Virology* 37:632, 1969.

105. Skehel JJ, Hay AJ, Armstrong JA: On the mechanism of inhibition of influenza virus replication by amantadine hydrochloride. *J Gen Virol* 38:97, 1977.

106. Richman DD, Yazaki P, Hostetler KY: The intracellular distribution and antiviral activity of amantadine. *Virology* 112:81, 1981.

107. Appleyard G: Amantadine-resistance as a genetic marker for influenza viruses. *J Gen Virol* 36:249, 1977.

108. Lubeck MD, Schulman JL, Palese P: Susceptibility of influenza A viruses to amantadine is influenced by the gene coding for M protein. *J Virol* 28:710, 1978.
109. Scholtissek C, Faulkner GP: Amantadine-resistant and -sensitive influenza A strains and recombinants. *J Gen Virol* 44:807, 1979.
109a. Heider H, Adamczyk B, Presber HW, et al: Occurrence of amantadine and rimantadine resistant influenza A virus strains during the 1980 epidemic. *Acta Virol* 25:395, 1981.
110. Bleidner WE, Harmon JB, Hewes WE, et al: Absorption, distribution and excretion of amantadine hydrochloride. *J Pharmocol Exp Ther* 150:484, 1965.
111. Hayden FG, Hoffman HE, Spyker DA: Differences in side effects of amantadine hydrochloride and rimantadine hydrochloride relate to differences in pharmocokinetics. *Antimicrob Agents Chemother* 23:458, 1983.
112. Biandrate P, Tognoni G, Belvedere G, et al: A gas chromatographic method for the determination of amantadine in human plasma. *J Chromatogr* 74:31, 1972.
113. Aoki FY, Sitar DS, Ogilvie RI: Amantadine kinetics in healthy young subjects after long-term dosing. *Clin Pharmacol Ther* 26:729, 1979.
114. Pacifici GM, Nardini M, Ferrari P, et al: Effect of amantadine on drug-induced parkisonism: Relationship between plasma levels and effect. *Br J Clin Pharmacol* 3:883, 1976.
114a. Wright PF, Khaw KT, Oxman MN, Schwachman H: Evaluation of the safety of amantadine HCl and the role of respiratory viral infections in children with cystic fibrosis. *J Infect Dis* 134:144, 1976.
115. Smith CB, Purcell RH, Chanock RM: Effect of amantadine hydrochloride on parainfluenza type 1 virus infections in adult volunteers. *Am Rev Respir Dis* 95:689, 1967.
115a. Fishaut M, Mostow S: Amantadine for severe influenza A pneumonia in infancy. *Am J Dis Child* 134:321, 1980.
116. Knight V, Bloom K, Wilson SZ, et al: Amantadine aerosol in humans. *Antimicrob Agents Chemother* 16:572, 1979.
117. Horadam VW, Sharp JG, Smilack JD, et al: Pharmacokinetics of amantadine hydrochloride in subjects with normal and impaired renal function. *Ann Intern Med* 94:454, 1981.
118. Montanari C, Ferrari P, Bavazzano A: Urinary excretion of amantadine by the elderly. *Eur J Clin Pharmacol* 8:349, 1975.
119. Ing TS, Daugirdas JT, Soung LS, et al: Toxic effects of amantadine in patients with renal failure. *CMA J* 120:1695, 1979.
120. Soung L-S, Ing TS, Daugirdas JT, et al: Amantadine hydrochloride pharmacokinetics in hemodialysis patients. *Ann Intern Med* 93:46, 1980.
121. Schwab RS, Poskanzer DC, England AC, et al: Amantadine in Parkinson's disease. *JAMA* 222:792, 1972.
122. Parkes JD, Marsden P, Zilkha KJ, et al: Amantadine dosage in treatment of Parkinson's disease. *Lancet* 1:1130, 1970.
123. Parkes JD, Marsden P, Price P: Amantadine-induced heart-failure. *Lancet* 1:904, 1977.
124. Pearlman JT, Kadish AH, Ramseyer JC: Vision loss associated with amantadine hydrochloride use. *JAMA* 237:1200, 1977.
125. Hayden FG, Gwaltney JM Jr, Van de Castle RL, et al: Comparative toxicity of amantadine hydrochloride and rimantadine hydrochloride in healthy adults. *Antimicrob Agents Chemother* 19:226, 1981.
126. Millet VM, Dreisbach M, Bryson YJ: Double-blind controlled study of central nervous system side effects of amantadine, rimantadine, and chlorpheniramine. *Antimicrob Agents Chemother* 21:1, 1982.
127. Kantor RJ, Stevens D, Potts DW, et al: Prevention of influenza A/USSR/77 (H1N1): An evaluation of the side effects and efficacy of amantadine in recruits at Fort Sam Houston. *Milit Med* May 1980, p 312,
128. Harper RW, Knothe BUC: Coloured lilliputian hallucinations with amantadine. *Med J Aust* 1:444, 1973.
129. Monto AS, Gunn RA, Bandyk MG, et al: Prevention of Russian influenza by amantadine. *JAMA* 241:1003, 1979.

130. Dolin R, Reichman RC, Madore HP, et al: A controlled trial of amantadine and rimantadine in the prophylaxis of influenza A infection. *N Engl J Med* 307:580, 1982.
131. Pettersson RF, Hellström P-E, Penttinen K, et al: Evaluation of amantadine in the prophylaxis of influenza A (H1N1) virus infection: A controlled field trial among young adults and high-risk patients. *J Infect Dis* 142:377, 1980.
132. Casey DE: Amantadine intoxication reversed by physostigmine. *N Engl J Med* 298:516, 1978.
133. Rawls WE, Melnick JL, Olson GB, et al: Effect of amantadine hydrochloride on the response of human lymphocytes to phytohemagglutinin. *Science* 158:506, 1967.
134. Mardiney MR Jr, Bredt AB: The immunosuppressive effect of amantadine upon the response of lymphocytes to specific antigens in vitro. *Transplantation* 12:183, 1971.
135. Dickinson PCT, Chang T-W, Weinstein L: Effects of amantadine on influenza B and measles virus infection in children. *Antimicrob Agents Chemother* 521, 1966.
136. Smorodintsev AA, Zlydnikov DM, Kiseleva AM, et al: Evaluation of amantadine in artificially induced A2 and B influenza. *JAMA* 213:1448, 1970.
137. Oker-Blom N, Hovi T, Leinikki P, et al: Protection of man from natural infection with influenza A2 Hong Kong virus by amantadine: A controlled field trial. *Br Med J* 3:676, 1970.
138. O'Donoghue JM, Ray CG, Terry DW Jr, et al: Prevention of nosocomial influenza infection with amantadine. *Am J Epidemiol* 97:276, 1973.
139. Galbraith AW, Oxford JS, Schild GC, et al: Protective effect of 1-adamantanamine hydrochloride on influenza A2 infections in the family environment. *Lancet* 2:1026, 1969.
139a. Payler DK, Purdham PA: Influenza A prophylaxis with amantadine in a boarding school. *Lancet* 1:502, 1984.
140. Muldoon RL, Stanley ED, Jackson GG: Use and withdrawal of amantadine chemoprophylaxis during epidemic influenz A. *Am Rev Respir Dis* 113:487, 1976.
141. Knight V, Fedson D, Baldini J, et al: Amantadine therapy of epidemic influenza A2 (Hong Kong). *Infect Immun* 1:200, 1970.
142. Wingfield WL, Pollack D, Grunert RR: Therapeutic efficacy of amantadine HC1 and rimantadine HC1 in naturally occurring influenza A2 respiratory illness in man. *N Engl J Med* 281:579, 1969.
143. Togo Y, Hornick RB, Felitti VJ, et al: Evaluation of therapeutic efficacy of amantadine in patients with naturally occurring A2 influenza. *JAMA* 211:1149, 1970.
144. Galbraith AW, Oxford JS, Schild GC, et al: Therapeutic effect of 1-adamantanamine hydrochloride in naturally occurring influenza A2/Hong Kong infection. *Lancet* 2:113, 1971.
145. Van Voris LP, Betts RF, Hayden FG, et al: Successful treatment of naturally occurring influenza A/USSR/77 H1N1. *JAMA* 245:1128, 1981.
146. Little JW, Hall WJ, Douglas RG Jr, et al: Amantadine effect on peripheral airways abnormalities in influenza. *Ann Intern Med* 85:177, 1976.
147. Little JW, Hall WJ, Douglas RG Jr, et al: Airway hyperreactivity and peripheral airway dysfunction in influenza A infection. *Am Rev Respir Dis* 118:295, 1978.
148. Younkin SW, Betts RF, Roth FK, et al: Reduction in fever and symptoms in young adults with influenza A/Brazil/78 H1N1 infection after treatment with aspirin or amantadine. *Antimicrob Agents Chemother* 23:577, 1983.
149. DeClercq E, Descamps J, DeSomer P, et al: (E)-5-(2-bromovinyl)-2′-deoxyuridine: A potent and selective anti-herpes agent. *Proc Natl Acad Sci* 76:2947, 1979.
150. DeClercq E, Descamps J, Verhelst G, et al: Comparative efficacy of antiherpes drugs against different strains of herpes simplex virus. *J Infect Dis* 141:563, 1980.
151. DeClercq E, Descamps J, Ogata M, et al: In vitro susceptibility of varicella-zoster virus to E-5-(2-bromovinly)-2′-deoxyuridine and related compounds. *Antimicrob Agents Chemother* 21:33, 1982.
152. Mayo DR: Differentiationof herpes simplex virus types 1 and 2 by sensitivity to (E)-5-(2-bromovinyl)-2′-deoxyuridine. *J Clin Microbiol* 15:733–736, 1982.
153. Park N-H, Pavan-Langston D, Boisjoly HM, et al: Chemotherapeutic efficacy of E-5:(2-

bromovinyl)-2′-deoxyuridine for orofacial infection with herpes simplex virus type 1 in mice. *J Infect Dis* 145:909, 1982.

154. DeClercq E, Zhang Z-X: Differential effects of E-5-(2-bromovinyl)-2′-deoxyuridine on infections with herpes simplex virus type 1 and type 2 in hairless mice. *J Infect Dis* 145:130, 1982.
155. Field HJ, DeClercq E: Effects of oral treatment with acyclovir and bromovinyldeoxyuridine on the establishment and maintenance of latent herpes simplex virus infection in mice. *J Gen Virol* 56:259, 1981.
156. Soike KF, Gibson S, Gerone PJ: Inhibition of simian varicella virus infection of African green monkeys by (E)-5-(2-bromovinyl)-2′-deoxyuridine (BVDU). *Antiviral Res* 1:325, 1981.
157. Cheng Y-C, Dutschman G, DeClercq E, et al: Differential affinities of 5-(2-halogenovinyl)-2′-deoxyuridines for deoxythymidine kinases of various origins. *Mol Pharmacol* 20:230, 1981.
158. Allaudeen HS, Kozarich JW, Bertino JR, et al: On the mechanism of selective inhibition of herpesvirus replication by (E)-5-(2-bromovinly)-2′-deoxyuridine. *Proc Natl Acad Sci* 78:2698, 1981.
159. Larsson A, Oberg B: Selective inhibition of herpesvirus deoxyribonucleic acid synthesis by acycloguanosine, 2′-fluoro-5-iodo-aracytosine, and (E)-5-(2-bromovinyl)-2′-deoxyuridine. *Antimicrob Agents Chemother* 19:927, 1981.

159a. Whitley RJ, Barton NH, Welchel J, Diethelm AG, et al: Plasma pharmacokinetics of bromovinyl deoxyuridine (BVDU) after oral adminstration to humans. Program and Abstracts of the Twenty-third Interscience Conference on Antimicrobial Agents and Chemotherapy, 1983, No. 145.

160. DeClercq E, Degreef H, Wildiers J, et al: Oral (E)-5-(2-bromovinyl)-2′-deoxyuridine in severe herpes zoster. *Br J Med* 281:1178, 1980.
162. Prusoff WH, Goz B: Halogenated pyrimidine deoxyribonucleosides, in Sartorelli AC, Johns DG (eds): *Handbook. Experimental Pharmocology.* New York, Springer-Verlag, 1975, Vol 3812, p 272.
163. Lerner AM, Bailey EJ: Concentrations of idoxuridine in serum, urine, and cerebrospinal fluid of patients with suspected diagnoses of Herpesvirus hominis encephalitis. *J Clin Invest* 51:45, 1972.
164. Wildenhoff KE, Ipsen J, Esmann V, et al: Treatment of herpes zoster with idoxuridine ointment, including a multivariate analysis of symptoms and signs. *Scand J Infect Dis* 11:1, 1979.
165. Boston Interhospital Virus Study Group and The NIAID-Sponsored Cooperative Antiviral Clinical Study: Failure of high dose 5-iodo-2′-deoxyuridine in the therapy of herpes simplex virus encephalitis. *N Engl J Med* 292:599, 1975.
166. McCallum DI, Johnston ENM, Raju BH: 5-iodo-2′-deoxyuridine in the treatment of herpes zoster. *Br J Dermatol* 76:459, 1964.
167. Kibrick S, Katz AS: Topical idoxuridine in recurrent herpes simplex, with a note on its effect on early varicella. *Ann NY Acad Sci* 173:83, 1970.
168. Juel-Jensen BE, MacCallum FO, Mackenzie AMR, et al: Treatment of zoster with idoxuridine in dimethyl sulphoxide. *Br Med J* 4:776, 1970.
169. Dawber R: Idoxuridine in herpes zoster: Further evaluation of intermittent topical therapy. *Br Med J* 2:526, 1974.
170. Silvestri DL, Corey L, Holmes KK: Ineffectiveness of topical idoxuridine in dimethyl sulfoxide for therapy of genital herpes. *JAMA* 248:953, 1982.
171. Jacob SW, Rosenbaum EE: The toxicology of dimethyl sulfoxide (DMSO). *Headache* October 1966, p 127.
172. Laibson PR, Leopoid IH: An evaluation of double-blind IDU therapy in 100 cases of herpetic keratitis. *Trans Am Acad Ophthalmol* 68:22, 1964.
173. Gold JA, Stewart RC, McKee J: The epidemiology and chemotherapy of herpes simplex keratitis and herpes simplex skin infections. *Ann NY Acad Sci* 130:209, 1965.
174. Woodson B, Joklik WK: The inhibition of vaccinia virus multiplication by isatin-b-thiosemicarbazone. *Proc Natl Acad Sci* 54:946, 1965.

175. Kucers A, Bennett NM: Methisazone, in Kucers A, Bennett NM (eds): *The Use of Antibiotics.* London, William Heinemann Medical Books LTD, 1979, p 965.

176. Bauer DJ, St. Vincent L, Kempe CH, et al: Prophylactic treatment of smallpox contacts with N-methylisatin b-thiosemicarbazone (compound 33T57, marboran). *Lancet* 2:494, 1963.

177. de Valle LAR, de Melo PR, de Salles Gomes LF, et al: Methisazone in prevention of variola minor among contacts. *Lancet* 2:976, 1965.

178. Heiner GG, Fatima N, Russell PK, et al: Field trials of methisazone as a prophylactic agent against smallpox. *Am J Epidemiol* 94:435, 1971.

179. Brainerd HD, Hanna L, Jawetz E: Methisazone in progressive vaccinia. *N Engl J Med* 276:620, 1967.

180. Jaroszynska-Weinberger B: Treatment with methisazone of complications following smallpox vaccination. *Arch Dis Child* 45:573, 1970.

181. Landsman JB, Grist NR: Controlled trial of marboran on group vaccinated against smallpox. *Lancet* 1:330, 1964.

182. Helgstrand E, Eriksson B, Johansson NG, et al: Trisodium phosphonoformate, a new antiviral compound. *Science* 201:819, 1978.

183. Reno JM, Lee LF, Boezi JA: Inhibition of herpesvirus replication and herpesvirus-induced deoxyribonucleic acid polymerase by phosphonoformate. *Antimicrob Agents Chemother* 13:188, 1978.

184. Datta AK, Hood RE: Mechanism of inhibition of Epstein-Barr virus replication by phosphonoformic acid. *Virology* 114:52, 1981.

185. Cheng Y-C, Grill S, Derse D, et al: Mode of action of phosphonoformate as an anti-herpes simplex virus agent. *Biochem Biophys Acta* 652:90, 1981.

186. Eriksson B, Oberg B: Characteristics of herpesvirus mutants resistant to phosphonoformate and phosphonoacetate. *Antimicrob Agents Chemother* 15:758, 1979.

187. Becker Y, Asher Y, Cohen Y, et al: Phosphonoacetic acid-resistant mutants of herpes simplex virus: Effect of phosphonoacetic acid on virus replication and in vitro deoxyribonucleic acid synthesis in isolated nuclei. *Antimicrob Agents Chemother* 11:919, 1977.

188. Alenius S, Dinter Z, Oberg B: Therapeutic effect of trisodium phosphonoformate on cutaneous herpesvirus infection in guinea pigs. *Antimicrob Agents Chemother* 14:408, 1978.

189. Bopp BA, Estep CB, Anderson DJ: Disposition of disodium phosphonoacetate-^{14}C in rat, rabbit, dog, and monkey. *Fed Proc* 36:939, 1977.

190. Oberg B, Eriksson B, Helgstrand E, et al: Trisodium phosphonoformate, antiviral activities, pharmacokinetics and safety evaluation, in Nahmias AJ, Dowdle WR, Schinazi RF (eds): *The Human Herpesviruses: An Interdisciplinary Perspective.* New York, Elsevier-North Holland Inc, 1981, p 679.

191. Klein RJ, DeStefano E, Brady E, et al: Latent infections of sensory ganglia as influenced by phosphonoformate treatment of herpes simplex virus-induced skin infections in hairless mice. *Antimicrob Agents Chemother* 16:266, 1979.

192. Wallin J, Lernestedt J-O, Lycke E: Therapeutic efficacy of trisodium phosphonoformate in treatment of recurrent herpes labialis. *Antimicrob Agents Chemother* 16:680, 1979.

193. Huffman JH, Sidwell RW, Khare GP, et al: In vitro effect of 1-b-D-ribofuranosyl-1,2,4-triazole-3-carboxamide (Virazole, ICN 1229) on deoxyribonucleic acid and ribonucleic acid viruses. *Antimicrob Agents Chemother* 3:235, 1973.

194. Sidwell RW, Robins RK, Hillyard IW: Ribavirin: An antiviral agent. *Pharmacol Ther* 6:123, 1979.

195. Hruska JF, Bernstein JM, Douglas RG Jr, et al: Effects of ribavirin on respiratory syncytial virus in vitro. *Pharmacol Ther* 6:770, 1980.

196. Stephen EL, Jones DE, Peters CJ, et al: Ribavirin treatment of toga-, arena- and bunyavirus infections in subhuman primates and other laboratory animal species, in Smith RA, Kirkpatric W (eds): *Ribavirin: A Broad Spectrum Antiviral Agent.* New York, Academic Press, 1980, p 169.

196a. Kirsi JJ, North JA, McKerran PA, Murray BK, et al: Broad-spectrum antiviral activity of

2-b-D ribofuronosyl-selenazole-4-carboxamide, a new antiviral agent. *Antimicrob Agents Chemother* 24:353–361, 1983.

197. Miller JP, Kigwana LJ, Streeter DG, et al: The relationship between the metabolism of ribavirin and its proposed mechanism of action. *Ann NY Acad Sci* 284:211, 1977.
198. Streeter DG, Witkowski JT, Khare GP, et al: Mechanism of action of 1-b-D-ribofuranosyl-1,2,4-triazole-3-carboxamide (Virazole), a new broad-spectrum antiviral agent. *Proc Natl Acad Sci* 70:1174, 1973.
199. Zimmerman TP, Deeprose RD: Metabolism of 5-amino-1-b-D-ribofuranosyl-imidazole-4-carboxamide and related five-membered heterocycles to 5′-triphosphates in human blood and L5178Y cells. *Biochem Pharmacol* 27:709, 1978.
200. Browne MJ: Mechanism and specificity of action of ribavirin. *Antimicrob Agents Chemother* 15:747, 1978.

200a. Browne MJ: Comparative inhibition of influenza and parainfluenza virus replication by ribavirin in MDCK cells. *Antimicrob Agents Chemother* 19:712, 1981.

201. Larsson A, Stenberg K, Oberg B: Reversible inhibition of cellular metabolism by ribavirin. *Antimicrob Agents Chemother* 13:154, 1978.
202. Muller WEG, Maidhof A, Taschner H, et al: Virazole (1-b-D-ribofuranosyl-1,2,4-triazole-3-carboxamide): A cytostatic agent. *Biochem Pharmacol* 26:1071, 1977.
203. Oxford JS: Inhibition of the replication of influenza A and B viruses by a nucleoside analogue (ribavirin). *J Gen Virol* 28:409, 1975.
204. Scholtissek C: Inhibition of influenza RNA synthesis by virazole (ribavirin). *Arch Virol* 50:349, 1976.
205. Sarver N, Stollar V: Virazole prevents production of sindbis virus and virus-induced cytopathic effect in *Aedes albopictus* cells. *Virology* 91:267, 1978.
206. Eriksson B, Helgstrand E, Johansson NG, et al: Inhibition of influenza virus ribonucleic acid polymerase by ribavirin triphosphate. *Antimicrob Agents Chemother* 11:946, 1977.
207. Goswami BB, Borek E, Sharma OK: The broad spectrum antiviral agent ribavirin inhibits capping of mRNA. *Biochem Biophys Res Commun* 89:830, 1979.
208. Allen LB, Fingal CM: Failure of type 1 herpesvirus to develop resistance to ribavirin. *Antimicrob Agents Chemother* 12:120, 1977.
209. Potter CW, Phair JP, Vodinelich L, et al: Antiviral, immunosuppressive and antitumour effects of ribavirin. *Nature* 259:496, 1976.
210. Peavy DL, Powers CN, Knight V: Inhibition of murine plaque-forming cell responses *in vivo* by ribavirin. *J Immunol* 126:861, 1981.
211. Peavy DL, Koff WC, Hyman DS, et al: Inhibition of lymphocyte proliferative responses by ribavirin. *Infect Immun* 29:583, 1980.
212. Smith CB, Charette RP, Fox JP, et al: Lack of effect of oral ribavirin in naturally occurring influenza A virus (H1N1) infection. *J Infect Dis* 141:548, 1980.
213. Newman H, Vodinelich L, Potter CW: The effects of 1-b-D ribofuranosyl-1,2,4-triazole-3-carboxamide (ribavirin) on the transplanted tumours of animals. *Eur J Cancer* 13:821, 1977.
214. Jolly WB, Chu WT, Slater JM, et al: Antitumor effects of ribavirin on L1210 leukemia in the DBA/2 mouse. *Ann NY Acad Sci* 284:585, 1977.
215. Klassen LW, Williams GW, Reinertsen JL, et al: Ribavirin treatment in murine autoimmune disease. I. Therapeutic efficacy and effect on the immune response. *Arthritis Rheum* 22:145, 1979.
216. Hillyard IW: The preclinical toxicology and safety of ribavirin, in Smith RA, Kirkpatric W (eds): *Ribavirin: A Broad Spectrum Antiviral Agent.* New York, Academic Press, 1980, p 59.
217. Catlin DH, Smith RA, Samuels AI, et al: ^{14}C-ribavirin: Distribution and pharmacokinetic studies in rats, baboons and man, in Smith RA, Kirpatric W (eds): *Ribavirin: A Broad Spectrum Antiviral Agent.* New York, Academic Press, 1980, p 59.
218. Van Dyke R, Hintz M, Connor JD: Pharmacology of ribavirin aerosol therapy in children. Abstracts of the Twenty-second Interscience Conference on Antimicrobial Agents and Chemotherapy, no. 424, 1982.

218a. Connor JD, Van Dyke R, Hintz M, et al: Pharmacokinetics of ribavirin small particle aerosol therapy in children and young adults. Abstracts of the Twenty-third Interscience Conference on Antimicrobial Agents and Chemotherapy, 1983. No. 932.

219. Minkoff DI, Connor JD: Clinical use of ribavirin and the treatment of herpes zoster in otherwise normal adults, in Smith RA, Kirkpatric W (eds): *Ribavirin: A Broad Spectrum Antiviral Agent.* New York, Academic Press, 1980, p 185.

220. Magnussen CR, Douglas RG Jr, Betts RF, et al: Double-blind evaluation of oral ribavirin (virazole) in experimental influenza A virus infection in volunteers. *Antimicrob Agents Chemother* 12:498, 1977.

221. Togo Y, McCracken EA: Chemoprophylaxis and therapy of respiratory viral infections, double-blind clinical assessment of ribavirin (Virazole) in the prevention of induced infection with type B influenza virus. *J Infect Dis* 133:A109, 1976.

222. Cohen A, Togo Y, Khakoo R, et al: Comparative clinical and laboratory evaluation of the prophylactic capacity of ribavirin, amantadine hydrochloride, and placebo in induced human influenza type A. *J Infect Dis* 133:A109, 1976.

223. Patki SA, Gupta P: Evaluation of ribavirin in the treatment of acute hepatitis. *Chemotherapy* 28:298, 1982.

224. Bierman SM, Kirkpatrick W, Fernandez H: Clinical efficacy of ribavirin in the treatment of genital herpes simplex virus infection. *Chemotherapy* 27:139, 1981.

225. Hruska JF, Morrow PE, Suffin SC, et al: In vivo inhibition of respiratory syncytial virus by ribavirin. *Antimicrob Agents Chemother* 21:125, 1982.

226. Hall CB, McBride JT, Walsh EE, et al: Aerosolized ribavirin treatment of infants with respiratory syncytial viral infection. *N Engl J Med* 308:1443, 1983.

226a. Taber LH, Knight V, Gilbert BE, et al: Ribavirin aerosol treatment of bronchiolitis associated with respiratory syncytial virus infection in infants. *Ped* 72:613, 1983.

227. Jahrling PB, Hesse RA, Eddy GA, et al: Lassa virus infection of rhesus monkeys: pathogenesis and treatment with ribavirin. *J Infect Dis* 141:580, 1980.

228. Tinsdale M, Bauer DJ: The relative potencies of antiinfluenza compounds. *Ann NY Acad Sci* 284:254, 1977.

229. Burlington DB, Meiklejohn G, Mostow SR: Anti-influenza A virus activity of amantadine hydrochloride and rimantadine hydrochloride in ferret tracheal ciliated epithelium. *Antimicrob Agents Chemother* 21:794, 1982.

230. Schulman JL: Effect of 1-amantanamine hydrochloride (amantadine HCl) and methyl-1-adamatanethylamine hydrochloride (rimantadine HCl) on transmission of influenza virus infection in mice (33222). *Proc Soc Exp Biol Med* 128:1173, 1968.

231. Scott GH, Stephen EL, Berendt RF: Activity of amantadine, rimantadine, and ribavirin against Swine influenza in mice and squirrel monkeys. *Antimicrob Agents Chemother* 13:284, 1978.

232. Bukrinskaya AG, Vorkunova NK, Narmanbetova RA: Rimantadine hydrochloride blocks the second step of influenza virus uncoating. *Arch Virol* 66:275, 1980.

232a. Bukrinskaya AG, Vorkunova NK, Kornilayeva GV, et al: Influenza virus uncoating in infected cells and effect of rimantadine. *J Gen Virol* 60:49, 1982.

233. Van Voris LP, Bartram J, Hoffman HE, et al: Comparative pharmacokinetics of rimantadine HCl and amantadine HCl. Program and Abstracts of the Twenty-third Interscience Conference on Antimicrobial Agents and Chemotherapy, 1983. No. 684.

233a. Patriarca PA, Kater NA, Kendal AP, et al: Safety of prolonged administration of rimantadine hydrochloride in the prophylaxis of influenza A infections in nursing homes. Program and Abstracts of the Twenty-third Interscience Conference on Antimicrobial Agents and Chemotherapy, 1983. No. 683.

234. Dawkins AT Jr, Gallager LR, Togo Y, et al: Studies on induced influenza in man. *JAMA* 203:93, 1968.

235. Quarles JM, Couch RB, Cate TR, et al: Comparison of amantadine and rimantadine for prevention of type A (Russian) influenza. *Antiviral Res* 1:149, 1981.

236. Zlydnikov DM, Kubar OI, Kovaleva TP, et al: Study of rimantadine in the USSR: A review of the literature. *Rev Infect Dis* 3:408, 1981.

236a. Dolin R, Betts RF, Treanor JJ, et al: Rimantadine prophylaxis in the elderly. Program and Abstracts of the Twenty-third Interscience Conference on Antimicrobial Agents and Chemotherapy, 1983. No. 691.

237. Hayden FG, Zylidnikov DM, Iljenko VI, et al: Comparative therapeutic effect of aerosolized and oral rimantadine HCl in experimental human influenza A virus infection. *Antiviral Res* 2:147, 1982.

238. Fujiwara Y, Heidelberger C: Fluorinated pyrimidines. XXXVIII. The incorporation of 5-trifluoromethyl-2′-deoxyuridine into the deoxyribonucleic acid of vaccinia virus. *Mol Pharmacol* 6:281, 1970.

239. Heidelberger C: On the molecular mechanism of the antiviral activity of trifluorothymidine. *Ann NY Acad Sci* 255:317, 1975.

240. Spector SA, Tyndall M, Kelly E: Inhibition of human cytomegalovirus by trifluorothymidine. *Antimicrob Agents Chemother* 23:133, 1983.

241. Van Bijsterveld OP, Post H: Trifluorothymidine versus adenine arabinoside in the treatment of herpes simplex keratitis. *Br J Ophthalmol* 64:33, 1980.

242. Coster DJ, McKinnon JR, McGill JI, et al: Clinical evaluation of adenine arabinoside and trifluorothymidine in the treatment of corneal ulcers caused by herpes simplex virus. *J Infect Dis* 133:A173, 1976.

243. Hyndiuk RA, Charlin RE, Alpren VPA, et al: Trifluridine in resistant human herpetic keratitis. *Arch Ophthalmol* 96:1839, 1978.

244. Coster DJ, Jones BR, McGill JI: Treatment of amoeboid herpetic ulcers with adenine arabinoside or thrifluorothymidine. *Br J Ophthalmol* 63:418, 1979.

245. Shannon WM: Adenine arabinoside: Antiviral activity in vitro, in Pavan-Langston D, Buchanan RA, Alford CA Jr (eds): *Adenine Arabinoside: An Antiviral Agent.* New York, Raven Press, 1975, p 1.

246. Bryson YJ, Connor JD: In vitro susceptibility of varicella zoster virus to adenine arabinoside and hypoxanthine arabinoside. *Antimicrob Agents Chemother* 9:540, 1976.

247. Coker-Vann M, Dolin R: Effect of adenine arabinoside on Epsein-Barr virus in vitro. *J Infect Dis* 135:447, 1977.

248. Field H, McMillan A, Darby G: The sensitivity of acyclovir-resistant mutants of herpes simplex virus to other antiviral drugs. *J Infect Dis* 143:281, 1981.

249. Gephart JF, Lerner AM: Comparison of the effects of arabinosyladenine, arabinosylhypoxanthine, and arabinosyladenine 5′-monophosphate against herpes simplex virus, varicella-zoster virus, and cytomegalovirus with their effects on cellular deoxyribonucleic acid synthesis. *Antimicrob Agents Chemother* 19:170, 1981.

250. Biron KK, Fyfe JA, Noblin JE, et al: Selection and primary characterization of acyclovir-resistant mutants of varicella zoster virus. *Am J Med* 73(suppl):383, 1982.

251. Muller WEG, Zahn RK, Bittlingmaier K, et al: Inhibition of herpesvirus DNA synthesis by 9-b-D-arabinofuranosyladenine in cellular and cell-free systems. *Ann NY Acad Sci* 284:34, 1977.

252. Pelling JC, Drach JC, Shipman C Jr: Internucleotide incorporation of arabinosyladenine into herpes simplex virus and mammalian cell DNA. *Virology* 109:323, 1981.

253. Muller WEG, Zahn RK, Beyer R, et al: 9-b-D-arabinofuranosyladenine as a tool to study herpes simplex virus DNA replication in vitro. *Virology* 76:787, 1977.

254. Champney KJ, Lauter CB, Bailey EJ, et al: Antiherpesvirus activity in human sera and urine after administration of adenine arabinoside. *J Clin Invest* 62:1142, 1978.

254a. Shannon WM, Westbrook L, Arrett G, et al: Comparison of the efficacy of vidarabine, its carbocyclic analog (cyclaradine), and cyclaradine-5′-methoxy-acetate in the treatment of herpes simplex type 1 encephalitis in mice. *Antimicrob Agents Chemother* 24:538, 1983.

254b. Vince R, Dalarge S, Lee H, et al: Carbocyclic arabinofuranosyladenine (cyclaradine): Efficacy against genital herpes in guinea pigs. *Science* 221:1405, 1983.

255. Sacks SL, Merigan TC, Kaminska J, et al: Inactivation of S-adenosylhomocysteine hydrolase during adenine arabinoside therapy. *J Clin Invest* 69:226, 1982.
256. Cantoni GL, Aksamit RR, Kim I-K: Methionine biosynthesis and vidarabine therapy. *N Engl J Med* 307:1079, 1982.
257. Hinrichs J, Kitz D, Kobayashi G, et al: Immune enhancement in mice by ARA-A. *J Immunol* 130:829, 1983.
258. Kinkel AW, Buchanan RA: Human pharmacology, in Pavan-Langston D, Buchanan RA, Alford CA Jr (eds): *Adenine Arabinoside: An Antiviral Agent.* New York, Raven Press, 1975, p 197.
259. Whitley R, Alford C, Hess F, et al: Vidarabine: A preliminary review of its pharmacological properties and therapeutic use. *Drugs* 20:267, 1980.
260. Brady TG, O'Donovan CI: A study of the tissue distribution of adenosine deaminase in six mammal species. *Comp Biochem Physiol* 14:101, 1965.
261. Buchanan RA, Kinkel AW, Alford CA Jr, et al: Plasma levels and urinary excretion of vidarabine after repeat dosing. *Clin Pharmacol Ther* 27:690, 1980.
262. Bryson Y, Connor J, Hebblewaite D: Pharmacology and efficacy of ara A in neonates and adults. Program and Abstracts of the Eleventh International Congress of Chemotherapy and Nineteenth Interscience Conference on Antimicrobial Agents and Chemotherapy, 1979. No. 974.
263. Shope TC, Kauffman RE, Bowman D, et al: Pharmacokinetics of vidarabine in infants and children with infections due to herpesviruses. *J Infect Dis* 148:721, 1983.
264. Aronoff GR, Szwed JJ, Nelson RL, et al: Hypoxanthine-arabinoside pharmacokinetics after adenine arabinoside administration to a patient with renal failure. *Antimicrob Agents Chemother* 18:212, 1980.
265. Ross AH, Julia A, Balakrishnan C: Toxicity of adenine arabinoside in humans. *J Infect Dis* 133:A192, 1976.
266. Ramos E, Timmons RF, Schimpff SC: Inappropriate antidiuretic hormone following adenine arabinoside administration. *Antimicrob Agents Chemother* 15:142, 1979.
267. Lauter CB, Bailey EJ, Lerner AM: Microbiologic assays and neurological toxicity during use of adenine arabinoside in humans. *J Infect Dis* 134:75, 1976.
268. Friedman HM, Grasela T: Adenine arabinoside and allopurinol: possible adverse drug interaction. *N Engl J Med* 304:423, 1981.
269. Etta LV, Brown J, Mastri A, et al: Fatal vidarabine toxicity in a patient with normal renal function. *JAMA* 246:1703, 1981.
270. Marker SC, Howard RJ, Groth KE, et al: A trial of vidarabine for cytomegalovirus infection in renal transplant patients. *Arch Intern Med* 140:1441, 1980.
271. Steele RW, Chapa IA, Vincent MM, et al: Effects of adenine arabinoside on cellular immune mechanisms in humans. *Antimicrob Agents Chemother* 7:203, 1975.
272. Pavan-Langston D, Buchanan RA: Vidarabine therapy of simple and idu-complicated herpetic keratitis. *Trans Acad Ophthalmol Otol* 81:813, 1976.
273. Whitley RJ, Soong S-J, Dolin R, et al: Adenine arabinoside therapy of biopsy-proven herpes simplex encephalitis. *N Engl J Med* 297:289, 1977.
274. Whitley RJ, Soong S-J, Hirsch MS, et al: Herpes simplex encephalitis, vidarabine therapy and diagnostic problems. *N Engl J Med* 304:313, 1981.
275. Whitley RJ, Nahmias AJ, Soong S-J, et al: Vidarabine therapy of neonatal herpes simplex virus infection. *Pediatrics* 66:495, 1980.
276. Whitley RJ, Spruance S, Hayden F, et al: Vidarabine therapy of mucocutaneous herpes simplex virus infections in the immunocompromised host. *J Infect Dis* 149:1, 1984.
277. Whitley R, Hilty M, Haynes R, et al: Vidarabine therapy of varicella in immunosuppressed patients. *J Pediatr* 101:125, 1982.
278. Bassendine MF, Chadwick RG, Salmeron J, et al: Adenine arabinoside therapy in HBsAg-positive chronic liver disease: A controlled study. *Gastroenterology* 80:1016, 1981.
279. Koplan JP, Monsur KA, Foster SO, et al: Treatment of variola major with adenine arabinoside. *J Infect Dis* 131:34, 1975.

280. Rand KH, Johnson KP, Rubinstein LJ, et al: Adenine arabinoside in the treatment of progressive multifocal leukoencephalopathy: Use of virus-containing cells in the urine to assess response to therapy. *Ann Neurol* 1:458, 1977.
281. Ch'ien LT, Cannon NJ, Whitley RJ, et al: Effect of adenine arabinoside on cytomegalovirus infections. *J Infect Dis* 130:32, 1974.
282. Kraemer KG, Neiman PE, Reeves WC, et al: Prophylactic adenine arabinoside following marrow transplantation. *Transplant Proc* X:237, 1978.
283. Pollard RB, Egbert PR, Gallagher JG, et al: Cytomegalovirus retinitis in immunosuppressed hosts. *Ann Intern Med* 93:655, 1980.
284. Kern ER, Richards JT, Overall JC Jr, et al: Alteration of mortality and pathogenesis of three experimental herpesvirus hominis infections in mice with adenine arabinoside 5′-monophosphate, adenine arabinoside, and phosphonoacetic acid. *Antimicrob Agents Chemother* 13:53, 1978.
285. Whitley RJ, Tucker BC, Kinkel AW, et al: Pharmacology, tolerance, and antiviral activity of vidarabine monophosphate in humans. *Antimicrob Agents Chemother* 18:709, 1980.
286. Preiksaitis JK, Lank B, Ng PK, et al: Effect of liver disease on pharmacokinetics and toxicity of 9-b-D-arabinofuranosyladenine-5′-phosphate. *J Infect Dis* 144:358, 1981.
287. Weller IVD, Bassendine MF, Murray AK, et al: HBsAg-positive chronic liver disease: Inhibition of viral replication by highly soluble adenine arabinoside 5′-monophosphate (ARA-AMP). *Gastroenterology* 79:1129, 1980.
288. Field AK, Davies ME, DeWitt C, et al: 9-{[2-hydroxy-1-(hydroxymethyl) ethoxy]methyl }guanine: A selective inhibitor of herpes group virus replication. *Proc Natl Acad Sci* 80:4139, 1983.
289. Smee DF, Martin JC, Verheyden PH, et al: Anti-herpesvirus activity of the acyclic nucleoside 9-(1,3-dihydroxy-2-propoxymethyl)guanine. *Antimicrob Agents Chemother* 23:676, 1983.
290. Smith KO, Galloway KS, Kennell WL, et al: A new nucleoside analog, 9-[[2-hydroxy-1-(hydroxymethyl)ethoxy]methyl] guanine, highly active in vitro against herpes simplex virus types 1 and 2. *Antimicrob Agents Chemother* 22:55, 1982.
291. Mar EC, Cheng YC, Huang ES: Effect of 9-(1,3 dihydroxy-2-propoxymethyl) guanine on human cytomegalovirus replication in vitro. *Antimicrob Agents Chemother* 24:518, 1983.
292. McSharry JJ, Caliguiri LA, Eggers HI: Inhibition of uncoating of poliovirus by arildone, a new antiviral drug. *Virology* 97:307, 1979.
293. Kuhrt MF, Fancher MJ, Jasty V, et al: Preliminary studies of the mode of action of arildone, a novel antiviral agent. *Antimicrob Agents Chemother* 15:813, 1979.
294. Kim KS, Sapienza VJ, Carp RI: Antiviral activity of arildone on deoxyribonucleic acid and ribonucleic acid viruses. *Antimicrob Agents Chemother* 18:276, 1980.
295. McKinlay MA, Miralles JV, Brisson CJ, et al: Prevention of human poliovirus-induced paralysis and death in mice by the novel antiviral agent arildone. *Antimicrob Agents Chemother* 22:1022, 1982.
296. DeLong DC, Reed SE: Inhibition of rhinovirus replication in organ culture by a potential antiviral drug. *J Infect Dis* 141:87, 1980.
297. Phillpotts RJ, DeLong DC, Wallace J, et al: The activity of enviroxime against rhinovirus infection in man. *Lancet* 1:1342, 1981.
298. Hayden FG, Gwaltney JM Jr: Prophylactic activity of intranasal enviroxime against experimentally induced rhinovirus type 39 infection. *Antimicrob Agents Chemother* 21:892, 1982.
299. Levandowski RA, Pachucki CT, Rubenis M, et al: Topical enviroxime against rhinovirus infection. *Antimicrob Agents Chemother* 22:1004, 1982.
300. Phillpotts RJ, Wallace J, Tyrrell DA, et al: Therapeutic activity of enviroxime against rhinovirus infection in volunteers. *Antimicrob Agents Chemother* 23:671, 1983.
301. Lopez C, Watanabe KA, Fox JJ: 2′-fluoro-5-iodo-aracytosine, a potent and selective antiherpesvirus agent. *Antimicrob Agents Chemother* 17:803, 1980.
302. Kreis W, Damin L, Colacino J, et al: In vitro metabolism of 1-b-D-arabinofuranosylcytosine and 1-b-2′-fluoroarabino-5-iodocytosine in normal and herpes simplex virus type 1 virus-infected cells. *Biochem Pharmacol* 31:767, 1982.

303. Chou T-C, Feinberg A, Grant AJ, et al: Pharmacological disposition and metabolic fate of 2′-fluoro-5-iodo-1-b-D-arabinofuranosylcytosine in mice and rats. *Cancer Res* 41:3336, 1981.

304. Trousdale MD, Nesburn AB, Su T-L, et al: Activity of 1-(2′-fluoro-2′-deoxy-b-D-arabinofuranosyl)thymine against herpes simplex virus in cell cultures and rabbit eyes. *Antimicrob Agents Chemother* 23:808, 1983.

305. Leyland-Jones B, Donnelly H, Myskowski P, et al: FIAC, a potent new antiviral agent: Therapeutic superiority over adenine arabinoside (ARA-A) against varicella zoster infections in immunosuppressed patients. *Clin Res* 31:369A, 1983.

306. Schinazi RF, Peters J, Sokol MK, et al: Therapeutic activities of 1(2-fluoro-2-deoxy-b-D-arabinofuranosyl)-5-iodocytosine and -thymine alone and in combination with acyclovir and vidarabine in mice infected intracerebrally with herpes simplex virus. *Antimicrob Agents Chemother* 24:95, 1983.

306a. Colcacino JM, Lopez C: Efficacy and selectivity of some nucleoside analogs as anti-human cytomegalovirus agents. *Antimicrob Agents Chemother* 24:505, 1983.

307. Subak-Sharpe JH, Timbury MC, Williams JF: Rifampicin inhibits the growth of some mammalian viruses. *Nature* 222:341, 1969.

308. Halsted CC, Minnefor AB, Lietman PS: Inhibition of cytomegalovirus by rifampin. *J Infect Dis* 125:552, 1972.

309. Furukawa T, Tanaka S, Plotkin SA: Inhibition of human cytomegalovirus by rifampin. *J Gen Virol* 28:355, 1975.

310. Moshkowitz A, Goldblum N, Heller E: Studies of the antiviral effect of rifampincin in volunteers. *Nature* 229:422, 1971.

311. Swick HM: Rifampin ineffective in treating SSPE. *N Engl J Med* 293:405, 1975.

312. Korant BD, Kauer JC, Butterworth BE: Zinc ions inhibit replication of rhinoviruses. *Nature* 248:588, 1971.

313. Fridlender B, Chejanovsky N, Becker Y: Selective inhibition of herpes simplex virus type 1 DNA polymerase by zinc ions. *Virology* 84:551, 1978.

314. Katz E, Margalith E: Inhibition of vaccinia virus maturation by zinc chloride. *Antimicrob Agents Chemother* 19:213, 1981.

315. Tennican PO, Carl GZ, Chvapil M: The diverse effects of topical and systemic administration of zinc on the virulence of herpes simplex genitalis. *Life Sciences* 24:1877, 1979.

316. Eby GA, Davis DR, Halcomb WW: Reduction in duration of common colds by zinc gluconate lozenges in a double-blind study. *Antimicrob Agents Chemother* 25:20, 1984.

18

ANTIPARASITIC AGENTS

J. JOSEPH MARR

Because parasites are diverse in their morphology, life cycles, and, to some extent, biochemistry, the therapeutic modalities used to manage parasitic diseases are diverse. In this chapter, drugs are grouped according to the kinds of organisms to which they apply even though a single drug may be used to counter a number of different organisms (Table 1). Some drugs, marked in the text with an asterisk, are manufactured abroad and are not yet approved by the U.S. Food and Drug Administration. These may be obtained from the Centers for Disease Control, Atlanta, Georgia 30333 (Table 2).

PROTOZOAN

Malaria

Antimalarial agents may be divided into two groups based on their presumed mechanisms of action. The 4- and 8-aminoquinolines appear to exert their effects, in part, by intercalation into the DNA of the parasite (1). The selective toxicity depends on the accumulation of the drug within the erythrocyte through mechanisms that are dependent on the presence of the parasite within the cell (2). Chloroquine, for example, appears to bind to protoporphyrin IX, which is a product of hemoglobin degradation by the parasite (3). It is relatively certain that intercalation with nucleic acid is not the only mechanism of action of these compounds since mefloquine does not intercalate (4). Primaquine is similar to mefloquine in that it produces much less change in the properties of native DNA than do the other 4-aminoquinolines. Undoubtedly, several mechanisms of action are common to this group of compounds.

The second group of antimalarials is characterized by inhibition of the synthesis of folic acid from para-aminobenzoic acid (PABA). These agents either interfere with the incorporation of PABA into folic acid, a reaction not found in mammals, or they inhibit dihydrofolate reductase. The capacity of these compounds to inhibit the parasite dihydrofolate reductase is much greater than

TABLE 1. Drugs for Treatment of Parasitic Infections

Infection	*Drug*	*Adult Dosage*	*Pediatric Dosage*
AMEBIASIS (Entamoeba histolytica)			
Asymptomatic			
Drug of choice:	Iodoquinol	650 mg tid × 20d	30–40 mg/kg/d in 3 doses × 20d
Alternatives:	Diloxanide furoate	500 mg tid × 10d	20 mg/kg/d in 3 doses × 10d
	Paromomycin	25–30 mg/kg/d in 3 doses × 7d	25–30 mg/kg/d in 3 doses × 7d
Mild to moderate intestinal disease			
Drug of choice:	Metronidazole plus	750 mg tid × 5–10d	35–50 mg/kg/d in 3 doses × 10d
	Iodoquinol	650 mg tid × 20d	30–40 mg/kg/d in 3 doses × 20d
Alternative:	Paromomycin	25–30 mg/kg/d in 3 doses × 7d	25–30 mg/kg/d in 3 doses × 7d
Severe intestinal disease			
Drug of choice:	Metronidazole plus	750 mg tid × 10d	35–50 mg/kg/d in 3 doses × 10d
	Iodoquinol	650 mg tid × 20d	30–40 mg/kg/d in 3 doses × 20d
Alternatives:	Dehydroemetine plus	1 to 1.5 mg/kg/d IM (max. 90 mg/d) for up to 5d	1 to 1.5 mg/kg/d (max. 90 mg/d) IM in 2 doses for up to 5d
	Iodoquinol	650 mg tid × 20d	30–40 mg/kg/d in 3 doses × 20d
OR			
	Emetine plus	1 mg/kg/d (max. 60 mg/d) IM for up to 5d	1 mg/kg/d in 2 doses (max. 60 mg/d) IM for up to 5d
	Iodoquinol	650 mg tid × 20d	30–40 mg/kg/d in 3 doses × 20d
Hepatic abscess			
Drug of choice:	Metronidazole plus	750 mg tid × 10d	35–50 mg/kg/d in 3 doses × 10d
	Iodoquinol	650 mg tid × 20d	30–40 mg/kg/d in 3 doses × 20d
Alternatives:	Dehydroemetine followed by	1 to 1.5 mg/kg/d (max. 90 mg/d) IM for up to 5d	1 to 1.5 mg/kg/d (max. 90 mg/d) IM in 2 doses for up to 5d
	chloroquine phosphate plus	600 mg base (1 g) daily × 2d, then 300 mg base (500 mg) daily × 2–3 wks	10 mg base/kg/d (max. 300 mg base/d) × 2–3 wks
	Iodoquinol	650 mg tid × 20d	30–40 mg/kg/d in 3 doses × 20d
OR			
	Emetine followed by	1 mg/kg/d (max. 60 mg/d) IM for up to 5d	1 mg/kg/d in 2 doses (max. 60 mg/d) IM for up to 5d
	chloroquine phosphate plus	600 mg base (1 g) daily × 2d, then 300 mg base (500 mg) daily × 2–3 wks	10 mg base/kg/d (max. 300 mg base/d) × 2–3 wks
	Iodoquinol	650 mg tid × 20d	30–40 mg/kg/d in 3 doses × 20d

TABLE 1. (Continued)

Infection	*Drug*	*Adult Dosage*	*Pediatric Dosage*
AMEBIC MENINGOENCEPHALITIS, PRIMARY (Naegleria sp. Acanthamoeba sp.)			
Drug of choice:	Amphotericin B	1 mg/kg/d IV, uncertain duration	1 mg/kg/d IV, uncertain duration
ANCYLOSTOMA duodenale (hookworm)			
Drug of choice:	Mebendazole	100 mg bid × 3d	100 mg bid × 3d for children > 2 years
ANISAKIASIS (Anisakis sp.)			
Treatment of choice:	Surgical removal		
Alternative:	Thiabendazole	25 mg/kg bid × 3d	25 mg/kg bid × 3d
ANGIOSTRONGYLUS CANTONENSIS			
Drug of choice:	Thiabendazole	25 mg/kg bid × 3d	25 mg/kg bid × 3d
OR	Mebendazole	100 mg bid × 5d	100 mg bid × 5d for children > 2 years
ASCARIS lumbricoides (roundworm)			
Drug of choice:	Mebendazole	100 mg bid × 3d	100 mg bid × 3d for children > 2 years
Alternative:	Piperazine citrate	75 mg/kg (max. 3.5 g)/d × 2d	75 mg/kg (max. 3.5 g)/d × 2d
BABESIA			
Drug of choice:	Clindamycin	1.2 grams bid parenteral or 600 mg tid oral × 7d	20–40 mg/kg/d in 3 doses × 7d
	plus		
	quinine	650 mg tid oral × 7d	25 mg/kg/d in 3 doses × 7d
BALANTIDIUM coli			
Drug of choice:	Tetracycline	500 mg qid × 10d	10 mg/kg qid × 10d (max. 2 grams/d)
Alternative:	Iodoquinol	650 mg tid × 20d	40 mg/kg/d in 3 doses × 20d
Brugia malayi, see FILARIASIS			
CAPILLARIA philippinensis			
Drug of choice:	Mebendazole	200 mg bid × 20d	200 mg bid × 20d
Alternative:	Thiabendazole	25 mg/kg/d × 30d	25 mg/kg/d × 30d
Chagas' disease, see TRYPANOSOMIASIS			
Clonorchis sinensis, see FLUKES			

COCCIDIOSIS (Isospora belli)			
Drug of choice:	Trimethoprim-sulfamethoxazole	160 mg trimethoprim, 800 mg sulfamethoxazole qid × 10d, then bid × 3 wks	
CUTANEOUS LARVA MIGRANS (creeping eruption)			
Drug of choice:	Thiabendazole	Topically and/or 25 mg/kg bid (max. 3 g/d) × 2–5d	Topically and/or 25 mg/kg bid (max. 3 g/d) × 2–5d
DIENTAMOEBA fragilis			
Drug of choice:	Iodoquinol	650 mg tid × 20d	40 mg/kg/d in 3 doses × 20d
OR	Tetracycline	500 mg qid × 10d	10 mg/kg qid × 10d (max. 2 g/d)
Diphyllobothrium latum, see TAPEWORMS			
DRACUNCULUS medinensis (guinea worm)			
Drug of choice:	Niridazole	25 mg/kg (max. 1.5 g)/d × 10d	12.5 mg/kg bid (max. 1.5 g/d) × 10d
Alternative:	Metronidazole	250 mg tid × 10d	25 mg/kg/d (max. 750 mg/d) in 3 doses × 10d
Echinococcus, see TAPEWORMS			
Entamoeba histolytica, see AMEBIASIS			
ENTEROBIUS vermicularis (pinworm)			
Drug of choice:	Mebendazole	A single dose of 100 mg; repeat after 2 weeks	A single dose of 100 mg for children > 2 years; repeat after 2 weeks
Alternative:	Piperazine citrate	65 mg/kg (max. 2.5 g)/d × 7d; repeat after 2 weeks	65 mg/kg (max. 2.5 g)/d × 7d; repeat after 2 weeks
Fasciola hepatica, see FLUKES			
FILARIASIS			
Wuchereria bancrofti, Brugia (W.) *malayi, Acanthocheilonema perstans,* Loa loa			
Drug of choice:	Diethylcarbamazine	Day 1: 50 mg Day 2: 50 mg tid Day 3: 100 mg tid Days 4 through 21: 2 mg/kg tid	Day 1: 25–50 mg Day 2: 25–50 mg tid Day 3: 50–100 mg tid Days 4 through 21: 2 mg/kg tid

TABLE 1. (Continued)

Infection	*Drug*	*Adult Dosage*	*Pediatric Dosage*
Tropical eosinophilia			
Drug of choice:	Diethylcarbamazine	2 mg/kg tid × 7–10d	2 mg/kg tid × 7–10d
Onchocerca volvulus			
Drug of choice:	Diethylcarbamazine	25 mg/d × 3d, then 50 mg/d × 5d, then 100 mg/d × 3d, then 150 mg/d × 12d	0.5 mg/kg tid × 3d (max. 25 mg/d), then 1.0 mg/kg tid × 3–4d (max. 50 mg/d), then 1.5 mg/kg tid × 3–4d (max. 100 mg/d), then 2.0 mg/kg tid × 2–3 wks (max. 150 mg/d)
	followed by Suramin	100–200 mg (test dose) IV, then 1 g IV at weekly intervals × 5 wks	10–20 mg (test dose) IV, then 20 mg/kg IV at weekly intervals × 5 wks
Alternative:	Mebendazole	1 g bid × 28d (data on this dose are limited)	
FLUKES, hermaphroditic			
Clonorchis sinensis (Chinese liver fluke)			
Drug of choice:	Praziquantel	25 mg/kg tid × 1d	25 mg/kg tid × 1d
Fasciola hepatica (sheep liver fluke)			
Drug of choice:	Praziquantel	25 mg/kg tid × 1d	25 mg/kg tid × 1d
Fasciolopsis buski (intestinal fluke)			
Drug of choice:	Praziquantel	25 mg/kg tid × 1d	25 mg/kg tid × 1d
Alternative:	Tetrachlorethylene	0.1 ml/kg (max. 5 ml)	0.1 ml/kg (max. 5 ml)
Heterophyes heterophyes (intestinal fluke)			
Drug of choice:	Praziquantel	25 mg/kg tid × 1d	25 mg/kg tid × 1d
Alternative:	Tetrachlorethylene	0.1 ml/kg (max. 5 ml)	0.1 ml/kg (max. 5 ml)
Metagonimus yokogawai (intestinal fluke)			
Drug of choice:	Praziquantel	25 mg/kg tid × 1d	25 mg/kg tid × 1d
OR	Tetrachlorethylene	0.1 ml/kg (max. 5 ml)	0.1 ml/kg (max. 5 ml)
Opisthorchis viverrini (liver fluke)			
Drug of choice:	Praziquantel	25 mg/kg tid × 1d	25 mg/kg tid × 1d
Paragonimus westermani (lung fluke)			
Drug of choice:	Praziquantel	25 mg/kg tid × 1–2d	25 mg/kg tid × 1–2d

GIARDIASIS (Giardia lamblia)			
Drug of choice:	Quinacrine HCl	100 mg tid p.c. × 7d	2 mg/kg tid p.c. × 5d (max. 300 mg/d)
Alternatives:	Metronidazole	250 mg tid × 7d	5 mg/kg tid × 5d
	Furazolidone	100 mg qid × 7d	1.25 mg/kg qid × 7d
GNATHOSTOMIASIS (Gnathostoma spinigerum)			
Drug of choice:	Surgical removal		
OR	Mebendazole	200 mg po q3h × 6d	
Hookworm, see ANCYLOSTOMA, NECATOR			
Hymenolepis nana, see TAPEWORMS			
Kala azar, see LEISHMANIASIS			
LEISHMANIASIS			
L. braziliensis (American mucocutaneous leishmaniasis) and *L. mexicana* (American cutaneous leishmaniasis)			
Drug of choice:	Stibogluconate sodium	10 mg Sb/kg (max. 600 mg) IM or IV/d × 10d (may be repeated)	10 mg Sb/kg/d IM or IV (max 600 mg/d) × 10d
Alternative:	Amphotericin B	0.25 to 1 mg/kg by slow infusion daily or every 2d up to 8 weeks	0.25 to 1 mg/kg by slow infusion daily or every 2d up to 8 wks
L. donovani (kala azar, visceral leishmaniasis)			
Drug of choice:	Stibogluconate sodium	10 mg Sb/kg/d (max 600 mg/d) IM or IV × 20d (may be repeated)	10 mg/kg/d IM or IV (max. 600 mg/d × 6–10d
Alternative	Pentamidine isethionate	2–4 mg/kg/d IM up to 15 doses	2–4 mg/kg/d IM up to 15 doses
	Amphotericin B	0.5–1 mg/kg/d; total dose, 1–2 g	
L. tropica (oriental sore, cutaneous leishmaniasis)			
Drug of choice:		Treatment varies with organism, see Chapter 233.	
LICE (Pediculus humanus, capitis, Phthirus pubis)			
Drug of choice:	Pyrethrins with piperonyl butoxide	Topically	Topically
Alternatives:	Malathion lotion 0.5%	Topically	Topically
	Lindane	Topically	Topically
	0.03% copper oleate	Topically	Topically

TABLE 1. (Continued)

Infection	*Drug*	*Adult Dosage*	*Pediatric Dosage*
Loa loa, see FILARIASIS			
MALARIA (Plasmodium falciparum, P. ovale, P. vivax, and P. malariae)			
Suppression or chemoprophylaxis of disease while in endemic area (all *Plasmodium* except chloroquine-resistant *P. falciparum*)			
Drug of choice:	Chloroquine phosphate	300 mg base (500 mg) once weekly beginning 2 wks before and continued for 6 wks after last exposure in endemic area	See text
Prevention of attack after departure from areas where *P. vivax* and *P. ovale* are endemic			
Drug of choice:	Primaquine phosphate	15 mg base (26.3 mg)/d × 14d (with last 2 wks of chloroquine prophylaxis)	0.3 mg base/kg/d × 14d (with last 2 wks of chloroquine prophylaxis)
Treatment of uncomplicated attack (all *Plasmodium* except chloroquine-resistant *P. falciparum*)			
Drug of choice:	Chloroquine phosphate	600 mg base (1 g), then 300 mg base (500 mg) in 6 hr, then 300 mg base (500 mg)/d × 2d	10 mg base/kg (max. 600 mg base), then 5 mg base/kg 6 hr later, then 5 mg base/kg/d × 2d
Treatment of severe illness, parenteral dosage— only if oral dose cannot be administered (regardless of severity) (all *Plasmodium* except chloroquine-resistant *P. falciparum*)			
Drug of choice:	Quinine dihydrochloride	600 mg in 300 ml normal saline IV over 8 hr, continued until oral therapy can be started (max. 1800 mg/d)	25 mg/kg/d; administer half of dose in 2-hr infusion, then other half 6–8 hr later if oral therapy still cannot be started (max. 1800 mg/d)
OR	Chloroquine HCl	200 mg base (250 mg) IM q6h	Not recommended; see text
Prevention of relapses (''radical'' cure after ''clinical'' cure) (*P. vivax* and *P. ovale* only)			
Drug of choice:	Primaquine phosphate	15 mg base (26.3 mg)/d × 14d	0.3 mg base/kg/d × 14d
P. falciparum (chloroquine-resistant) suppression or chemoprophylaxis			
Drug of choice:	Pyrimethamine plus sulfadoxine	1 tablet (25 mg pyrimethamine, 500 mg sulfadoxine) once weekly from one wk before until 6 wks after exposure	6–11 mos: 1/8 tablet; 1–3 yrs: 1/4 tablet; 4–8 yrs: 1/2 tablet; 9–14 yrs: 3/4 tablet once weekly from one day before until 6 wks after exposure

Treatment of uncomplicated attack (chloroquine-resistant *P. falciparum*)			
Drug of choice:	Quinine sulfate	650 mg tid × 3d	25 mg/kg/d in 3 doses × 10 d
	plus pyrimethamine	25 mg bid × 3d	< 10 kg: 6.25 mg/d; 10–20 kg: 12.5 mg/d; 20–40 kg: 25 mg/d
	plus sulfadiazine	500 mg qid × 5d	100–200 mg/kg/d in 4 doses × 5d (max. 2 g/d)
Alternative:	Quinine sulfate	650 mg tid × 3d	25 mg/kg/d in 3 doses × 3d
	plus tetracycline	250 mg qid × 7d	5 mg/kg qid × 7d
OR	plus clindamycin	900 mg tid × 3d	20–40 mg/kg/d in 3 doses × 3d
Treatment of severe illness, parenteral dosage (chloroquine-resistant *P. falciparum*)			
Drug of choice:	Quinine dihydrochloride	600 mg in 300 ml normal saline IV over 8 hr, continued until oral therapy can be started (max. 1800 mg/d)	25 mg/kg/d; administer half of dose in 2-hr infusion, then other half 6–8 hr later if oral therapy still cannot be started (max. 1800 mg/d)
MITES (Sarcoptes scabiei)			
Drug of choice:	10% crotamiton	Topically	Topically
Alternatives:	Lindane	Apply topically once	Apply topically once
	Benzyl benzoate	Topically	Topically
	Sulfur in petrolatum	Topically	Topically
Naegleria species, see AMEBIC MENINGOENCEPHALITIS, PRIMARY			
NECATOR americanus (hookworm)			
Drug of choice:	Mebendazole	100 mg bid × 3d	100 mg bid × 3d for children > 2 yrs

Onchocerca volvulus, see FILARIASIS

Opisthorchis viverrini, see FLUKES

Paragonimus westermani, see FLUKES

Pediculus capitis, humanus, Phthirus pubis, see LICE

Pinworm, see ENTEROBIUS

TABLE 1. (Continued)

Infection	*Drug*	*Adult Dosage*	*Pediatric Dosage*
PNEUMOCYSTIS carinii			
Drug of choice:	Trimethoprim-sulfamethoxazole	Trimethoprim 20 mg/kg/d, sulfamethoxazole 100 mg/kg/d in 4 doses × 14d	Trimethoprim 20 mg/kg/d, sulfamethoxazole 100 mg/kg/d in 4 doses × 14d
Alternative:	Pentamidine isethionate	4 mg/kg/d IM × 12–14d	4 mg/kg/d IM × 12–14d
Roundworm, see ASCARIS			
Scabies, see MITES			
SCHISTOSOMIASIS			
S. haematobium			
Drug of choice:	Praziquantel	40 mg/kg once	40 mg/kg once
Alternative:	Metrifonate	7.5–10 mg/kg every other wk × 3 doses	10 mg/kg every other wk × 3 doses
S. japonicum			
Drug of choice:	Praziquantel	20 mg/kg three times in one day	20 mg/kg three times in one day
S. mansoni			
Drug of choice:	Praziquantel	40 mg/kg once	40 mg/kg once
Alternative:	Oxamniquine	15 mg/kg once	15–20 mg/kg once
S. mekongi			
Drug of choice:	Praziquantel	20 mg/kg three times in one day	20 mg/kg three times in one day
Sleeping sickness, see TRYPANOSOMIASIS			
STRONGYLOIDES stercoralis			
Drug of choice:	Thiabendazole	25 mg/kg bid (max. 3 g/d) × 2d	25 mg/kg bid (max. 3 g/d) × 2d
TAPEWORMS—Adult or intestinal stage			
Diphyllobothrium latum (fish), *Taenia saginata* (beef), *Taenia solium* (pork), *Dipylidium caninum* (dog)			
Drug of choice:	Niclosamide	A single dose of 4 tablets (2 g) chewed thoroughly	11–34 kg: a single dose of 2 tablets (1 g); > 34 kg: a single dose of 3 tablets (1.5 g)
OR	Praziquantel	10–20 mg/kg once	10–20 mg/kg once

Hymenolepis nana (dwarf tapeworm)			
Drug of choice:	Niclosamide	A single daily dose of 4 tablets (2 g) chewed thoroughly × 5d	11–34 kg: a single dose of 2 tablets (1 g) × 5d; > 34 kg: a single dose of 3 tablets (1.5 g) × 5d
OR	Praziquantel	15–20 mg/kg once	15–20 mg/kg once
Larval or tissue stage			
Echinococcus granulosus (Hydatid cysts)			
Drug of choice:	Surgical resection of cysts is the treatment of choice. When surgery is contraindicated, or cysts rupture spontaneously during surgery, mebendazole (experimental for this purpose in the USA) can be tried (JF Wilson and RL Rausch, *Ann Trop Med Parasitol* 76:165, 1982).		
Cysticercus cellulosae			
Drug of choice:	Praziquantel	50 mg/kg/d in 3 divided doses × 14d	50 mg/kg/d in 3 divided doses × 14d
Alternative:	Surgery		
Toxocariasis, see VISCERAL LARVA MIGRANS			
TOXOPLASMOSIS (Toxoplasma gondii)			
Drug of choice:	Pyrimethamine	25 mg/d × 3–4 wks	2 mg/kg/d × 3d (max. 25 mg/d), then 1 mg/kg/d × 4 wks
	plus		
	Sulfadiazine	75–100 mg/kg/d × 3–4 wks	100–150 mg/kg/d in 4 divided doses × 3–4 wks
Alternative:	Spiramycin	2–4 g/d × 3–4 wks	50–100 mg/kg/d × 3–4 wks
TRICHINOSIS (Trichinella spiralis)			
Drug of choice	Steroids for severe symptoms		
	plus thiabendazole	25 mg/kg bid × 5d	25 mg/kg bid × 5d
Alternative:	Mebendazole	200–400 mg tid × 3d, then 400–500 mg tid × 10d	
TRICHOMONAS vaginalis			
Drug of choice:	Metronidazole	250 mg tid × 7d	15 mg/kg/d in 3 doses × 7d
TRICHOSTRONGYLUS species			
Drug of choice:	Thiabendazole	25 mg/kg bid (max. 3 g/d) × 2d	25 mg/kg bid × 2d
Alternative:	Pyrantel pamoate	A single dose of 11 mg/kg (max. 1 g)	A single dose of 11 mg/kg (max. 1 g)

TABLE 1. (Continued)

Infection	*Drug*	*Adult Dosage*	*Pediatric Dosage*
TRICHURIS trichiura (whipworm)			
Drug of choice:	Mebendazole	100 mg bid × 3d	100 mg bid × 3d
TRYPANOSOMIASIS			
T. cruzi (South American trypanosomiasis, Chagas' disease)			
Drug of choice:	Nifurtimox	8–10 mg/kg/d in 4 divided doses	See ch. 234
T. gambiense; T. rhodesiense (African trypanosomiasis, sleeping sickness) hemolymphatic stage			
Drug of choice:	Suramin	100–200 mg (test dose) IV, then 1 g IV on days 1,3,7,14,21	20 mg/kg on days 1,3,7,14 and 21
Alternative:	Pentamidine isethionate	4 mg/kg/d IM × 10d	4 mg/kg/d IM × 10d
Late disease with CNS involvement			
Drug of choice:	Melarsoprol	2–3.6 mg/kg/d IV × 3 doses; after 1 wk 3.6 mg/kg/d IV × 3 doses; repeat again after 10–21 days	18–25 mg/kg total over 1 mo. Initial dose of 0.36 mg/kg IV, increasing gradually to max. 3.6 mg/kg at intervals of 1–5d for total of 9–10 doses
Alternatives:	Tryparsamide	One injection of 30 mg/kg IV every 5d to total of 12 injections; may be repeated after 1 mo.	Unknown
	plus suramin	One injection of 10 mg/kg IV every 5d to total of 12 injections; may be repeated after 1 mo.	Unknown
VISCERAL LARVA MIGRANS			
Drug of choice:	Thiabendazole	25 mg/kg bid × 5d	25 mg/kg bid × 5d
Whipworm, see TRICHURIS			
Wuchereria bancrofti, see FILARIASIS			

SOURCE: Modified from the *Medical Letter* 26:27 1984, with permission.

TABLE 2. Drugs for Parasitic Diseases Available from the Drug Service, Centers for Disease Control[a]

Investigational new drugs	*Indications*
Bayer 205 (Suramin)	African trypanosomiasis, onchocerciasis
Bithionol, N.F.	Paragonimiasis, *Fasciola hepatica*
Dehydroemetine	Amebiasis
Diloxanide furoate (Furamide)	Amebiasis
Melarsoprol (Mel B)	African trypanosomiasis
Nifurtimox (Lampit, Bayer 2502)	American trypanosomiasis
Pentamidine isethionate (Lomidine)	Pneumocystosis, African trypanosomiasis
Sodium antimony gluconate (Pentostam)	Leishmaniasis
Commercially licensed, but difficult-to-obtain drugs:	
Quinine (parenteral)	Malaria

[a] Drug Service, Centers for Disease Control, 1600 Clifton Road, Bld 1, room 1347, Atlanta, GA 30333. Telephone (day) (404) 329–3670, 8:00 AM to 4:30 PM, Monday through Friday; emergency (404) 329–2888.

for the corresponding mammalian enzyme. This group includes chloroguanide, pyrimethamine, and their derivatives, as well as the sulfonamides and sulfones.

Chloroquine Phosphate. Chloroquine phosphate is a white crystalline powder, 7-chloro-4-(4-diethylamino-1-methylbutylamino)-quinoline. It is the best known of the 4-aminoquinolines (Fig. 1) and remains the primary drug for the management of malaria. It is rapidly and completely absorbed from the GI tract, and one-half is bound to protein in the plasma. It concentrates in the liver, spleen, and kidney at levels 200–700 times the plasma concentration. The brain and spinal cord contain 10–30 times the plasma concentration. Because of the avidity for tissues, loading doses are needed when prophylaxis is given. Prolonged suppressive therapy causes few side effects, but use in acute malaria may cause nausea, vomiting, visual disturbances, and pruritus. It does not discolor the skin as does the closely related quinicrine. It should be used cautiously in persons with liver disease. Its primary use is for the suppression and treatment of malaria due to susceptible strains of *Plasmodium,* but it is also used in the treatment of amebic liver abscess, clonorchiasis, and certain other fluke infections. In

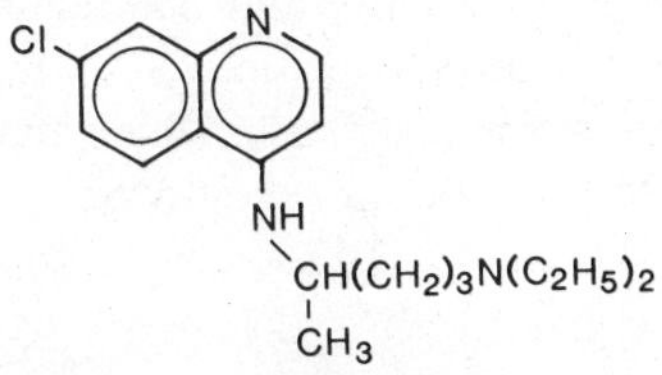

Chloroquine

FIGURE 1. Chloroquine.

the United States, it is marketed in 250 and 500 mg tablets (equal to 150 and 300 mg of base). It is also a component (500 mg) of the combination Aralen phosphate with Primaquine phosphate, used for the causal prophylaxis of all susceptible strains of malaria. A chloroquine hydrochloride salt, Aralen hydrochloride, is a parenteral solution for intramuscular use (each milliliter contains 50 mg of the dihydrochloride salt equivalent to 40 mg of chloroquine base), which can be substituted for the oral phosphate salt when severe nausea or vomiting is present, when absorption of the drug is in question, or when an infection is particularly severe. Great caution must be exercised in using the parenteral form in children, and oral administration should be substituted as soon as practicable. Its action is on the asexual erthrocytic forms of malaria parasites, but it does not affect the pre- or exoerythrocytic plasmodia and, therefore, does not prevent relapses of those malaria species with an exoerythrocytic stage. Irreversible retinal damage, seen when chloroquine is used in high daily doses for prolonged periods for collagen diseases, has not occurred in the usual recommended doses for malaria suppression and treatment (5). Chloroquine is considered safe in recommended doses for nonnursing mothers and pregnant women at risk from malaria. Acute overdosage of chloroquine can cause convulsions, acute circulatory failure, respiratory and cardiac arrest, and death. Chloroquine should not be used in patients with psoriasis or porphyria or in those with retinal changes of any etiology. An alternative drug should be used in areas of known chloroquine resistance for both suppression and treatment of this form of malaria. For suppression of sensitive malarial strains in adults, 300 mg of base is taken weekly, beginning 2 weeks before entering a malarious area, while in the malarious area, and for at least 6 weeks after leaving the malarious area. For infants and children, a weekly dose of 5 mg/kg base is given, not to exceed the adult dose regardless of weight. For oral treatment of acute malaria in adults, 600 mg of base is given initially, followed by 300 mg 6 hours later, and 300 mg at 24 hours and 48 hours. For children, 10 mg/kg base is given initially, followed by 5 mg/kg in 6 hours, and 5 mg/kg daily for the next 2 days. When treating malaria due to *Plasmodium vivax* and *Plasmodium ovale* or for the radical cure of these species following exposure, primaquine should follow after chloroquine doses. When chloroquine hydrochloride is used in treating severe acute malaria, adults should receive an initial dose of 160–200 mg IM to be repeated in 6 hours if necessary. The total parenteral dosage in the first 24 hours should not exceed 800 mg of base. Oral treatment should be started as soon as possible and should be continued until a total dose of 1.5 g of base over 3 days is completed. For infants and children, the recommended single dose is 5 mg/kg base, which may be repeated in 6 hours. The total dose in any 24-hour period should not exceed 10 mg/kg of base, and oral therapy should be started as soon as possible. Chloroquine has been used in *Babesia* infections (6).

Mefloquine. This compound is a representative of a new class of antimalarial agents, the quinolinemethanols (Fig. 2) and is promising for the treatment and

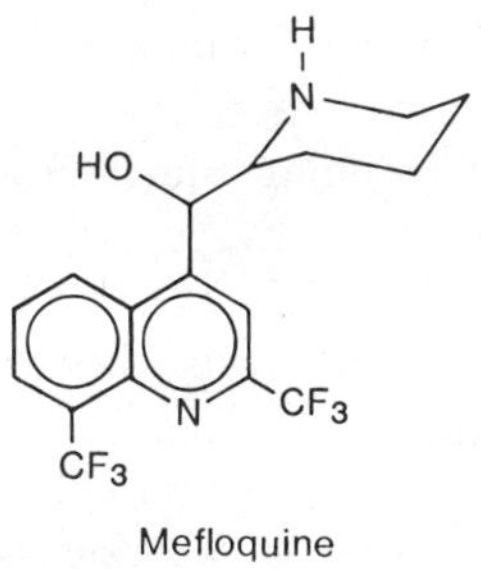

FIGURE 2. Mefloquine.

chemoprophylaxis of Fansidar-resistant *Plasmodium falciparum* (7). It is effective against almost all known strains of human plasmodia, including those resistant to chloroquine. Although this compound is not available commercially, it is being field tested in the Far East. It has a long half-life and appears to be an efficacious agent for chemoprophylaxis and therapy when given weekly or even every 2 weeks (8). Animal studies have shown that it is well absorbed after an oral dose and is extensively bound to plasma proteins. The concentration in the liver is high and prolonged. Most of the drug is excreted in the feces with only small amounts excreted in the urine. The half-life after a single dose averages 17 days (9). It is well tolerated in humans, but there is insufficient information regarding its long-term toxicity. Currently, the drug remains experimental but is the only single agent that is capable of providing suppression and cure of infections due to multidrug-resistant strains.

Primaquine Phosphate. Primaquine phosphate is an 8-aminoquinoline, 8-(4-amino-1-methylbutylamino)-6-methoxyquinoline phosphate (Fig. 3). It is used to prevent relapses and to provide radical cure of malaria due to *P. vivax* and *P. ovale* by acting on the exoerythrocytic stage of these species. It also has a gametocyticidal effect against malaria parasites (10). The drug has some activity against the asexual blood forms of *P. vivax,* but is not active against the comparable forms of *P. falciparum.* All of the 8-aminoquinolines are absorbed rapidly and metabolized rapidly. Plasma concentrations reach a peak in 6 hours and decline to nondetectable levels in 24 hours. Minor side effects include nausea,

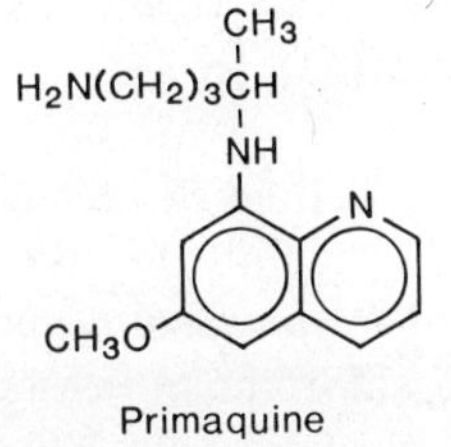

FIGURE 3. Primaquine.

abdominal discomfort, and headache. The major toxic effect occurs as a result of the oxidant action of primaquine and its metabolic derivatives. These agents can accelerate the transfer of reducing equivalents from NADPH, hemoglobin, reduced glutathione, and sulfhydryl groups to various acceptors. This may result in methemoglobinemia, impairment of all reductive processes dependent directly or indirectly on NADPH, and hemolysis (due to alterations in the membrane (11,12). There are many drugs that can cause such hemolysis; the most important of these are the other antimalarials of a similar chemical configuration, sulfonamides, nitrofurans, sulfones, vitamin K analogues, antipyretics, and analgesics.

In normal erythocytes, an oxidant stress is counterbalanced by increased activity of glucose-6-phosphate dehydrogenase (G6PD), generating a correspondingly increased amount of NADPH. By this mechanism, there is sufficient reducing power generated to reduce the oxidized glutathione, methemoglobin, and sulfhydryl-containing enzymes. Cells with a deficiency in this enzyme cannot respond to oxidant stress.

The severity of the hemolytic reaction depends largely on the genetic constitution of the patient. Persons with a G6PD deficiency of the type found in those of Mediterranian ancestry (Sephardic Jews, Greeks, Iranians) and some Orientals are more severely affected because the enzyme deficiency occurs in erythrocytes of all ages. Most blacks have the enzyme deficiency confined to older erythrocytes, and the hemolytic reaction is less severe. Since the gene is X-linked, the reaction is usually more severe in men. The reaction in women is variable since it depends on which X chromosome is expressed in the erythrocytes. There is a screening test available, and the results correlate well with the clinical severity of hemolysis. Primaquine should not be given to patients receiving at the same time other potentially hemolytic drugs, agents capable of depressing the myeloid elements of the bone marrow, or quinacrine.

Primaquine is marketed as the phosphate in 26.3 mg salt (15 mg of base) tablets and as a component (45 mg of base) of the combination Aralen phosphate with Primaquine phosphate.

As terminal treatment of acute malaria to prevent relapses, adults should receive 15 mg of base daily for 14 days after completing the 4-aminoquinoline course. Children should receive 0.3 mg/kg base daily for 14 days in broken tablets. The combination chloroquine-primaquine tablet may be used alternatively for radical cure of malaria in a dose of one tablet weekly for 8 weeks in adults. A daily dose of 30 mg of base for 14 days is occasionally necessary for adults exposed to so-called Chesson-strain *P. vivax* malaria in parts of Southwest Pacific and Southeast Asia (13).

Quinine. Quinine is a natural alkaloid extracted from the bark of the cinchona tree (Fig. 4) and is used today mainly for the treatment of malaria due to certain multiresistant strains of *P. falciparum* and for the emergency treatment of severe malaria (14). Since chloroquine-resistant malaria is increasing, this agent is having a resurgence of clinical use. The drug is available as quinine

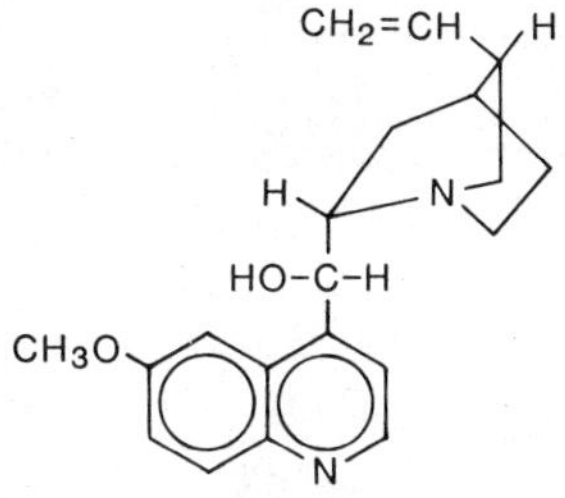

FIGURE 4. Quinine.

sulfate in 650-mg oral tablets, in capsules of 130, 200, and 325 mg, and as quinine dihydrochloride powder for intravenous use. The primary action of quinine is schizontocidal, and no lethal effect is exerted on sporozoites. It cannot be given by intramuscular injection due to tissue necrosis produced. Peak concentrations occur in 1–3 hours, and a dose of 10 mg/kg provides plasma levels of 7–17 μg/ml in the steady state. Concentrations above 10 μg/ml may be associated with side effects (15). Rapid intravenous infusion may cause cardiotoxicity; as discussed below. In one study, concentrations up to 20 μg/ml were not associated with cardiac toxicity. Vomiting is common but not clearly correlated with plasma or CSF drug levels. In plasma, 70 percent of the quinine is protein bound. CSF concentrations are 2–10 percent that of serum (1).

The half-life of quinine in the plasma is 16–18 hours. The drug is largely metabolized in the liver, with inactive metabolites excreted in the urine (16). Only 20 percent of unchanged drug is excreted in the urine (17). Nevertheless, in severe renal failure, quinine dosage should be reduced (18).

Usual therapeutic doses of quinine sulfate frequently cause symptoms of cinchonism (tinnitus, headache, nausea, abdominal pain, blurred vision, and altered auditory acuity), but these are seldom severe enough to necessitate cessation of treatment. Intravenous administration of quinine dihydrochloride may lead to arrhythmias, hypotension, and acute circulatory failure. It must be given slowly in dilute solutions with constant monitoring of the pulse and blood pressure; oral quinine sulfate should be substituted as soon as possible. For oral treatment of resistant *P. falciparum* in adults, quinine 650 mg tid is given for 10 days, along with pyrimethamine 25 mg bid for 3 days. In children, quinine is given as 25 mg/kg/day in three divided doses for 10 days, along with pyrimethamine 6.25–25 mg daily for 3 days. Sulfadiazine 500 mg qid for the first 5 days is also sometimes added. For intravenous use in severe *P. falciparum* malaria in adults, quinine dihydrochloride is administered as 600 mg in 300 ml of normal saline over 8 hours and continued until oral medication can be taken (maximum 1800 mg/day). For children 25 mg/kg/day is given (1800 mg maximum daily dose), half of the dose in a 2-hour infusion and then the other half 6–8 hours later if oral therapy still cannot be started.

Pyrimethamine. Pyrimethamine is the best known of the many 2,4-diaminopyrimidines synthesized for antimicrobial activity (Fig. 5). A closely related compound, trimethoprim, is active against many microorganisms including the malarial parasite. Of the various aminopyrimidines, pyrimethamine, 2,4-diamino-5-(*p*-chlorophenyl)-6-ethyl-pyrimidine, is the most active against plasmodia. It is used for the suppression of sensitive malaria (19), in the treatment of resistant *P. falciparum* malaria with quinine (19), and in the treatment of toxoplasmosis (20). The therapeutic action of the various diaminopyrimidines is due to their different affinities for the dihydrofolate reductases of mammals and parasites and because mammals can synthesize folate but protozoans and bacteria cannot. Pyrimethamine has a remarkable affinity for the enzyme of plasmodia, whereas trimethoprim is similarly active against several bacterial enzymes. Neither has a high affinity for the mammalian enzyme. Diaminopyrimidines are generally of low toxicity to humans, although high doses of pyrimethamine may cause a macrocytic anemia that responds to folinic acid.

Pyrimethamine is absorbed well after oral administration and has a half-life of 4 days. It is excreted in breast-milk and may be deleterious to infants. The relatively small doses used in malaria suppression appear to be safe in pregnancy, but benefit must be weighed against the potential risk when treating toxoplasmosis for 3–4 weeks.

Pyrimethamine is marketed as Daraprim in a 25 mg tablet. By itself it has little value in treating acute malaria with the exception of its use with quinine in resistant *P. falciparum* malaria. For malaria suppression in adults and children above 10 years of age, 25 mg is taken once weekly and continued for 6 weeks after leaving the malarious area. For children 2 years and under, 6.25 mg weekly is given, and for children 3–10 years, the dose is 12.5 mg weekly. Pyrimethamine-sulfadoxine combination (25:500 mg) has been available for many years outside this country and recently was licensed for sale in the United States under the name Fansidar. Similar combinations have been tried in the past with variable results (21,22), but the long half-life of sulfadoxine (7–9 days) has made this particular combination very effective. Its primary use is as a chemoprophylactic and therapeutic regimen for chloroquine-resistant malaria. For suppression, it is taken in a manner similar to chloroquine, one tablet each week. It has been used in the treatment of *P. falciparum* malaria and has provided cure rates of 80–90 percent (23). Fansidar is expected to achieve increasing usage since there are now many countries reporting chloroquine-resistant malaria (8). In some of these areas, Fansidar resistance has already emerged (24–26). To suppress

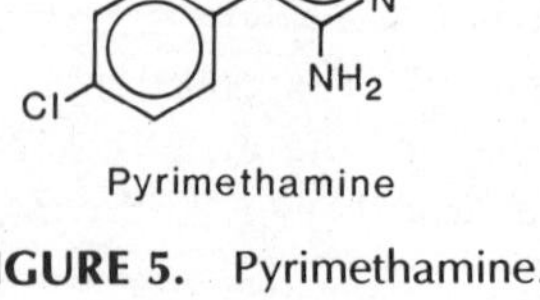

Pyrimethamine

FIGURE 5. Pyrimethamine.

malaria in adults, one tablet is taken weekly in the malarious area and for 6 weeks after leaving. For children under 4 years, the weekly dose is a one-quarter Fansidar tablet; for children 4–8 years, a one-half tablet; for children 9–14 years, a three-quarters tablet. Use of Fansidar for more than 6 months is discouraged until more information becomes available on possible toxicity associated with long-term use. To prevent relapsing malaria, a terminal 14-day course of primiquine should follow the use of both pyrimethamine and Fansidar. There is widespread resistance and often cross-resistance between pyrimethamine and chloroguanide in many parts of the world.

Amebiasis

Metronidazole. Metronidazole is a nitroimidazole compound, 2-methyl-5-nitroimidazole-1-ethanol, used in the treatment of trichomoniasis, amebiasis, and giardiasis (Fig. 6). The compound is active by virtue of the reduction of the 5-nitro group to the amine through a sequence of intermediate steps (27). This develops a concentration gradient across the membrane of the parasite that permits the accumulation of high concentrations of the reduced compounds within the cell. Metronidazole has a redox potential similar to that of ferredoxin and other electron carriers of anaerobic organisms. It acts as an artificial electron acceptor to divert electrons from the normal pathways of these organisms. The mechanism appears to apply to the protozoans mentioned above as well as anaerobic bacteria. For this reason, it is inactive against obligate aerobes (27). There is some evidence that metronidazole also interacts with DNA to impair its function as a template (27–29). The drug is absorbed well after oral administration and has a half-life of 8 hours. It achieves high concentrations in the CSF (30,31). The major route of excretion is the urine. Low concentrations are present in breast-milk and saliva. Side effects are uncommon, and those encountered relate to gastrointestinal toxicity and include nausea, epigastric discomfort, vomiting, and a metallic taste. An overgrowth of *Candida* may occur due to suppression of the anaerobic flora of the mouth and gastrointestinal tract. Stomatitis or glossitis also may occur. Rarely, dizziness, vertigo, ataxia, or sensory neuropathies may appear. The urine of some patients may become red or brown due to the presence of metabolic products of the drug. All of the above are temporary and disappear when the drug is discontinued. Metronidazole is known to produce a disulfuram-like effect, and patients should be cautioned not to take alcohol while receiving the drug. It may potentiate the anticoagulant effect of coumarin (32). Metronidazole has caused lung tumors in mice and is mutagenic to some bacteria (33). Metronidazole is not known to be carcinogenic in humans, but

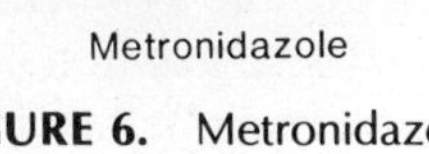

Metronidazole

FIGURE 6. Metronidazole.

human urine contains metabolites that are carcinogenic in rodents and mutagenic to bacteria. The drug should not be used in pregnancy (34).

Metronidazole is marketed as Flagyl in 250 mg tablets and as a 0.5 percent solution for intravenous administration. It is trichomonacidal and giardicidal. Metronidazole is also amebicidal at both intestinal and extraintestinal sites. It is more effective in symptomatic or invasive amebiasis than in the asymptomatic cyst-passer (35). Metronidazole continues to be the drug of choice for *Trichomonas vaginalis* infections in a dose of 250 mg tid for 7 days. For symptomatic nondysenteric intestinal amebiasis, adults should receive 750 mg tid for 10 days, and children 35–50 mg/kg/day in three divided doses for 10 days. For acute amebic dysentary and amebic liver abscess, adults should receive 750 mg tid for 10 days and children, 35–50 mg/kg/day in three dividend doses. When used in amebiasis, metronidazole should always be followed by a luminal-active drug such as diiodohydrodroxyquin (36). Although not approved as yet by the Food and Drug Administration for treatment of giardiasis, metronidazole is often used for this condition, being somewhat less effective but usually better tolerated than quinacrine (37) at a dosage of 250 mg tid for 7 days.

Emetine Hydrochloride. Emetine hydrochloride is prepared from ipecac. It has a direct action in *E. histolytica,* being more active against trophozoites than against cysts. Emetine inhibits protein synthesis in eukaryotes by blocking the translocation of peptidyl-tRNA from the acceptor to the donor site (38). Since oral administration causes gastrointestinal irritation, the drug is given by deep subcutaneous or intramuscular injection. It is well absorbed from parenteral sites of administration and is excreted slowly. It appears in the urine within an hour after injection. Excretion continues for 1 or 2 months after treatment has been halted. The persistence of the alkaloid is the reason for its toxicity (39). The greatest concentrations are found in the liver. It is probably for this reason that, like chloroquine, emetine has a greater efficacy in hepatic than in intestinal amebiasis.

The toxic effects of emetine are manifold. The most common are gastrointestinal. These include diarrhea, which may occur in one-half of the patients treated, and is due to the increased peristalsis caused by a direct action of the drug on the intestinal smooth muscle. Nausea and vomiting occur in one-third of patients and probably are central in origin. Dizziness, weakness, and prostration may also occur. Other neuromuscular toxic effects are not common but include weakness, myalgias, and stiffness of skeletal muscles. Mild sensory disturbances and tremor may occur. There is some evidence that emetine can block the neuromuscular junction (40); a direct effect on the skeletal muscle of animals has been shown (41). Weakness and muscular pain tend to appear before serious symptoms and may serve as a guide to prevent overdosage.

Cardiovascular toxicity is the most important side effect. Emetine causes a wide range of symptoms, which include hypotension, precordial pain, arrhythmias, tachycardia, and dyspnea. These manifestations may mimic a myocardial infarction. A direct toxic effect of emetine has been shown on cardiac muscle in both animals and humans. Electrocardiographic changes occur in one-fourth to one-half of patients and may serve as an index of cardiac toxicity; the major changes are flattening and inversion of the T waves in all leads and prolongation of the QT interval. Some of these alterations may persist for several weeks after emetine is discontinued. The drug must be stopped as soon as significant electrocardiographic changes occur. Patients receiving this drug should be monitored carefully for such toxicity and should be hospitalized. Emetine is contraindicated in those with heart and kidney disease.

Local reactions to emetine are common and include pain, tenderness, and weakness of the muscles in the area of the injection site. A course of emetine therapy should not be continued for more than 5 days. The daily dose should not exceed 60 mg or the total dose 300 mg. A course should not be repeated until a rest period of at least 6 weeks has intervened. In the treatment of acute amebic dysentery and amebic liver abscess, adults should receive 1 mg/kg/day for 5 days (up to maximum of 60 mg/day) and children should receive 0.5 mg/kg/bid for up to 5 days. When used in amebic liver abscess, it should be given along with chloroquine (42). When used for invasive intestinal amebiasis, it should always be followed by a luminal drug such as diiodohydroxyquin. Its major use is as an alternative to metronidazole. The latter is the preferred agent.

Dehydroemetine Dihydrochloride.* Dehydroemetine dihydrochloride is identical to emetine except for the lack of hydrogen atoms at positions 2 and 3 and is also used in the treatment of invasive amebiasis. It is rarely used in the United States but is available from the Centers for Disease Control. The compound is supplied in a 2-ml ampule containing 30 mg/ml of dehydroemetine dihydrochloride in solution for intramuscular injection. It has the amebicidal properties of emetine but may be somewhat less toxic. Cardiovascular changes have been less frequent and less severe with dehydroemetine (43), but it should nevertheless be used with the same caution as emetine. Its indications and the need for combined or sequential use of other antiamebic drugs are similar to emetine. The dose for adults is 1–1.5 mg/kg/day for up to 5 days (maximum 90 mg/day) and for children 1–1.5 mg/kg/day in two divided doses for up to 5 days with the same maximum daily dose.

Iodoquinol. Iodoquinol (diidohydroxyquin) is a halogenated oxyquinoline (5,7-diiodo-8-hydroxyquinoline) used in the treatment of amebiasis and *Dientamoeba fragilis* and *Balantidium coli* infection. It is available generically in 650 mg tablets and as Yodoxin in both 210 and 650 mg tablets. Iodoquinol is directly amebicidal against both trophozoites and cysts. The mechanism of action in unknown. The drug is not well absorbed and, for this reason, is ineffective against extraintestinal sites of amebiasis.

A related compound, iodochlorhydroxyquin, is absorbed much more readily and has been incriminated as a cause of myelooptic atrophy. As a result, iodochlorhydroxyquin has been removed from use in the United States and should not be prescribed. This syndrome of subacute myelooptic neuropathy was first described in Japan and became almost epidemic before it was discovered to be related to the use of iodochlorhydroxyquin. The discontinuance of the sale of the drug led to an almost immediate reduction in cases of this syndrome. A similar syndrome can occur with other 8-hydroxyquinolines (44), and, for this reason, the drug should not be given for long periods of time.

In the doses recommended for intestinal amebiasis iodoquinol has not been shown to cause optic atrophy. Because it is only slightly absorbed, it has a low order of toxicity and rarely causes abdominal pain, diarrhea, or rash. As with other iodine-containing compounds, it may interfere with the results of thyroid function tests for several months and can cause iodine dermatitis. It is contraindicated in patients with iodine intolerance or hepatic damage.

Because of chemical relationship to iodochlorhydroxyquin some authorities believe that iodoquinol should not be used and diloxanide furoate should be substituted (see below). Iodoquinol is used in the treatment of asymptomatic amebiasis by itself or to follow a more potent drug in symptomatic amebiasis. The dose of iodoquinol in adults is 650 mg tid for 20 days. Children should receive 30–40 mg/kg/day in three doses for 20 days. Similar doses are used for *Dientamoeba fragilis* and *Balantidium coli,* either alone or after a course of tetracycline.

Tetracycline Hydrochloride. Tetracycline hydrochloride is used in the treatment of intestinal amebiasis. It is active against amoebas in the intestinal lumen and wall and is effective by virtue of its modification of the intestinal anaerobic bacterial flora necessary for the amoeba to live. Tetracycline is discussed in Chapter 21. It should not be used alone since relapses are frequent (45). As initial treatment, 250 mg are given qid for 10 days. This usually is followed by a drug that is active against intestinal amoeba. For *Dientamoeba* and *Balantidium* infections, 500 mg qid is given for 10 days.

Diloxanide Furoate*. Diloxanide furoate is a substituted acetanilide, 4(*N*-methyldichloroacetamido)-phenyl-2-furoate. The furoate ester is hydrolyzed after oral ingestion to diloxanide and furoic acid. The former is directly amebicidal in vitro, and the ester is more potent than emetine, being active at concentrations of 0.01–0.1 μg/ml. Its mechanism of action is unclear. Most of an oral dose is excreted in the urine within 48 hours, and peak drug concentrations appear in the plasma within 1 hour. Since most of an oral dose is rapidly absorbed and rapidly excreted in the urine, blood levels fall within 6 hours. There are few serious side effects from this compound. The most commonly observed effect is flatulence or mild abdominal discomfort (46).

Diloxanide furoate is produced in England as Furamide in 500 mg tablets and is regarded as an agent of first choice in the treatment of asymptomatic passers of cysts (47) or in the treatment of invasive and extraintestinal amebiasis only if administered with other appropriate drugs. It is ineffective alone in the treatment of extraintestinal amebiasis. It is only recommended for the asymptomatic or mildly symptomatic intestinal infection and is given in a dose of 500 mg tid for 10 days.

Leishmaniasis

The pentavalent antimonials are less toxic than the formerly used trivalent antimonials, perhaps because the trivalent compounds have a high affinity for cells and leave the plasma very rapidly. Some of the drug is bound to erythrocytes, where it interferes with the function of hemoglobin. The pentavalent antimonials are not bound to erythrocytes and achieve high plasma concentrations. They are excreted more rapidly by the kidney. Up to half of the dose may appear in the urine in 24 hours. When the pentavalent antimonials are given over several days, the plasma concentration and urinary excretion levels of the drug both rise. Increasing amounts of the drug are retained by the patient.

The toxic effects of pentavalent antimonials are less than those that have been associated with the trivalent compounds; however, as the antimony accumulates within the body, the probability of toxic side effects increases. Subsequent courses of therapy also increase the probability of toxic effects, including nausea and vomiting, headache, fainting, abdominal pain, and various rashes. More serious reactions include liver dysfunction, probably because some pentavalent antimony is reduced to trivalent antimony in this organ. Bradycardia and other arrhythmias may occur due to toxic effects of antimony on the myocardium and conducting system. Renal failure is not infrequent and may require discontinuance of the drug. These compounds should be used cautiously in people who have received antimony therapy within 2 months. Antimonials should not be used in patients who manifest cardiac, liver, or renal disease.

Sodium antimony gluconate (Pentostam*, Glucantime) is a powder that is readily soluble in water and contains approximately 30 percent pentavalent antimony. The antimony content varies from one batch to another, and the dose for a patient must be calculated on the basis of the amount of antimony in the material being used. The drug is available in an aqueous solution for parenteral administration and, in the United States, may be obtained from the Centers for Disease Control. The compound may be given either intravenously or by the intramuscular route. The dose is based on antimony content and varies from one form of the disease to another. Treatment is discussed extensively in Chapter 233.

Since the toxicity of pentavalent antimonials is related to the duration of therapy, attempts have been made to shorten the course of therapy (48). This has met with some success but cannot yet be recommended for general use. The current treatment of leishmaniasis has been reviewed by Marsden (49) and, more recently, by Marr (50).

Amphotericin B is a second-line drug and is discussed in Chapter 16.

Trypanosomiasis

American trypanosomiasis, Chagas' disease, is treated quite differently from the African trypanosomiasis. The compounds used for the former are not active in the latter and vice versa. All agents used for the treatment of trypanosomiasis are quite toxic to the host and often must be discontinued because of their inherent toxicity.

American Trypanosomiasis (Chagas' Disease). Nifurtimox* is a nitrofuran derivative that has been shown to be effective in acute Chagas' disease. There have been a significant number of failures in the treatment of acute Chagas' disease with this drug. The results of therapy depend on the South American region that is studied. This is undoubtedly due to variations of both parasite and the host (51). In certain areas, progression from the acute to the chronic disease is uncommon, and in others it is commonplace. For this reason, reports on effectiveness of treatment must be considered carefully. In some areas, treatment results in disappearance of parasitemia and amelioration of symptoms in 80 percent or more of those treated. These results have been described in Argentina, southern Brazil, Chile, and Venezuela. In the central sections of Brazil, the results have been much poorer. Efficacy in chronic Chagas' disease has not been established.

Nifurtimox is manufactured in Germany under the name Lampit. Only low concentrations are found in the blood and tissues. It has many toxic effects, and the incidence of these is high, 40–70 percent of patients. Most of the symptoms are related to the central nervous system and the gastrointestinal tract. Nausea and vomiting are common, as are weight loss and significant myalgias with stiffness and weakness. Convulsions may occur. The drug may have to be given with anticonvulsants.

Therapy must be monitored carefully and patients given symptomatic treatment for relief of side effects. It is not uncommon for treatment to be halted because of the severity of these effects. Unfortunately, since the disease is often progressive, the toxic effects must be suppressed and treatment continued.

African Trypanosomiasis. Melarsoprol* (Mel B) is an organic compound of arsenic, melarsen oxide, coupled to dimercaprol (BAL) to reduce toxicity, and is the drug of choice in late African trypanosomiasis with central nervous system involvement (52). It is a trivalent arsenical and the mechanism of action is presumed to be the inactivation of enzymes of glycolysis by combining with sulfhydryl groups of these proteins. Its differential toxicity may be due to the fact that it penetrates the parasite more readily than host cells. The drug is administered intravenously by slow injection and penetrates the central nervous system and cerebrospinal fluid. Side effects are common (53), with encephalopathy being the most frequent. Clinical manifestations of encephalopathy appear rapidly during the first 3–4 days of treatment. Agents that bind heavy metals, such as dimercaprol, do not reverse this process. The encephalopathy occurs more often and to a greater degree in patients with more severe infection of the CSF. Other toxic effects include myocardial damage, renal failure, hypertension, and peripheral neuropathy (52). Hypersensitivity reactions are not uncommon and occur during subsequent courses of treatment. It may be necessary to desensitize the patient for a second course of therapy by using small doses and increasing them gradually. Corticosteroids may be needed to control the hypersensitivity reaction.

Because of its ability to penetrate the CSF, melarsoprol is the drug of choice in the treatment of meningoencephalitis caused by the African trypanosomes. It is active against both East and West African varieties. But, because of its toxicity, it is usually reserved for the management of patients in the later and more severe stages of the disease. For this same reason it is not used for prophylaxis. In the severely debilitated patient pretreatment with Suramin is indicated to decrease toxicity (52). For adults, 3.6 mg/kg/day intravenously is given for three doses; after 1 week this course is repeated and is repeated again after 10–21 days. Children should receive a 18–25 mg/kg total dose over 1 month; an initial dose of 0.36 mg/kg IV, increasing gradually to max 3.6 mg/kg; a total of 9–10 doses IV is then given at 1- to 5-day intervals, depending on reactions.

Suramin.* Suramin is a synthetic urea compound, that is the drug of choice for therapy of early Rhodesian sleeping sickness when the central nervous system is not involved (52) and for the destruction of adult worms in onchocerciasis (54). It is a dye known to inhibit a variety of enzyme systems although its mechanism of action is unclear. Since it is a polyanion, it forms complexes with some proteins. Exposure of trypanosomes to suramin results in the loss of intracellular membranes (55) (Fig. 7).

The compound is given by slow intravenous injection and achieves high concentrations in the plasma. There is a rapid distribution and then a slow elimination phase. Low concentrations are present for as long as 3 months. The persistence of the drug in the plasma is due to its binding to proteins. For this reason, it is effective in prophylaxis of both East and West African trypanosomiasis, since the protein-bound drug dissociates slowly to yield effective concentra-

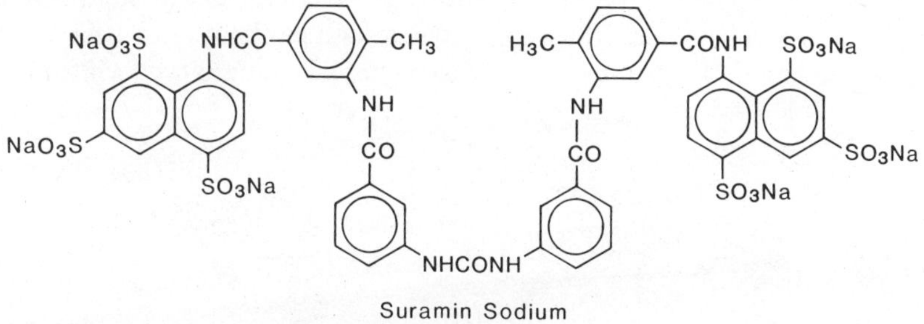

FIGURE 7. Suramin sodium.

tions over a long period of time. The compound enters tissues very poo ly and does not enter the CSF in any appreciable concentration. For this reason, it is not used for treatment of African trypanosomiasis when there is CSF involvement. The kidneys retain more suramin than other organs (in experimental animals), and this may account for the relatively common occurrence of acute renal failure when the drug is used in humans. In addition to its renal toxicity, suramin has a variety of other toxic effects. These are more pronounced in malnourished populations. The most serious reactions are nausea and vomiting, shock, and loss of consciousness. It also can give rise to pruritus, urticaria, fever, paresthesias, and hyperesthesia of the palms and soles (54).

Surimin is used in the treatment of both East and West African sleeping sickness and is effective only in the early stages of the disease. In the late stages, when central nervous system involvement has occurred, suramin is used before a course of arsenical treatment since it is less toxic, and then melarsoprol is given, since it penetrates the CSF.

The drug powder must be mixed into a solution with 5 ml of distilled water immediately before use and should not be stored for more than 30 minutes. A 100- to 200-mg intravenous dose to test for sensitivity should be given initially. Idiosyncracy may lead to circulatory collapse, and deaths have occurred from immediate hypersensitivity (54). In the hemolymphatic stage of African trypanosomiasis, 1 g is given IV on days 1,3,7,14, and 21. Children receive 20 mg/kg on the same schedule. In late disease with CNS involvement, adults are given 10 mg/kg IV every 5 days for a total of 12 injections. A second course of treatment should not be given earlier than 3 months after the first. For treatment of onchocerciasis after a test dose, the dose is 1 g IV in adults and 20 mg/kg IV in children once weekly for 5–6 weeks after initial treatment with diethylcarbamazine. In the United States, the risk of severe toxicity from suramin in the face of usually light onchocerciasis infections (without ocular involvement) makes suramin very rarely indicated.

Pentamidine Isethionate*. Pentamidine isethionate is effective in the treatment of early cases of East and West African sleeping sickness and has been used for prophylaxis against *Trypanosoma gambiense.* This compound is the most valuable member of the diamidine group of drugs because of its stability, relative low toxicity (compared to the others in this group), and ease of administration (Fig. 8). A closely related compound, hydroxystilbamidine, has been used in the management of North American blastomycosis. Pentamidine is white powder

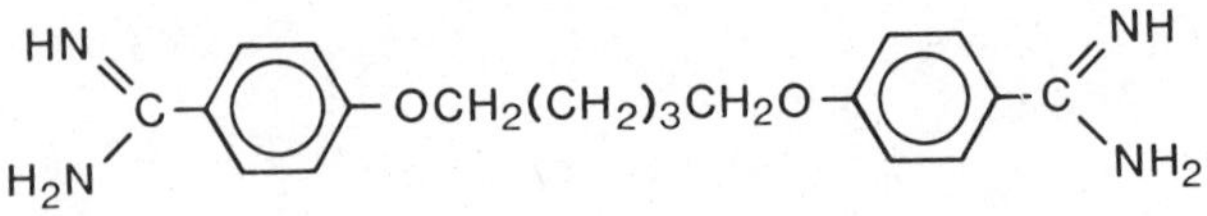

Pentamidine

FIGURE 8. Pentamidine.

marketed in ampules containing 200 mg of the isethionate or as methanesulfonate in ampules with 120 mg base. The diamidines are toxic to a variety of protozoans, although there is a remarkable variation in susceptibility across species lines. The mechanism of action of pentamidine is unclear, but diamidines are known to bind to DNA, particularly that of the trypanosomal kinetoplast, where they may inhibit its replication (56). The major uses of pentamidine are in the management of African trypanosomiasis and *Pneumocystis carinii* pneumonitis.

The administration of pentamidine is associated with significant adverse effects, which include renal failure, liver dysfunction, profound hypoglycemia, hypotension, hypocalcemia, rashes, and a variety of hematologic disorders (57). It must be used with caution and under close medical supervision. The drug is well absorbed from intramuscular sites but is detected in the blood for only a relatively short time. It does not enter the CSF and cannot be given intrathecally. For this reason it is not used to treat the neurologic stage of African trypanosomiasis nor in the treatment of trypanosomiasis caused by *Trypanosoma rhodesiense* because of the rapidity with which the organism may invade the CNS. In the management of African trypanosomiasis caused by *T. gambiense,* the drug is given by intramuscular injection in doses of 4 mg/kg (or, with methanesulfonate, 3 mg base/kg) daily or on alternate days. In the treatment of early disease, 10 injections usually are given. Pentamidine has a greater use as a prophylactic agent in endemic areas. When used in this fashion, it is given as a single intramuscular injection at 6-month intervals at a dose of 3–5 mg/kg.

In the management of *Pneumocystis* pneumonitis, the drug usually is administered as an intramuscular injection of 4 mg/kg per day for 2 weeks. In severe cases, it may be given as a slow intravenous injection, but this is associated with a high proportion of adverse reactions.

Coccidiosis

Human coccidiosis is an inflammatory disease of the small bowel caused by *Isospora belli.* This parasite is a sporozoan which undergoes asexual reproduction in the intestinal epithelial cells and has a life cycle analogous to the malarial parasite. Many therapeutic agents have been used, generally with little success. Furazolidone, 100 mg qid for 10 days, has been used for treatment, although it is considered an experimental drug for this purpose. Furazolidone is discussed in the section on giardiasis. Trimethoprim-sulfamethoxazole is also recommended; the dosage is given in Table 1.

Giardiasis

This ubiquitous protozoan organism is a major cause of waterborne gastrointestinal disease throughout the world. Like the amoeba, it has both a trophozooite and a cyst form. Unlike the amoeba, only the trophozooite form is addressed therapeutically.

Quinacrine Hydrochloride. Quinacrine hydrochloride is a bright yellow acridine dye, 3-chloro-7-methoxy-9-(1-methyl-4-diethylamino-butylamino) acridine (Fig. 9). It was originally used as an antimalarial, but its primary indication now is for treatment of giardiasis (37). The mechanism of action is unclear, but this compound, like many similar antimalarials, intercalates into DNA. It is absorbed readily from the intestinal tract and is distributed widely in the tissues. Since it is lost from the body very slowly, it accumulates when administered chronically. Quinacrine can be detected in the urine for at least two months after therapy is discontinued. It may color the urine yellow and, in larger doses, may color the skin and sclerae as well. The drug has been available since World War II and was used extensively at that time as an antimalarial agent. For this reason data on its toxicity are well documented. Quinacrine hydrochloride commonly causes headache, dizziness, and vomiting. Skin rashes, including urticaria and exofoliative dermatitis, may occur. In the larger doses used in the past for the treatment of cestode infections, transitory toxic psychoses were seen. In the smaller doses used for the treatment of giardiasis this reaction is uncommon. Toxic psychoses may occur in 1–2 percent of those receiving quinacrine for giardiasis, but this side effect is self-limited and lasts usually 2–4 weeks. Quinacrine should not be given to patients receiving antimalarial therapy with primaquine, since concurrent administration results in a greatly increased drug concentration of the latter (or any other 8-aminoquinoline) in the plasma and enhances its toxicity. Since quinacrine crosses the the placenta, it should not be given to pregnant women. Quinacrine and other antimalarial compounds should be used cautiously in patients with psoriasis. Exacerbations of the underlying disease occur in the presence of these drugs and exofoliative dermatitis can develop. Quinacrine is also known as mepracrine hydrochloride and has the trade name Atabrine, which is produced in 100 mg tablets. For treatment of giardiasis in adults and children above 8 years of age, the dose is 100 mg tid for 7 days. For younger children who often do not tolerate it well, the dose is 2 mg/kg tid for 5 days.

Furazolidone. Furazolidone is a nitrofuran derivative, 3-[(5-nitrofurfurylidene)amino]-2-oxazolidinone, used in the treatment of giardiasis (37). It is marketed as Furoxone in 100-mg tablets and as a liquid in combination with colloidal kaolin and citrus pectin. The latter is particularly useful in treating infants

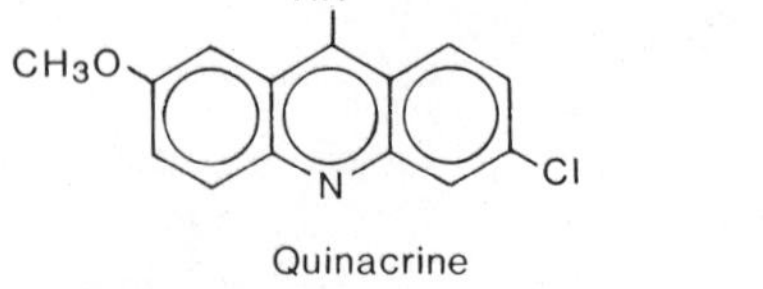

FIGURE 9. Quinacrine.

and young children with giardiasis since it is the only available antigiardia drug in the United States produced as a liquid. Furazolidone can produce a disulfiram-type reaction when taken with alcohol and is also a monamine oxidase inhibitor. Occasional hypersensitivity reactions may occur: hypotension, urticaria, fever, arthralgia, nausea, vomiting, and headache. Furazolidone may cause mild hemolysis in glucose-6-phosphate-dehydrogenase-deficient persons. Metabolic degradation products may give a brown color to the urine. The dosage for adults is 100 mg qid for 7 days. Children should receive 1.25 mg/kg four times a day, but the drug should not be given to nursing mothers or infants under 1 month of age. Furazolidone has shown some beneficial effect in symptomatic intestinal coccidiosis infections, in doses similar to those used in giardiasis. Because of furazolidone's toxicity, metronidazole (discussed in the section on amebiasis) or quinacrine are preferred to furazolidone in the treatment of giardiasis.

Pneumocystis

Pneumocystis carinii is a poorly understood pathogen which is considered, on morphologic grounds, to be a protozoan. The organism, as encountered in hospitalized patients, causes pneumonitis in the immunocompromised host. This is considered to represent activation of a pathogen already present in a dormant state; however, the organism clearly is transmissible from human to human as demonstrated by outbreaks in Europe among malnourished infants and children following World War II (58).

Pentamidine isethionate was the first drug used to treat pneumonitis caused by this organism (59). Although it is a toxic compound, it is quite effective. This agent is discussed in the section on trypanosomiasis.

Trimethoprim-sulfamethoxazole (TMP-SMZ) has been shown to be efficacious (60–64) and is discussed in Chapter 27. TMP 20 mg/kg per day; SMZ, 100 mg/kg per day in 3–4 divided doses is given orally or intravenously. This regimen provides cures in 70–80 percent of patients (63,64). Hughes and coworkers (65) have shown that this combination is effective in chemoprophylaxis of leukemic and other immunosuppressed cancer patients against *P. carinii* infections. Long-term therapy with 150 mg/M^2 of TMP and 750 mg/M^2 SMZ daily in two divided doses virtually eliminated this infection from a population of children with leukemia.

Toxoplasmosis

Toxoplasmosis is caused by an obligate intracellular protozoan, *Toxoplasma gondii.* It is a coccidian and is classified among the Sporozoa. The cyst form of *T. gondii* in the brain is resistant to available chemotherapeutic agents. Pyrimethamine and sulfonamides both are active against the trophozoite and are synergistic (66). Pyrimethamine is discussed in the section on malaria. When used in the treatment of toxoplasmosis, a loading dose of 100–200 mg po of pyrimethamine is given in two divided doses to adults. This provides high blood levels quickly. The maintenance dose for adults is 25 mg given every 12, 24, or 48 hours, depending on severity of the infection (67).

In children twice the daily dose (2 mg/kg) is given as a loading dose for the first 2–3 days of treatment and 1 mg/kg per day thereafter. Administration at 3-to 4-day intervals has been suggested in neonates and infants since the half-life of the drug is 4–5 days. Patients treated with this drug should have peripheral blood cell and platelet counts to anticipate bone marrow suppression. Should this occur, it is a reversible, dose-related effect and may be treated with folinic acid IM or po in doses of 2–10 mg per day.

Sulfadiazine is the most active sulfonamide against this organism and is given in conjunction with pyrimethamine. The reader is referred to Chapter 13 for a discussion of this agent. The usual dose of sulfadiazine for the treatment of this infection in adults is 75–100 mg/kg per day in four divided doses. A loading dose of 50–75 mg/kg is used. In infants, the dose is 100–150 mg/kg per day in four equal doses with a loading dose of 75–100 mg/kg.

Trichomoniasis

See metronidazole in the section on amebiasis.

METAZOANS

Many of the agents used in the past for the treatment of metazoan infestations have been superseded by relatively few newer drugs.

Intestinal Nematodes

The intestinal roundworms generally are treated with agents that are relatively nontoxic. There are three drugs in common use in the United States.

Mebendazole. Mebendazole is a synthetic benzimidazole, methyl 5-benzoyl-5-benzoyl benzimidazole-2-carbamate, and is a broad-spectrum antihelmintic used in the treatment of trichuriasis (68), ascariasis (68), enterobiasis (69), and hookworm (70) infections. It is effective in strongyloidiasis (71) and in tapeworm infections (72) (Fig. 10). Mebendazole is a very effective and broad-spectrum antihelminthic agent. It appears to act through its ability to inhibit glucose uptake in the parasite, since it does not affect glucose concentration in the host, even at high doses (73). The parasites are immobilized and are cleared from the gastrointestinal tract. This clearance does not take place rapidly and may not be complete until several days after treatment. It is known to inhibit the development of hookworm larvae in vitro but has no effect on fully formed larvae. The eggs of hookworms and of *Trichuris* do not develop to the larval

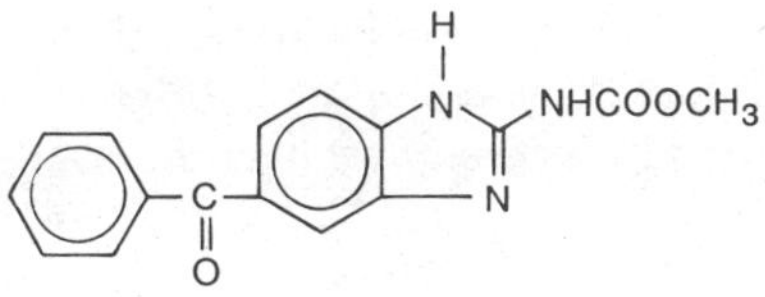

Mebendazole

FIGURE 10. Mebendazole.

stage after exposure to this drug (74). Mebendazole is given in 100 mg tablets, but only a small proportion of the dose is absorbed. Most of that is recovered in the urine within 24–48 hours as a decarboxylated metabolic product. It has little systemic toxicity, probably as a result of its poor absorption. Abdominal pain and diarrhea may occur, especially in cases of massive infestation. Since it has teratogenic effects in pregnant animals, it should not be given to pregnant women nor to children under the age of 2. For the treatment of trichuriasis, ascariasis, and hookworm infections, both adults and children receive a dose of 100 mg bid for 3 days. For enterobiasis, a single 100-mg tablet is taken, and a similar dose is repeated 2 weeks later.

Thiabendazole. Thiabendazole is one of the most potent antihelminthic agents known and is active against both larvae and adult worms. It is a broad-spectrum antihelminthic compound, 2-(4′-thiazolyl)-1H-benzimidazole (75), used in the treatment of strongyloidiasis (76), trichostrongyliasis (76), cutaneous larva migrans (77), and visceral larva migrans (77) (Fig. 11).

Although it possesses a high degree of activity against many nematodes, its mechanism of action is unknown. The compound inhibits the helminth fumarate reductase, and this may be important in preventing the organism from eliminating reducing equivalents as succinic acid. It is larvicidal in vitro at very low concentrations (as low as one ppm) (78–80). It is marketed in 500-mg tablets and as a suspension of 500 mg/5 ml. After oral administration, it is rapidly absorbed and achieves peak concentrations in the plasma within about 1 hour. Most of the drug is excreted in the urine within 24 hours as an hydroxylated derivative. The most frequently encountered side effects are nausea, vomiting, dizziness, and anorexia. Occasionally epigastric pain and diarrhea occur. Much less common side effects occur that may be related to the central nervous system, including tinnitus, paresthesias of the eyes, numbness, and drowsiness. For these rea-

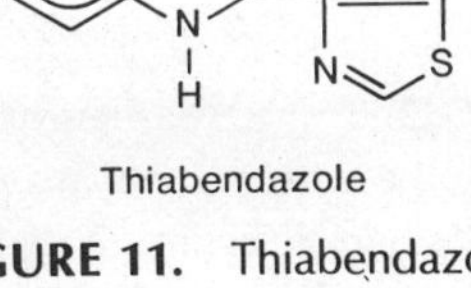

Thiabendazole

FIGURE 11. Thiabendazole.

sons, people taking this drug should avoid activities that require mental alertness. Since there may be changes in liver function tests while taking this drug, it should be used with caution in persons with liver disease. Symptoms of hypersensitivity reactions include fever, conjunctival injection, angioneurotic edema, perianal rash, and skin rashes. It is unclear whether these represent hypersensitivity to the drug or hypersensitivity to the parasite.

The drug should be given after meals and the maximum daily recommended dose is 3 g. The usual dose for strongyloidiasis and trichostrongyliasis is 25 mg/kg given twice a day for 2 days. In disseminated strongyloidiasis, therapy should be continued for at least 5 days. For cutaneous larva migrans, similar oral doses are taken for 2 days. Alternatively, thiabendazole suspension may be applied locally to the lesion (77). In visceral larva migrans, 25 mg/kg bid is given for 5 days. Thiabendazole has been used in trichinosis infections, but its effect on larvae in muscle is thought to be more anti-inflammatory than lethal (81,82).

Piperazine Citrate. Piperazine citrate is a salt of piperazine (diethylenediamine) and is used in the treatment of ascariasis and enterobiasis. It has been replaced by other drugs (see above), but, because of its effect on the worms, it is useful in certain situations. The predominant effect of piperazine on *Ascaris* is to produce a flaccid paralysis so that intestinal peristalsis can eliminate it. This property may be useful when the worms create an obstructing lesion either in the upper intestine or the biliary tract. Piperazine blocks the action of acetylcholine on the muscle of the worm by producing hyperpolarization and suppression of spontaneous action potentials (83). It is readily absorbed from the gastrointestinal tract and excreted as unchanged drug and as metabolic products. Piperazine has a wide therapeutic index and shows only occasional gastrointestinal upset. Transient neurologic effects have been described. Epilepsy may be exaggerated, and alternative drugs should be used in epileptic patients (84). Visual disturbances, ataxia, and hypotonia have occurred rarely (85).

Piperazine salts are available as 500-mg tablets and suspensions of 100 mg/ml. For treatment of ascariasis, both adults and children receive 75 mg/kg/day (maximum of 3.5 g) for 2 days.

Blood and Tissue Nematodes

A single agent, diethylcarbamazine, is effective for most of the blood and tissue nematodes. *Onchocera volvulus,* in certain severe cases, may require supplemental therapy with suramin (see above). Trichinosis is managed with thiabendazole (see above).

Diethlycarbamazine Citrate. Diethlycarbamazine citrate is a piperazine derivative, *N,N*-diethyl-4-methyl-1-piperazinecarboxamide dihydrogen citrate, used in the treatment of filariasis and as an alternative drug in the treatment of visceral larva migrans (Fig. 12). It is readily absorbed from the gastrointestinal tract,

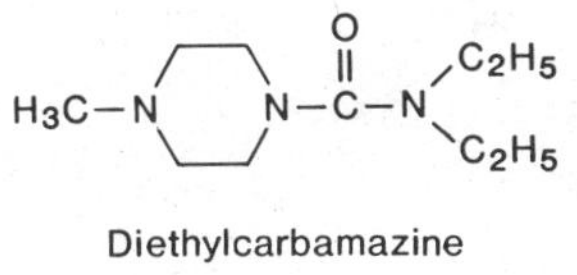

FIGURE 12. Diethylcarbamazine.

and after a single oral dose, peak blood concentration occurs within 3 hours. The drug disappears from the circulation within 48 hours, primarily in the urine and generally as metabolic products. It is distributed equally throughout all body compartments, except for fat, and there is little accumulation even with repeated dosage.

Diethylcarbamazine kills microfilariae of all species found in humans. There is presumptive evidence that it kills adult worms of *Wuchereria bancrofti* and *Brugia malayi.* Repeated courses are often necessary to kill *Loa-loa* and *Acanthocheilonema perstans* adult worms. It has relatively little action on adult *Onchocerca volvulus.* A 50- to 100-mg dose of diethylcarbamazine is used as a provocative test for onchocerciasis, the Mazzotti reaction (86), and a 200-mg dose has been used to increase the number of circulating microfilariae of *W. bancrofti* for diagnosis (87). Common side effects include headache, dizziness, nausea, and fever. Rapid destruction of microfilariae in the early days of treatment may cause allergic reactions, including exacerbation of rash and pruritus in onchocerciasis (86), lymphadenopathy and nodular swellings along the course of lymphatics in bancroftian and Malayan filariasis, and, rarely, encephalopathy in patients with heavy *Loa-loa* infections (88).

In order to decrease these initial reactions, particularly in onchocerciasis with ocular involvement, the initial daily dose should be small and should be increased gradually to the maximum daily recommended dose. Symptoms tend to persist for 3–7 days and then subside; after this, normal doses of the drug can be tolerated without further reaction. Leukocytosis and eosinophilia may appear or be intensified during the early stages of drug treatment. In the treatment of onchocerciasis, an initial 25 mg/day dose is given for 3 days and then increased to 50 mg/day for 5 days, then 100 mg/day for 3 days, then 150 mg/day for 12 days. In the treatment of *Loa loa* infection and *A. perstans,* the regimen is as follows: Day 1, 50 mg; day 2, 50 mg tid; day 3, 100 mg tid; days 4–21, 2 mg/kg tid. In other forms of filariasis and in tropical pulmonary eosinophilia, 2 mg/kg tid for 7–10 days is given to both adults and children. Antihistamines or corticosteroids may be required to control allergic reactions, particularly in onchocerciasis and bancroftian filariasis. Diethylcarbamazine in a dose of 2–4 mg/kg tid for 4 weeks has been used as an alternative treatment for visceral larva migrans with variable success (89).

Tapeworms

Although other agents are available, a single drug, niclosamide, has become the drug of choice for all of the tapeworms.

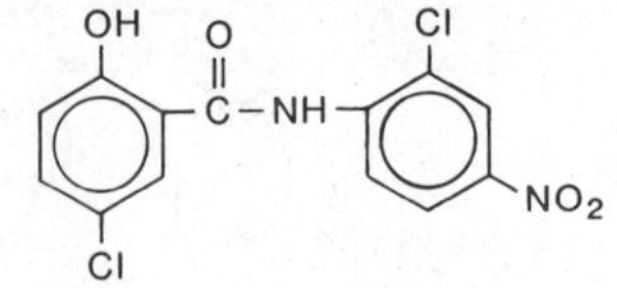

Niclosamide

FIGURE 13. Niclosamide.

Niclosamide. Niclosamide is *N*-(2′-chloro-4′-nitrophenyl)-5-chlorosalicylamide (90) (Fig. 13). The drug is available as Niclocide (Yomesan) from Miles Pharmaceuticals, 400 Morgan Lane, West Haven, CT, 06516. Niclosamide inhibits oxidative phosphorylation in the mitochondria of cestodes and kills, on contact, the scolices and proximal segments. The scolex is often disintegrated and difficult to identify. The worm is released and rapidly passed, often partially disintegrated and yellow-stained. Niclosamide is very well tolerated, rarely causing minor gastrointestinal disturbances. There are no contraindications to its use. As niclosamide does not kill cestode ova, cysticercosis is theoretically possible after treatment of *Taenia solium* infections, but as yet no cases have been recognized. To prevent this theoretic possibility, some authorities recommend a purge 2 hours after treatment of *Taenia solium* infections to eliminate all mature segments before ova can be released. For treatment of *T. saginata, T. solium,* and *Diphyllobothrium latum* infections, adults take a single dose of 2 g (4 tablets chewed thoroughly). Children weighing 11–34 kg take a single dose of 1 g, and those children above 34 kg take a single dose of 1.5 g. For *Hymenolepis nana* infections, these same doses are taken for 5 consecutive days.

Flukes

The drug of choice for the treatment of liver and intestinal flukes is praziquantel. This agent is discussed in the section on schistosomiasis.

Schistosomiasis

Current therapy for schistosomiasis rests on three compounds: metrifonate, oxamniquine, and praziquantel. The first is active only against *Schistosoma haematobium;* the second is active against *Schistosoma mansoni;* the last, praziquantel, is active against *Schistosoma japonicum* as well as the other two species.

Metrifonate. Metrifonate (Fig. 14) is an organophosphate that is metabolized in humans to dichlorvos (91). The latter is a cholinesterase inhibitor and probably acts by inhibiting this enzyme in the schistosome. It is active only against *S. haematobium.* When given to humans, this drug causes a decrease of 95 percent in plasma cholinesterase activity within 6 hours of administration. This usually returns to normal relatively quickly. Erythrocyte cholinesterase is inhibited to approximately 50 percent of pretreatment values but takes much longer to return

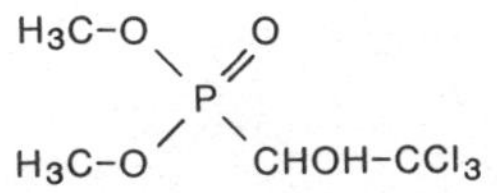

Metrifonate

FIGURE 14. Metrifonate

to normal levels, approximately 2 or 2½ months. Although tolerance to the drug usually is good, nausea, vomiting, and, occasionally, bronchospasm have been reported. Metrifonate is given in three doses at intervals of 2 weeks. Each dose is7.5–10 mg/kg. The cure rate is 70–80 percent.

Oxamniquine. Oxamniquine (Fig. 15) is a tetrahydroquinoline active against *S. mansoni* and appears to be more effective against strains of the worm present in the western hemisphere (92,93). The side effects are usually mild and may be decreased by giving the drug after meals. These effects include dizziness, which may occur in as many as 40 percent of the treated population. Seizures occasionally have been reported, so any patient with a history of a seizure disorder should be controlled before oxamniquine is given. The drug is given as a single oral dose of 15 mg/kg in adults; in children a slightly higher dose of 20 mg/kg has been shown to be more effective. Some strains of *S. mansoni* found in Africa are less sensitive, and a total dosage of 60 mg/kg, given over 2 days, is necessary to achieve the same effects as the lower dose used in treating strains in the western hemisphere (94,95). Oxamniquine has received wide use in Brazil, where a control program based on community therapy was quite successful (96).

Praziquantel. Praziquantel (Fig. 16) is the newest antischistosomal agent and may develop into the most important drug (97,98). Unlike metrifonate and oxamniquine, each of which is active against a single species of schistosome, it is active against all three species. In addition, it is active against cestodes and other flukes that are usually found in Asian populations: *Clonorchis sinensis (Opisthorchis sinensis), Opisthorchis viverrini,* and the lung fluke *Paragonimus westermani.* The use of praziquantel in treating diseases caused by these flukes is experimental, and the dosages for the drug, given here are estimates based on experimental studies and may be changed in the future. This agent is a mixture of the stereoisomers of prazinoisoquinolines. The mode of action is unknown, but praziquantel causes a tetanic contraction of the musculature of

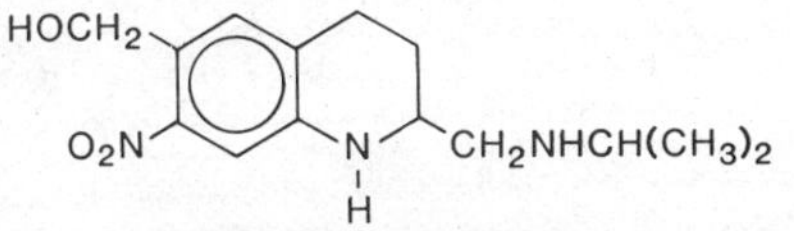

Oxamniquine

FIGURE 15. Oxamniquine.

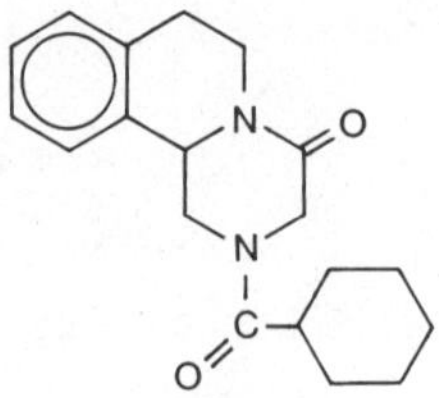

FIGURE 16. Praziquantel.

the fluke within minutes after exposure. The available evidence indicates that this reaction is due to a rapid influx of calcium into the worm (JL Bennett, personal communication). For treatment of *S. mansoni* and *S. haematobium*, praziquantel is given in a single dose of 40 mg/kg; treatment of *S. japonicum* requires higher doses, usually 20 mg/kg given three times at 4 hour intervals (99,100). The side effects occur shortly after therapy, often within 1 hour, and resolve within 48 hours. These side effects include nausea, vomiting, and abdominal pain. Since these discomforts are relatively mild, the drug can be used in community control efforts (100). Praziquantel is available from Miles Pharmaceuticals, West Haven, CT 06516.

Niridazole. Niridazole is a nitrothiazole derivative, 1-(5-nitro-2-thiazolyl)-2-imidazolidinone, used orally for the treatment of *S. haematobium* and *S. mansoni* infections (101) (Fig. 17). It is somewhat more effective for the former than for the latter (102). It is also effective in the treatment of dracunculiasis (guinea worm disease) (101), where it acts by reducing swelling and pain and permits relatively easy extraction of worms. It acts after concentration in the adult worms, by inhibiting phosphorylase inactivation, which causes glycogen depletion in the parasite. Niridazole also causes depletion of egg-shell substance in the vitelline glands of the female worm. Ultimately the size of the ovary decreases. In the male, spermatogenesis is halted, and obstruction of the testes follows (103).

Minor side effects occur more commonly in adults than in children. These include gastrointestinal disturbance, headache, rash, myalgia, and arthralgias. ECG changes may occur. The urine may become dark brown from a metabolite, and an unpleasant odor may be noticed. Hemolysis can be provoked in glucose-

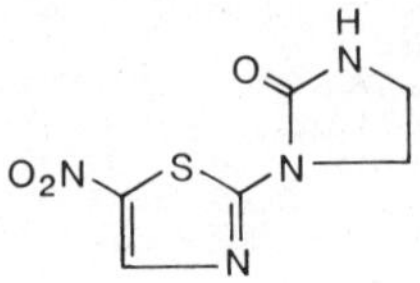

FIGURE 17. Niridazole.

6-phosphate dehydrogenase-deficient persons (104). Niridazole should not be used in patients with hepatic dysfunction or neuropsychiatric disorders, since hallucinations or psychosis may develop (105). For treatment of schistosomiasis, both adults and children should receive 25 mg/kg/day orally, divided into morning and evening doses taken after meals, with a maximum daily dose of 1500 mg. The same dose is used for the treatment of dracunculiasis and continued 10 days.

REFERENCES

1. Thompson PE, Werbel LM: *Antimalarial Agents: Chemistry and Pharmacology*. New York, Academic Press, 1972, p 172.
2. Warhurst DC, Thomas SC: The chemotherapy of rodent malaria. XXXI. The effect of some metabolic inhibitors upon chloroquine-induced pigment clumping in *Plasmodium berghei*. *Ann Trop Med Parasitol* 72:203, 1978.
3. Banyal HS, Fitch CD: Ferriprotoporphyrin IX-binding substances in the mode of action of chloroquine against malaria. *Life Sci* 31:1141, 1982.
4. Davidson MW, Griggs BG Jr, Boykin DW, et al: Mefloquine: A clinically useful quinolinemethanol antimalarial which does not significantly bind to DNA. *Nature* 254:632, 1975.
5. Appleton B, Wolfe MS, Mishtowt GI: Chloroquine as a malarial suppressive. Absence of visual effects. *Milit Med* 138:225, 1973.
6. Miller LH, Neva F, Gill F: Failure of chloroquine in human babesiosis (*Babesia microti*): Case report and chemotherapeutic trial in hamsters. *Ann Intern Med* 88:200, 1978.
7. Trenholme GM, Williams RL, Desjardins RE, et al: Mefloquine in the treatment of human malaria. *Science* 190:792, 1975.
8. Wyler DJ: Malaria-resurgence, resistance, and research. *N Engl J Med* 308:875, 1983.
9. Desjardins RE, Pamplin CL, von Bredow J, et al: Kinetics of a new antimalarial, mefloquine. *Clin Pharmacol Ther* 26:372, 1979.
10. Berman SJ, Holmes KK: Gametocytemia in falciparum malaria. Eradication of gametocytemia with primaquine. *JAMA* 215:291, 1971.
11. Tarlov AR, Brewer GJ, Carson PE, and Alving AS: Primaquine sensitivity. *Arch Intern Med* 109:209, 1962.
12. Beutler E: Drug-induced hemolytic anemia. *Pharmacol Rev* 21:73, 1969.
13. Clyde DE, McCarthy VC: Radical cure of Chesson strain vivax malaria in man by 7, not 14, days of treatment with primaquine. *Am J Trop Med Hyg* 26:562, 1977.
14. Hall AP: The treatment of malaria. *Br Med J* 1:323, 1976.
15. Powell RD, McNamara JV: Quinine side effects and plasma levels. *Proc Helminth Soc Wash* 39:331, 1972.
16. Brodie BB, Baer, JE, Craig LC: Metabolic products of the cinchona alkaloids in human urine. *J Biol Chem* 188:567, 1951.
17. White NJ, Looareesuwan S, Warrell DA, et al: Quinine pharmacokinetics and toxicity in cerebral and uncomplicated falciparum malaria. *Am J Med* 73:564, 1982.
18. Canfield CJ, Miller LH, Bastelloni PJ, et al: Acute renal failure in Plasmodium falciparum malaria. *Arch Intern Med* 122:199, 1968.
19. Centers for Disease Control: Chemoprophylaxis of malaria. *Morbid Mortal Weekly Rep* 27(suppl):82, 1978.
20. Frenkel JK, Weber RW, Lunde MN: Acute toxoplasmosis: Effective treatment with pyrimethamine, sulfadiazine, leucovorin calcium, and yeast. *JAMA* 173:1471, 1960.
21. Lucas AO, Hendrickse RG, Okubadego OA, et al: The suppression of malarial parasitemia by pyrimethamine in a combination with dapsone or sulphormethoxine. *Trans Roy Soc Trop Med Hyg* 63:216, 1969.

22. Hitchings GH, Burchall JJ: Inhibition of folate biosynthesis and function as a basis for chemotherapy. *Adv Enzymol* 27:417, 1965.
23. Doberstyn EB, Phintuyothin P, Noeypatimanondh S, et al: Single-dose therapy of falciparum malaria with mefloquine or pyrimethamine-sulfadoxine. *Bull WHO* 57:275, 1979.
24. Hurwitz ES, Johnson D, Campbell CC: Resistance of *Plasmodium falciparum* malaria to sulfadoxine-pyrimethamine (Fansidar) in a refugee camp in Thailand. *Lancet* 1:1068, 1981.
25. Darlow B, Vrbova H, Stace J, et al: Fansidar-resistant falciparum malaria in Papua, New Guinea. *Lancet* 2:1243, 1980.
26. Rumans LW, Dennis DT, Atmosoedjono S: Fansidar-resistant falciparum malaria in Indonesia. *Lancet* 2:580, 1979.
27. Lindmark DG, Muller M: Antitrichomonad action, mutagenicity, and reduction of metronidazole and other nitroimadazoles. *Antimicrob Agents Chemother* 10:476, 1976.
28. Knight RC, Skolimowski IM, Edwards DI. The interaction of reduced metronidazole with DNA. *Biochem Pharmacol* 27:2089, 1978.
29. LaRusso NF, Tomaz M, Muller M, Lipman R: Interaction of metronidazole with nucleic acids in vitro. *Mol Pharmacol* 13:872, 1977.
30. Ralph ED, Clarke JT, Libke RD, et al: Pharmacokinetics of metronidazole as determined by bioassay. *Antimicrob Agents Chemother* 6:691, 1974.
31. Schwartz DE, Jeunet F: Comparative pharmacokinetic studies of ornidazole and metronidazole in man. *Chemotherapy* 22:19, 1976.
32. Kazmier FJ: A significant interaction between metronidazole and warfarin. *Mayo Clin Proc* 51:782, 1976.
33. Speck WT, Stein AB, Rosenkranz HS: Mutagenicity of metronidazole: Presence of several active metabolites in human urine. *J Natl Cancer Inst* 56:283, 1976.
34. Roe FJC: Metronidazole: Review of its uses and toxicity. *J Antimicrob Chemother* 3:205, 1977.
35. Spillman R, Ayala S, DeSanchez CE: Double-blind test of metronidazole and tinidazole in the treatment of asymptomatic *Entamoeba histolytica* and *Entamoeba hartmanni* carriers. *Am J Trop Med Hyg* 25:549, 1976.
36. Wolfe MS: Treatment of intestinal amebiasis in United States, Foreign Service personnel. Proceedings of the International Conference on Amebiasis, Mexico City, 1977, Instituto Mexicano del Seguro Social, p 842.
37. Wolfe MS: Giardiasis. *JAMA* 233:1362, 1975.
38. Huang T, Grollman AP: Novel inhibitors of protein synthesis in animal cells. *Fed Proc* 29:609, 1970.
39. Klatskin G, Friedman H: Emetine toxicity in man: Studies on the nature of early toxic manifestations, their relation to the dose level and their significance in determining safe dosage. *Ann Intern Med* 28:892, 1948.
40. Ng KKF: Blockade of adrenergic and cholinergic transmissions by emetine. *Br J Pharmacol Chemother* 28:228, 1966.
41. Bradley WG, Fewlings JD, Harris JB, Johnson MA: Emetine myopathy in the rat. *Br J Pharmacol* 57:29, 1976.
42. Scragg JN, Powell SJ: Emetine hydrochloride and dehydroemetine combined with chloroquine in the treatment of children with amoebic liver abscess. *Arch Dis Child* 43:121, 1968.
43. Powell SJ, Wilmot AJ, MacLeod IN, et al: A comparative trial of dehydroemetine and emetine hydrochloride in identical dosage in amebic liver abscess. *Ann Trop Med Parasitol* 61:26, 1967.
44. Oakley GP Jr: The neurotoxicity of the halogenated hydroxyquinolines. *JAMA* 225:395, 1973.
45. Powell SJ: Short-term followup studies in amoebic dysentery. *Trans Roy Soc Trop Med Hyg* 61:765, 1967.
46. Wolfe MS: Nondysenteric intestinal amebiasis. Treatment with dioxanide furoate. *JAMA* 224:1601, 1973.
47. Krogstad DJ, Spencer HC Jr, Healy GR: Amebiasis. *N Engl J Med* 298:262, 1978.
48. Chulay JD, Bhatt SM, Muigai R, et al: A comparison of three dosage regimens of sodium

stibogluconate in the treatment of visceral leishmaniasis in Kenya. *J Infect Dis* 148:148, 1983.
49. Marsden PD: Current concepts in parasitology. *N Engl J Med* 300:350, 1979.
50. Marr JJ: The chemotherapy of leishmaniasis, in Mansfield J (ed): *Parasitic Diseases, The Chemotherapy.* New York, Marcel Dekker, vol 2, p. 201, 1984.
51. Dvorak JA, Howe CL: The effects of Lampit (Bayer 2502) on the interaction of *Trypanosoma cruzi* with vertebrate cells in vitro. *Am J Trop Med Hyg* 26:58, 1977.
52. Robertson DHH: Chemotherapy of African trypanosomiasis. *Practitioner* 188:80, 1962.
53. Robertson DHH: A trial of Mel-B in the treatment of *Trypanosoma rhodesiense* sleeping sickness. *Trans Roy Soc Trop Med Hyg* 57:274, 1963.
54. Duke BOL, Anderson J: Onchocerciasis and its treatment. *Trop Doct* 2:107, 1972.
55. Findley GM: *Recent Advances in Chemotherapy.* London, J & A Churchill, vol 2, 1951.
56. Brack C, Delain E, Riou G: Replicating, covalently closed, circular DNA from kinetoplasts of *Trypansoma cruzi. PNAS* 69:1642, 1972.
57. Walzer PD, Perl DP, Krogstad DJ, et al: *Pneumocystis carinii* pneumonia in the United States. *Ann Intern Med* 80:83, 1974.
58. Bommer W: Die interstitielle plasma cellulare Pneumonie and *Pneumosystis carinii. Ergeb Mikrobiol* 38:116, 1977.
59. Ivady G, Paldy L, Kolty M, et al: *Pneumocystis carinii* pneumonia. *Lancet* 1:616, 1967.
60. Vandermeer G, Brug SL: Infection a *Pneumocystis* chez l'homme et chez les animaux. *Ann Soc Belg Med Trop* 22:301, 1942.
61. Vanek J, Jirovec O: Parasitäre Pneumonie "Interstitielle" Plas mazelle-pneumonie der Frühgeboren, verwisacht durch *Pneumocystis carinii. Zentralbl f Bakt* 158:210, 1952.
62. Dauzier G, Willis T, Barnett RN: *Pneumocystis carinii* in an infant. *Am J Clin Pathol* 26:787, 1956.
63. Hughes WT, Feldman S, Sanyal SK: Treatment of *Pneumocystis carinii* pneumonitis with trimethoprim-sulfamethoxazole. *Can Med Assoc J* 12:47S, 1975.
64. Lau WK, Young LS: Trimethoprim-sulfamethoxazole treatment of *Pneumocystis carinii* pneumonia in adults. *New Engl J Med* 295:716, 1976.
65. Hughes WT, Kuhn S, Chaudhary S, et al: Successful chemoprophylaxis for *Pneumocystis carinii* pneumonitis. *New Engl J Med* 276:1419, 1977.
66. Frankel JK, Weber RW, Lunde MN: Acute toxoplasmosis. Effective treatment with pyrimethamine, sulfadiazine, leucovorin calcium, and yeast. *JAMA* 173:1471, 1960.
67. Remington JS, Anderson SE: Diagnosis and treatment of pneumocystosis and toxoplasmosis in the immunosuppressed host. *Transplant Proc* 5:1263, 1973.
68. Wolfe MS, Wershing JM: Mebendazole. Treatment of trichuriasis and ascariasis in Bahamian children. *JAMA* 230:1408, 1974.
69. Fierlafijan E: Mebendazole in enterobiasis. *JAMA* 218:1051, 1971.
70. Partono F, Purnomo, Tangkilisan A: The use of mebendazole in the treatment of polyparasitism. *Southeast Asian J Trop Med Public Health* 5:258, 1974.
71. Islam N, Chowdhury NA: Mebendazole and pyrantel pamoate as broad-spectrum antihelminthics. *Southeast Asian J Trop Med Public Health* 7:81, 1976.
72. Peña-Chavarria A, Villarejos VM, Zeledon R: Mebendazole in the treatment of Taeniasis Solium and Taeniasis Saginata. *Am J Trop Med Hyg* 26:118, 1977.
73. Van den Bossch H: Biochemical effects of the antihelminthic drug Mebendazole, in Van den Bossch H (ed): *Comparative Biochemistry of Parasites.* New York Academic Press, 1972, p 139.
74. Wagner ED, Chavarria AP: In vivo effects of a new antihelminthic Mebendazole (R-17, 635) on the eggs of *Trichiura* and hookworm. *Am J Trop Med Hyg* 23:151, 1974.
75. Brown HD, Matzuk AR, Ilves IR, et al: Antiparasitic drugs. IV. 2-(4′-thiazolyl)-benzimidazole: A new antihelminthic. *J Am Chem Soc* 83:1764, 1961.
76. Cuckler AC, Mezey KC: The therapeutic efficacy of thiabendazole for helminthic infections in man. A literature review. *Drug Res* 16:411, 1966.
77. Stone OJ: Systemic and topical thiabendazole for creeping eruption. *Texas Rep Biol Med* 27(suppl 2):659, 1969.

78. Standen OD: Chemotherapy of helminthic infections, in Schnitzer RJ, Hawking F (eds): *Experimental Chemotherapy.* New York Academic Press, 1963 vol 1, 701.
79. Egerton JR: The effect of thiabendazole upon *Ascaris* and *Stephanurus* infections. *J Parasitol* 47(Sect II):37, 1961.
80. Saz HJ, Bueding E: Relationships between antihelminthic effects and biochemical and physiological mechanisms. *Pharmacol Rev* 18:871, 1966.
81. Campbell WC: Thiabendazole effects in visceral larva migrans. Letter, JAMA 217:342, 1971.
82. Most H: Current Concepts in Parasitology: Trichinosis-preventable yet still with us. *N Engl J Med* 298:1178, 1978.
83. Saz HJ, Bueding E: Relationships between antihelminthic effects and biochemical and physiological mechanisms. *Pharmacol Rev* 18:871, 1966.
84. Nickey LN: Possible precipitation of petit mal seizures with piperazine citrate. *JAMA* 195:1069, 1966.
85. Parsons AC: Piperazine neurotoxicity: "Worm Wobble." *Br Med J* 4:792, 1971.
86. Wolfe MS, Petersen JL, Neafie RC, et al: Onchocerciasis presenting with swelling of limb. *Am J Trop Med Hyg* 23:361, 1974.
87. Sullivan TJ, Hembree SC: Enhancement of the density of circulating microfilariae with diethylcarbamazine. *Trans Roy Soc Trop Med Hyg* 64:787, 1970.
88. Downie CGB: Encephalitis during treatment of loiasis with diethylcarbamazine. *J Roy Army Med Corp* 112:46, 1966.
89. Wiseman RA, Woodruff AW, Pettitt LE: The treatment of toxocaral infection: Some experimental and clinical observations. *Trans Roy Soc Trop Med Hyg* 65:591, 1971.
90. Perera DR, Western KA, Schultz MG: Niclosamide treatment of cestodiasis: Clinical trials in the United States. *Am J Trop Med Hyg* 19:610, 1970.
91. Davis A, Bailey DR: Metrifonate in urinary schistosomiasis. *Bull WHO* 41:209, 1969.
92. Katz N, Zicker F, Pereira JP: Field trials with oxaminiquine in a schistosomiasis mansoni-epidemic area. *Am J Trop Med Hyg* 26:234, 1977.
93. Katz N: Chemotherapy of schistosomiasis mansoni. *Adv Pharmacol Chemother* 14:1, 1977.
94. Omer AHS: Oxamniquine for treating *Schistosoma mansoni* infection in Sudan. Br Med J 163:178.
95. Kilpatrick ME, Farid Z, Bassily S, et al: Treatment of schistosomiasis mansoni with oxamiquine—5 years' experience. *Am J Trop Med Hyg* 30:1219, 1981.
96. Machado PA: The Brazilian program for schistomiasis control, 1975–1979. *Am J Trop Med Hyg* 31:76, 1982.
97. Davis A, Wagner DHG: Multicenter trials of praziquantel in human schistosomiasis. *Bull WHO* 57:767, 1979.
98. Katz N, Rocha RS, Chaves A: Preliminary trials with praziquantel in human infections due to Schistosoma mansoni. *Bull WHO* 57:781, 1979.
99. Ishizaki T, Kamo E, Boehme K: Double blind studies of tolerance to praziquantel in Japanese patients with *Schistosoma japonicum* infections. *Bull WHO* 57:787, 1979.
100. Cook JA: Schistosome infection in humans: Perspectives and recent findings. *Ann Intern Med* 97:740, 1982.
101. Goble FC (ed): The pharmacological and chemotherapeutic properties of niridazole and other anti-schistosomal compounds. *Ann NY Acad Sci* 160:423, 1969.
102. Farid Z, Bassily S, Lehman JS, et al: A comparative evaluation of the treatment of *Schistosoma mansoni* with niridazole and potassium antimony tartrate. *Trans Roy Soc Trop Med Hyg* 66:119, 1972.
103. Goble FC (ed): The pharmacological and chemotherapeutic properties of niridazole and other antischistosomal compounds. *Ann NY Acad Sci* 160:423, 1969.
104. McCaffrey RP, Farid Z, Kent DC: Acute hemolysis with Ambilhar treatment in glucose-6-phosphate dehydrogenase deficiency. *Trans Roy Soc Trop Med Hyg* 63:795, 1969.
105. Davidson JC: Neuropsychiatric effects and EEG changes in niridazole therapy. *Trans Roy Soc Trop Med Hyg* 63:579, 1969.

19

PROBLEMS IN ANTIBIOTIC USAGE

CALVIN M. KUNIN

The general problem of appropriate use of drugs has existed for a long time. Osler could assume a position of therapeutic nihilism in the early 1900s since there were few effective agents available to him. The antibiotic era, which began less than 40 years ago, is much more complex. There are a wealth of excellent agents from which to choose, each with its own special benefits and economic, toxic, and ecologic costs. We now have the luxury of debating the value of using antibiotics to prevent complications of relatively simple problems such as the common cold or a sore throat, and we can more readily deal with serious surgical and life-threatening infections.

Soon after antibiotics were introduced, it was recognized that they were being overused and misused. A review of the subject by Jawetz in 1956 (1) eloquently stated the problems of the attractiveness of new antibiotics to physicians, exaggerated claims, and the enormous impact of promotion by the drug companies on medical practice. The following year, based on a nationwide study, Welch et al. (2) described the relatively high frequency of severe reactions to antibiotics. In 1959, Finland et al. (3) documented the increasing occurrence of serious bacterial infections since the introduction of antibacterial agents. Reimann and D'Ambola (4) conducted one of the earliest surveys on appropriate use of antibiotics in 1966 and clearly demonstrated that antibiotics were often used inappropriately. In 1974, Lockwood (5) described the syndrome of compulsive antibiotic prescribing (CAP) and advocated formation of an organization called Antibiotics Anonymous to deal with the problem. It is therefore appropriate that a chapter appear in this book to examine the problem and explore potential solutions.

The aim of this chapter is to examine the extent of the current problem, outline methods by which it can be assessed, and propose tentative solutions. In addition we will consider the role of antibiotics in animal feed and for veterinary purposes. Use of antibiotics in developing countries will also be considered, since they have created major problems worldwide in the emergence of resistant strains of microorganisms.

MAGNITUDE OF THE USE OF ANTIMICROBIAL AGENTS IN THE UNITED STATES

Antimicrobial drugs are the second most commonly used class of drugs; they are second to agents used for central nervous system disorders. According to data from the *US Industrial Outlook* published by the Department of Commerce, it is estimated that about 2 billion dollars worth of anti-infectives were shipped in 1982. This accounted for about 18 percent of the total cost of all ethical drug products. This does not include the costs of markup or administration of the agents, which could readily double the expenditure to about 4 billion dollars. There are about 185 million prescriptions written for oral antibiotics each year. Anti-infectives accounted for 15.4 percent of all drugs prescribed in office-based practice in 1980. Much of this expenditure is for treatment of conditions such as sinusitis, bronchitis, and respiratory infections. Since most of these are caused by viruses, much of this expenditure is wasted (6).

In hospitals, antimicrobial agents are given to 23.0–37.8 percent of patients and account for about 25 percent of total drug acquisition costs (7). We will later show that much of this is not only unnecessary but also a waste of resources and is potentially harmful to the patient and society.

REASONS FOR CONCERN ABOUT APPROPRIATE USE OF ANTIMICROBIAL AGENTS

Selection of Resistant Bacteria

Development of resistant organisms was recognized by Paul Ehrlich as a potential problem during his early studies of organic arsenicals almost 100 years ago. The overall problem of emergence of resistant strains is discussed elsewhere (Chapter 1) and is a persistent theme throughout the sections on antimicrobial chemotherapy. It must be emphasized, however, that multiple drug-resistant organisms derived through transfer of plasmids or through transduction by bacteriophage have amplified the magnitude of the problem. At first, most emphasis was focused on emergence of resistant bacteria in hospitals in which antimicrobial agents are used most heavily. More recently, common virulent organisms resistant to previously effective agents have been encountered in office practice as well. This has forced physicians to alter their cost/benefit equation and to use expensive and potentially toxic drugs for treatment of infections due to staphylococci, gonococci, *Hemophilus influenzae, Shigella,* and possibly the pneumococci.

Three approaches to the problem of emerging resistant strains are being explored. The simplest and least costly measure is to decrease the selective pressure exerted by antibiotics. Several groups have presented evidence that control of usage will result in reversion of the bacterial population to sensitive organisms (8–10). A second approach is to develop immunogens that can enhance host resistance to virulent organisms. Development of a polyvalent pneumococcal vaccine is an example of this approach. The major difficulty with the use of vaccines is the complex problems of effective delivery to the target high-risk population and the multiplicity of immunogens needed to deal with an expanding number of microorganisms for which vaccines are being developed. The third and most costly approach is to develop and exploit new antimicrobial agents or alter the chemical structure of older agents to circumvent mechanisms of resistance developed by the microorganisms. This has been the major path taken by the pharmaceutical industry and is most accepted by the medical community.

Rising Costs of Medical Care: Emergence of the "Drugs of Fear"

A new antimicrobial era emerged during the 1970's, the era of the "drugs of fear" (11). By this is meant fear on the part of physicians of failing to provide patients with the very best drug for a presumed infection. Although many lives have been saved by these drugs, the underlying conditions that precipitate infection with "difficult hospital bacteria" have not been resolved, and therefore in many cases, the drugs have been used without effect or have simply delayed death. Widespread use of these agents ensures their own phased obsolescence as new resistant organisms emerge, and it also increases the costs of medical care. We can expect costs to increase with only modest improvement in therapeutic efficacy. A large group of new β-lactam antibiotics is being introduced. These agents are designed for therapy for multiresistant gram-negative bacteria in immunosuppressed and granulocytopenic patients. Thus far, they are only marginally superior to currently available agents, but they cost several times as much. Ordinarily they would be welcome additions to therapy, but they are being promoted for conditions that can be equally well or better treated with older, less-expensive drugs. Physicians, by their control over prescriptions and diagnostic procedures, generate costs to the patient or third-party payers. Therefore, physicians must consider the economic, as well as medical, consequences of their decisions.

Adverse Reactions to Antimicrobial Agents

Untoward toxic effects of antibiotics are well known; they range from death from anaphylaxis or aplastic anemia, with penicillin and chloramphenicol, respectively, to severe diarrhea from lincosamides, rash from ampicillin, nephrotoxicity and ototoxicity from the aminoglycosides, and bleeding disorders with some of the new β-lactam antibiotics. Cluff (12) and Seidl et al. (13) reported that approximately 5 percent of the hospitalized patients who are given an antibiotic will experience some adverse reaction to the drug, and about 20 percent of patients requiring medical care have a history of adverse reaction(s) to an antibiotic.

EVIDENCE OF INAPPROPRIATE USE OF ANTIMICROBIAL AGENTS

Office Practice

Drug prescribing was examined in a careful epidemiologic study by Stolley et al. (14). They reported that market research data indicated that about 95 percent of physicians will issue one or more prescriptions to a patient whom they diagnose as having the "common cold." Almost 60 percent of these prescriptions are for antibiotics, with the tetracyclines and penicillins being the most popular choices. In their own study in a U.S. community, they found that antibiotics were the most commonly dispensed drugs (15.3 percent of all prescriptions). Another analysis by the same group of investigators (15) showed that prescribing patterns are largely determined by educational experiences. Higher ratings for appropriate drug use and lower frequency of chloramphenicol use in particular were found among more recently trained physicians who had more postgraduate training.

We can roughly estimate the magnitude of overusage. Approximately 750 million dollars is spent annually on prescriptions for sinusitis, bronchitis, and respiratory infections. If 60 percent of these prescriptions are for antimicrobial agents (14), the cost for these drugs is 450 million dollars. Assuming that at least one-half of the prescriptions are inappropriate, about 225 million dollars are wasted each year.

It has been argued that antibiotics should be used more often to treat the bacterial complications of upper respiratory infections (16), but carefully conducted clinical studies have clearly demonstrated the lack of efficacy with this approach in otherwise healthy adults (17). It has also been argued that the major reason for the marked decrease in rheumatic fever may be due to widespread use of antibiotics in office practice, but Stollerman (18) has presented forceful arguments that this is more closely associated with changes in the pathogenetic characteristics of the group A streptococci. There is still considerable disagreement among practitioners of various specialties concerning the proper use of antibiotics to treat respiratory infections (19). In one study of usage in an emergency room (20), 31 percent of infections encountered were respiratory. Antibiotic prescribing was appropriate in 78 percent of cases.

The problem of antibiotics overusage in office practice has been compounded in recent years by the promotion of new high-cost proprietary agents such as oral cephalosporins and new derivatives of ampicillin. These agents rarely cure more patients, but do cost more.

Despite the widespread use of new antibiotics in office practice, there are still practitioners who continue to prescribe chloramphenicol, mostly for upper respiratory infections, and tetracycline to children under the age of 8 years, despite repeated recommendations against this practice by the Committee on Drugs of the American Academy of Pediatrics. According to the studies of Ray et al. (21,22), a small group of physicians located in rural, primary care settings account for most of these inappropriate prescriptions. The most alarming finding is that physicians who recently finished training also take part in these poor practices.

Hospital Practice

There are now numerous studies in representative hospital populations that document that antimicrobial agents are used for unjustifiable reasons or that the wrong drug, dose, or duration of therapy is selected *about half the time* (Table 1). One of the remarkable findings of all these studies is that even though criteria for justified or acceptable usage may differ, the results are generally the same.

Virtually all the studies identify the same reasons for overuse and excessive costs of antimicrobial agents in hospitals. These are (*1*) inappropriate use of agents for prophylaxis of surgical infections and (*2*) high cost of parenteral agents, particularly the cephalosporin and aminoglycoside antibiotics, which account for 70 percent of total antibiotic costs (7,23–25).

In recent years the proportion of costs for cephalosporins has increased because of the introduction of many new expensive agents. They have tended to replace the portion of usage occupied by aminoglycosides. The most representative study of use of antimicrobial drugs in general hospitals in the United States was conducted by Shapiro et al. (26). They studied 20 short-stay general hospitals in Pennsylvania selected by a stratified random-sampling technique. Approximately 30 percent of patients received an antimicrobial drug during hospitalization, and about 30 percent received the drugs for prophylaxis in operations or invasive nonsurgical procedures. Despite indications that prophylaxis, when useful at all, is effective only when given concurrently with and for 24–48 hours after an operation, it was usually continued throughout hospitalization. Almost 80 percent of prophylactic antimicrobial agents were administered at least 48 hours after an operation or procedure (Fig. 1). It is apparent that most of the costs were for periods when the drugs would not be helpful to the patient. Similar results were obtained in a survey of 27 hospitals in Minnesota (27). Savings of 18–50 percent could be achieved by limiting duration of drug administration. A benefit cost analysis of antimicrobial prophylaxis in abdominal and vaginal hysterectomy demonstrated that using three doses of cefazolin would markedly reduce costs. (28) The benefits would be eroded by use of newer, more expensive cephalosporins.

Self-Administration

It is quite common to learn from patients that they often treat themselves with drugs prescribed in the past or given to them by friends or relatives. Chretien et al. (29), in a study of students going to a university health service, have reported that this is a frequent practice, especially for the treatment of respiratory symptoms.

TABLE 1. Summary of Studies Evaluating Appropriate Use of Antimicrobial Agents in Hospitals

Hospitals	*Investigators*	*No. Patients*	*Findings*
Community (7 hospitals surveyed)	Scheckler and Bennett (49)[a]	2094	62% of patients treated had no evidence of infection
Community	Roberts and Visconti (50)	340	13% rational, 21% questionable, 66% irrational
Pediatric	Gibbs et al. (51)	167	32% rational, 49% questionable, 19% irrational
University	Kunin et al. (11)	500	52% inappropriate[d]
University	Castle et al. (25)	50	64% inappropriate[d]
University	Petrello et al. (52)	65	42.6% rational, 48% irrational, 9.3% insufficient data
University	Maki and Schuna (53)	549	41% inappropriate
VA	Jones et al. (36) Before	145	64% inappropriate
	After[c]	200	51% inappropriate NS
Community	Achong et al. (24) Before	219	42%[e] 50%[f] irrational
	After	240	24%[e] 25%[f] irrational 0.02[g]

[a] Reference number.
[b] Use of clindamycin only.
[c] Education program in appropriate use of antimicrobial agents.
[d] Judged inappropriate according to criteria in Table 3.
[e] Surgical service.
[f] Gynecologic service.
[g] Degree of significant difference.

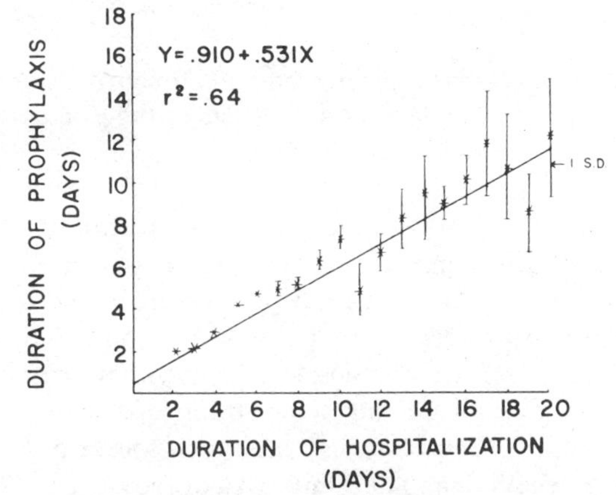

FIGURE 1. Duration of antimicrobial prophylaxis in relation to duration of hospitalization. [Reproduced with permission from Shapiro et al. (26).].

Usage in Other Countries

Misuse of antibiotics is a major problem all over the world. In many Asian and South American countries, potent antibiotics are sold without prescription. A review of antibiotics marketed in Central America (30) revealed that in most countries more than 200 different antibiotic drug products were sold. At least one-third of these were drug combinations of questionable value. Most of the drugs used in the Third World originate from the major Western pharmaceutical companies that promote agents unacceptable in their own countries. Large-scale epidemics of typhoid fever, gonorrhea, and meningococcal meningitis may be traced to resistant strains originating in Third World countries in which antibiotic use is poorly controlled. A study in Israel (31) revealed that 30 percent of pharmacy costs could be accounted for by antibiotics (as in the United States), but that Israeli physicians tend to use less expensive agents, such as ampicillin, more widely than cephalosporins. In the United Kingdom, a study of antibiotic usage for prophylaxis in surgery revealed enormous variation among London teaching hospitals in regard to choice of drug, dose, and timing of administration (32). In a district general hospital in London, ampicillin, cloxacillin, and other penicillins accounted for 61 percent of all antibiotic usage (33). This is quite different from the United States in which much more expensive agents are used. Nevertheless, most of the patients were treated without bacteriologic evidence of the infecting agent, and only 7 percent of antibiotics prescribed for surgical prophylaxis fulfilled reasonable criteria for their use. Similar results were obtained in a National Prevalence Survey conducted in 43 hospitals in England (34). Although oral agents were most commonly used, parenteral agents accounted for 72 percent of the costs.

Antibiotic Use in Animals

Antibiotics are commonly used in farm animals for growth promotion and for therapeutic and prophylactic purposes. The magnitude of use in the world is highly variable. It is somewhat less in Europe than in the United States and is more sporadic and uncontrolled in Third World countries. The major fear is that plasmid-mediated multiple-resistant strains originating in farm animals will spread to the human population. The issues of control of use of antibiotics in animals as they relate to human health are complex and controversial. Not all animal pathogens cause disease in humans. For example, staphylococci (in cattle, poultry, and dogs) are distinct from those that present a problem in humans. In contrast, *Salmonella* and some strains of *Campylobacter* infect humans as well as animals. *Escherichia coli* are a rich source of R plasmids potentially transferable in the human gut. Outbreaks of food-borne *Salmonella* infections due to multiple-resistant strains may present a major problem, particularly when they produce invasive disease in compromised hosts (35).

There is very little evidence that the major problem of antibiotic resistance observed in hospitals can be attributed to use in animals, but rather it is the result of excessive use of therapeutic or prophylactic antibiotics in humans. Experts agree, however, that antibiotics important to treat human infections should not be used for animals.

Methods to Define the Problem and Evaluate Appropriate Usage

As awareness of excessive use of antimicrobial agents increases, demand for accountability will require development of clear-cut methods to evaluate the problem. Most of the studies reported in the literature use different criteria for appropriateness of use. This makes it difficult to compare data gathered in different institutions. Broad categories of surveillance methods are presented in Table 2 together with a brief list of the advantages and disadvantages of each. The simplest and least expensive method is to obtain gross utilization data from hospital pharmacies. This method can often identify a special problem such as overuse of chloramphenicol or a newly introduced agent. Attention can then be focused on individual services, particularly on patterns of use in a major problem area such as surgical prophylaxis. Drug orders can also be audited in relation to specific indications, such as use of antibiotics for upper respiratory infections. Case reviews can be conducted using broad judgmental criteria established by specialists in the field. Examples of evaluation categories proposed by Kunin et al. (11) and modified by Jones and his group (36) are presented in Table 3.

An advisory committee on infectious disease to the Veterans Administration (VA) established specific guidelines and audits for antibiotic use to aid individual hospital staffs in conducting their own programs of surveillance (37). The guidelines were prepared for 18 common problem areas including prophylaxis in

TABLE 2. Methods of Surveillance of Antimicrobial Agent Usage in Hospitals

Gross use data based on pharmacy records

Inexpensive; provides secular trends on usage of individual agents and costs; may be used for interhospital comparisons when adjusted for patient hospital days; may identify unusual practices that may lead to more detailed studies

Utilization by services

Inexpensive if pharmacy record system is on unit dose system or can identify shipment to specific wards; will provide data on problems of use by different groups of physicians and may lead to detailed studies of potential problem areas; will refine gross utilization for more appropriate interhospital comparisons

Survey of routine orders for prophylaxis in surgery

Requires chart review of all cases for specific operations; provides data on actual practices of individual surgeons; permits comparison of practices in different hospitals; identifies unusual practices and can be used for feedback to the surgical service

Survey of orders for specific infectious diseases

Based on discharge diagnosis such as pneumonia, bronchitis, urinary tract infection; provides data on actual practices of individual physicians; permits comparison of practice according to specialty groups and can be used for feedback in education programs

Case review by independent experts

Requires establishment of strict criteria to avoid subjective or varying standards; requires establishment of feedback loops to practicing physicians; may identify specific problems of individual physicians

Guidelines audit

Hospital staffs establish standards of practice and guidelines based on national criteria; audit is used to evaluate compliance with self-imposed standards; enables peer pressure to provide checks and balances; mutes external judgmental evaluations; must be altered as new knowledge of new agents is introduced. Audits may be used for interhospital comparisons.

surgery, evaluation of high-cost or potentially toxic agents, criteria for obtaining blood and other cultures, and services that should be available in a competent clinical microbiology laboratory to perform antibiotic sensitivity testing. It is important to emphasize that these are guidelines, not commandments written in stone. They can potentially be used to establish policy for individual hospitals after they have been thoroughly reviewed and debated by the staff. Some, such as the guideline on surgical prophylaxis, may have to be modified to meet special local problems. Others, such as indications for bacteriologic culture, can be applied without much adaptation. The essential point, however, is that once these guidelines are adopted, the physicians and surgeons should be expected to adhere to them and to respond to questions that will arise when actual practices are audited.

Several groups have experimented with methods to evaluate appropriate use of antimicrobial agents in ambulatory practice. This is somewhat more difficult to assess than in hospitals because of the widely dispersed nature of office practice. Nevertheless, useful data are being gathered by the Kaiser-Permanente group in California and by others. Ray et al. (21,22) have reported that Medicaid data can be used as a surveillance method of individual practitioners. As third-party payment for drugs becomes more extensive, excellent data should be gener-

TABLE 3. Suggested Categories for Determining Appropriate Use of Antimicrobial Agents by Peer Review

Categories	
Kunin et al.	*Jones et al.*
Appropriate Use	
I. Agree with the use of antimicrobial therapy/prophylaxis	I. Appropriate
II. Agree with the use of antimicrobial therapy/prophylaxis, but a potentially fatal bacterial infection cannot be ruled out or prophylaxis is probably appropriate, advantages derived remain controversial	II. Probably Appropriate
Inappropriate Use	
III. Agree with the use of antimicrobial therapy/prophylaxis, but a different (usually less expensive or toxic) antimicrobial is preferred	III. More effective drug recommended IV. Less expensive/toxic drug recommended V. Improper dosage or dosage interval VI. Unjustified, length of treatment excessive
IV. Agree with the use of antimicrobial therapy/prophylaxis, but a modified dose is recommended	VII. Unjustified, use of any antimicrobial not indicated VIII. Records insufficient for categorization
V. Disagree with the use of antimicrobial therapy/prophylaxis, administration is unjustified	

SOURCE: Kunin et al. (11); Jones et al. (36).

ated by using this approach. The major advantage is the ability to detect a small group of aberrant physicians who appear to account for most of the inappropriate usage.

CONSTRAINTS OF MEDICAL PRACTICE THAT LEAD TO INAPPROPRIATE USAGE

To solve the problem of inappropriate usage, we must understand the constraints under which the physician works and the pressures that are exerted on him or her to prescribe drugs. An overall scheme of the elements that motivate the patient to seek help and to comply with the physician and the forces that lead the physician to prescribe drugs are outlined in Figure 2. Each of the factors leading to misuse of antimicrobial agents is described in Table 4. They begin with the desire of physicians to help their patients and end with the ready solution offered by the pharmaceutical manufacturers to satisfy these needs.

The pharmaceutical manufacturers are keenly aware of the needs of the practicing physician. Dr. Donald Kennedy, the former FDA commissioner, estimated that in 1977 the industry spent $4000 per physician on direct drug advertising. IMS America Limited, reported that advertising by U.S. drug companies in 1981 cost $742,200,000 (*New York Times,* January 21, 1981). This does not

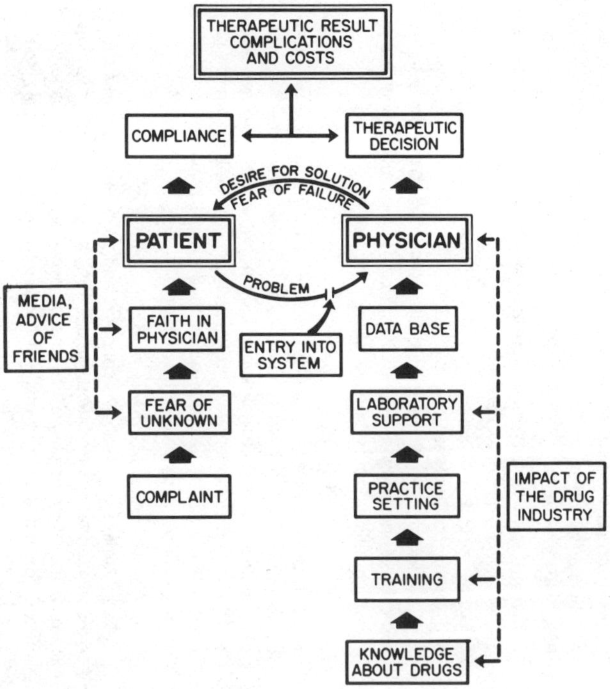

FIGURE 2. Outline of the elements and complex interrelationships that influence the patient and physician to use drugs.

include funds spent for premarketing evaluation of new drugs by clinical investigators. It is apparent that enormous pressure is exerted on the physician. Not all these funds are spent directly on individual physicians but are often invested in medical education programs. Some of the methods of promotional attack and their objectives are presented in Table 5. We must realize that every step in the medical educational process, beginning with the undergraduate years and upward, is subjected to heavy pharmaceutical promotion, including pressure on academic physicians who tend to set standards of practice (38, 39).

PROPOSALS FOR IMPROVEMENT OF ANTIBIOTIC USE

Methods to improve the use of antibiotics have been proposed in several editorials and reviews. Most emphasize the need for improved education of physicians in the diagnosis and treatment of infectious diseases. Some institutions have developed effective programs by requiring consultation for high-cost oral cephalosporins (40), compulsory prospective antibiotic control (41), antibiotic prescription forms that justify the reason for antibiotic use (41a), or routine surveillance

TABLE 4. Factors That Lead to Inappropriate Use of Antimicrobial Agents

Motivation of the physician to give the best treatment

Desire to provide the patient with the very best drug available without regard to outside influences such as cost; fear of failure to provide patient with the most appropriate drugs; desire to prevent infection before it may occur

Belief that if a small amount of drug will be effective, higher and more prolonged usage might be better

For example, use of high dose intravenous penicillin for pneumococcal infections rather than equally effective smaller doses of procaine penicillin

Use of multiple antimicrobial agents or "broad-spectrum agents" to "cover" unusual organisms

Often appropriate in patients with severe leukopenia, but usually used as a substitute for diagnostic judgment

Inappropriate use of resources of clinical microbiology laboratory

Failure to obtain appropriate cultures; delay in transport of specimens and receiving needed information; poor interpersonal relations with the diagnostic laboratory; lack of explanation of results of tests by the laboratory; resistance of the laboratory to use simple culture methods in wards and clinics; need for consultant for interpretation of stained specimens; availability of rapid tests such as penicillinase production, Quellung reactions, tube dilution sensitivities, serum bactericidal levels; inappropriate sensitivity testing of ineffective agents, e.g., nitrofurantoin for systemic gram-negative infection

Pressure from the patient to be treated with an antimicrobial agent

Desire to get rid of infection as soon as possible to avoid interference with life-style; concern of parents about febrile illness in their child; enhanced expectation for solution of problems by drugs; fear of the unknown

Cost and availability of x-ray film studies and diagnostic tests in relation to ready solution offered by drugs

Depends on practice setting, availability and costs of x-ray film studies and diagnostic tests, policy of third-party payors and distribution of physicians and other health care providers

Adequacy of the physician's knowledge of diagnostic and management of patients with infectious disease

Depends on extent of exposure to these disciplines in medical school and during postgraduate training; number of years since graduation, medical discipline, continuing education, self-instruction from literature, source(s) of information, experience in caring for patients with simple versus complicated infectious disease

Malpractice considerations

Have forced physicians to practice defensive medicine by ordering excessive tests and using drugs to solve anticipated problems; explain in part, overuse of oral cephalosporins in the hope that these new more expensive, but relatively safe, drugs will prevent embarrassment later on; the threat of malpractice tends to decrease usage of more toxic agents such as aminoglycoside antibiotics

Solution provided by pharmaceutical manufacturers

Take advantage of the above concerns and problems by offering often expensive and inappropriate panaceas using heavy promotion; exploitation of the "fear of failure" by the physician to help his patient and of the concept that "if it might do some good, and probably will do little harm why not try it?"

TABLE 5. Methods Used by the Pharmaceutical Industry to Influence Physician Prescribing Habits

Group	*Objectives*	*Methods*
Medical students	Develop confidence in industry	Gifts of books, equipment, drugs for family; visits to plant; distribution of learning aids
House staff and fellows	Develop confidence in specific products	Same as for students, plus free samples for patients; advice on products by representatives, support for travel to meetings, throw-away journals
Practicing physicians	Create image of common goal of the physician and industry	Same as above plus special emphasis on personal contact with firm representatives; small medical-related gifts, stationery, forms
Hospital and medical societies	General goodwill to case entry of representatives of the firm	Support for outside speakers, often product oriented; support of meetings, entertainment, educational aids films, books—usually product oriented
General media	Raise public expectation for new drugs	News releases timed with development or release of a new agent
Academic physicians	Influence leaders to introduce new drugs to students and physicians	Support of directed studies of new agents; general research support; support for trainees; consultant arrangements, provide teaching aids; travel to national and international meetings
Medical media	Increase awareness of new products; blunt attack of critics	Direct advertising; throw-away journals (totally supported by advertising), published proceedings of symposia on new drugs; planted articles in throw-away news media, *Physicians' Desk Reference*
Diagnostic labs	Increase awareness of new agents	Special diagnostic tests that are related to selection of new drugs

(41b). The efficacy of each of the proposed methods to control the misuse of antibiotics (Table 6) depends on whether they meet the needs of the practicing physician.

The first method is education (42). Neu and Howrey (43) demonstrated that there were major deficiencies in the physician's knowledge of antibiotic use, and they emphasized the need for further postgraduate education in this field. However, even though continued medical education is expanding in the United States, there is no concrete evidence that it improves actual practice. One study evaluating the effect of education was conducted by Jones et al. (36). Staff at a VA hospital did not show improvement in antibiotic use after an intensive educational program (Table 1). Gilbert and Jackson (44) reported success in improving use by targeting their campaign for one drug, gentamicin. Achong et al. (24) reported remarkable success, which in large part was attributable to improved use of antibiotics in surgical prophylaxis.

Another method, control of contact between pharmaceutical representatives and staff physicians, is only sporadically successful in a few institutions. The representative is usually visualized as a helpful colleague who provides quick information and favors and is properly obsequious. His or her entry is aided by advertising gimmicks and gifts, provision of funds for education, guest speakers, and funds for research or fellowship training. It is extremely difficult even for the academic physician to restrict these people since the information they bring is often valuable and the companies do develop many excellent antimicrobial agents. However, I believe that contact with drug representatives should be limited and restricted only to providing new information in a physician–hospital controlled setting. Some have proposed that "counterdetailing" by clinical pharmacists may help (45), but this remains to be proven.

The hospital formulary committee can be extremely useful in examining the claims and need for new agents. It is in this area that the clinical pharmacist may be of greatest help by advising the committee on the relative benefits of adding or deleting agents from the formulary.

In many ways, the diagnostic laboratory also plays a key role in selection of antimicrobial agents by physicians. So it is exceedingly important that antibiotic sensitivity tests results be reported by generic name and class and be tailored to the best agents according to the organism and site of infection (46).

Another way to control antibiotic usage is to use automatic "stop" orders for specific high-cost agents.

Written justification for use of antibiotics on the prescription is an effective method to decrease inappropriate usage. This forces physicians to explain their actions, and the requirement to write even a brief justification tends to blunt unnecessary prescribing. McGowan and Finland (47) have demonstrated that removal of this requirement has been followed by increased use of these agents.

Required consultations and control of high-cost or toxic agents by experts have been shown to work well in an institution in which there is an active training program in infectious disease and a strong infectious disease group interested in antimicrobial therapy. However, these measures are not applicable

TABLE 6. Methods Used to Control Use of Antimicrobial Agents in Hospitals

Education programs on use of antimicrobial agents
- Staff conferences
- Lectures by outside authorities
- Audio-visual programs
- Clinical pharmacist consultants
- Hospital–Pharmacy Committee newsletters
- Independent sources of information (Medical Letter, AMA Drug Evaluations)

Control of contact between pharmaceutical representatives and staff physicians
- Registration in the pharmacy
- Visits to staff physicians by appointment only
- Policy concerning entry of salesmen to patient care areas
- Restricted time and place of displays
- Policy on free samples, gifts
- Policy on sponsoring speakers, distribution of literature, and advertising note paper

Hospital formulary
- Restriction of formulary to minimum number of agents needed for most effective therapy
- Elimination of duplicative agents
- Substitution rules for least expensive, most effective agent among a given class of agents
- Generic terminology required for all orders and labels

Diagnostic microbiology laboratory sensitivity tests
- Appropriate selction of sensitivity tests for organism and site
- Use of generic class disks
- Restriction of reports on "specialized" agents unless specifically requested or indicated
- Print own resort forms with generic terminology

Automatic "stop" orders for specific high-cost agents

Written justification for high-cost agents:
- In cases where alternative, equally effective, less expensive or toxic agents may be used, e.g., oral cephalosporins, new parenteral aminoglycosides, and cephalosporins, lincosamides, chloramphenicol

Required consultation
- This is to be done after first three doses of specific high-cost agents are ordered, e.g., aminoglycosides, parenteral cephalosporins, carbenicillin-ticarcillin, lincosamides

Controlled agents
- Release of specific agents which may alter ecology of hospital flora requires approval by infectious disease consultants, e.g., amikacin, carbenicillin-ticarcillin

Guidelines and audits of antimicrobial usage
- These permit the hospital staff to set standards of use based on local needs and judgments, guided by independent criteria. Audit is based on compliance with these standards, but requires a well-structured, authoritative feedback loop

at this time to many hospitals in the United States. Nevertheless, the results of these two approaches are instructive. They clearly demonstrate that most antibiotic usage is wasteful and unnecessary. For example, we have been able to reduce overusage markedly by generating an automatic consultation through the hospital pharmacy once the first three doses of an expensive, potentially toxic agent are ordered. This avoids denying the patient a needed drug but permits early appraisal of the appropriateness of the antibiotic. As the program continues, less consultation is required, since physicians soon become aware that their practice will be reviewed with them. Cephalosporin antibiotic use fell dramatically during the period of control. In most cases, a less-expensive agent such as penicillin G was used instead, or postsurgical use of a cephalosporin was curtailed. Evaluation of patient records revealed that no patient was denied adequate therapy during the control period. The difference between use of this class of drugs before and after control measures indicates the amount of this drug unnecessarily prescribed in the hospital.

Since most hospital staffs must function without the aid of experts in antimicrobial therapy, independent guidelines for appropriate use are needed (48). These guidelines potentially offer a basis for local discussion of the issues and modifications that best suit the judgment and needs of the practicing physicians. The most critical guidelines are for prophylaxis in surgery and for use of oral and parenteral cephalosporin antibiotics. It is in these areas that the highest cost and greatest waste occurs. The guidelines are not excessively restrictive since they are based on the best available data from the surgical literature that emphasize short perioperative courses of the most effective agents. This auditing function measures compliance with local standards and provides feedback to the hospital staff who fail to adhere to guidelines accepted by their peers. The report of success in controlling overuse by Achong et al. (24) supports the idea that a well-informed and concerned staff can reduce inappropriate use of antibiotics.

SUMMATION AND COMMENTARY

This chapter has described the problem of overuse of antibiotics. It is part of a larger problem of overuse of medical care facilities, diagnostic tests, and other drugs. The problem and its solution depend on knowledge of the constraints in medical practice that tend to lead the physician to overprescribe antibiotics. Instruction in infectious disease and antimicrobial therapy has been severely curtailed recently in most medical schools. This error, in my view, must be redressed by greater, rather than less, formal instruction. The problem, however, extends well beyond the formative years of the physician's education and cannot be solved by a punitive approach to the pharmaceutical industry. The industry simply exploits the constraints of medical practice to sell its products.

Overuse of antibiotics is not simply an economic problem, even though it is easily measured by these standards; nor is it just poor practice because of the heavy price paid for ecologic changes with new, resistant microbial strains. Most importantly, in my view, it reveals how effectively we as physicians use scientific technology to help our patients. The solution to the problem rests on our willingness to use this technology wisely.

REFERENCES

1. Jawetz E: Antimicrobial chemotherapy. *Annu Rev Microbiol* 10:85, 1956.
2. Welch H, Lewis CN, Weinstein HI, et al: Severe reactions to antibiotics: A nationwide survey. *Antibiot Med Chem Ther* 4:800, 1957.
3. Finland M, Jones WF, Barnes MW: Occurrence of serious bacterial infections since introduction of antibacterial agents. *JAMA* 170:84, 1959.
4. Reimann HA, D'Ambola J: The use and cost of antimicrobics in hospitals. *Arch Environ Health* 13:631, 1966.
5. Lockwood, WR: Antibiotics anonymous. *N Engl J Med* 290:465, 1974.
6. Simmons HE, Stolley PD: This is medical progress? Trends and consequences of antibiotic use in the United States. *JAMA* 227:1023, 1974.
7. Craig WA, Sarver KP: Antimicrobial usage in the USA, in Williams JD, Geddes AM (eds): *Chemotherapy,* vol 4. New York, Plenum, 1976, p 293.
8. Bulger RJ, Roberts CE, Sherris JC: Changing incidence of antibiotic resistance among *Staphylococcus aureus, Escherichia coli, Aerobacter–Klebsiella,* and *Pseudomonas* encountered in a teaching hospital over a 7-year period, in Hobby GL (ed): *Antimicrobial Agents and Chemotherapy—1966,* Proceedings of the Sixth Interscience Conference on Antimicrobial Agents and Chemotherapy. Philadelphia, 1966, p 42.
9. Sogaard H, Zimmerman-Nielsen C, Sibioni K: Antibioticresistant gram-negative bacilli in a urological ward for male patients during a 9-year period: Relationship to antibiotic consumption. *J Infect Dis* 130:646, 1974.
10. Bulger RJ, Sherris JC: Decreased incidence of antibiotic resistance among *Staphylococcus aureus.* A study in a university hospital over a 9-year period. *Ann Intern Med* 69:1099, 1968.
11. Kunin CM, Tupasi T, Craig WA: Use of antibiotics: A brief exposition of the problem and some tentative solutions. *Ann Intern Med* 79:555, 1973.
12. Cluff LE: The prescribing habits of physicians. *Hosp Prac* 2:100, 1967.
13. Seidl LG, Thornder GF, Smith SW, et al: Studies on epidemiology of adverse drug reactions. III. Reactions in patients on general medical service. *Bull Johns Hopkins Hosp* 119:299, 1966.
14. Stolley PD, Becker MH, McEvilla JB, et al: Drug prescribing and use in an American community. *Ann Intern Med* 76:537, 1972.
15. Becker MH, Stolley PD, Lasagna L, et al: Differential education concerning therapeutics and resultant physician prescribing patterns. *J Med Educ* 47:118, 1972.
16. Antibiotics for common colds? editorial. *Lancet* 1:132, 1976.
17. Stott NCH, West RR: Randomized controlled trial of antibiotics in patients with cough and purulent sputum. *Lancet* 2:556, 1976.
18. Stollerman GH: The relative rheumatogenicity of strains of group A streptococci. *Mod Concepts Cardiovasc Dis* 44:35, 1975.
19. Greenberg RA, Wagner EH, Wolf SH, et al: Physician opinions on the use of antibiotics in respiratory infections. *JAMA* 240:650, 1978.
20. Bernstein LR, Barriere SL, Conte JE: Utilization of antibiotics: Analysis of appropriateness of use. *Ann Emergency Med* 11:400, 1982.
21. Ray WA, Federspiel CF, Schaffner W: Prescribing of chloramphenicol in ambulatory practice. An epidemiologic study among Tennessee Medicaid recipients. *Ann Intern Med* 84:266, 1976.

22. Ray WA, Federspiel CF, Schaffner W: Prescribing of tetracycline to children less than 8 years old. *JAMA* 237:2069, 1977.
23. McGowan JE Jr, Finland M: Effects of monitoring the usage of antibiotics: An interhospital comparison. *South Med J* 69:193, 1976.
24. Achong MR, Theal HK, Wood J, et al: Changes in hospital antibiotic therapy after a quality-of-use study. *Lancet* 2:1118, 1977.
25. Castle M, Wilfert CM, Cate TR, et al: Antibiotic use at Duke University Medical Center. *JAMA* 237:2819, 1977.
26. Shapiro M, Townsend TR, Rosner B, et al: Use of antimicrobial drugs in general hospitals. *N Engl J Med* 301:351, 1979.
27. Crossley K, Gardner LC: Antimicrobial prophylaxis in surgical patients. *JAMA* 245:722, 1981.
28. Shapiro M, Schoenbaum SC, Tager IB, et al: Benefit–cost analysis of antimicrobial prophylaxis in abdominal and vaginal hysterectomy. *JAMA* 249:1290, 1983.
29. Chretien JH, McGarvey M, de Stowlinski A, et al: Abuse of antibiotics, a study of patients attending a university clinic. *Arch Intern Med* 135:1063, 1975.
30. Gustafsson LL, Wide K: Marketing of obsolete antibiotics in Central America. *Lancet* 1:31, 1981.
31. Levy M, Nir I, Superstine E, et al: Antimicrobial therapy in patients hospitalized in a medical ward. A report from the Boston collaborative drug surveillance program. *Israel J Med Sci* 11:322, 1975.
32. Study group in the use of antimicrobial drugs: Prophylactic antimicrobial drug therapy at five London teaching hospitals. *Lancet* 1:1351, 1977.
33. Cook D, Salter AJ, Phillips I: Antimicrobial misuse, antibiotic policies and information responses. *J Antimicrob Chemother* 6:435, 1980.
34. Leigh DA: Antimicrobial usage in forty-three hospitals in England. *J Antimicrob Chemother* 9:75, 1982.
35. Cherubin CE: Antibiotic resistance of Salmonella in Europe and the United States. *Rev Infect Dis* 3:1105, 1981.
36. Jones SR, Bratton T, McRee E: The effect of an educational program upon hospital use. *Am J Med Sci* 273:79085, 1977.
37. Kunin CM: Guidelines and audits for use of antimicrobial agents in hospitals. *J Infect Dis* 135:335, 1977.
38. Musher DM: Correspondence, Antibiotics: The medium is the message. *Rev Infect Dis* 5:809, 1983.
39. Kass EH: Editorial, seduction in a grand hotel. *Rev Infect Dis* 5:973, 1983.
40. Seligman SJ: Reduction in antibiotic costs by restricting use of an oral cephalosporin. *Am J Med* 71:941, 1981.
41. Recco RA, Gladstone JL, Friedman SA, et al: Antibiotic control in a municipal hospital. *JAMA* 241:2283, 1979.
41a. Durbin WA, Lapidas B, Goldmann DA: Improved antibiotic usage following introduction of a novel prescription system. *JAMA* 246:1796, 1981.
41b. Feldman L, Lamson M, Gallelli JF, et al: Surveillance of nosocomial infections by antibiotic monitoring. *JAMA* 241:2806, 1979.
42. Counts GW: Review and control of antimicrobial usage. *JAMA* 238:2170, 1977.
43. Neu HC, Howrey SP: Testing the physician's knowledge of antibiotic use: self-assessment and learning via videotape. *N Engl J Med* 293:1291, 1975.
44. Gilbert DN, Jackson J: Effect of an education program on the proper use of gentamicin in a community hospital. *Clin Res* 24:112A, 1976.
45. Hendeles L: Need for "counter-detailing" antibiotics. *Am J Hosp Pharm* 33:918, 1976.
46. Kunin CM: Antibiotic sensitivity tests: how to get the most out of them. *Wis Med J* 70:206, 1971.
47. McGowan JE Jr, Finland M: Usage of antibiotics in a general hospital: effect of requiring justification. *J Infect Dis* 130:165, 1974.

48. Kunin CM, Efron HY: Audits of antimicrobial guidelines for peer review. *JAMA* 237:1001, 1003, 1134, 1241, 1243, 1366, 1367, 1481, 1482, 1605, 1607, 1723, 1724, 1725, 1859, 1860, 1967, 1968, 1969, 1977.
49. Scheckler WE, Bennett JV: Antibiotic usage in seven community hospitals. *JAMA* 213:264, 1970.
50. Roberts AW, Visconti JA: The rational and irrational use of systemic antimicrobial drugs. *Am J Hosp Pharm* 29:1054, 1972.
51. Gibbs CW Jr, Gibson JT, Newton DS: Drug utilization review of actual versus preferred pediatric antibiotic therapy. *Am J Hosp Pharm* 30:892, 1973.
52. Petrello MA, Linkewich JA, Gluckman SJ, et al: Clindamycin prescribing patterns in a university hospital. *Am J Hosp Pharm* 32:1111, 1975.
53. Maki DG, Schuna AA: A study of antimicrobial misuse in a university hospital. *Am J Med Sci* 275:271, 1978.
54. Adler JL, Shulman JA: Nosocomial infection and antibiotic usage at Grady Memorial Hospital. *South Med J* 63:102, 1970.
55. Moody ML, Burke JP: Infections and antibiotic usage in a large private hospital. *Arch Intern Med* 130:261, 1972.
56. Shoji Kt, Axnick K, Rytel MW: Infections and antibiotic use in a large municipal hospital 1970–72. A prospective analysis of the effectiveness of a continuous surveillance program. *Health Lab Sci* 11:283, 1974.

20

TABLES OF ANTIMICROBIAL AGENT PHARMACOLOGY

SANDRA M. NORRIS
GERALD L. MANDELL

INTRODUCTION

The selection of an appropriate dose of an antimicrobial agent is based on information such as the site of infection, the identity and known or presumed antibiotic susceptibility of the infecting organism, dose-related drug toxicity, and the patient's ability to eliminate the drug. This chapter serves as a centralized source of pharmacologic information frequently sought for antimicrobial agents. For more detailed information about specific agents, see the appropriate chapter.

Generic and trade name tables for antimicrobial agents are provided. The antimicrobial "family" classification is also included to help the reader locate specific information in subsequent tables.

Dosing Guidelines

Generally, *dosage* selections from the upper end of the dosage range are recommended for severe, life-threatening infections (sepsis, meningitis). The lowest dosages are used for urinary tract infections. A sizable range in dosing *intervals* exists for some antimicrobial agents, with the longer duration between doses appropriate for less severe infections in which a critical threshold level in serum or other site of infection (e.g., central nervous system) is not mandatory or the drug concentrates significantly at the site of infection (urine, bile).

Dosing recommendations for the following drugs result from preliminary, premarketing clinical trials and at the time of publication have not been officially approved by the U.S. Food and Drug Administration: apalcillin, aztreonam, amdinocillin (mecillinam), imipenem, temocillin, fusidic acid, cefotiam, cefotetan, cefmenoxime, cefsulodin, ceftazidime, ceftriaxone, and sulbactam.

To prevent errors, the dosing recommendations should be checked with recent package inserts or current reference sources.

Dosage Adjustment for Renal Impairment

Drug half-life in *adults* with impaired renal function and changes related to dialysis procedures (HD = hemodialysis, PD = peritoneal dialysis) are summarized for the user. An alternative to the elongation of the interval between doses is reduction of the daily dose given at the "usual" dosing interval (Bennett et al., 1983). Antimicrobial serum levels should be determined and patient-specific dosage adjustments made on the basis of these determinations.

Unless otherwise stated, the doses indicated for hemodialysis should supplement "anuric doses." The "usual, adult dose" is for parenteral therapy unless designated oral (po).

With the increasing use of chronic ambulatory peritoneal dialysis (CAPD), drug addition to the dialysate solution with direct instillation into the peritoneal cavity is becoming a widely used method of drug delivery. Generally, one adds an amount of drug to dialysate solution to mimic the target serum concentration. For example, add 5 mg gentamicin per liter of dialysate solution for a desired serum level of 5 μg/ml.

Body Fluid Concentrations

In determining the appropriateness of a particular antibiotic for a given site of infection, the ultimate concentration of a drug as compared with the minimum inhibitory concentration for the infecting organism is critical, rather than percent penetration as compared to serum. For example, the aminoglycosides are ineffective therapy for meningitis although they penetrate into the cerebrospinal fluid to a higher percentage than penicillin G, which is effective therapy for certain organisms. Percent penetration (relationship between peak concentration in a specific body fluid to serum) is, however, a valuable tool for comparisons among similar agents.

TABLE 1. Generic–Trade Names

Generic	*Trade*	*Family*
Acyclovir	Zovirax	Antiviral agents
Amantadine	Symmetrel	Antiviral agents
Amdinocillin	—	Penicillins
Amikacin	Amikin	Aminoglycosides
Aminosalicylic acid	PAS	Antimycobacterial agents
	Para	Antimycobacterial agents
	Parasal	Antimycobacterial agents
	Rezipas	Antimycobacterial agents
Amoxicillin	Amoxil	Penicillins
	Larotid	Penicillins
	Polymox	Penicillins
	Robamox	Penicillins
	Trimox	Penicillins
Amphotericin B	Fungizone	Antifungal agents
Ampicillin	Ampen	Penicillins
	Amcill	Penicillins
	Omnipen	Penicillins
	Omnipen N	Penicillins
	PenA	Penicillins
	Penbritin	Penicillins
	Pensyn	Penicillins
	Polycillin	Penicillins
	Polycillin N	Penicillins
	Principen	Penicillins
	Probampacin	Penicillins
	Supen	Penicillins
	Totacillin	Penicillins
Ampicillin probenecid	Polycillin-PRB	Penicillins
	Trojacillin-Plus	Penicillins
Ansamycin	—	Antimycobacterial agents
Apalcillin	—	Penicillins
Azlocillin	Azlin	Penicillins
Aztreonam	Azactam	Other β-lactams
Bacampicillin	Spectrobid	Penicillins
Benzathine penicillin	Bicillin	Penicillins
	Permapen	Penicillins
Bithionol	Bitin	Antiparasitic agents
Capreomycin	Capastat	Antimycobacterial agents
Carbenicillin	Geopen	Penicillins
	Pyopen	Penicillins
Carbenicillin indanyl sodium	Geocillin	Penicillins
Cefaclor	Ceclor	Cephalosporins
Cefadroxil	Duricef	Cephalosporins
Cefamandole	Mandol	Cephalosporins
Cefazolin	Ancef	Cephalosporins
	Kefzol	Cephalosporins
Cefmenoxime	Cefmax	Cephalosporins
Cefonicid	Monocid	Cephalosporins
Cefoperazone	Cefobid	Cephalosporins
Ceforanide	Precef	Cephalosporins
Cefotaxime	Claforan	Cephalosporins
Cefotetan	Apace	Cephalosporins
Cefotiam	—	Cephalosporins
Cefoxitin	Mefoxin	Cephalosporins
Cefsulodin	Cefomonil	Cephalosporins

Ceftazidime	Fortaz	Cephalosporins
Ceftizoxime	Cefizox	Cephalosporins
Ceftriaxone	Rocephin	Cephalosporins
Cefuroxime	Zinacef	Cephalosporins
Cephalexin	Keflex	Cephalosporins
Cephaloglycine	Kafocin	Cephalosporins
Cephaloridine	Loridine	Cephalosporins
Cephalothin	Keflin	Cephalosporins
Cephapirin	Cefadyl	Cephalosporins
Cephradine	Anspor	Cephalosporins
	Velosef	Cephalosporins
Chloramphenicol	Chloromycetin	Chloramphenicol
Chloroquine	Aralen	Antiparasitic agents
Chlortetracycline	Aureomycin	Tetracyclines
Cinoxacin	Cinobac	Other urinary tract agents
Clavulanic acid + amoxicillin	Augmentin	β-lactamase inhibitors
Clavulanic acid + ticarcillin	Timentin	β-lactamase inhibitors
Clindamycin	Cleocin	Lincosamides
Clofazimine	Lamprene	Antimycobacterial agents
Clotrimazole	Canesten	Antifungal agents
	Lotrimin	Antifungal agents
Cloxacillin	Tegopen	Penicillins
Colistimethate	Colymycin M	Polymyxins
Colistin	Colymycin S	Polymyxins
Cotrimoxazole	—	Sulfonamides + trimethoprim
Cyclacillin	Cyclapen	Penicillins
Cycloserine	Oxamycin	Antimycobacterial agents
	Seromycin	Antimycobacterial agents
Dapsone	Avlosulfon	Antimycobacterial agents
Demeclocycline	Declomycin	Tetracyclines
Dicloxacillin	Dycill	Penicillins
	Dynapen	Penicillins
	Pathocil	Penicillins
	Veracillin	Penicillins
Diethylcarbamazine	Hetrazan	Antiparasitic agents
Diiodohydroxyquin	Panaquin	Antiparasitic agents
Diloxanide furoate	Furamide	Antiparasitic agents
Doxycycline	Doxy II	Tetracyclines
	Doxychel	Tetracyclines
	Vibramycin	Tetracyclines
Emetine	—	Antiparasitic agents
Erythromycin	E-mycin	Erythromycins
	Erypar	Erythromycins
	Ethril	Erythromycins
	Ilotycin	Erythromycins
	Kesso-mycin	Erythromycins
	Robimycin	Erythromycins
Erythromycin estolate	Ilosone	Erythromycins
Erythromycin ethyl succinate	E.E.S.	Erythromycins
	Pediamycin	Erythromycins
Erythromycin ethyl succinate plus sulfisoxazole	Pediazole	
Erythromycin stearate	Bristamycin	Erythromycins
	Erythrocin	Erythromycins
	Pfizer-E	Erythromycins

TABLE 1. (Continued)

Generic	*Trade*	*Family*
Ethambutol	Myambutol	Antimycobacterial agents
Ethionamide	Trecator-SC	Antimycobacterial agents
Flucytosine	Ancobon	Antifungal agents
Furazolidone	Furoxone	Antiparasitic agents
Fusidic acid	—	Fusidic acid
Gentamicin	Garamycin	Aminoglycosides
Griseofulvin	Fulvicin P-G	Antifungal agents
	Fulvicin U-F	Antifungal agents
	Grifulvin V	Antifungal agents
	Gris-PEG	Antifungal agents
	Grisactin	Antifungal agents
Hetacillin	Versapen	Penicillins
	Versapen K	Penicillins
Idoxuridine	Dendrid	Antiviral agents
	Herplex	Antiviral agents
	Stoxil	Antiviral agents
Imipenem + cilastatin	Primaxin	Other β-lactams
Iodoquinol (diiodohydroxyquin)	Yodoxin	Antiparasitic agents
Isoniazid	Hyzyd	Antimycobacterial agents
	INH	Antimycobacterial agents
	Niadox	Antimycobacterial agents
	Niconyl	Antimycobacterial agents
	Nydrazid	Antimycobacterial agents
Kanamycin	Kantrex	Aminoglycosides
Ketoconazole	Nizoral	Antifungal agents
Lincomycin	Lincocin	Lincosamides
Mafenide	Sulfamylon	Sulfonamides + trimethoprim
Mebendazole	Vermox	Antiparasitic agents
Melarsoprol	Arsobal	Antiparasitic agents
	Mel B	Antiparasitic agents
Methacycline	Rondomycin	Tetracyclines
Methenamine hippurate	Hiprex	Other urinary tract agents
	Urex	Other urinary tract agents
Methenamine mandelate	Mandelamine	Other urinary tract agents
Methicillin	Celbenin	Penicillins
	Dimocillin RT	Penicillins
	Staphcillin	Penicillins
Metrifonate	Bilarcil	Antiparasitic agents
Metronidazole	Flagyl	Metronidazole
Mezlocillin	Mezlin	Penicillins
Miconazole	Micatin	Antifungal agents
	Monistat	Antifungal agents
Minocycline	Minocin	Tetracyclines
	Vectrin	Tetracyclines
Moxalactam	Moxam	Cephalosporins
Nafcillin	Nafcil	Penicillins
	Unipen	Penicillins
Nalidixic acid	Cybis	Quinolones
	NegGram	Quinolones
Neomycin	Mycifradin	Aminoglycosides
Netilmicin	Netromycin	Aminoglycosides

Niclosamide	Niclocide	Antiparasitic agents
	Yomesan	Antiparasitic agents
Nifurtimox	Lampit	Antiparasitic agents
Niridazole	Ambilhar	Antiparasitic agents
Nitrofurantoin	Cyantin	Other urinary tract agents
	Furadantin	Other urinary tract agents
	Macrodantin	Other urinary tract agents
	Trantoin	Other urinary tract agents
Norfloxacin	Noraxin	Other urinary tract agents
Novobiocin	Albamycin	—
Nystatin	Mycostatin	Antifungal agents
	Nilstat	Antifungal agents
Oxacillin	Bactocill	Penicillins
	Prostaphlin	Penicillins
	Resistopen	Penicillins
Oxamniquine	Vansil	Antiparasitic agents
Oxolinic acid	Utibid	Quinolones
Oxytetracycline	Terramycin	Tetracyclines
	Uri-Tet	Tetracyclines
Para-aminosalicylic acid, *see* aminosalicylic acid		
Paromomycin	Humatin	Antiparasitic agents
Penicillin G	Pentids	Penicillins
	Pfizerpen	Penicillins
Penicillin G procaine	Crysticillin	Penicillins
	Duracillin AS	Penicillins
	Wycillin	Penicillins
Penicillin G sodium + penicillin G procaine	Duracillin FA	Penicillins
Penicillin G + phenoxymethyl penicillin	Kesso-pen	Penicillins
Penicillin V potassium (phenoxymethyl penicillin)	Betopen VK	Penicillins
	Ledercillin VK	Penicillins
	Penapar VK	Penicillins
	Pen Vee K	Penicillins
	Robicillin VK	Penicillins
	Uticillin VK	Penicillins
	V-Cillin K	Penicillins
	Veetids	Penicillins
Pentamidine	Pentam 300	Antiparasitic agents
Phenazopyridine	Azo Gantrisin	—
Phenethicillin	Darcil	Penicillins
	Maxipen	Penicillins
	Synicillin	Penicillins
Piperacillin	Pipracil	Penicillins
Piperazine	Antepar	Antiparasitic agents
Pivmecillinam	Selexid	Penicillins
Polymyxin B	Aerosporin	Polymyxins
Praziquantel	Biltricide	Antiparasitic agents
Primaquine phosphate	Primaquine	Antiparasitic agents
Pyrantel pamoate	Antiminth	Antiparasitic agents
Pyrazinamide	—	Antimycobacterial agents
Pyrimethamine	Daraprim	Antiparasitic agents
Pyrimethamine-sulfadoxine	Fansidar	Antiparasitic agents

TABLE 1. (Continued)

Generic	*Trade*	*Family*
Pyrivinium pamoate	Povan	Antiparasitic agents
Quinacrine	Atabrine	Antiparasitic agents
Quinine sulfate	—	Antiparasitic agents
Rifampin	Rifadin	Antimycobacterial agents
	Rimactane	Antimycobacterial agents
Rifampin-isoniazid	Rifamate	Antimycobacterial agents
Silver sulfadiazine	Silvadine	Sulfonamides + trimethoprim
Spectinomycin	Trobicin	Aminoglycosides
Stibogluconate	Pentostam	Antiparasitic agent
Succinylsulfathiazole	Rolsul	Sulfonamides + trimethoprim
	Sulfasuxidine	Sulfonamides + trimethoprim
Sulbactam + ampicillin	—	β-lactamase inhibitors
Sulbactam + cefoperazone	—	β-lactamase inhibitors
Sulfacetamide	Bleph	Sulfonamides + trimethoprim
	Isopto cetamide	Sulfonamides + trimethoprim
	Sulamyd sodium	Sulfonamides + trimethoprim
Sulfachlorpyridazine	Sonilyn	Sulfonamides + trimethoprim
Sulfacytine	Renoquid	Sulfonamides + trimethoprim
Sulfadiazine	Sulfadyne	Sulfonamides + trimethoprim
Sulfamethizole	Thiosulfil	Sulfonamides + trimethoprim
	Urifon	Sulfonamides + trimethoprim
Sulfamethoxazole	Gantanol	Sulfonamides + trimethoprim
Sulfasalazine	Azulfidine	Sulfonamides + trimethoprim
Sulfisoxazole	Gantrisin	Sulfonamides + trimethoprim
Sultamicillin	—	β-lactamase inhibitors
Suramin	Germanin	Antiparasitic agents
Teichomycin	—	—
Temocillin	—	Penicillins
Tetracycline	Achromycin	Tetracyclines
	Kesso-tetra	Tetracyclines
	Panmycin	Tetracyclines
	Polycycline	Tetracyclines
	Robitet	Tetracyclines
	Steclin	Tetracyclines
	Sumycin	Tetracyclines
	Tetracyn	Tetracyclines
	Tetrex	Tetracyclines
Thiabendazole	Mintezol	Antiparasitic agents
Ticarcillin	Ticar	Penicillins
Tobramycin	Nebcin	Aminoglycosides
Tolnaftate	Tinactin	Antifungal agents
Trimethoprim	Proloprim	Sulfonamides + trimethoprim
	Trimpex	Sulfonamides + trimethoprim
Trimethoprim-sulfamethoxazole	Bactrim	Sulfonamides + trimethoprim
	Septra	Sulfonamides + trimethoprim
Trisulfapyrimidines	Terfonyl	Sulfonamides + trimethoprim
Troleandomycin	TAO	—
Vancomycin	Vancocin	Vancomycin
Vidarabine	Vira-A	Antiviral agents
Viomycin	Vinactane	Antimycobacterial agents
	Viocin	Antimycobacterial agents

TABLE 2. Trade–Generic Names

Trade	Generic	Family	Trade	Generic	Family
Achromycin	Tetracycline	Tetracyclines	Bactocill	Oxacillin	Penicillins
Aerosporin	Polymyxin B	Polymyxins	Bactrim	Trimethoprim-sulfamethoxazole	Sulfonamides + trimethoprim
Albamycin	Novobiocin	—	Betopen VK	Penicillin V potassium	Penicillins
Ampen	Ampicillin	Penicillins	Bicillin	Benzathine penicillin G	Penicillins
Ambilhar	Niridazole	Antiparasitic agents	Bilarcil	Metrifonate	Antiparasitic agents
Amcill	Ampicillin	Penicillins	Biltricide	Praziquantel	Antiparasitic agents
Amikin	Amikacin	Aminoglycosides	Bitin	Bithionol	Antiparasitic agents
Amoxil	Amoxicillin	Penicillins	Bleph	Sulfacetamide	Sulfonamides + trimethoprim
Ancef	Cefazolin	Cephalosporins	Bristamycin	Erythromycin stearate	Erythromycins
Ancobon	Flucytosine	Antifungal agents	Canesten	Clotrimazole	Antifungal agents
Anspor	Cephradine	Cephalosporins	Capastat	Capreomycin	Antimycobacterial agents
Antepar	Piperazine citrate	Antiparasitic agents	Ceclor	Cefaclor	Cephalosporins
Antiminth	Pyrantel pamoate	Antiparasitic agents	Cefadyl	Cephapirin	Cephalosporins
Apace	Cefotetan	Cephalosporins	Cefizox	Ceftizoxime	Cephalosporins
Aralen	Chloroquine	Antiparasitic agents	Cefmax	Cefmenoxime	Cephalosporins
Arsobal	Melarsoprol	Antiparasitic agents	Cefobid	Cefoperazone	Cephalosporins
Atabrine	Quinacrine	Antiparasitic agents	Cefomonil	Cefsulodin	Cephalosporins
Augmentin	Clavulanic acid + amoxicillin	β-lactamase inhibitors	Celbenin	Methicillin	Penicillins
Aureomycin	Chlortetracycline	Tetracyclines	Chloromycetin	Chloramphenicol	Chloramphenicol
Avlosulfon	Dapsone	Antimycobacterial agents	Cinobac	Cinoxacin	Other urinary tract agents
Azactam	Aztreonam	Other β-lactams	Claforan	Cefotaxime	Cephalosporins
Azlin	Azlocillin	Penicillins	Cleocin	Clindamycin	Lincosamides
Azo Gantrisin	Phenazopyridine	—	Colymycin M	Colistimethate	Polymyxins
Azulfidine	Sulfasalazine	Sulfonamides + trimethoprim	Colymycin S	Colistin	Polymyxins

TABLE 2. (Continued)

Trade	*Generic*	*Family*
Crysticillin	Penicillin G procaine	Penicillins
Cyantin	Nitrofurantoin	Other urinary tract agents
Cybis	Nalidixic acid	Quinolones
Cyclapen	Cyclacillin	Penicillins
Daraprim	Pyrimethamine	Antiparasitic agents
Darcil	Phenethicillin	Penicillins
Declomycin	Demeclocycline	Tetracyclines
Dendrid	Idoxuridine	Antiviral agents
Dimocillin RT	Methicillin	Penicillins
Doxy II	Doxycycline	Tetracyclines
Doxychel	Doxycycline	Tetracyclines
Duracillin AS	Penicillin G procaine	Penicillins
Duracillin FA	Penicillin G sodium + penicillin G procaine	Penicillins
Duricef	Cefadroxil	Cephalosporins
Dycill	Dicloxacillin	Penicillins
Dynapen	Dicloxacillin	Penicillins
E-mycin	Erythromycin	Erythromycins
E.E.S.	Erythromycin ethyl succinate	Erythromycins
Erypar	Erythromycin	Erythromycins
Erythrocin	Erythromycin stearate	Erythromycins
Ethril	Erythromycin	Erythromycins
Fansidar	Pyrimethamine-sulfadoxine	Antiparasitic agents
Flagyl	Metronidazole	Metronidazole
Fortaz	Ceftazidime	Cephalosporins
Fulvicin P-G	Griseofulvin	Antifungal agents
Fulvicin U-F	Griseofulvin	Antifungal agents
Fungizone	Amphotericin B	Antifungal agents
Furadantin	Nitrofurantoin	Other urinary tract agents
Furamide	Diloxanide furoate	Antiparasitic agents
Furoxone	Furazolidone	Antiparasitic agents
Gantanol	Sulfamethoxazole	Sulfonamides + trimethoprim
Gantrisin	Sulfisoxazole	Sulfonamides + trimethoprim
Garamycin	Gentamicin	Aminoglycosides
Geocillin	Carbenicillin indanyl sodium	Penicillins
Geopen	Carbenicillin	Penicillins
Germanin	Suramin	Antiparasitic agents
Grifulvin V	Griseofulvin	Antifungal agents
Gris-PEG	Griseofulvin	Antifungal agents
Grisactin	Griseofulvin	Antifungal agents
Herplex	Idoxuridine	Antiviral agents
Hetrazan	Diethylcarbamazine	Antiparasitic agents
Hiprex	Methenamine hippurate	Other urinary tract agents
Humatin	Paromomycin	Antiparasitic agents
Hyzyd	Isoniazid	Antimycobacterial agents
Ilosone	Erythromycin estolate	Erythromycins
Ilotycin	Erythromycin	Erythromycins
INH	Isoniazid	Antimycobacterial agents

Isopto cetamide	Sulfacetamide	Sulfonamides + trimethoprim
Kafocin	Cephaloglycine	Cephalosporins
Kantrex	Kanamycin	Aminoglycosides
Keflex	Cephalexin	Cephalosporins
Keflin	Cephalothin	Cephalosporins
Kefzol	Cefazolin	Cephalosporins
Kesso-mycin	Erythromycin	Erythromycins
Kesso-pen	Penicillin G + phenoxymethyl penicillin	Penicillins
Kesso-tetra	Tetracycline	Tetracyclines
Lampit	Nifurtimox	Antiparasitic agents
Lamprene	Clofazimine	Antimycobacterial agents
Larotid	Amoxicillin	Penicillins
Ledercillin VK	Penicillin V potassium	Penicillins
Lincocin	Lincomycin	Lincosamides
Loridine	Cephaloridine	Cephalosporins
Lotrimin	Clotrimazole	Antifungal agents
Macrodantin	Nitrofurantoin	Other urinary tract agents
Mandelamine	Methenamine mandelate	Other urinary tract agents
Mandol	Cefamandole	Cephalosporins
Maxipen	Phenethicillin	Penicillins
Mefoxin	Cefoxitin	Cephalosporins
Mel B	Melarsoprol	Antiparasitic agents
Mezlin	Mezlocillin	Penicillins
Micatin	Miconazole	Antifungal agents
Minocin	Minocycline	Tetracyclines
Mintezol	Thiabendazole	Antiparasitic agents
Monocid	Cefonicid	Cephalosporins
Monistat	Miconazole	Antifungal agents
Moxam	Moxalactam	Cephalosporins
Myambutol	Ethambutol	Antimycobacterial agents
Mycifradin	Neomycin	Aminoglycosides
Mycostatin	Nystatin	Antifungal agents
Nafcil	Nafcillin	Penicillins
Nebcin	Tobramycin	Aminoglycosides
NegGram	Nalidixic acid	Quinolones
Netromycin	Netilmicin	Aminoglycosides
Niadox	Isoniazid	Antimycobacterial agents
Niclocide	Niclosamide	Antiparasitic agents
Niconyl	Isoniazid	Antimycobacterial agents
Nilstat	Nystatin	Antifungal agents
Nizoral	Ketoconazole	Antifungal agents
Noraxin	Norfloxacin	Other urinary tract agents
Nydrazid	Isoniazid	Antimycobacterial agents
Omnipen	Ampicillin	Penicillins
Omnipen-N	Ampicillin	Penicillins
Oxamycin	Cycloserine	Antimycobacterial agents
PAS	Aminosalicylic acid	Antimycobacterial agents
Panaquin	Diiodohydroxyquin	Antiparasitic agents
Panmycin	Tetracycline	Tetracyclines
Para	Aminosalicylic acid	Antimycobacterial agents
Parasal	Aminosalicylic acid	Antimycobacterial agents
Pathocil	Dicloxacillin	Penicillins

TABLE 2. (Continued)

Trade	*Generic*	*Family*	*Trade*	*Generic*	*Family*
Pediamycin	Erythromycin ethyl succinate	Erythromycins	Principen	Ampicillin	Penicillins
Pediazole	Erythromycin ethyl succinate plus sulfisoxazole		Probampacin	Ampicillin	Penicillins
			Proloprim	Trimethoprim	Sulfonamides + trimethoprim
			Prostaphlin	Oxacillin	Penicillins
Pen Vee K	Penicillin V potassium	Penicillins	Pyopen	Carbenicillin	Penicillins
PenA	Ampicillin	Penicillins	Renoquid	Sulfacytine	Sulfonamides + trimethoprim
Penapar VK	Penicillin V potassium	Penicillins	Resistopen	Oxacillin	Penicillins
Penbritin	Ampicillin	Penicillins	Rezipas	Aminosalicylic acid	Antimycobacterial agents
Pensyn	Ampicillin	Penicillins	Rifadin	Rifampin	Antimycobacterial agents
Pentam 300	Pentamidine	Antiparasitic agents	Rifamate	Rifampin-isoniazid	Antimycobacterial agents
Pentids	Penicillin G	Penicillins	Rimactane	Rifampin	Antimycobacterial agents
Pentostam	Stibogluconate	Antiparasitic agents	Robamox	Amoxicillin	Penicillins
Permapen	Benzathine penicillin G	Penicillins	Robicillin VK	Penicillin V potassium	Penicillins
Pfizer-E	Erythromycin stearate	Erythromycins	Robimycin	Erythromycin	Erythromycins
Pfizerpen	Penicillin G	Penicillins	Robitet	Tetracycline	Tetracyclines
Pipracil	Piperacillin	Penicillins	Rocephin	Ceftriaxone	Cephalosporins
Polycillin	Ampicillin	Penicillins	Rolsul	Succinylsulfathiazole	Sulfonamides + trimethoprim
Polycillin N	Ampicillin	Penicillins	Rondomycin	Methacycline	Tetracyclines
Polycillin-PRB	Ampicillin probenecid	Penicillins	Selexid	Pivmecillinam	Penicillins
Polycycline	Tetracycline	Tetracyclines	Septra	Trimethoprim-sulfamethoxazole	Sulfonamides + trimethoprim
Polymox	Amoxicillin	Penicillins			
Povan	Pyrivinium pamoate	Antiparasitic agents	Seromycin	Cycloserine	Antimycobacterial agents
Precef	Ceforanide	Cephalosporins	Silvadine	Silver sulfadiazine	Sulfonamides + trimethoprim
Primaquine	Primaquine phosphate	Antiparasitic agents	Sonilyn	Sulfachlorpyridazine	Sulfonamides + trimethoprim
Primaxin	Imipenem + cilastatin	Other β-lactams	Spectrobid	Bacampicillin	Penicillins
			Staphcillin	Methicillin	Penicillins

Steclin	Tetracycline	Tetracyclines
Stoxil	Idoxuridine	Antiviral agents
Sulamyd sodium	Sulfacetamide	Sulfonamides + trimethoprim
Sulfadyne	Sulfadiazine	Sulfonamides + trimethoprim
Sulfamylon	Mafenide	Sulfonamides + trimethoprim
Sulfasuxidine	Succinylsulfathiazole	Sulfonamides + trimethoprim
Sumycin	Tetracycline	Tetracyclines
Supen	Ampicillin	Penicillins
Symmetrel	Amantadine	Antiviral agents
Synicillin	Phenethicillin	Penicillins
TAO	Troleandomycin	—
Tegopen	Cloxacillin	Penicillins
Terfonyl	Trisulfapyrimidines	Sulfonamides + trimethoprim
Terramycin	Oxytetracycline	Tetracyclines
Tetracyn	Tetracycline	Tetracyclines
Tetrex	Tetracycline	Tetracyclines
Thiosulfil	Sulfamethizole	Sulfonamides + trimethoprim
Ticar	Ticarcillin	Penicillins
Timentin	Clavulanic acid + ticarcillin	β-lactamase inhibitors
Tinactin	Tolnaftate	Antifungal agents
Totacillin	Ampicillin	Penicillins
Trantoin	Nitrofurantoin	Other urinary tract agents
Trecator-SC	Ethionamide	Antimycobacterial agents
Trimox	Amoxicillin	Penicillins
Trimpex	Trimethoprim	Sulfonamides + trimethoprim
Trobicin	Spectinomycin	Aminoglycosides
Trojacillin-Plus	Ampicillin probenecid	Penicillins
Unipen	Nafcillin	Penicillins
Urex	Methenamine hippurate	Other urinary tract agents
Uri-Tet	Oxytetracycline	Tetracyclines
Urifon	Sulfamethizole	Sulfonamides + trimethoprim
Utibid	Oxolinic acid	Quinolones
Uticillin VK	Penicillin V potassium	Penicillins
V-Cillin K	Penicillin V potassium	Penicillins
Vancocin	Vancomycin	Vancomycin
Vansil	Oxamniquine	Antiparasitic agents
Vectrin	Minocycline	Tetracyclines
Veetids	Penicillin V potassium	Penicillins
Velosef	Cephradine	Cephalosporins
Veracillin	Dicloxacillin	Penicillins
Vermox	Mebendazole	Antiparasitic agents
Versapen	Hetacillin	Penicillins
Versapen K	Hetacillin	Penicillins
Vibramycin	Doxycycline	Tetracyclines
Vinactane	Viomycin	Antimycobacterial agents
Viocin	Viomycin	Antimycobacterial agents
Vira-A	Vidarabine	Antiviral agents
Wycillin	Penicillin G procaine	Penicillins
Yodoxin	Iodoquinol	Antiparasitic agents
Yomesan	Niclosamide	Antiparasitic agents
Zinacef	Cefuroxime	Cephalosporins
Zovirax	Acyclovir	Antiviral agents

TABLE 3a. Antimicrobial Agent Pharmacology: Penicillins—Absorption, Serum and Urine Concentrations, and Dosage

	Serum and Urine Concentration for Selected Doses		
		Peak Serum	*Peak or Range Urine*
Drug (Oral Absorption %)	*Dose (g)*	*(μg/ml)*	
Amdinocillin	10 mg/kg IV[a]	50	1260
Amoxicillin (89)	0.25 po[b] 0.5 po[b]	4.7 (avg) 7.5 (avg)	 600–2000
Ampicillin (50 avg)	0.25 po[b] 0.5 po[b] 1 po[b] 0.5 IV 0.5 IM 1 IV	1.8–2.9 2.5–4 2–6 2.9–7.1 8 40	90 100–700 100–1450 130–610 500–1000
Apalcillin	0.5 IM 1 IV[e,f] 2 IV[f]	28–37 47–58 208	 835
Azlocillin[g] (minimal)	2 IV[a] 2 IV[f] 3 IV[a] 3 IV[f]	300 165 350 214	2200–8100
Bacampicillin[j] (60–90)	0.4 po 0.8 po	6–8 11–14	
Carbenicillin (minimal)	1 IM 2 IM 1 IV 1 g/hr IV 3 IV[a]	15–20 47 45–71 160 278	 2500 1000 4165
Carbenicillin indanyl sodium (30–50)	0.382 po (1 tablet)	6.5	1130
Cloxacillin (50)	0.5 po	7–14	410–1080
Cyclacillin	0.25 po 0.5 po	6–7 11–12	
Dicloxacillin (37–74)	0.5 po	15–18	

Dosage Recommendations						
Adults			*Children*		*Newborn (Parenteral)*	
Oral	*Parenteral*	*Maximum Daily Dose (g)*	*Oral*	*Parenteral*	*Up to 1 wk*	*1 to 4 wk*
Dose/Interval			*Dose/Interval*			
0.25–0.5 g q8h		3	6.6–13.3 mg/kg q8h		Not recommended	
0.5–1 g q6h	1–2 g q4–6h[c]	12	12.5–25 mg/kg q6h	25–50 mg/kg q6h[d]	50–100 mg/kg/day q12h	100–200 mg/kg/day q6–8h
	2–4 g q4–6h[h]	24		50 mg/kg q4–6h[i] (not approved)	Not recommended	
0.4–0.8 g q12h		1.6	12.5–25 mg/kg q12h			
	5–6.5 g q4–6h[k]	40		25–100 mg/kg q4–6h	200–300 mg/kg/day q8h	400 mg/kg/day q6–8h
1–2 tablets q6h		3	12.5–16.25 mg/kg q6h			
0.5–1 g q6h		4	12.5–25 mg/kg q6h		Not recommended	
0.25–0.5 g q6h		2	12.5–25 mg/kg q6h		Not recommended	
0.25–0.5 g q6h		4	3.125–6.25 mg/kg q6h		Not recommended	

Table 3a. (Continued)

Drug (Oral Absorption %)	Serum and Urine Concentration for Selected Doses		
	Dose (g)	*Peak Serum* (μg/ml)	*Peak or Range Urine* (μg/ml)
Hetacillin[l]	0.225 po	1.7–2.1	
	0.45 po	2.5–2.7	
Methicillin (minimal)	1 IV[a]	60	
	1 IM	18	
	2 IV[f]	80	
Mezlocillin[g] (minimal)	1 IM	15	
	2 IV[a]	199	
	3 IV[a]	310	
	3 IV[f]	263	>4000
Nafcillin (10–20 erratic)	0.5 IV[f]	11	
Oxacillin (33)	0.5 po	5–6	
	0.5 IM	11	200–2000
Penicillin G (15–30)	0.25 po	0.6	85
	0.5 po	1.5–2.7	
	3 IV[f] (4.8 × 10⁶ U)	400	
	12 g/day IV (19.2 × 10⁶ U)[n]	16	
Penicillin V (60) (phenoxymethyl penicillin)	0.5 po	3–5	
Procaine penicillin G	600,000 U IM	1	
Penicillin G benzathine	1.2 × 10⁶ U IM	0.12 U/ml	20 U/ml
Piperacillin[g] (minimal)	2 IV[a]	220	
	4 IV[f]	244	1,000–8,500
	4 IV[a]	412	

Dosage Recommendations						
Adults			*Children*		*Newborn (Parenteral)*	
Oral	*Parenteral*	*Maximum Daily Dose (g)*	*Oral*	*Parenteral*	*Up to 1 wk*	*1 to 4 wk*
Dose/Interval			*Dose/Interval*			
0.225–0.45 g q6h			5.6–11.25 mg/kg q6h			
	1–2 g q4–6h	12		25–33.3 mg/kg q4–6h	50–75 mg/kg/day q8–12h	100–150 mg/kg/day q6–8h
	3 g q4h or 4 g q6h	24		50 mg/kg q4–6h	150 mg/kg/day q12h	300 mg/kg/day q6h[m]
0.5–1 g q6h	0.5–1.5 g q4–6h	9	12.5–25 mg/kg q6h	25–33.3 mg/kg q4–6h	40 mg/kg/day q12h	60–80 mg/kg/day q6–8h
0.5–1 g q6h	0.5–2 g q4–6h	12	12.5–25 mg/kg q6h	25–33.3 mg/kg q4–6h	50–75 mg/kg/day q8–12h	100–150 mg/kg/day q6–8h
0.5–1 g q6h	1.2–24 × 10^6 U/day q2–12h[o]	24 × 10^6 U	6.25–12.5 mg/kg q6h	100,000–250,000 U/kg/day q2–12h[o]	50,000–150,000 U/kg/day q8–12h	75,000–250,000 U/kg/day q6–8h
0.25–0.5g q6h		4	6.25–12.5 mg/kg q6h		Not recommended	
	0.3–4.8 × 10^6 U/day IM					
	2.4 × 10^6 U IM[p]	2.4 × 10^6 U IM		300,000–600,000 U IM	50,000 U/kg IM	50,000 U/kg IM
	3–4 g q4–6h	24		50 mg/kg q4–6h (Not approved)		

TABLE 3a. (Continued)

Drug (Oral Absorption %)	Serum and Urine Concentration for Selected Doses		
	Dose (g)	Peak Serum (μg/ml)	Peak or Range Urine (μg/ml)
Ticarcillin (minimal)	1 IM 3 IV 5 IV	35 190 327	2000
Temocillin (minimal)	0.5 IV[a] 1 IV[a] 2 IV[a]	78 160 236	100–500

[a] IV push (over 2–5 min).
[b] Fasting.
[c] Meningitis should be treated q4h.
[d] Up to 400 mg/kg/day for *Hemophilus influenzae* type b meningitis in children.
[e] Remarkable differences in peak serum levels measured immediately after a 2-minute bolus (1 gram: 825 μg/ml) as compared to a 2-hour infusion.
[f] Infusion (over 30 min).
[g] Dose-dependent pharmacokinetics.
[h] For severe, life-threatening infections: 4 g q4h.
[i] Up to 450 mg/kg/day for patients with cystic fibrosis.
[j] 100% of a dose of bacampicillin is metabolized to ampicillin.
[k] 4–8 g/day usually sufficient for urinary tract infections.

TABLE 3b. Antimicrobial Agent Pharmacology: Penicillins—Dosage Adjustment for Renal Insufficiency, Serum Half Life, and Body Fluid Levels

Drug (Oral Absorption %)	Usual Adult Dose and Interval Adjustment					Dosage for Dialysis	
	Dose	For Creatinine Clearance (ml/min)				Dose after HD Supplemental to Anuric	Daily Dose during PD
		>80	80–50	50–10	<10 (Anuric)		
Amdinocillin							
Amoxicillin (89)	0.25–0.5 g po	8 h	8 h	12 h	12–24 h	0.25 g	
Ampicillin (50 avg)	1–2 g	4–6 h	6 h	8 h	12 h	0.5 g	
Apalcillin							
Azlocillin[e] (minimal)	2–4 g	4–6 h	4–6 h	8 h	12 h	3 g	

Dosage Recommendations						
Adults			*Children*		*Newborn (Parenteral)*	
Oral	*Parenteral*	*Maximum Daily Dose (g)*	*Oral*	*Parenteral*	*Up to 1 wk*	*1 to 4 wk*
Dose/Interval			*Dose/Interval*			
	3 g q4–6h	24–30		37.5–50 mg/kg q4–6h	150–225 mg/kg/day q8–12h[q]	225–300 mg/kg/day q6–8h[q]

[l] The antibiotic activity of hetacillin is provided by its rapid conversion to ampicillin.
[m] 75 mg/kg q8h for infants weighing less than 2000 g.
[n] By continuous infusion.
[o] The interval between parenteral doses is variable: it can be as frequent as every 2 hours for initial therapy of meningococcemia or as long as 12 hours between IM doses of procaine penicillin G.
[p] Patients with latent syphilis of more than 1 year's duration should be treated with penicillin G benzathine, 2.4 million units weekly for 4 weeks.
[q] For infants <2000 g: 75 mg/kg q12h for first week and 75 mg/kg q8h for 1–4 wks old. Those >2000 g: 75 mg/kg q8h for first week and 100 mg/kg q8h for 1–4 wks old.

Serum Half-life (hr)								
For Creatinine Clearance (ml/min)		*With Dialysis*		*CSF/Serum (%) Inflamed Meninges[a]*	*Newborn Serum/ Maternal Serum (%)*	*Breast Milk/ Maternal Serum[b] (%)*	*Bile/ Serum (%)*	*Aqueous Humor/ Serum (%)*
>80	*<10*	*HD*	*PD*					
0.8–1	3.4	1.8						
1	16	2.2–4.5		5–10	100	5		
0.5–1	8–20	2–5	10.9	8–13[c]	100	11[d]	100–1000	2–8
1.5–2								
1	5	1.5–2.6	Minimal	13.3[c]				

TABLE 3b. (Continued)

	Usual Adult Dose and Interval Adjustment					*Dosage for Dialysis*	
		For Creatinine Clearance (ml/min)					
Drug (Oral Absorption %)	*Dose*	*>80*	*80–50*	*50–10*	*<10 (Anuric)*	*Dose after HD Supple-mental to Anuric*	*Daily Dose during PD*
Bacampicillin[f] (60–90)	0.4–0.8 g po	12 h	12 h	12 h	24 h		
Carbenicillin (minimal)	5–6.5 g	4–6 h	6 h	2–3 g q6–8h	2 g q12h	2 g	2 g q6h
Carbenicillin indanyl sodium (30–50)							
Cloxacillin (50)	0.5–1 g po	6 h	6 h	6 h	6 h		
Cyclacillin	0.25–0.5 g po	6 h	6 h	12–24 h	24 h		
Dicloxacillin (37–74)	0.25–0.5 g po	6 h	6 h	6 h	6 h		
Hetacillin[g]	0.225–0.45 g po	6 h					
Methicillin (minimal)	1–2 g	4–6 h	6 h	8 h	12 h	2 g	
Mezlocillin[e] (minimal)	3–4 g	4–6 h	4–6 h	6–8 h	8–12 h	2–3 g	
Nafcillin (10–20 erratic)	0.5–1.5 g	4–6 h	4–6 h	4–6 h	4–6 h		
Oxacillin (33)	0.5–2 g	4–6 h	4–6 h	4–6 h	4–6 h		
Penicillin G (15–30)	1.2–24 × 10^6 U/day	2–12 h	2–12 h	2–12 h	⅓–½ maximum daily dose[h]	0.5 × 10^6 U	
Penicillin V (60) (phenoxymethyl penicillin)	0.25–0.5 g po	6 h	6 h	8 h	12 h	0.25 g	
Procaine penicillin G							
Penicillin G benzathine							
Piperacillin[e] (minimal)	3–4 g	4–6 h	4–6 h	6–12 h	12 h	2 g q8h + 1 g after HD	

Serum Half-life (hr)								
For Creatinine Clearance (ml/min)		*With Dialysis*		*CSF/Serum (%) Inflamed Meninges*[a]	*Newborn Serum/ Maternal Serum (%)*	*Breast Milk/ Maternal Serum*[b] *(%)*	*Bile/ Serum (%)*	*Aqueous Humor/ Serum (%)*
>80	*<10*	*HD*	*PD*					
1	8–20	2–5			65–75	1.7–3.6	17	
0.5–1	12.5	6	4.2–7.4	9.4[c]	50–100	0.4	50–75	up to 3
0.5	0.8	Minimal	Minimal					
0.5	3.5							
0.7	1–2	1.6	Minimal	Minimal	0–10		5–8	
0.3								
0.5	4	Minimal	Minimal	3–12	50–100		20–50	1–2
1.1[e]	1.6–2.6	1.2–1.4	Minimal	14[c]	100		1000	
0.5	1.2	Minimal	Minimal	9–20	10–15		4000	1–2
0.5	2	Minimal	1.4		10–15	<or = 3.5	20–40	0–20
0.5	7–10	5		2–6	100	6 avg	200–800	
1	4							
1.3–1.5	2.1–5	1.2–2.4	3.6	15.7[c]		1	1000	

TABLE 3b. (Continued)

Drug (Oral Absorption %)	Usual Adult Dose and Interval Adjustment: Dose	For Creatinine Clearance (ml/min): >80	80–50	50–10	<10 (Anuric)	Dosage for Dialysis: Dose after HD Supple-mental to Anuric	Daily Dose during PD
Ticarcillin (minimal)	3 g	4–6 h	4–6 h	2–3 g q6–8h	2 g q12h	3 g	3 g q12h
Temocillin (minimal)							

[a] Penicillins penetrate minimally across uninflamed meninges into the CSF.

[b] Penicillins do not appear in sufficient quantities to treat infections in the infant, but do appear in quantities which could lead to allergic sensitization.

[c] Mean concentration.

[d] Candidiasis and diarrhea in infants may result from ampicillin administration to nursing mothers (*Pharm J* 217:219, 1976).

TABLE 4a. Antimicrobial Agent Pharmacology: Cephalosporins—Absorption, Serum and Urine Concentrations, and Dosage

Drug (Oral Absorption %)	Serum and Urine Concentration for Selected Doses: Dose (g)	Peak Serum (μg/ml)	Peak or Range Urine (μg/ml)
First Generation			
Cefadroxil[a]	0.25 po	9	
	0.5 po	18	1200
	1 po	35	
Cefazolin	0.5 IM	40	2460
	1 IM	59–68	4010
	1 IV	188	
Cephalexin[a] (80–100)	0.25 po[b]	8	
	0.50 po[b]	15–40	1000
Cephaloridine	0.5 IM	20	
	1 IV[c]	60	400–1000
Cephalothin	1 IV[d]	40–60	2500
	2 IV[d]	80–100	

Serum Half-life (hr)								
For Creatinine Clearance (ml/min)		*With Dialysis*		*CSF/Serum (%) Inflamed Meninges*[a]	*Newborn Serum/ Maternal Serum (%)*	*Breast Milk/ Maternal Serum*[b] *(%)*	*Bile/ Serum (%)*	*Aqueous Humor/ Serum (%)*
>80	*<10*	*HD*	*PD*					
1–1.5	13	6	Minimal	9.5[c]				
4.5–5	18–27	4.5						

[e] Dose-dependent pharmacokinetics.

[f] 100% of a dose of bacampicillin is metabolized to ampicillin.

[g] The antibiotic activity of hetacillin is provided by its rapid conversion to ampicillin.

[h] Patients on low daily doses usually tolerate full dosage. Upper dosage limit approximation: dose (10^6 U/day) = 3.2 + CLCR (*Ann Intern Med* 82:194, 1975).

Dosage Recommendations						
Adults			*Children*		*Newborn (Parenteral)*	
Oral	*Parenteral*	*Maximum Daily Dose (g)*	*Oral*	*Parenteral*	*Up to 1 wk*	*1 to 4 wk*
Dose/Interval			*Dose/Interval*			
1 g q12h or 2 g q24h		2	15 mg/kg q12h			
	0.5–1.5 g q6–8h	6		8.3–25 mg/kg q6–8h	15 mg/kg q12h	15–20 mg/kg q8–12h
0.25–1 g q6h		4	6.25–12.5 mg/ kg q6h		Not recommended	
	0.5–1.5 g q6–8h	6				
	0.5–2 g q4–6h	12		75–125 mg/ kg/day q4–6h	20 mg/kg q12h	20 mg/kg q8h

Table 4a. (Continued)

Drug (Oral Absorption %)	Serum and Urine Concentration for Selected Doses		
	Dose (g)	*Peak Serum* (μg/ml)	*Peak or Range Urine* (μg/ml)
Cephapirin	1 IV[c]	70	2560
	1 IM	25	1280
Cephradine			
oral (90–100)	0.5 po[b]	15	1000
parenteral	1 IV	85	1975
Second Generation			
Cefaclor[a,e]	0.25 po	5–7	600
	0.5 po	15	900
	1 po	35	
Cefamandole	1 IM	20–35	
	1 IV[d]	90	
	2 IV	165	5000
Cefonicid	7.5 mg/kg IV[c]	95–155	100–1000
	0.5 IM	60	
	1 IV[d]	150	
Ceforanide	1 IV[d]	135	
	1 IM	70	
	2 IV[d]	220	
Cefotiam	1 IV[d]	50	
	2 IV[d]	135	
Cefoxitin	1 IM	20	450–7200
	1 IV[d]	110–125	
Cefuroxime	0.5 IM	25	
	1 IM	40	
	1 IV[c]	100	5000–7000
	1.5 IV[d]	65	
Third Generation			
Cefmenoxime	1 IV[d]	40	1740
	1 IM	15	
	2 IV[d]	95	3620
Cefoperazone	1 IV[d]	100–125	1600
	2 IV	200	2000

Dosage Recommendations						
Adults			*Children*		*Newborn (Parenteral)*	
Oral	*Parenteral*	*Maximum Daily Dose (g)*	*Oral*	*Parenteral*	*Up to 1 wk*	*1 to 4 wk*
Dose/Interval			*Dose/Interval*			
	0.5–2 g q4–6h	12		10–20 mg/kg q6h		
0.25–1 g q6h		4	6.25–12.5 mg/kg q6h			
	1–2 g q6h	8		12.5–25 mg/kg q6h	Not recommended	
0.25–0.5 g q8h		4	6.6–13.3 mg/kg q8h			
	0.5–2 g q4–6h	12		16.6–25 mg/kg q4–6h		
	0.5–2 g q24h	2				
	0.5–1 g q12h	2		10–20 mg/kg q12h	Not recommended	
	1–2 g q4–6h or 3 g q6h	12		20–26.6 mg/kg q4–6h		
	0.75–1.5 g q8h[f]	9		16.6–25 mg/kg q6–8h[g]	Not recommended	
	0.5–2 g q4–6h	12				
	1–4 g q8h or 0.5–3 g q6h	12		50 mg/kg q8h (not approved)		

Table 4a. (Continued)

Drug (Oral Absorption %)	*Serum and Urine Concentration for Selected Doses* *Dose (g)*	*Peak Serum* ($\mu g/ml$)	*Peak or Range Urine* ($\mu g/ml$)
Cefotaxime	1 IM	10–15	2010
	1 IV[d]	40	
	2 IV[d]	80–90	
(Desacetyl cefotaxime)	2 IV[c]	9.8	
Cefotetan	0.5 IM	35	1000
	1 IV[c]	255	3500
	2 IV[d]	200	
Cefpiramide	1 IV[d]	165	300
	2 IV[d]	320	
Cefsulodin	1 IM	20	
	1 IV[d]	65	1500–3500
	2 IV[d]	140	
Ceftazidime	1 IV[d]	85	4000–6000
	2 IV[c]	180	
Ceftizoxime	0.5 IM		1120
	1 IV[d]	90	
	2 IV[d]	120	
Ceftriaxone[h]	0.5 IM	50	
	1 IV[d]	150	995
	2 IV[d]	270	2700
Moxalactam	1 IV[d]	60–100	2100
	2 IV	150	4200

[a] Oral.
[b] Fasting.
[c] IV push (over 2–5 min).
[d] Infusion (over 30 min).
[e] Dose dependent pharmacokinetics.
[f] Up to 3 g every 8 hours for meningitis.
[g] Up to 240 mg/kg/day divided every 6–8 hours for meningitis.
[h] Nonlinear kinetics; 35 $\mu g/ml$ at 12 h and 15 $\mu g/ml$ at 24 h.
[i] For the treatment of uncomplicated gonococcal infections, 0.125 to 0.25 g as a single intramuscular dose is effective.

Dosage Recommendations						
Adults			*Children*		*Newborn (Parenteral)*	
Oral	*Parenteral*	*Maximum Daily Dose (g)*	*Oral*	*Parenteral*	*Up to 1 wk*	*1 to 4 wk*
Dose/Interval			*Dose/Interval*			
	1–2 g q4–6h	12		25–33 mg/kg q4–6h	50 mg/kg q12h	50 mg/kg q8h
	0.5–3 g q6h	12				
	0.5–2 g q8–12h	6		30–50 mg/kg q8h	30 mg/kg q12h	30 mg/kg q12h
	1–4 g q8–12h	12				
	0.5–1 g q12–24h[i]	2[j]		25–50 mg/kg q12h[k]		
	0.5–4 g q8–12 h[l]	12[l]		50 mg/kg q6–8h[l,m]	50 mg/kg q12h[l,m]	50 mg/kg q8h[l,m]

[j] The maximum recommended daily dose is currently 2 g; however, data for adult meningitis is incomplete.

[k] For gram-negative meningitis in children, manufacturer recommends an initial loading dose of 75 mg/kg.

[l] Bleeding time should be monitored in patients receiving more than 4 g/day for more than 3 days. Prophylactic vitamin k, 10 mg per week, should be given to patients treated with moxalactam.

[m] For gram-negative meningitis in children, manufacturer recommends an initial loading dose of 100 mg/kg.

TABLE 4b. Antimicrobial Agent Pharmacology: Cephalosporins—Dosage Adjustment for Renal Insufficiency, Serum Half Life, and Body Fluid Levels

	Usual Adult Dose and Interval Adjustment					*Dosage for Dialysis*	
		For Creatinine Clearance (ml/min)					
Drug (Oral Absorption %)	*Dose*	*>80*	*80–50*	*50–10*	*<10 (Anuric)*	*Dose after HD Supplemental to Anuric*	*Daily Dose during PD*
First Generation							
Cefadroxil[c]	1 g po	12–24 h	12–24 h	24 h	36 h	1 g	
Cefazolin	0.5–1.5 g	6–8 h	8h	0.5–1 g q8–12h	0.5–1 g q24h	0.25–0.5 g	
Cephalexin[c] (80–100)	0.25–1 g po	6 h	6 h	8–12 h	24–48 h	0.25–1 g	
Cephaloridine	0.5–1.5 g	6–8 h	1 g q12h	0.5 g q12h	0.5 g q24h	1 g	1 g
Cephalothin	0.5–2 g	4–6 h	6 h	8 h	12 h	Supplemental dose	No supplemental dose[f]
Cephapirin	0.5–2 g	4–6 h	6 h	8 h	12 h	7.5–15 mg/kg before dialysis	
Cephradine oral (90–100)							
parenteral	1–2 g	6 h[h]	6 h	8 h	12–24 h	1–2 g	
Second Generation							
Cefaclor[c,d]	0.25–0.5 g po	8 h	8 h	8 h	8 h	Repeat dose after HD	
Cefamandole	0.5–2 g	4–6 h	1–2 g q6h	1–2 g q8h	0.5–1 g q12h	No supplemental dose	No supplemental dose
Cefonicid	0.5–2 g	24 h	0.5–1.5 g q24h	0.5–1 g q24h	0.5–1 g q3–5 days	No extra dose	
Ceforanide	0.5–1 g	12 h	12 h	24–48 h	48–72 h	0.5–1 g	
Cefotiam							

Serum Half-life (hr)								
For Creatinine Clearance (ml/min)		*With Dialysis*		*CSF/Serum (%) Inflamed Meninges*[a]	*Newborn Serum/ Maternal Serum (%)*	*Breast Milk/ Maternal Serum*[b] *(%)*	*Bile/ Serum (%)*	*Aqueous Humor/ Serum (%)*
>80	*<10*	*HD*	*PD*					
1.2–1.6[d]	approx. 20	2.5–3.4			50	8	100	
1.5–2	20–70	6.5–9.0	20–46[e]	1–4	35–69	3	100–300	<1–10
1–1.5	20–40	4.5–6		Minimal	60	2		11
1–1.5	23	3–4	8–9	17	50			Minimal
0.5–1	3–18	2.5–3	5.1	1.2–5.6	10	2–4.7[g]	40–80	4
0.5–1	1.5–2.4	1.8			60			
1–1.5	8–15				22		10–200	
0.5–1	2.9	1.5				2	60	3
0.5–1	11	6.6	7.2	0.5–20		2.4	300–400	1.5
4.4	50–65	33–46				0.5	8.5 avg	<1
2.9–3.2	20–40	5					270	
0.7–1				10			20	

Table 4b. (Continued)

Drug (Oral Absorption %)	*Usual Adult Dose and Interval Adjustment* Dose	*For Creatinine Clearance (ml/min)* >80	80–50	50–10	<10 (Anuric)	*Dosage for Dialysis* Dose after HD Supplemental to Anuric	Daily Dose during PD
Cefoxitin	1–3 g	4–6 h	1–2 g q8h	1–2 g q12h	0.5–1 g q12–24h	1–2 g	
Cefuroxime	0.75–1.5 g	8 h	8 h	8–12 h	24 h	Supplemental dose	No supplemental dose
Third Generation							
Cefmenoxime	0.5–2 g	4–6 h					
Cefoperazone	1–4 g	6–8 h	6–8 h	6–8 h	6–8 h[j]	No supplemental dose	
Cefotaxime	1–2 g	4–6 h	4–6 h	6–12 h	12 h	Maintenance dose X 50%	
(Desacetyl cefotaxime)							
Cefotetan							
Cefpiramide							
Cefsulodin	0.5–3 g	6 h	8 h	0.25–1.5 g q6h	0.5 g q12h	0.25 g	
Ceftazidime	0.5–2 g	8–12 h	8–12 h	1 g q12–24h	0.5 g q24–48h		1 g then 0.5 g q24h

Serum Half-life (hr)								
For Creatinine Clearance (ml/min)		*With Dialysis*		*CSF/Serum (%) Inflamed Meninges*[a]	*Newborn Serum/ Maternal Serum (%)*	*Breast Milk/ Maternal Serum*[b] *(%)*	*Bile/ Serum (%)*	*Aqueous Humor/ Serum (%)*
>80	*<10*	*HD*	*PD*					
0.75–1	10–22	4	Minimal (7.8–CAPD)	50	33–50	Up to 3	280	4
1–2	15	3.75	5.4–13.6[i]	6–10	20–33	Up to 3	35–80	1
1	8				30		250	2.6
1.8–2[d]	2.5	2.2		5–9	20–50	Up to 1.5	800–1200	1–3
1.1	2.5	1.6	2.9	10–25	25[k]	Up to 3	50	0.5–4
1.6	11	3.2						
3–4.6	12–35.1	5.6–7.5			<1.4[l]	17[l]	2100	
1.6–1.9	10–13	2.1–3.3		15	40		30–40	5.5
1.8	16.1–25	2.8	8.7	21.5		7		3–5

Table 4b. (Continued)

Drug (Oral Absorption %)	Usual Adult Dose and Interval Adjustment					Dosage for Dialysis	
		For Creatinine Clearance (ml/min)				Dose after HD Supplemental to Anuric	Daily Dose during PD
	Dose	>80	80–50	50–10	<10 (Anuric)		
Ceftizoxime	1–4 g	8–12 h	0.5–1.5 g q8h	0.25–1 g q12h	0.25–1 g q24–48h	Give scheduled dose after dialysis	3 g q48h
Ceftriaxone[m]	0.5–1 g	12–24 h	12–24 h	12–24 h	12–24 h[n]	No supplemental dose	
Moxalactam	0.5–4 g	8–12 h	0.5–3 g q8h	0.25–2 g q8h or 0.25–3 g q12h	0.25 g q12h to 1 g q24h	1–2 g	

[a] Cephalosporins penetrate minimally across uninflamed meninges into the CSF.

[b] Cephalosporins do not appear in sufficient systemic quantities via breast milk to treat infections in the infant but could theoretically sensitize the newborn.

[c] Oral.

[d] Dose dependent pharmacokinetics.

[e] Only two patients studied.

[f] Peritoneal dialysis is reported to diminish the mean peak concentration of cephalothin by 24% as well as reducing the subsequent cephalothin levels by as much as 50% from baseline. Despite this enhanced elimination during peritoneal dialysis, the cephalothin serum level persisted above 16 μg/ml for 12 hours (*Am J Med Sci* 257:116–24, 1969).

[g] Data from rabbits.

[h] Parenteral doses can be divided q4–6h.

TABLE 5a. Antimicrobial Agent Pharmacology: Other Beta-Lactams and Beta-Lactamase Inhibitors—Absorption, Serum and Urine Concentrations, and Dosage

Drug (Oral Absorption %)	Serum and Urine Concentration for Selected Doses		
	Dose (g)	Peak Serum (μg/ml)	Peak or Range Urine (μg/ml)
Other β-lactams			
Aztreonam (minimal)	0.5 IV[a]	58	1400
	0.5 IM	22	
	1 IV[a]	125	3000
	1 IM	47	
	2 IV[a]	245	6500

Serum Half-life (hr) For Creatinine Clearance (ml/min) >80	<10	With Dialysis HD	PD	*CSF/Serum (%) Inflamed Meninges*[a]	*Newborn Serum/ Maternal Serum (%)*	*Breast Milk/ Maternal Serum*[b] *(%)*	*Bile/ Serum (%)*	*Aqueous Humor/ Serum (%)*
1.7	25–36	4.9	8.3 (10–14.1-CAPD)	21–22	33	1–6	10–31 avg	3.6–5.5
8[d]	11.9–15.4	16.1		7–11	25	2–3	Up to 1000	
2	19–22	4	Minimal	10–20[o]	30–40	2.7	100–200	1.5

[i] Limited number of patients studied.

[j] From manufacturer's data: "When hepatic function is essentially normal, cefoperazone generally does not require adjustment of usual dosages in cases of renal impairment, including end-stage renal failure." Antibiotic serum concentrations are recommended, however, to assess drug accumulation for patients with renal compromise receiving greater than 4 g/day.

[k] From fetal samples after abortion.

[l] From investigator's brochure: fetal rat data.

[m] Nonlinear kinetics; 35 μg/ml at 12 h and 15 μg/ml at 25 h.

[n] Serum levels of ceftriaxone should be monitored in patients with severe renal impairment or concomitant renal and hepatic compromise.

[o] Data from clinical studies have reported CSF penetration up to 40%.

Dosage Recommendations Adults: Oral (Dose/Interval)	Adults: Parenteral (Dose/Interval)	Adults: Maximum Daily Dose (g)	Children: Oral (Dose/Interval)	Children: Parenteral (Dose/Interval)	Newborn (Parenteral): Up to 1 wk	Newborn (Parenteral): 1 to 4 wk
	0.5–2 g q6–12h	8				

Table 5a. (Continued)

Drug (Oral Absorption %)	*Dose (g)*	*Serum and Urine Concentration for Selected Doses* — *Peak Serum* (*μg/ml*)	*Peak or Range Urine* (*μg/ml*)
Imipenem (minimal)	0.25 IV	22	50
	0.5 IV	43	100[b]
	1 IV	68–78	> or = 100
β-lactamase inhibitors			
Clavulanic acid	0.125 po	4	380
	0.25 po	6	680
	0.2 IV[d]	13.4	
Sulbactam (60–80)	0.5 IV[d]	20–30	
	1 IV[d]	40–60	
	0.25 po[f]	3.6	
	0.5 po	4.4–5.1	

[a] IV push.

[b] Urine concentrations are obtained with concomitant administration of dehydropeptidase inhibitor, cilastatin.

[c] For children 3 years of age or less: 25 mg/kg/dose; for children over 3 years: 15 mg/kg/dose to a maximum of 3 g/day.

TABLE 5b. Antimicrobial Agent Pharmacology: Other Beta-Lactams and Beta-Lactamase Inhibitors—Dosage Adjustment for Renal Insufficiency, Serum Half Life, and Body Fluid Levels

Drug (Oral Absorption %)	*Usual Adult Dose and Interval Adjustment* — *Dose*	*For Creatinine Clearance (ml/min)* — *>80*	*80–50*	*50–10*	*<10 (Anuric)*	*Dosage for Dialysis* — *Dose after HD Supplemental to Anuric*	*Daily Dose during PD*
Other β-lactams							
Aztreonam (minimal)	0.5–2 g	6–12 h	8–12 h	12–24 h	24–36 h		
Imipenem (minimal)	0.5–1 g	6–8 h	6–8 h	6–12 h	12–24 h	2 g/day max and one dose after HD	

Adults: Oral (Dose/Interval)	Adults: Parenteral (Dose/Interval)	Adults: Maximum Daily Dose (g)	Children: Oral (Dose/Interval)	Children: Parenteral (Dose/Interval)	Newborn (Parenteral): Up to 1 wk	Newborn (Parenteral): 1 to 4 wk
	0.5–1 g q6–8 h	4		15–25 mg/kg q6h[c]	16.6–33.3 mg/kg q8h (preliminary)	
0.25–0.5 g q8h[e]		1.5[e]	6.6–13.3 mg/kg q8h[e]			

Dosage Recommendations

[d] IV infusion over 30 min.

[e] Based on amoxicillin content. 250 mg and 500 mg tablets contain 125 mg clavulanic acid.

[f] As sultamicillin, a double ester of ampicillin and the β-lactamase inhibitor, sulbactam.

Serum Half-life (hr): For Creatinine Clearance (ml/min) >80	Serum Half-life (hr): For Creatinine Clearance (ml/min) <10	Serum Half-life (hr): With Dialysis HD	Serum Half-life (hr): With Dialysis PD	CSF/Serum (%) Inflamed Meninges	Newborn Serum/Maternal Serum (%)	Breast Milk/Maternal Serum (%)	Bile/Serum (%)	Aqueous Humor/Serum (%)
1.7–2	6–8.7	[a]	3	8[b]			46	
1	4			30[b]			Minimal	46[b]

Table 5b. (Continued)

Drug (Oral Absorption %)	*Usual Adult Dose and Interval Adjustment*					*Dosage for Dialysis*	
	Dose	*For Creatinine Clearance (ml/min)*				*Dose after HD Supple-mental to Anuric*	*Daily Dose during PD*
		>80	*80–50*	*50–10*	*<10 (Anuric)*		
β-lactamase inhibitors							
Clavulanic acid						Supplemental dose	
Sulbactam (60–80)							

[a] Hemodialysis removes up to 50% of aztreonam.
[b] Animal data.
[c] Data obtained 1 hour after dose of oral Augmentin (amoxicillin plus clavulanic acid).

TABLE 6a. Antimicrobial Agent Pharmacology: Aminoglycosides—Absorption, Serum and Urine Concentrations, and Dosage

Drug (Oral Absorption %)	*Serum and Urine Concentrations for Selected Doses*		
	Dose	*Peak Serum* (μg/ml)	*Peak or Range Urine* (μg/ml)
Amikacin	5 mg/kg IM	16	830
	7.5 mg/kg IM	21	700
	7.5 mg/kg IV	38	
Gentamicin (minimal)	1.25 mg/kg IM	5–7	5–100
Kanamycin	0.5 g IM	14–29	140–250
Neomycin (minimal)	4.0 g po[c]	4	
Netilmicin	2 mg/kg IM	6	
	2.5 mg/kg IM	7.5	

Serum Half-life (hr) For Creatinine Clearance (ml/min) >80	<10	With Dialysis HD	PD	*CSF/Serum (%) Inflamed Meninges*	*Newborn Serum/ Maternal Serum (%)*	*Breast Milk/ Maternal Serum (%)*	*Bile/ Serum (%)*	*Aqueous Humor/ Serum (%)*
0.7–1.4	2.9	1.6			100	Minimal	50[c]	
0.7–1	8.1	2.4						

Dosage Recommendations						
Adults			*Children*		*Newborn (Parenteral)*	
Oral	*Parenteral*[a]	*Maximum Daily Dose*	*Oral*	*Parenteral*	*Up to 1 wk*	*1 to 4 wk*
Dose/Interval			*Dose/Interval*			
	5 mg/kg q8h or 7.5 mg/kg q12h	1.5 g		5 mg/kg q8h or 7.5 mg/kg q12h	7.5 mg/kg q12h	7.5 mg/kg q12h
	1–1.7 mg/kg q8h[b]	5 mg/kg		1–2.5 mg/kg q8h[b]	2.5 mg/kg q12h	2.5 mg/kg q8h
	5 mg/kg q8h or 7.5 mg/kg q12h	1.5 g		5 mg/kg q8h or 7.5 mg/kg q12h	7.5–10 mg/kg q12h	Same as children's
6.6 mg/kg q4h < or = 3 days[d]		3 g po	12.5 mg/kg q6h			
	1.5–3.25 mg/kg q12h or 1.3–2.2 mg/kg q8h	6.5 mg/kg		1.8–2.7 mg/kg q8h or 2.7–4 mg/kg q12h	2.5 mg/kg q12h	2.5 mg/kg q8h

Table 6a. (Continued)

Drug (Oral Absorption %)	*Serum and Urine Concentrations for Selected Doses*		
	Dose	*Peak Serum* ($\mu g/ml$)	*Peak or Range Urine* ($\mu g/ml$)
Spectinomycin	2 g IM 4 g IM	74 199	9000
Streptomycin	0.5 g IM 1 g IM	6–42 25–50	300–400 1000
Tobramycin	1 mg/kg IM 2 mg/kg IV	4 3.1–14	75–100 320

[a] The dosing strategy for aminoglycosides involves the use of ideal (lean) body weight (IBW) for dosage calculation. In obese patients, this approach would result in serum antibiotic concentrations less than expected. Alternative dosing recommendations have been proposed that account for the change in drug distribution volume with obesity.

[b] For meningitis, aminoglycosides may be administered intraventricularly in single, supplemental daily doses until CSF cultures are negative. (Gentamicin and tobramycin dose: 5–10 mg for adults; 1–2 mg for infants; not recommended for the newborn.)

TABLE 6b. Antimicrobial Agent Pharmacology: Aminoglycosides—Dosage Adjustment for Renal Insufficiency, Serum Half Life, and Body Fluid Levels

Drug (Oral Absorption %)	*Usual Adult Dose and Interval Adjustment*[a]					*Dosage for Dialysis*	
		For Creatinine Clearance (ml/min)					
	Dose	*>80*	*80–50*	*50–10*	*<10 (Anuric)*	*Dose after HD Supplemental to Anuric*	*Daily Dose during PD*
Amikacin	5–7.5 mg/kg	8–12 h	12 h	24–36 h	36–48 h	2.5–3.75 mg/kg	3–4 mg/2 liters dialysate removed
Gentamicin (minimal)	1.5 mg/kg	8 h	8–12 h	12–24 h	24–48 h	1–1.5 mg/kg	1 mg/2 liters dialysate removed
Kanamycin	5–7.5 mg/kg	8–12 h	24 h	24–72 h	72–96 h	5 mg/kg	3.5 mg/kg q day
Neomycin (minimal)	6.6 mg/kg po	4 h					

Dosage Recommendations						
Adults			*Children*		*Newborn (Parenteral)*	
Oral	*Parenteral*[a]	*Maximum Daily Dose*	*Oral*	*Parenteral*	*Up to 1 wk*	*1 to 4 wk*
Dose/Interval			*Dose/Interval*			
	2 g once[e]	4 g		40 mg/kg once	Not recommended	
	0.5–1g q12h	2 g		10–15 mg/kg q12h	Not recommended	
	1–1.7 mg/kg q8h	5 mg/kg		2–2.5 mg/kg q8h[f]	2.5 mg/kg q12h	2.5 mg/kg q8h

[c] Although neomycin is classified as nonabsorbable, some absorption from the GI tract does occur. A review of neomycin-induced deafness has identified ototoxicity as a consequence of all modes of administration—parenteral, aerosol, oral, wound and bowel irrigation, and cutaneous.

[d] The recommended dosage schedule for bowel evacuation; as adjunctive therapy for hepatic coma: 25 mg/kg q6h × 24 hours, then 12.5 mg/kg q6h thereafter.

[e] For disseminated gonococcal infections, spectinomycin may be administered 2 g every 12 hours for 3 days.

[f] Daily dosage may also be divided q6h per manufacturer.

Serum Half-life (hr)				*CSF/Serum (%) Inflamed Meninges*[b]	*Newborn Serum/ Maternal Serum (%)*	*Breast Milk/ Maternal Serum (%)*	*Bile/ Serum*[c] *(%)*	*Aqueous Humor/ Serum (%)*
For Creatinine Clearance (ml/min)		*With Dialysis*						
>80	*<10*	*HD*	*PD*					
2–2.5	44–86[d]	3.75–5.6	17.9–29	15–24	16		30	0–4
2–3	48–72	8–10	5–15[e]	10–30	30–40		30–60	<8
2.2–3	30–80[f]	4.9	5[g]	43	50	35	100	
3								

Table 6b. (Continued)

Drug (Oral Absorption %)	Usual Adult Dose and Interval Adjustment[a]					Dosage for Dialysis	
		For Creatinine Clearance (ml/min)					
	Dose	>80	80–50	50–10	<10 (Anuric)	Dose after HD Supple-mental to Anuric	Daily Dose during PD
Netilmicin	1.3–2.2 mg/kg	8 h	8–12 h	12–24 h	24–48 h	2 mg/kg	
Spectinomycin	2 g once[g]						
Streptomycin	0.5–1 g	12 h	24 h	24–72 h	72–96 h	5 mg/kg	
Tobramycin	1.5 mg/kg	8 h	8–12 h	12–24 h	24–48 h	1 mg/kg	1 mg/2 liters dialysate removed

[a] Or calculate the dosage interval in hours as nine times the serum creatinine concentration in mg/100 ml (amikacin, kanamycin) or eight times the serum creatinine concentration in mg/100 ml (gentamicin, netilmicin, tobramycin). Alternatively, refer to nomogram in FA Sarubbi, Jr, et al., *Ann Intern Med* 89:612–18, 1978. The simplicity of these predictive methods make them useful for establishing initial dosing schedules, but serum antimicrobial concentrations should be determined subsequently to ensure therapeutic, nontoxic blood levels.

TABLE 7a. Antimicrobial Agent Pharmacology: Tetracyclines—Absorption, Serum and Urine Concentrations, and Dosage

Drug (Oral Absorption %)	Serum and Urine Concentration for Selected Doses		
	Dose (g)	Peak Serum (μg/ml)	Peak or Range Urine (μg/ml)
Chlortetracycline (30)	0.25 po	1.5–2.5	320
	0.5 po	7	
Demeclocycline (66)	0.3 po	2	
Doxycycline (90–100[b])	0.1 po	1.8–2.9	
	0.2 po	3.7–6.7	
	0.2 IV[c]	4	
Methacycline (58)	0.3 po	1–2	

Serum Half-life (hr)								
For Creatinine Clearance (ml/min)		*With Dialysis*		*CSF/Serum (%) Inflamed Meninges*[b]	*Newborn Serum/ Maternal Serum (%)*	*Breast Milk/ Maternal Serum (%)*	*Bile/ Serum*[c] *(%)*	*Aqueous Humor/ Serum (%)*
>80	*<10*	*HD*	*PD*					
2.2–2.5	33	5.5		21–26				
1.7	18.5–29.3							
2–3	100–110			20	10–40	<25	40–300	
2–2.75	50–70	2.9–10	12–16	14–23	15		13–20	18

[b] Mean percent penetration into CSF of aminoglycoside antibiotics in normal rabbits has been reported less than 10%.

[c] Aminoglycosides do not penetrate the biliary tree in the presence of obstruction.

[d] Half-life of 86.5 h in anephric patients and 44.3 h in patients with minimal residual kidney function.

[e] In the absence of an inflammatory response, peritoneal clearance is diminished; t½ reported as approximately 29 hours. The elimination half-life during CAPD is 36 hours.

[f] The serum half-life of kanamycin in severely uremic patients may be prolonged to 70–80 hours.

[g] As dialysis continues, removal of drug is slower and the half-life is reportedly prolonged to 48 hours.

Dosage Recommendations						
Adults			*Children*[a]		*Newborn (Parenteral)*	
Oral	*Parenteral*	*Maximum Daily Dose (g)*	*Oral*	*Parenteral*	*Up to 1 wk*	*1 to 4 wk*
Dose/Interval			*Dose/Interval*			
see tetracycline			*see* tetracycline		Not recommended	
0.15 g q6h or 0.3 g q12h		0.6	6.6–13.2 mg/kg/day q6–12h		Not recommended	
0.1 g q12–24h	0.1 g q12–24h	0.2	2 mg/kg q12–24h		Not recommended	
0.15 g q6h or 0.3 g q12h		1.2	2.5 mg/kg q6h or 5 mg/kg q12h		Not recommended	

Table 7a. (Continued)

Drug (Oral Absorption %)	Serum and Urine Concentration for Selected Doses		
	Dose (g)	Peak Serum (μg/ml)	Peak or Range Urine (μg/ml)
Minocycline (95–100[b])	0.2 po	0.7–4.5	15[d]
	0.1 IV[c]	8.8	
Oxytetracycline (59)	0.25 po	0.9	300
Tetracycline (75[b])	0.25 po	2–4	300
	0.5 IV[c]	8	

[a] The tetracyclines cause brown discoloration of the teeth and may retard growth of bone in the human fetus and children. They are not recommended for use in patients younger than 12 years of age.

TABLE 7b. Antimicrobial Agent Pharmacology: Tetracyclines—Dosage Adjustment for Renal Insufficiency, Serum Half Life, and Body Fluid Levels

Drug (Oral Absorption %)	Usual Adult Dose and Interval Adjustment					Dosage for Dialysis	
	Dose	For Creatinine Clearance (ml/min) >80	80–50	50–10	<10 (Anuric)	Dose after HD Supple-mental to Anuric	Daily Dose during PD
Chlortetracycline (30)	0.25–0.5 g po	6h	Not recommended				
Demeclocycline (66)	0.15–0.3 g po	6–12 h	Not recommended				
Doxycycline (90–100[d])	0.1 g po	12–24 h	12–24 h	12–24 h	12–24 h		
Methacycline (58)	0.15–0.3 g po	6–12 h	Not recommended				
Minocycline (95–100[d])	0.1 g po	12–24 h	Not recommended				
Oxytetracycline (59)	0.25–0.5 g po	6 h	Not recommended				
Tetracycline (75[d])	0.25–0.5 g po	6 h	Not recommended				

[a] Patients in convalescent stage of poliomyelitis.

[b] Not detected at dose of 300 mg/day.

[c] Biliary levels determined after IV injection of 500 mg of the antibiotic.

[d] Serum levels of doxycycline are reduced by 20% if given with food, whereas serum levels of tetracycline are reduced up to 50%. The oral absorption of minocycline is not significantly impaired by food or milk.

Dosage Recommendations						
Adults			*Children*[a]		*Newborn (Parenteral)*	
Oral	*Parenteral*	*Maximum Daily Dose (g)*	*Oral*	*Parenteral*	*Up to 1 wk*	*1 to 4 wk*
Dose/Interval			*Dose/Interval*			
0.1 g q12h	0.1 g q12–24h	0.2	4 mg/kg once then 2 mg/kg q12h		Not recommended	
see tetracycline			*see* tetracycline		Not recommended	
0.25–0.5 g q6h	0.125–0.5 g q6–12h	2	6.25–12.5 mg/kg q6h	2.5–5 mg/kg q6h	Not recommended	

[b] Serum levels of doxycycline are reduced by 20% if given with food, whereas serum levels of tetracycline are reduced up to 50%. The oral absorption of minocycline is not significantly impaired by food or milk.

[c] Infused over 30 min

[d] Urine concentration of minocycline approximates 5 to 10 times serum concentration (lowest of tetracyclines).

Serum Half-life (hr)								
For Creatinine Clearance (ml/min)		*With Dialysis*		*CSF/Serum (%) Inflamed Meninges*	*Newborn Serum/ Maternal Serum (%)*	*Breast Milk/ Maternal Serum (%)*	*Bile/ Serum (%)*	*Aqueous Humor/ Serum (%)*
>80	*<10*	*HD*	*PD*					
5.6	6.8–11	Minimal		2–6[a]		40		
15						70[b]	2000[c]	10–30
18.5	19.5–25	18.8		12–20		30–40	1000–2000	
14								
12.6–16	13.6–20.4[e]				77	8	3000	10–14[f]
9	48–66	12					600–1000	
8.5	57–108	[g]		25	50–100	70	500–1000	

[e] Little accumulation in renal failure but aggravation of uremia reported even with reduced dosage.

[f] Data from dogs and rabbits.

[g] Tetracycline plasma level decreased by 14 to 27% with hemodialysis.

TABLE 8a. Antimicrobial Agent Pharmacology: Erythromycin, Lincosamides, Chloramphenicol, and Metronidazole—Absorption, Serum and Urine Concentrations, and Dosage

Drug (Oral Absorption %)	*Serum and Urine Concentration for Selected Doses*		
	Dose (g)	*Peak Serum* (μg/ml)	*Peak or Range Urine* (μg/ml)
Erythromycin (18–45[a])			
base	0.25 po[b]	0.4–1.3	13–46[c]
stearate	0.5 po[b]	0.4–1.9	30
ethyl succinate[d]			
lactobionate	0.5 IV	9.9	
gluceptate	1 IV	9.9	
estolate	0.5 po	4.2[e]	
Clindamycin (approx. 90[f])	0.15 po	2.5	3–4
	0.3 IM	4.8–6	
	0.6 IV[g]	10	
Lincomycin (20–30)	0.3 IV	8–22	
Chloramphenicol (75–90)	0.5 po	3–4	70–150[j]
	1 IV	5–12[i]	200
Metronidazole[l] (80[m])	0.25 po	6.2 avg	50–390
	0.5 po	11.5 avg	
	0.5 IV[g]	20–25	
(67–82 rectal[n])	0.5 rectal suppository	5.1	

[a] The extent of gastrointestinal absorption of erythromycin formulations relates to the chemical structure and their susceptibility to gastric acid, the protective enteric coating, and concomitant presence of food (*Am J Hosp Pharm* 37:1119–1205, 1980.)

[b] Fasting.

[c] Alkalinization of urine pH to 8 increases the amount of nonionized drug that remains in the urine and enhances the local antibacterial activity.

[d] Absorption of the ethylsuccinate preparation is enhanced by food. After absorption, 45% of the ethylsuccinate preparation is present in serum as the inactive ester and 55% as the active base.

[e] Erythromycin estolate total drug concentration with 500 mg dosing is 4.2 μg/ml (ester plus base) or 1.1 μg/ml free base.

[f] Absorption is not decreased by food.

[g] IV infusion (over 20 minutes).

[h] Total daily dose may be divided every 8 hours.

Dosage Recommendations						
Adults			*Children*		*Newborn (Parenteral)*	
Oral	*Parenteral*	*Maximum Daily Dose*	*Oral*	*Parenteral*	*Up to 1 wk*	*1 to 4 wk*
Dose/Interval		*(g)*	*Dose/Interval*			
0.25–0.5 g q6h	0.25–1 g q6h	4	7.5–12.5 mg/kg q6h	3.75–12.5 mg/kg q6h	Not recommended	
0.15–0.45 g q6h	0.15–0.9 g q6h	4.8	2–5 mg/kg q6h	2.5–10 mg/kg q6h[h]	Unknown	
0.5 g q6–8h	0.6–1 g q8–12h	8	10–15 mg/kg q6–8h	2.5–5 mg/kg q6h[h]	Not recommended	
12.5–25 mg/kg q6h	12.5–25 mg/kg q6h	4	12.5–25 mg/kg q6h	12.5–25 mg/kg q6h	25 mg/kg q24h[k]	25 mg/kg q12–24h[k]
7.5 mg/kg q6h	7.5 mg/kg q6h	4	7.5 mg/kg q6h	7.5 mg/kg q6h	15 mg/kg once, then 7.5 mg/kg q12h	15 mg/kg once, then 7.5 mg/kg q12h

[i] IM administration may produce a plasma level of active drug that is but one-half that achieved with a comparable oral dose and is therefore not recommended. The intravenous preparation (succinate ester) produces serum chloramphenicol levels 30% less than those achieved with a comparable oral dose.

[j] Urine concentration of unmetabolized chloramphenicol is inversely correlated with renal function. When the creatinine clearance is below 20 ml/min, less than 1% of the dose is excreted in the active form, compared to 5–10% in patients with normal renal function.

[k] Initial dosage. Subsequent dosage should be based on the determination of serum concentrations (10 to 25 μg/ml, desired). For premature infants throughout the first month of life, initial dosage is 25 mg/kg/day.

[l] Dosage for anaerobic bacterial infections. First dose (loading dose) should be 15 mg/kg. Dosage should be reduced with severe hepatic disease.

[m] Absorption of metronidazole is not significantly decreased by food.

[n] Rectal absorption is inversely dependent on dose.

TABLE 8b. Antimicrobial Agent Pharmacology: Erythromycin, Lincosamides, Chloramphenicol, and Metronidazole—Dosage Adjustment for Renal Insufficiency, Serum Half Life, and Body Fluid Levels

	Usual Adult Dose and Interval Adjustment					*Dosage for Dialysis*	
		For Creatinine Clearance (ml/min)					
Drug (Oral Absorption %)	Dose	*>80*	*80–50*	*50–10*	*<10 (Anuric)*	*Dose after HD Supple-mental to Anuric*	*Daily Dose during PD*
Erythromycin (18–45[a])	0.25–1 g	6 h	6 h	6 h	6 h	No change	No change
base stearate ethyl succinate[b]							
lactobionate							
gluceptate							
estolate							
Clindamycin (approx. 90[c])	0.15–0.9 g	6 h	6h	6 h	6 h[d]	No change	No change
Lincomycin (20–30)	0.5 g po	6 h	6 h	6–8 h	8–12 h	No change	No change
Chloramphenicol (75–90)	12.5–25 mg/kg	6 h	6 h	6 h	6 h	No change	No change
Metronidazole[e] (80[f]) (67–82 rectal[g])	7.5 mg/kg	6 h[h]	6 h	6 h	6 h	No change	No change

[a] The extent of gastrointestinal absorption of erythromycin formulations relates to the chemical structure and their susceptibility to gastric acid, the protective enteric coating, and concomitant presence of food (*Am J Hosp Pharm* 37:1119–1205, 1980.)

[b] Absorption of the ethylsuccinate preparation is enhanced by food. After absorption, 45% of the ethylsuccinate preparation is present in serum as the inactive ester and 55% as the active base.

[c] Absorption is not decreased by food.

[d] Dose modification should be made with coexisting renal and hepatic disease.

[e] Dosage for anaerobic bacterial infections. First dose (loading dose) should be 15 mg/kg. Dosage should be reduced with severe hepatic disease.

[f] Absorption of metronidazole is not significantly decreased by food.

[g] Rectal absorption is inversely dependent on dose.

[h] Clinical work with metronidazole completed outside the United States supports the use of an 8-hour dosing interval.

[i] The hydroxy metabolite may accumulate in anuric patients.

Serum Half-life (hr)								
For Creatinine Clearance (ml/min)		*With Dialysis*		*CSF/Serum (%) Inflamed Meninges*	*Newborn Serum/ Maternal Serum (%)*	*Breast Milk/ Maternal Serum (%)*	*Bile/ Serum (%)*	*Aqueous Humor/ Serum (%)*
>80	*<10*	*HD*	*PD*					
1.4	5.6	No change	No change	7–25	2–10	50	800–2500	25–30
2.4	3.4–6	1.9	4.6	Minimal	6–46	50	250–300	
4–5	13			Minimal	25–36	13–17	250–400	75
2.7	3.7	No change	No change	90	100	50	20–50	40
6–14	8–15[i]	2.6	5.6	100		100	100	33–50

TABLE 9a. Antimicrobial Agent Pharmacology: Polymyxins, Vancomycin, and Fusidic Acid—Absorption, Serum and Urine Concentrations, and Dosage

	Serum and Urine Concentration for Selected Doses		
		Peak Serum	*Peak or Range Urine*
Drug (Oral Absorption %)	*Dose*	*(μg/ml)*	
Colistimethate (minimal)	75 mg IM	1–2	50
	150 mg IM	6–8	
	150 mg IV	10–13	200–270
Polymyxin B (minimal[a])	50 mg IM	2–8	
Vancomycin (minimal)	0.5 g IV	6–10	
	1 g IV	20–50	100–300
	0.125 g q6h po	<1 [d]	
Fusidic acid	0.5 g po	14–38[f]	<1

[a] The only significant absorption from the gastrointestinal tract has been observed in newborn animals and small infants.

[b] Although not recommended, the IM dosage of polymyxin B for adults is 2.5–3.0 mg/kg/day given in 4 to 6 divided doses.

[c] Although not recommended, daily dose may be divided and given by the IM route.

TABLE 9b. Antimicrobial Agent Pharmacology: Polymyxins, Vancomycin, and Fusidic Acid—Dosage Adjustment for Renal Insufficiency, Serum Half Life, and Body Fluid Levels

	Usual Adult Dose and Interval Adjustment					*Dosage for Dialysis*	
		For Creatinine Clearance (ml/min)					
Drug (Oral Absorption %)	*Dose*	*>80*	*80–50*	*50–10*	*<10 (Anuric)*	*Dose after HD Supple-mental to Anuric*	*Daily Dose during PD*
Colistimethate (minimal)	0.8–1.7 mg/kg	8 h	2.5 mg/kg on day 1, then 1–1.5 mg/kg q24h	2.5 mg/kg on day 1, then 1–1.5 mg/kg q24–72h	2.5 mg/kg on day 1, then 1–1.5 mg/kg q48–72h[a]	[b]	[c]

Dosage Recommendations						
Adults			*Children*		*Newborn (Parenteral)*	
Oral	*Parenteral*	*Maximum Daily Dose*	*Oral*	*Parenteral*	*Up to 1 wk*	*1 to 4 wk*
Dose/Interval			*Dose/Interval*			
	0.8–1.7 mg/kg q8h	5 mg/kg		0.8–1.7 mg/kg q8h	Not recommended	
	1.5–2.5 mg/kg/day continuous IV infusion[b]	2.5 mg/kg		up to 4–4.5 mg/kg/day continuous IV infusion[c]	Not recommended	
0.125–0.5 g q6h	15 mg/kg q12h or 6.5–8 mg/kg q6h	2 g	12.5 mg/kg q6h	10 mg/kg q6h[e]	15 mg/kg q12h	15 mg/kg q8h
0.5–1 g q8h	580 mg q8h IV[g]		6.6–16.6 mg/kg q8h	6.6 mg/kg q8h		

[d] Stool concentration ranges from 100 to 800 μg/ml.

[e] Doses as high as 60 mg/kg/day may be necessary for staphylococcal CNS infections.

[f] Accumulation occurs with multiple doses of 0.5 g given every 8 hours; a mean serum level of 71 μg/ml has been reported after 96 hours of therapy.

[g] 580 mg diethanolamine fusidate = 500 mg sodium fusidate.

Serum Half-life (hr)								
For Creatinine Clearance (ml/min)		*With Dialysis*		*CSF/Serum (%) Inflamed Meninges*	*Newborn Serum/ Maternal Serum (%)*	*Breast Milk/ Maternal Serum (%)*	*Bile/ Serum (%)*	*Aqueous Humor/ Serum (%)*
>80	*<10*	*HD*	*PD*					
2–3	10–20	1.5	Poor	Minimal	50	18	Not detectable	25–30

Table 9b. (Continued)

Drug (Oral Absorption %)	*Usual Adult Dose and Interval Adjustment*					*Dosage for Dialysis*	
		For Creatinine Clearance (ml/min)					
	Dose	*>80*	*80–50*	*50–10*	*<10 (Anuric)*	*Dose after HD Supplemental to Anuric*	*Daily Dose during PD*
Polymyxin B (minimal[d])	1.5–2.5 mg/kg/day	24 h	3 mg/kg on day 1, then 1.5–2.5 mg/kg q24h	3 mg/kg on day 1, then 1.5–2.5 mg/kg q24–72h	3 mg/kg on day 1, then 1.5–2.5 mg/kg q48–72h[a]		
Vancomycin (minimal)	15 mg/kg q12h or 6.5–8 mg/kg q6h	6–12 h	See nomogram, Chapter 11			No change	[f]
Fusidic acid	0.5–1 g po	8 h	8 h	8 h	8 h		

[a] The interval is extended to every 5 to 7 days for the anuric patient.

[b] The rate of removal of colistimethate by hemodialysis or peritoneal dialysis remains controversial. Studies using a Kollf twin coil dialyzer demonstrate no removal (*N Engl J Med* 270:394–7, 1964, *Ann Intern Med* 68:984–94, 1968), whereas studies using the Kiil type dialyzer recommend the dose be adjusted so that the patient receives a 2–3 mg/kg dose following dialysis (*B. Med J* 1:484–5, 1968, *Antimicrob Agents Chemother* 373–8 1964).

[c] Small quantities of colistimethate are removed by PD with clearance rates ranging from 5.8–11.3 ml/min. Supplemental doses may be considered based on the duration of dialysis and the need to maintain target serum levels.

[d] The only significant absorption from the gastrointestinal tract has been observed in newborn animals and small infants.

TABLE 10a. Antimicrobial Agent Pharmacology: Sulfonamides and Trimethoprim—Absorption, Serum and Urine Concentrations, and Dosage

Drug (Oral Absorption %)	*Serum and Urine Concentration for Selected Doses*		
	Dose (g)	*Peak Serum* (μg/ml)	*Peak or Range Urine* (μg/ml)
Trimethoprim-sulfamethoxazole (TMP-SMX) (85–90)	0.16/0.8 po	2–4/80–100[b]	120/300[c]
	0.16/0.8 IV[a]	3.4/47.3	

Serum Half-life (hr)								
For Creatinine Clearance (ml/min)		*With Dialysis*						
>80	*<10*	*HD*	*PD*	*CSF/Serum (%) Inflamed Meninges*	*Newborn Serum/ Maternal Serum (%)*	*Breast Milk/ Maternal Serum (%)*	*Bile/ Serum (%)*	*Aqueous Humor/ Serum (%)*
6	48–72			Minimal[e]			Not detectable	
4–8[g]	240	Negligible effect	18	7–21	20[h]	33–66[i]	50	Minimal

[e] Although rarely used the daily intrathecal dose of polymyxin B is 5–10 mg for adults and 2 mg for children over 2 years. Intrathecal therapy should be administered on a daily basis for the first 3 to 5 days and then every other day for 3 weeks or for 2 weeks following negative CSF cultures and a normal CSF glucose.

[f] Conflicting opinion exists with regard to dosage alteration of vancomycin during PD. The regimen chosen will depend upon the frequency and duration of dialysis as well as the nature of the infection being treated. One can elect to treat with systemic doses, supplementing an anuric dosage schedule with a dose after dialysis (based on the change in drug elimination during the dialytic period). Another approach is the intraperitoneal administration of 25–50 mg of vancomycin per liter of peritoneal dialysate following an initial IV loading dose (*Nephron* 24:274–7, 1979).

[g] The elimination half-life of vancomycin varies with age: 5.9–9.8 hours in newborns; 4.1 hours in older infants; 2.2–3 hours in children.

[h] Data from animals (rabbits).

[i] Data from animals (cats).

Dosage Recommendations						
Adults			*Children*		*Newborn (Parenteral)*	
Oral	*Parenteral*	*Maximum Daily Dose (g)*	*Oral*	*Parenteral*	*Up to 1 wk*	*1 to 4 wk*
Dose/Interval			*Dose/Interval*			
2 tablets q12h or 1 tablet q6h[d]	4–5 mg/kg q6–12h (as TMP)[d]	4 tablets orally or 1.2 g TMP, 6 g SMX intravenously (usual)	4–5 mg/kg q6–12h (as TMP)[d]	4–5 mg/kg q6–12h (as TMP)[d]	Not recommended[e]	

Table 10a. (Continued)

Drug (Oral Absorption %)	Serum and Urine Concentration for Selected Doses		
	Dose (g)	Peak Serum (μg/ml)	Peak or Range Urine (μg/ml)
Trimethoprim (80)	0.32 po 0.1 po	5.5 1	 30–160[f]
Sulfonamides (70–90)			
sulfisoxazole	2 po	40–50 (free)	
sulfamethoxazole	2 po	80–100 (free)	
sulfamethizole	2 po	60	
sulfacytine	0.25 po	17	420
sulfadiazine	0.5 po	20–40[b]	
sulfadoxine[j]	2 po	50–75 (free)	
sulfasalazine (10–15)	2 po	14 sulfasalazine 21 sulfapyridine (total)	
sulfaphenazole	2 po	100–150	

[a] Infused over 60 minutes.

[b] Active (unmetabolized).

[c] The urine concentrations of the drugs depend on the urine flow rate, urine pH, and the time of collection. The approximate urine concentration for trimethoprim is 100 times the plasma concentration. For sulfamethoxazole the level is 5 times the concentration in plasma. Alkalinization of urine increases renal excretion of sulfonamides. See footnote f.

[d] Each tablet contains 80 mg trimethoprim and 400 mg sulfamethoxazole. Double-strength tablets are also available and are usually administered 1 tablet q12h. The suspension contains 40 mg trimethoprim and 200 mg sulfamethoxazole per 5 ml. Parenteral dosage ranges from 8 to 20 mg/kg/day trimethoprim and 40 to 100 mg/kg/day sulfamethoxazole.

Dosage Recommendations

Adults			*Children*		*Newborn (Parenteral)*	
Oral	*Parenteral*	*Maximum Daily Dose (g)*	*Oral*	*Parenteral*	*Up to 1 wk*	*1 to 4 wk*
Dose/Interval			*Dose/Interval*			
0.1 g q12h		0.2	2 mg/kg q12h (not approved in children less than 12 years old)			
0.5–1 g q6h[g]	25 mg/kg q6h[g]	8	37.5 mg/kg q6h[g]	25 mg/kg q6h[g]	Not recommended	
1 g q8–12h[h]		3	25–35 mg/kg q12h[i]		Not recommended	
0.5–1 g q6–8h		6	7.5–11.25 mg/kg q6h		Not recommended	
0.5 g initial dose, then 0.25 g q6h		1	Not recommended		Not recommended	
2–4 g initial dose, then 0.5–1 g q4–6h	Not recommended	6	16.25–25 mg/kg q4–6h[g]		Not recommended	
1 tablet every week or 2 tablets every other week[k]		1.5	By age[l]		Not recommended	
0.5–1 g q4–6h		8	10 mg/kg q4–8h			
2–3 g, then 1 g q12h		2	66 mg/kg, then 33 mg/kg q12h			

[e] Unsuitable for newborn because appropriate dosage requires a ratio of trimethoprim : sulfamethoxazole = 1 : 3 and the only formulation available is a 1 : 5 combination (*J Ped* 100:647–50, 1982).

[f] Renal clearance of trimethoprim is increased with acidification of urine.

[g] Administer one-half of the daily dose as the initial, loading dose.

[h] Administer 2 g loading dose = 4 regular strength tablets or 2 double-strength tablets.

[i] Administer 50–60 mg/kg loading dose. The maximum dose for children should not exceed 75 mg/kg/24 h.

[j] For malaria prophylaxis. The first dose should be given 1–2 days before departure to an endemic area and the course continued throughout the stay and 4–6 weeks thereafter.

[k] 1 tablet = 500 mg sulfadoxine and 25 mg pyrimethamine.

[l] Under 4 years: ¼ tablet weekly or ½ tablet every other week; 4 to 6 years: ½ tablet weekly or 1 tablet every other week; 9 to 14 years: ¾ tablet weekly or 1½ tablet every other week.

TABLE 10b. Antimicrobial Agent Pharmacology: Sulfonamides and Trimethoprim—Dosage Adjustment for Renal Insufficiency, Serum Half Life, and Body Fluid Levels

Drug (Oral Absorption %)	*Usual Adult Dose and Interval Adjustment*					*Dosage for Dialysis*	
		For Creatinine Clearance (ml/min)					
	Dose	*>80*	*80–50*	*50–10*	*<10 (Anuric)*	*Dose after HD Supple-mental to Anuric*	*Daily Dose during PD*
Trimethoprim-sulfamethoxazole (TMP-SMX) (85–90)	4–5 mg/kg (as TMP)	6–12 h	12 h	18 h	24–48 h	4–5 mg/kg (as TMP)	0.16/0.8 g q48h
Trimethoprim (80)	0.1 g po	12 h	12 h	24 h	24–48 h		
Sulfonamides (70–90)							
sulfisoxazole	0.5–1 g po	6 h	6–8 h	8–12 h	12–24 h		
sulfamethoxazole	1 g po	8–12 h					
sulfamethizole	0.5–1 g po	6–8 h					
sulfacytine	0.25 g po	6 h					
sulfadiazine	0.5–1 g po	4–6 h					
sulfadoxine[d]	0.5 g po or 1 g po	every wk every other wk					
sulfasalazine (10–15)	0.5–1 g po	4–6 h					
sulfaphenazole	1 g po	12 h					

[a] Nonacetylated SMX.

[b] Under normal conditions the $T_{1/2}$ of elimination was determined as 6 hours, whereas under alkaline conditions the half-life approached 4 hours.

[c] Under acidic conditions, the $T_{1/2}$ of elimination is slightly longer (11 h) than under alkaline conditions (9 h).

[d] For malaria prophylaxis. The first dose should be given 1–2 days before departure to an endemic area and the course continued throughout the stay and 4–6 weeks thereafter.

Serum Half-life (hr)								
For Creatinine Clearance (ml/min)		*With Dialysis*		*CSF/Serum (%) Inflamed Meninges*	*Newborn Serum/ Maternal Serum (%)*	*Breast Milk/ Maternal Serum (%)*	*Bile/ Serum (%)*	*Aqueous Humor/ Serum (%)*
>80	*<10*	*HD*	*PD*					
11/9	25/27	9.4/ 11.7[a]		30–50/25–30	100/70–90	125/10	200/40–70	10–45/ 20–30
7.5	14–46	9.4		30–50	100	100	100	10
				30–80	70–90	10	40–70	20–30
4–6[b]	12			30–50				
10–12[c]	27			25–30				
2	58							
4								
10–12	34			50–80				
150–200								
7.6								

TABLE 11a. Antimicrobial Agent Pharmacology: Quinolones and Other Urinary Tract Agents—Absorption, Serum and Urine Concentrations, and Dosage

	Serum and Urine Concentration for Selected Doses		
		Peak Serum	*Peak or Range Urine*
Drug (Oral Absorption %)	*Dose (g)*	*(μg/ml)*	
Quinolones			
Cinoxacin (97)	0.25 po	8	400
	0.5 po	16	
Ciprofloxacin	0.5 po	2.4	
Nalidixic acid (96)	1 po	25–35	>OR = 275
Norfloxacin (50)	0.2 po	0.75	200
	0.4 po	1.6	480
	0.8 po	2.4	700
Oxolinic acid (poor)	0.75 po	0.9–3.6	45–100 avg
Other urinary tract agents			
Indanyl carbenicillin (30–40)	0.382 po (1 tablet)	6.5	1130
	1 po	6–17	
Methenamine mandelate[a] (70[b])	1 po		40 (formaldehyde)
Methenamine hippurate[a] (100)	1	70–100 μmol/liter[c]	1100–1500 (methenamine) approx 50 (formaldehyde)
Nitrofurantoin (good but variable)	0.1 po	<1	150[d]

[a] Usually coadministered with an acidifying agent to convert methenamine salts in urine to ammonia and bactericidal formaldehyde (pH < OR = 5.5). Mandelic and hippuric acids are mildly antiseptic and contribute to urine acidification.

[b] Oral absorption is decreased 30% by enteric coating.

[c] Serum concentration of methenamine has no clinical significance.

[d] Alkaline conditions reduce tubular reabsorption, yielding higher nitrofurantoin concentrations in urine.

Dosage Recommendations						
Adults			*Children*		*Newborn (Parenteral)*	
Oral	*Parenteral*	*Maximum Daily Dose (g)*	*Oral*	*Parenteral*	*Up to 1 wk*	*1 to 4 wk*
Dose/Interval			*Dose/Interval*			
0.25 g q6h or 0.5 g q12h		1	Not recommended			
1 g q6h		4	Not recommended		Not recommended	
0.2–0.4 g q12h		0.8				
0.75 q12h		2	Not recommended		Not recommended	
1–2 tablets q6h		3	12.5–16.25 mg/kg q6h			
1 g q6h		4	12.5–18.75 mg/kg q6h		Not recommended	
1 g q12h		4	12.5–25 mg/kg q12h		Not recommended	
0.05–0.1 g q6h		0.4	1.25–1.75 mg/kg q6h		Not recommended	

TABLE 11b. Antimicrobial Agent Pharmacology: Quinolones and Other Urinary Tract Agents—Dosage Adjustment for Renal Insufficiency, Serum Half Life, and Body Fluid Levels

	Usual Adult Dose and Interval Adjustment					*Dosage for Dialysis*	
		For Creatinine Clearance (ml/min)					
Drug (Oral Absorption %)	*Dose*	*>80*	*80–50*	*50–10*	*<10 (Anuric)*	*Dose after HD Supplemental to Anuric*	*Daily Dose during PD*
Quinolones							
Cinoxacin (97)	0.25–0.5 g po	6–12 h	0.25 g q8h	0.25 g q12-24h	Not recommended		
Ciprofloxacin							
Nalidixic acid (96)	1 g po	6 h	6 h	6 h	Not recommended[c]		
Norfloxacin (50)	0.2–0.4 g po	12 h					
Oxolinic acid (poor)	0.75 g po	12 h		Not recommended[c]	Not recommended[c]		
Other urinary tract agents							
Indanyl carbenicillin (30–40)	1–2 tablets po	6 h	6 h	6 h	Not recommended[c]		
Methenamine mandelate[e] (70[f])	1 g po	6 h	6 h	Not recommended[c]	Not recommended[c]		
Methenamine hippurate[e] (100)	1 g po	12 h	12 h	Not recommended[c]	Not recommended[c]		
Nitrofurantoin (good but variable)	0.05–0.1 g po	6 h	6 h	Not recommended[c,h]	Not recommended[c,h]		

[a] Use during pregnancy not recommended.

[b] Animal pharmacology studies indicate the presence of drug in the milk of lactating rats receiving oral doses of cinoxacin. Human data is currently unavailable.

[c] Ineffective urinary concentrations expected with compromised renal function.

[d] Breast milk percentage extrapolated from data indicating 4 μg/ml breast milk concentration in four patients (*Lancet* 2:691, 1965). Hemolytic anemia has been described in one nursing infant whose mother received nalidixic acid.

[e] Usually coadministered with an acidifying agent to convert methenamine salts in urine to ammonia and bactericidal formaldehyde (pH < OR = 5.5). Mandelic and hippuric acids are mildly antiseptic and contribute to urine acidification.

[f] Oral absorption is decreased 30% by enteric coating.

[g] Methenamine penetrates a number of body fluids, including bile and cerebrospinal fluid. This penetration proves clinically inconsequential since negligible amounts of formaldehyde are generated at physiological pH (*see* Chapter 14).

[h] Nitrofurantoin accumulates in the serum of patients with a creatinine clearance <60 ml/min, leading to systemic toxicity.

[i] Although only small amounts of nitrofurantoin have been detected in breast milk, the drug could cause hemolytic anemia in a G6PD-deficient infant exposed in this manner.

Serum Half-life (hr)								
For Creatinine Clearance (ml/min)		*With Dialysis*		*CSF/Serum (%) Inflamed Meninges*	*Newborn Serum/ Maternal Serum (%)*	*Breast Milk/ Maternal Serum (%)*	*Bile/ Serum (%)*	*Aqueous Humor/ Serum (%)*
>80	*<10*	*HD*	*PD*					
2.7	8.4	3–4.4			[a]	<100 (18–78)[b]		
3.9								
1.5	21					13[d]		
4.3–7								
6–7						Not recommended		
0.5–1	12.5							
3–6				[g]			[g]	[g]
4				[g]	50	70–100	[g]	[g]
0.3	1				100	<25[i]	200–400	

TABLE 12a. Antimicrobial Agent Pharmacology: Antimycobacterial Agents—Absorption, Serum and Urine Concentrations, and Dosage

	Serum and Urine Concentration for Selected Doses		
		Peak Serum	*Peak or Range Urine*
Drug (Oral Absorption %)	*Dose*	*(μg/ml)*	
Ansamycin			
Capreomycin[a] (minimal)	1 g	30	1685
Clofazimine			
Cycloserine	0.25 g po q6h 0.5 g po	15–25	 55–340
Ethambutol (80)	25 mg/kg po	2–5	
Ethionamide	1 g po	20	
Isoniazid[e]	5 mg/kg	1–5	
Paraamino salicylic acid	4 g po (free acid)	75 7–8	
Pyrazinamide	1 g po	45	60
Rifampin (100)	0.6 g po (fasting)	7	240
Streptomycin	1 g IM	25–50	1000
Viomycin			

[a] Pharmacokinetics similar to streptomycin.

[b] The dosage is 1 g IM daily for 2 to 4 months and is reduced to 1 g 2 to 3 times weekly thereafter.

[c] In combination therapeutic regimens, 300 mg monthly to 50–100 mg daily is recommended.

[d] Doses as high as 25 mg/kg/day are occasionally administered during the first 2 to 3 months of therapy. Intermittent therapy consists of 50 mg/kg/day, administered twice weekly.

[e] To minimize the risk of polyneuritis from isoniazid-induced pyridoxine deficiency, pyridoxine (15–50 mg) is often given concurrently.

Dosage Recommendations						
Adults			*Children*		*Newborn (Parenteral)*	
Oral	*Parenteral*	*Maximum Daily Dose*	*Oral*	*Parenteral*	*Up to 1 wk*	*1 to 4 wk*
Dose/Interval			*Dose/Interval*			
0.15–0.3 g/day		0.3 g				
	0.75–1 g q24h 15–20 mg/kg/day IM[b]	20 mg/kg/day				
0.1 g/day[c]		0.6 g				
0.25–0.5 g q12h		1 g	3.5–5 mg/kg q12h			
15 mg/kg/day[d]		15 mg/kg/day[d]	Not recommended (15 mg/kg/day)			
0.25–0.5 g q12h		1 g				
5 mg/kg/day (0.3 g)[f]	5 mg/kg/day	0.6 g	10–20 mg/kg/day[g]			
3 g q6–8h		12 g	66.6–75 mg/kg q6–8h			
25 mg/kg/day[h]		3 g	10–15 mg/kg q12h or 5–7.5 mg/kg q6h			
0.6 g/24 h[i]		1.2 g[i]	10–20 mg/kg/day			
	15 mg/kg/day[j]	2 g		10–15 mg/kg q12h		
	1 g q12h twice weekly	2 g				

[f] For noncompliant patients, 15 mg/kg can be given twice weekly under supervision. For prophylaxis, isoniazid is usually given for a year in a daily dose of 300 mg for adults and 10 mg/kg (up to 300 mg max) for children.

[g] In children with tuberculosis meningitis, some clinicians use 30 mg/kg/day for the first few weeks.

[h] When given intermittently, the adult dosage is 50 mg/kg twice weekly. The daily dosage is divided in 2 to 4 equally spaced doses.

[i] For noncompliant patients, supervised therapy with 600 mg rifampin twice a week can be given. Dose for prophylaxis of meningococcal meningitis is 600 mg twice daily for 2 days.

[j] An alternative dosage schedule is 25–30 mg/kg twice weekly.

TABLE 12b. Antimicrobial Agent Pharmacology: Antimycobacterial Agents—Dosage Adjustment for Renal Insufficiency, Serum Half Life, and Body Fluid Levels

Drug (Oral Absorption %)	*Usual Adult Dose and Interval Adjustment*					*Dosage for Dialysis*	
	Dose	*For Creatinine Clearance (ml/min)*				*Dose after HD Supplemental to Anuric*	*Daily Dose during PD*
		>80	*80–50*	*50–10*	*<10 (Anuric)*		
Ansamycin	0.15–0.3 g po	24 h	24 h	0.15 g q24h	0.075 g q72h		
Capreomycin[a] (minimal)	0.75–1 g	24 h					
Clofazimine	0.1 g po	24 h					
Cycloserine	0.25–0.5 g po	12 h					
Ethambutol (80)	15 mg/kg/day po	15 mg/kg/day	15 mg/kg/day	7.5–15 mg/kg/day	5 mg/kg/day	15 mg/kg/day on dialysis day	15 mg/kg/day during PD
Ethionamide	0.25–0.5 g po	12 h					
Isoniazid[b]	5 mg/kg po	24 h	24 h	24 h	24 h[c]	5 mg/kg	[d]
Paraamino salicylic acid	3 g po	6–8 h					
Pyrazinamide	25 mg/kg/day po	6–12 h					
Rifampin (100)	0.6 g po	24 h	24 h	24 h	24 h	No supplemental dose	No supplemental dose
Streptomycin	15 mg/kg/day	24 h	24 h	24–72 h	72–96 h	5 mg/kg	
Viomycin	1 g	12 h twice weekly					

[a] Pharmacokinetics similar to streptomycin.

[b] To minimize the risk of polyneuritis from isoniazid-induced pyridoxine deficiency, pyridoxine (15–50 mg) is often given concurrently.

[c] For slow acetylators (at least ½ of Caucasian Americans), the daily dose should be reduced to 200 mg.

[d] In cases where peritoneal dialysis has been used for the management of acute isoniazid intoxication, the procedure decreased INH serum concentration by 68% over 24 hours (*N Engl J Med* 269:852 1963).

[e] Specific elimination kinetics of isoniazid depend on acetylator phenotype of the individual; half-life for rapid acetylators is 0.5–1.5 h and for slow acetylators, 2–4 h.

[f] There is a progressive shortening of the half-life of rifampin by about 40% during the first 14 days of treatment, due to increased biliary excretion.

Serum Half-life (hr)								
For Creatinine Clearance (ml/min)		*With Dialysis*		*CSF/Serum (%) Inflamed Meninges*	*Newborn Serum/ Maternal Serum (%)*	*Breast Milk/ Maternal Serum (%)*	*Bile/ Serum (%)*	*Aqueous Humor/ Serum (%)*
>80	*<10*	*HD*	*PD*					
70 days								
				100	100	72		
4–6	7–32			25				
2–4				100				
0.5–4[e]	8 (avg)	3.4		20		100		
1	Increased			poor				
9–10				100				
1.5–5[f]	2–5	Minimal	Minimal	10–15	33	20–60	10,000	
2–3	100–110			20	10–40	<25	40–300	
				poor				

TABLE 13a. Antimicrobial Agent Pharmacology: Antifungal Agents—Absorption, Serum and Urine Concentrations, and Dosage

Drug (Oral Absorption %)	Dose	Serum and Urine Concentration for Selected Doses: Peak Serum (μg/ml)	Peak or Range Urine (μg/ml)
Amphotericin (poor)	0.1–1 mg/kg	0.5–5.5	
Flucytosine (90)	150 mg/kg/day po	100–500	5800
Griseofulvin (50[d])	1 g po	1–2.8[e]	Minimal
Ketoconazole	0.2 g po 0.4 g po	2 4	0.4
Miconazole (25–30)	0.5 g IV[g]	2–9	
Nystatin (minimal)[i]	all doses	Minimal	

[a] See Chapter 16 for details.

[b] Or up to 1.5 mg/kg every other day.

[c] With severe infections, such as meningitis, even higher doses (62.5 mg/kg q6h) have been suggested.

[d] Dose for conventional microsize griseofulvin. Significant interindividual variation exists with griseofulvin absorption. Bioavailability studies have demonstrated 150% greater absorption of ultramicrosize products (Fulvicin P-G, Gris-PEG). Dosing guidelines for ultramicrosize griseofulvin are 330–660 mg daily for adults and 7.25 mg/kg/day for children (*J Pharmacokinet Biopharm* 8:347–62, 1980).

[e] Serum level is increased with high-fat meal and decreased in the absence of acid (concomitant antacid or H2 blocker therapy).

[f] Less than 20 kg: 50 mg; 20 to 40 kg: 100 mg; greater than 40 kg: 200 mg.

[g] Over 15 minutes.

[h] The manufacturer recommends an initial test dose of 200 mg.

[i] Dosage for oral candidiasis. Nystatin suspension = 100,000 U/ml.

Dosage Recommendations						
Adults			*Children*		*Newborn (Parenteral)*	
Oral	*Parenteral*	*Maximum Daily Dose*	*Oral*	*Parenteral*	*Up to 1 wk*	*1 to 4 wk*
Dose/Interval			*Dose/Interval*			
	0.25–1 mg/kg q24h[a]	1 mg/kg[b]		0.25–1 mg/kg q24h[a]	0.1–1 mg/kg/day[a]	0.1–1 mg/kg/day[a]
12.5–37.5 mg/kg q6h[c]		150 mg/kg	12.5–37.5 mg/kg q6h		Not recommended	
0.5–1 g/day in single or 2–4 doses[d]		2 g	11 mg/kg/day in single or 2–4 doses[d]			
0.2–0.4 g q24h		1 g	5–10 mg/kg q24h[f]			
	0.066–1.2 g q8h[h]	3.6 g		6.6–13.3 mg/kg q8h		
400,000–600,000 U q6h (4–6 ml)		4×10^6 U	250,000–500,000 U q6h (2.5–5 ml)		100,000 U q6h (0.25 ml) po	100,000 U q6h (0.25 ml) po

TABLE 13b. Antimicrobial Agent Pharmacology: Antifungal Agents—Dosage Adjustment for Renal Insufficiency, Serum Half Life, and Body Fluid Levels

Drug (Oral Absorption %)	*Usual Adult Dose and Interval Adjustment*: Dose	For Creatinine Clearance (ml/min): >80	80–50	50–10	<10 (Anuric)	*Dosage for Dialysis*: Dose after HD Supplemental to Anuric	Daily Dose during PD
Amphotericin (poor)	0.25–1 mg/kg IV	24 h	24 h	24 h	24 h	No change	
Flucytosine (90)	12.5–37.5 mg/kg po	6 h	6 h	12–24 h	15–25 mg/kg q24h or by plasma level = 50–75	37.5 mg/kg	
Griseofulvin (50[a])	0.5–1 g po	24 h	24 h	24 h	24 h		
Ketoconazole	0.2–0.4 g po	24 h	24 h	24 h	24 h		
Miconazole (25–30)	0.066–1.2 g IV	8 h	8 h	8 h	8 h		
Nystatin (minimal)[e]	400,000–600,000 U po	6 h	6 h	6 h	6 h		

[a] Dose for conventional microsize griseofulvin. Significant interindividual variation exists with griseofulvin absorption. Bioavailability studies have demonstrated 150% greater absorption of ultramicrosize products (Fulvicin P-G, Gris-PEG). Dosing guidelines for ultramicrosize griseofulvin are 330–660 mg daily for adults and 7.25 mg/kg/day for children (*J Pharmacokinet Biopharm* 8:347–62, 1980).

[b] Ketoconazole has dose-dependent elimination with half-lives of 6.5, 8.1, and 9.6 hours after doses of 100, 200, and 400 mg, respectively.

[c] Triphasic half-life with 0.4 hour absorption half-life and 2.1 and 24 hour elimination half-lives.

[d] Neither renal impairment nor hemodialysis affects elimination, although plasma concentrations are greater in patients with azotemia due to decreased distribution volume.

[e] Dosage for oral candidiasis. Nystatin suspension = 100,000 U/ml.

Serum Half-life (hr)								
For Creatinine Clearance (ml/min)		*With Dialysis*						
>80	*<10*	*HD*	*PD*	*CSF/Serum (%) Inflamed Meninges*	*Newborn Serum/ Maternal Serum (%)*	*Breast Milk/ Maternal Serum (%)*	*Bile/ Serum (%)*	*Aqueous Humor/ Serum (%)*
24	24 or more	Minimal		2–3	50			25
4–6	30–70	5–6		60–100				20
20	20				80			
6.5–9.6[b]	1.8	Minimal	Minimal	6.5–10			Minimal	
2.1/24.1[c]	24[d]	Minimal	Minimal	<3–48				

TABLE 14a. Antimicrobial Agent Pharmacology: Antiviral Agents—Absorption, Serum and Urine Concentrations, and Dosage

Drug (Oral Absorption %)	*Serum and Urine Concentration for Selected Doses*		
	Dose	*Peak Serum* (μg/ml)	*Peak or Range Urine* (μg/ml)
Acyclovir	2.5 mg/kg[a]	6.8	
	5 mg/kg[a]	9.8	
	0.2 po q4h	0.3–0.9	
Amantadine (85–90)	0.1 po	0.3–0.4	
Vidarabine	10–15 mg/kg/day (12 h)	0.2 vidarabine 6–8 arahypoxanthine	

[a] IV over 1 hour.

[b] The dose for children 1 to 9 years old should not exceed 150 mg per day.

TABLE 14b. Antimicrobial Agent Pharmacology: Antiviral Agents—Dosage Adjustment for Renal Insufficiency, Serum Half Life, and Body Fluid Levels

Drug (Oral Absorption %)	*Usual Adult Dose and Interval Adjustment*					*Dosage for Dialysis*	
		For Creatinine Clearance (ml/min)					
	Dose	*>80*	*80–50*	*50–10*	*<10 (Anuric)*	*Dose after HD Supplemental to Anuric*	*Daily Dose during PD*
Acyclovir	5 mg/kg	8 h	8 h	12–24 h	24 h	Give daily dose after HD	
Amantadine (85–90)	200 mg q24h or 100 mg q12h po	12 h	100 mg q12–24h	200 mg/day alternate days to alternating q7 days[b]		None	
Vidarabine	10–15 mg/kg/day	10–15 mg/kg/day	10–15 mg/kg/day	10–15 mg/kg/day	7.5–15 mg/kg/day	Give daily dose after HD	

[a] Data from manufacturer's product information using animals.

[b]Creatinine clearance (mL/min • 1.73 meter²)	Suggested Maintenance Regimen
50	100 mg daily
40	100 mg daily
30	200 mg twice weekly
20	100 mg thrice weekly
10	200 mg/100 mg alternating every 7 days

(From *Ann Intern Med* 94:954–8, 1981.)

Dosage Recommendations						
Adults			*Children*		*Newborn (Parenteral)*	
Oral	*Parenteral*	*Maximum*	*Oral*	*Parenteral*	*Up to 1 week*	*2 to 4 wk*
Dose/Interval		*Daily Dose*	*Dose/Interval*			
	5 mg/kg q8h	30 mg/kg		5–10 mg/ kg q8h	10 mg/kg q8h	10 mg/kg q8h
0.1 g q12h or 0.2 g q24h		0.2 g	2.2–4.4 mg/ kg q12h[b]			
	10–15 mg/ kg/day over 12 h	15 mg/kg		15–30 mg/ kg/day over 12 hours	15–30 mg/ kg/day over 12 hours	15–30 mg/ kg/day over 12 hours

Serum Half-life (hr)								
For Creatinine Clearance (ml/min)		*With Dialysis*		*CSF/Serum (%) Inflamed Meninges*	*Newborn Serum/ Maternal Serum (%)*	*Breast Milk/ Maternal Serum (%)*	*Bile/ Serum (%)*	*Aqueous Humor/ Serum (%)*
>80	*<10*	*HD*	*PD*					
2.2–5	20	5.7		50	100[a]			
12–17	Decreased	Minimal		50–60				
1.5	Decreased			50				

TABLE 15. Adverse Drug Interactions Involving Antimicrobial Agents†

Interacting Drugs	*Adverse Effect*	*Probable Mechanism*
Acyclovir, with:		
probenecid	Possible increased acyclovir toxicity	Decreased renal excretion
Amantadine, with:		
anticholinergics	Hallucinations, confusion, nightmares	Mechanism not established
Aminoglycoside antibiotics, with:		
amphotericin B	Nephrotoxocity	Synergism
bumetanide	Increased ototoxicity	Additive
carbenicillin	Decreased aminoglycoside effect in patients with renal failure and high serum concentration of carbenicillin	Inactivated by carbenicillin
cephalosporins	Increased nephrotoxicity	Mechanism not established
digoxin	Probable decreased digoxin effect with neomycin or kanamycin;	Decreased absorption
	increase in digoxin effect in those patients (<10%) who convert large portion of digoxin to inactive reduction products in GI tract	Increased bioavailability
ethacrynic acid	Increased ototoxicity	Additive
furosemide	Increased ototoxicity and nephrotoxicity	Additive
magnesium sulfate	Increased neuromuscular blockade	Additive
methotrexate	Possible increased methotrexate toxicity with kanamycin;	Mechanism not established
	decreased methotrexate effect with oral aminoglycosides	Decreased absorption
neuromuscular blocking agents	Neuromuscular blockade	Additive

Aminoglycoside antibiotics, with: (continued)		
polymyxins	Increased nephrotoxicity; neuromuscular blockade	Additive
ticarcillin	Decreased aminoglycoside effect in patients with renal failure and high concentration of ticarcillin	Inactivation by ticarcillin
Aminosalicylic acid (PAS), with:		
digoxin	Possible decreased digoxin effects	Decreased absorption
probenecid	Increased PAS toxicity	Decreased renal excretion
rifampin	Rifampin effectiveness may be decreased; separate doses by 8 to 12 hours	Decreased GI absorption due to excipient, bentonite
Amphotericin B, with:		
aminoglycoside antibiotics	Nephrotoxicity	Synergism
digitalis glycosides	Increased digitalis toxicity	Hypokalemia
miconazole	Decreased anticandidal effect	Mechanism not established
neuromuscular blocking agents	Increased neuromuscular blocking effect	Hypokalemia
Cephalosporins, with:		
alcohol	Disulfiram-like effect with cefamandole, cefoperazone, and moxalactam	Mechanism not established
aminoglycoside antibiotics	Increased nephrotoxicity	Mechanism not established
anticoagulants, oral	Possible increased anticoagulant effect with moxalactam	Mechanism not established
aspirin	Possible increased bleeding risk with moxalactam	Additive
ethacrynic acid	Increased nephrotoxicity	Mechanism not established
furosemide	Increased nephrotoxicity	Mechanism not established
heparin	Possible increased bleeding risk with moxalactam	Additive
Chloramphenicol, with:		
acetaminophen	Possible increased chloramphenicol toxicity	Decreased metabolism

TABLE 15. (Continued)

Interacting Drugs	*Adverse Effect*	*Probable Mechanism*
Chloramphenicol, with: (continued)		
alcohol	Minor disulfiram-like symptoms	Decreased metabolism
barbiturates	Increased barbiturate effect; decreased chloramphenicol effect	Decreased metabolism Increased metabolism
cimetidine	Aplastic anemia	Possibly additive or synergism
dicumarol	Increased anticoagulant effect	Decreased metabolism
etomidate	Prolonged anesthesia	Decreased metabolism
hypoglycemics, sulfonylurea	Increased hypoglycemic effect	Decreased metabolism
iron salts	Hematologic response to iron may be decreased	Delayed clearance of iron from plasma and iron incorporation into red blood cell
phenytoin	Increased phenytoin toxicity; decreased chloramphenicol effect	Decreased metabolism Increased metabolism
Clindamycin, with:		
neuromuscular blocking agents	Increased neuromuscular blockade	Additive
Colistimethate, same as polymyxin B		
Cycloserine, with:		
alcohol	Increased convulsions with chronic abuse	Mechanism not established
isoniazid	CNS effects, dizziness, drowsiness	Mechanism not established
Erythromycins, with:		
anticoagulant, oral	Hypoprothrombinemia potentiated	Possible decreased warfarin clearance
carbamazepine	Increased carbamazepine toxicity	Possibly decreased metabolism
digoxin	Increased digoxin effect	Decreased gut metabolism and increased absorption
theophylline	Increased theophylline effect	Decreased metabolism
Griseofulvin, with:		
anticoagulants, oral	Decreased anticoagulant effect	Increased metabolism

Griseofulvin, with: (continued)		
barbiturates	Decreased griseofulvin blood concentration	Increased metabolism and/or decreased absorption
Hydroxychloroquine, with:		
digoxin	Increased digoxin effect	Mechanism not established
Isoniazid, with:		
alcohol	Increased incidence of hepatitis; decreased isoniazid effect in some alcoholic patients	Mechanism not established Increased metabolism
aluminum antacids	Decreased isoniazid effect	Decreased absorption
anticoagulants, oral	Possible increased anticoagulant effect	Decreased metabolism
benzodiazepines	Pharmacologic effects of benzodiazepines may be increased; documented with diazepam and triazolam	Probable inhibition of hepatic metabolism
carbamazepine	Increased toxicity of both drugs	Altered metabolism
corticosteroids	Decreased isoniazid serum concentration	Increased hepatic metabolism and/or renal clearance
cycloserine	CNS effects, dizziness, drowsiness	Mechanism not established
diazepam	Possible increased IV diazepam effect	Decreased metabolism
disulfiram	Psychotic episodes, ataxia	Altered dopamine metabolism
phenytoin	Increased phenytoin toxicity	Decreased metabolism
rifampin	Possible increased isoniazid hepatotoxicity	Possible increased toxic metabolites
Ketoconazole, with:		
antacids, oral	Possible decreased antifungal effect	Decreased absorption
cimetidine	Possible decreased antifungal effect	Decreased absorption
rifampin	Possible decreased fungistatic activity	Increased metabolism
Lincomycin, with:		
kaolin-pectin	Decreased lincomycin effect	Decreased absorption
neuromuscular blocking agents	Increased neuromusuclar blockade	Additive

TABLE 15. (Continued)

Interacting Drugs	*Adverse Effect*	*Probable Mechanism*
Metronidazole, with:		
alcohol	Mild disulfiram-like symptoms	Possible inhibition of intermediary metabolism of alcohol
anticoagulants, oral	Increased anticoagulant effect	Decreased metabolism
disulfiram	Organic brain syndrome	Mechanism not established
phenobarbital	Decreased metronidazole effect	Probably increased metabolism
Miconazole, with:		
amphotericin B	Decreased antifungal effect	Mechanism not established
anticoagulants, oral	Increased anticoagulant effect	Mechanism not established
Nalidixic acid, with:		
anticoagulants, oral	Increased anticoagulant effect	Displacement from binding sites
Para-aminosalicylic acid, *see* aminosalicylic acid		
Polymyxin B, with:		
aminoglycoside antibiotics	Increased nephrotoxicity; increased neuromuscular blockade	Additive
neuromuscular blocking agents	Increased neuromuscular blockade	Additive
Quinacrine, with:		
alcohol	Minor disulfiram-like symptoms; theoretical, no clinical reports	Inhibition of intermediary metabolism of alcohol
Quinine, with:		
anticoagulants, oral	Increased anticoagulant effect	Mechanism not established
digoxin	Increased digoxin effect	Mechanism not established
Rifampin, with:		
aminosalicylic acid	Rifampin effectiveness may be decreased; separate doses by 8 to 12 hours	Decreased GI absorption due to excipient, bentonite
anticoagulants, oral	Decreased anticoagulant effect	Increased metabolism

Rifampin, with: (continued)		
barbiturates	Decreased barbiturate effect	Increased metabolism
β-adrenergic blockers	Decreased β-blocker effect	Mechanism not established
clofibrate	Pharmacologic effects of clofibrate may be decreased	Increased metabolism–enzyme induction
contraceptives, oral	Decreased contraceptive effect	Increased metabolism
corticosteroids	Decreased corticosteroid effect	Increased metabolism
diazepam	Possible decreased diazepam effect occurs with IV diazepam	Increased metabolism
digitoxin	Decreased digitoxin effect	Increased metabolism
disopyramide	Decreased disopyramide effect	Probably increased metabolism
hypoglycemics, sulfonylurea	Decreased hypoglycemic effect	Increased metabolism
isoniazid	Possible increased hepatotoxicity	Possible increased toxic metabolites
ketoconazole	Possible decreased fungistatic activity	Increased metabolism
methadone	Methadone withdrawal symptoms	Increased metabolism
mexiletene	Decreased antiarrhythmic effect	Increased metabolism
progestins	Decreased half-life, area under the concentration vs time curve, and plasma level	Increased metabolism
quinidine	Decreased quinidine effect	Increased metabolism
Spectinomycin, with:		
lithium	Increased lithium toxicity	Decreased renal excretion
Sulfonamides, with:		
anticoagulants, oral	Increased anticoagulant effect	Decreased metabolism and displacement from binding sites
digoxin	Possible decreased digoxin effect with sulfasalazine	Decreased digoxin absorption
hypoglycemics, sulfonylurea	Increased hypoglycemic effect	Mechanism not established
methotrexate	Possible increased methotrexate toxicity	Decreased renal clearance
phenytoin	Increased phenytoin effect, except possibly sulfisoxazole	Decreased metabolism

TABLE 15. (Continued)

Interacting Drugs	*Adverse Effect*	*Probable Mechanism*
Sulfonamides, with: (continued)		
thiopental sodium	Increased pental effects	Decreased albumin binding
Tetracyclines, with:		
antacids, oral	Decreased oral tetracycline effects	Decreased tetracycline absorption
anticoagulants, oral	Increased anticoagulant effect	Mechanism not established
barbiturates	Decreased doxycycline effect	Increased metabolism
bismuth subsalicylate	Decreased tetracycline effect	Decreased absorption
carbamazepine	Decreased doxycycline effect	Decreased metabolism
contraceptives, oral	Decreased contraceptive effect	Possible decreased enterohepatic circulation of estrogen
digoxin	Increased digoxin effect	Decreased gut metabolism and increased absorption
iron, oral	Decreased tetracycline effect	Decreased absorption
lithium	Increased lithium toxicity	Decreased renal excretion
phenformin	Increased lactic acidosis	Possible decreased phenformin excretion
phenytoin	Decreased doxycycline effect	Increased metabolism
zinc sulfate	Decreased tetracycline effect	Decreased absorption
Thiabendazole, with:		
theophyllines	Increased theophylline toxicity	Decreased metabolism
Trimethoprim, with:		
cyclosporin	Increased nephrotoxicity	Synergism
Troleandomycin, with:		
carbamazepine	Increased carbamazepine toxicity	Decreased metabolism
contraceptives, oral	Jaundice	Additive
ergot alkaloids	Increased ergot toxicity	Mechanism not established
methylprednisolone	Increased steroid effect	Decreased metabolism
theophyllines	Increased theophylline toxicity	Decreased metabolism
Vancomycin, *see* aminoglycoside antibiotics		
Vidarabine, with:		
allopurinol	Increased vidarabine toxicity	Decreased metabolism

†SOURCE: Primarily from Rizack MA, Hillman CDM: *The Medical Letter Handbook of Drug Interactions,* ed 1. New York, The Medical Letter, Inc., 1983, pp 5–132.

BIBLIOGRAPHY

Abramowicz M: *Handbook of Antimicrobial Therapy,* Revised Edition 1982. New York, The Medical Letter, Inc., 1982, pp 36–45, 87–99.

Anderson PO: Drugs and breast feeding: A review. *Drug Intell Clin Pharmacy* 11:208–223, 1977.

Bennett WM, Aronoff GR, Morrison G, et al: Drug prescribing in renal failure: Dosing guidelines for adults. *Am J Kidney Dis* 3:155–193, 1983.

Cunha BA: Symposium on antimictorial therapy, in *Med Clin North Am* 66:1–312, 1982.

Kucers A, Bennett N McK: *The Use of Antibiotics,* ed 3. London, William Heinemann Medical Books Ltd, 1979, pp 3–970.

Manuel MA, Paton TW, Cornish WR: Drugs and peritoneal dialysis. *Peritoneal Dialysis Bulletin* July–September: 117–125, 1983.

Platzker ACD, Lew CD, Stewart D: Drug administration via breast milk. *Hosp Pract* 15:111–122, 1980.

Richards ML, Prince RA, Kenaley KA, et al: Antimicrobial penetration into cerebrospinal fluid. *Drug Intell Clin Pharmacy* 15:341–368, 1981.

Rollins DE, Klaassen DC: Biliary excretion of drugs in man. *Clin Pharmacokinet* 4:368–379, 1979.

Sanford JP: *Guide to Antimicrobial Therapy,* ed 12. United States of America, J.P. Sanford, M.D., 1983, pp 3–113.

Schönfeld H (ed): Pharmacokinetics, in *Antibiot Chemother* 25:1–320, 1978.

Schönfeld H (ed): Pharmacokinetics II, in *Antibiot Chemother* 31:1–224, 1982.

Wilson JT, Brown RD, Cherek DR, et al: Drug excretion in human breast milk: Principles, pharmacokinetics and projected consequences. *Clin Pharmacokinet* 5:1–65, 1980.

INDEX